CDC

HEALTH INFORMATION FOR
INTERNATIONAL TRAVEL

THE YELLOW BOOK

2014

Emergency Preparedness and
Occupational Health Directorate (EPOHD)
NCR, Occupational Health Clinic
171 Slater Street, 12th floor, PL 3712M
Ottawa, ON, K1A 0K9

CDC

HEALTH INFORMATION FOR INTERNATIONAL TRAVEL

THE YELLOW BOOK

2014

Editor in Chief
Gary W. Brunette, MD, MS

Chief Medical Editor
Phyllis E. Kozarsky, MD

Medical Editors
Nicole J. Cohen, MD, MS
Mark D. Gershman, MD
Alan J. Magill, MD
Stephen M. Ostroff, MD
Edward T. Ryan, MD
David R. Shlim, MD
Michelle Weinberg, MD, MPH
Mary Elizabeth Wilson, MD

Managing Editor
Amanda Whatley Lee, MPH

US DEPARTMENT OF HEALTH AND HUMAN SERVICES
Public Health Service
Centers for Disease Control and Prevention
National Center for Emerging and Zoonotic Infectious Diseases
Division of Global Migration and Quarantine
Atlanta, Georgia

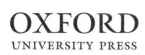

OXFORD
UNIVERSITY PRESS

Oxford University Press is a department of the University of Oxford.
It furthers the University's objective of excellence in research, scholarship,
and education by publishing worldwide.

Oxford   New York
Auckland   Cape Town   Dar es Salaam   Hong Kong   Karachi
Kuala Lumpur   Madrid   Melbourne   Mexico City   Nairobi
New Delhi   Shanghai   Taipei   Toronto

With offices in
Argentina   Austria   Brazil   Chile   Czech Republic   France   Greece
Guatemala   Hungary   Italy   Japan   Poland   Portugal   Singapore
South Korea   Switzerland   Thailand   Turkey   Ukraine   Vietnam

Oxford is a registered trademark of Oxford University Press in the UK
and certain other countries.

Published in the United States of America by
Oxford University Press
198 Madison Avenue, New York, NY 10016

ISSN 0095-3539
ISBN 978-0-19-994849-9

1 2 3 4 5 6 7 8 9
Printed in the United States of America
on acid-free paper

Oxford University Press is proud to pay a portion of its sales for this book to the CDC Foundation. Chartered
by Congress, the CDC Foundation began operations in 1995 as an independent, nonprofit organization fostering support for CDC through public-private partnerships. Further information about the CDC Foundation
can be found at www.cdcfoundation.org. The CDC Foundation did not prepare any portion of this book and
is not responsible for its contents.

Suggested Citation

Centers for Disease Control and Prevention. CDC Health Information for International Travel 2014. New York: Oxford University Press; 2014.

Readers are invited to send comments and suggestions regarding this publication to Gary W. Brunette, Editor in Chief, Centers for Disease Control and Prevention, Division of Global Migration and Quarantine (E-03), Travelers' Health Branch (*proposed*), 1600 Clifton Road NE, Atlanta, GA 30333, USA.

Disclaimers

Both generic and trade names (without trademark symbols) are used in this text. In all cases, the decision to use one or the other was made based on recognition factors and was done for the convenience of the intended audience. Therefore, the use of trade names and commercial sources in this publication is for identification only and does not imply endorsement by the US Department of Health and Human Services, the Public Health Service, or CDC.

References to non-CDC Internet sites are provided as a service to readers and do not constitute or imply endorsement of these organizations or their programs by the US Department of Health and Human Services, the Public Health Service, or CDC. CDC is not responsible for the content of these sites. URL addresses were current as of the date of publication.

Notice

This material is not intended to be, and should not be considered, a substitute for medical or other professional advice. Treatment for the conditions described in this material is highly dependent on the individual circumstances. While this material is designed to offer accurate information with respect to the subject matter covered and to be current as of the time it was written, research and knowledge about medical and health issues are constantly evolving, and dose schedules for medications and vaccines are being revised continually, with new side effects recognized and accounted for regularly. Readers must, therefore, always check the product information and clinical procedures with the most up-to-date published product information and data sheets provided by the manufacturers and the most recent codes of conduct and safety regulation. Oxford University Press and the authors make no representations or warranties to readers, express or implied, as to the accuracy or completeness of this material, including without limitation that they make no representations or warranties as to the accuracy or efficacy of the drug dosages mentioned in the material. The authors and the publishers do not accept, and expressly disclaim, any responsibility for any liability, loss, or risk that may be claimed or incurred as a consequence of the use and/or application of any of the contents of this material.

The Publisher is responsible for author selection and the Publisher and the Author(s) make all editorial decisions, including decisions regarding content. The Publisher and the Author(s) are not responsible for any product information added to this publication by companies purchasing copies of it for distribution to clinicians.

For additional copies, please contact Oxford University Press. Order online at www.oup.com/us.

Contents

1 INTRODUCTION 2

2 THE PRE-TRAVEL CONSULTATION 26

③INFECTIOUS DISEASES RELATED TO TRAVEL 148

4 SELECT DESTINATIONS 406

5 POST-TRAVEL EVALUATION

6 CONVEYANCE & TRANSPORTATION ISSUES

7 INTERNATIONAL TRAVEL WITH INFANTS & CHILDREN

List of Boxes, Figures, Maps, & Tables, by Topic

DISEASES, CONDITIONS, & VACCINES

Influenza

Injury

Japanese Encephalitis

Malaria

Measles

RESOURCES

General Resources

Insect Avoidance

Pre-Travel Consultation

Water Treatment

SPECIAL POPULATIONS

Cruise Ship Passengers

Immigrants and Migrants

Immunocompromised

Infants and Children

Long-Term Travelers

Medical Tourists

Military

Pregnant Travelers

Returning Travelers

Students

Travelers with Chronic Illnesses

Travelers Visiting Friends and Relatives

LIST OF MAPS

Disease Maps

Destination and Reference Maps

Other Maps

Editorial Staff

Editor in Chief: Gary W. Brunette
Chief Medical Editor: Phyllis E. Kozarsky
Medical Editors: Nicole J. Cohen, Mark D. Gershman, Alan J. Magill, Stephen M. Ostroff, Edward T. Ryan, David R. Shlim, Michelle Weinberg, and Mary Elizabeth Wilson
Managing Editor: Amanda Whatley Lee
Design and Production Editor: Kelly Holton
Technical Writer-Editors: Ronnie Henry and Ava W. Navin
Editorial Assistant: Julie Ephgrave
Cartographer: Kevin Liske

CDC Contributors

Alexander, James P.
Allen, Jessica
Anderson, Alicia
Ansari, Armin
Arguin, Paul M.
Averhoff, Francisco
Bair-Brake, Heather
Balaban, Victor
Ballesteros, Michael F.
Barskey IV, Albert E.
Barzilay, Ezra J.
Batts, Dahna
Benenson, Gabrielle A.
Bern, Caryn
Bhan, Ashika Devi
Bialek, Stephanie R.
Blaney, David D.
Bowen, Anna
Bresee, Joseph
Brogdon, William G.
Brooks, John T.
Brown, Clive M.
Brunette, Gary W.
Brunkard, Joan M.
Buff, Ann M.
Cantey, Paul T.
Chai, Shua J.
Chiller, Tom M.
Ciesielski, Carol
Cohen, Nicole J.
Cohn, Amanda

Czarkowski, Alan G.
Dasch, Gregory A.
De, Barun K.
Dhara, V. Ramana
Dunne, Eileen F.
Dykewicz, Clare A.
Eidex, Rachel B.
Erskine, Stefanie
Fagan, Ryan P.
Fiebelkorn, Amy Parker
Fischer, Marc
Fox, LeAnne M.
Gaines, Joanna
Gallagher, Nancy M.
Galland, G. Gale
Gargano, Julia Warner
Garrison, Laurel E.
Gee, Jay E.
Gershman, Mark D.
Goodson, James L.
Gould, L. Hannah
Grant, Althea
Green, Michael D.
Greenbaum, Adena
Griffin, Patricia M.
Grosse, Scott
Guerra, Marta A.
Hall, Aron J.
Heiman, Katherine E.
Henry, Ronnie
Herwaldt, Barbara L.

Hicks, Lauri A.
Hills, Susan L.
Hlavsa, Michele C.
Holtzman, Deborah
Iademarco, Michael F.
Illig, Petra A.
Imanishi, Maho
Jentes, Emily S.
Johnson, Katherine J.
Jones, Jeffrey L.
Kapella, Bryan K.
Khan, Ali S.
Kidd, Sarah
Knust, Barbara
Kozarsky, Phyllis E.
Kroger, Andrew T.
Kutty, Preeta K.
Lankau, Emily W.
Lee, Amanda Whatley
Lee, C. Virginia
Liang, Jennifer L.
LoBue, Philip
Lopman, Ben
MacNeil, Jessica R.
Mahon, Barbara E.
Malilay, Josephine
Maloney, Susan A.
Marano, Nina
Margolis, Harold S.
Marienau, Karen J.
Marin, Mona

Markowitz, Lauri
Marston, Chung K.
Mathieu, Els
McLean, Huong Q.
McQuiston, Jennifer
Mead, Paul S.
Meites, Elissa
Miller, Charles W.
Mintz, Eric
Mitruka, Kiren
Mody, Rajal
Montgomery, Susan
Moore, Anne
Moro, Pedro L.
Mullan, Robert J.
Nasci, Roger S.
Naughton, Mary P.
Navin, Ava W.
Nelson, Christina A.
Newton, Anna E.
Novak, Ryan T.
Olson, Christine K.
O'Reilly, Ciara

Ortega, Luis S.
O'Sullivan, Megan Crawley
Powers, Ann M.
Reef, Susan E.
Reyes, Nimia
Reynolds, Mary G.
Roehler, Douglas R.
Rollin, Pierre E.
Roy, Sharon L.
Rupprecht, Charles E.
Schneider, Eileen
Shadomy, Sean V.
Sharapov, Umid M.
Shealy, Katherine
Skoff, Tami H.
Slaten, Douglas D.
Sleet, David A.
Smith, Nicole M.
Smith, Theresa L.
Sommers, Theresa E.
Sotir, Mark J.
Spruit-McGoff, Kathryn
Staples, J. Erin

Steele, Stefanie F.
Stoddard, Robyn A.
Strikas, Raymond A.
Tan, Kathrine R.
Teo, Chong-Gee
Teshale, Eyasu H.
Tiwari, Tejpratap S. P.
Tomashek, Kay M.
Wallace, Gregory S.
Wassilak, Steven G. F.
Waterman, Stephen H.
Watson, John C.
Weber, Ingrid B.
Weinberg, Michelle
Weinberg, Nicholas
Wilson, Todd W.
Wirtz, Robert A.
Workowski, Kimberly
Yanni, Emad A.
Yendell, Stephanie J.
Yoder, Jonathan S.
Zielinski-Gutierrez, Emily

External Contributors

Ahmed, Qanta	State University of New York, Stony Brook, NY; Glasgow Caledonian University School of Public Health, Scotland, UK; and Templeton-Cambridge Journalism Fellow, England, UK
Ansdell, Vernon E	University of Hawaii, Honolulu, HI
Backer, Howard D.	California Emergency Medical Services Authority, Sacramento, CA
Barbeau, Deborah Nicolls	Tulane University, New Orleans, LA
Barnett, Elizabeth D.	Boston University School of Medicine and Boston Medical Center, Boston, MA
Borwein, Sarah T.	TravelSafe Medical Centre, Hong Kong, China
Brownstein, John S.	Boston Children's Hospital Informatics Program at the Harvard-MIT Division of Health Sciences and Technology; Division of Emergency Medicine, Boston Children's Hospital; and Department of Pediatrics, Harvard Medical School, Boston, MA
Carroll, I. Dale	The Pregnant Traveler, Spring Lake, MI
Chen, Lin H.	Mount Auburn Hospital—Travel Medicine Center, Cambridge, MA, and Harvard Medical School, Boston, MA
Connor, Bradley A.	Weill Medical College of Cornell University, New York, NY
DeRomana, Ines	University of California System, Education Abroad Program, Santa Barbara, CA
Dupont, Herbert L.	University of Texas Health Science Center, School of Public Health, Houston, TX
Ebner, Jodi	Chapman University, Center for Global Education, Orange, CA
Eremeeva, Marina E.	Georgia Southern University, Statesboro, GA
Fairley, Jessica K.	Emory University School of Medicine, Atlanta, GA

Forgione, Michael A.	Keesler Medical Center—Infectious Diseases Consultant to the Surgeon General, Keesler Air Force Base, MS
Freedman, David O.	University of Alabama at Birmingham, Birmingham, AL
Freifeld, Clark C.	Boston Children's Hospital Informatics Program at the Harvard-MIT Division of Health Sciences and Technology; Division of Emergency Medicine, Boston Children's Hospital; and Department of Biomedical Engineering, Boston University, Boston, MA
Fukuda, Mark M.	Armed Forces Health Surveillance Center—Global Emerging Infections Malaria Program, Silver Spring, MD
Gushulak, Brian D.	Migration Health Consultants, Cheltenham, Canada
Hackett, Peter H.	Institute for Altitude Medicine, Telluride, CO, and Altitude Research Center, University of Colorado Denver School of Medicine, Denver, CO
Hansen, Amy L. Sonricker	Boston Children's Hospital Informatics Program at the Harvard-MIT Division of Health Sciences and Technology and Division of Emergency Medicine, Boston Children's Hospital, Boston, MA, and Department of Epidemiology and Biostatistics, State University of New York, Albany, NY
Howard, Cynthia R.	University of Minnesota, Minneapolis, MN
John, Chandy C.	University of Minnesota, Minneapolis, MN
Kain, Kevin C.	University of Toronto, Toronto, Canada
Keystone, Jay S.	University of Toronto, Toronto, Canada
Kotton, Camille Nelson	Massachusetts General Hospital and Harvard University, Boston, MA
LaRocque, Regina C.	Massachusetts General Hospital and Harvard Medical School, Boston, MA
Libassi, Lisa	Swedish Medical Center, Seattle, WA
Libman, Michael	McGill University, Centre for Tropical Disease, Montreal, Canada
Mackell, Sheila M.	Mountain View Pediatrics, Flagstaff, AZ
Magill, Alan J.	Walter Reed Army Institute of Research, Experimental Therapeutics, Silver Spring, MD
Maguire, Jason D.	Naval Medical Center Portsmouth—Infectious Diseases Division and Travelers' Health Clinic, Portsmouth, VA
McCarthy, Anne E.	Ottawa Hospital and University of Ottawa, Ottawa, Canada
Neumann, Karl	Weill Medical College of Cornell University and New York Presbyterian Hospital/ Cornell Medical Center, New York, NY
Nord, Daniel A.	Divers Alert Network, Durham, NC
Offit, Paul	The Children's Hospital of Philadelphia, Philadelphia, PA
Ostroff, Stephen M.	Pennsylvania Department of Health, Harrisburg, PA
Reisenauer, Amy K.	Hawaii Permanente Medical Group, Wailuku, HI
Rhodes, Gary	Center for Global Education, University of California, Los Angeles, CA
Rosselot, Gail	Travel Well of Westchester, Inc., Briarcliff Manor, NY
Ryan, Edward T.	Massachusetts General Hospital and Harvard University, Boston, MA
Shlim, David R.	Jackson Hole Travel and Tropical Medicine, Jackson Hole, WY
Stauffer, William M.	University of Minnesota, Minneapolis, MN, and CDC, Atlanta, GA
Valk, Thomas H.	VEI Inc., Marshall, VA
Walker, Patricia F.	University of Minnesota, Minneapolis, MN, and HealthPartners, Center for International Health and Travel and Tropical Medicine Center, St. Paul, MN
Wilson, Mary Elizabeth	Harvard School of Public Health, Boston, MA
Wu, Henry M.	Emory University, Department of Medicine, Atlanta, GA
Youngster, Ilan	Children's Hospital Boston and Harvard University, Boston, MA

All contributors have signed a statement indicating that they have no conflicts of interest with the subject matter or materials discussed in the document(s) that they have written or reviewed for this book and that the information that they have written or reviewed for this book is objective and free from bias.

Acknowledgments

The *CDC Health Information for International Travel 2014* editorial team gratefully acknowledges all the authors and reviewers for their commitment to this new edition. We extend sincere thanks to the following people for their contributions to the production of this book:

- Elise Beltrami and Clive Brown for their extensive review of the text.
- Stefanie Erskine, Nomana Khan, C. Virginia Lee, Megan Crawley O'Sullivan, Crystal Polite, and Kate Spruit-McGoff for their assistance in preparing the text for publication.

Preface

To stay on the cutting edge of travel health information, this latest edition of *CDC Health Information for International Travel* has been extensively revised. The book serves as a guide to the practice of travel medicine, as well as the authoritative source of US government recommendations for immunizations and prophylaxis for foreign travel. As international travel continues to become more common in the lives of US residents, having at least a basic understanding of the medical problems that travelers face has become a necessary aspect of practicing medicine. The goal of this book is to be a comprehensive resource for clinicians to find the answers to their travel health–related questions.

CENTERS FOR DISEASE CONTROL AND PREVENTION
Thomas R. Frieden, MD, MPH, Director

NATIONAL CENTER FOR EMERGING AND ZOONOTIC INFECTIOUS DISEASES
Beth P. Bell, MD, MPH, Director

DIVISION OF GLOBAL MIGRATION AND QUARANTINE
Martin S. Cetron, MD, Director
Gary W. Brunette, MD, MS, Chief, Travelers' Health Branch *(proposed)*
Phyllis E. Kozarsky, MD, Expert Consultant, Travelers' Health Branch *(proposed)*
Amanda Whatley Lee, MPH, MCHES, Health Communications Specialist, Travelers' Health Branch *(proposed)*

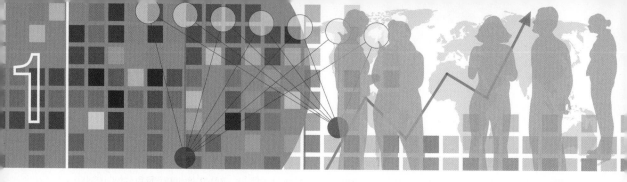

Introduction

INTRODUCTION TO TRAVEL HEALTH & THE YELLOW BOOK

Amanda Whatley Lee, Phyllis E. Kozarsky

TRAVEL HEALTH

The number of people traveling internationally has continued to grow substantially in the past decade. According to the World Tourism Organization (WTO), there were an estimated 990 million international tourist arrivals in 2011 throughout the world. In 2010, US residents made nearly 60 million trips with at least 1 night outside the United States. International travel takes on many forms, including tourism, business, study abroad, research, visiting friends and relatives, ecotourism, adventure, medical tourism, mission work, and responding to international disasters. Travelers are as unique as their itineraries, covering all age ranges and having a variety of health concerns and conditions. The infectious disease risks that travelers face are dynamic—some travel destinations have become safer, while in other areas, new diseases have emerged and other diseases have reemerged.

The risk of becoming ill or injured during international travel depends on many factors, such as the region of the world visited, a traveler's age and health status, the length of the trip, and the diversity of planned activities. The Centers for Disease Control and Prevention (CDC) provides international travel

health information to address the range of health risks a traveler may face, with the aim of assisting travelers and clinicians to better understand the measures necessary to prevent illness and injury during international travel. This publication and the CDC Travelers' Health website (www.cdc.gov/travel) are the 2 primary avenues of communicating CDC's travel health recommendations.

HISTORY AND ROLES OF THE YELLOW BOOK

CDC Health Information for International Travel ("The Yellow Book") has been a trusted resource since 1967. Originally, it was a small pamphlet published to satisfy the International Sanitary Regulations' requirements and the International Health Regulations (IHR), adopted by the World Health Organization (WHO) in 1951 and 1969, respectively; the IHR were completely revised in 2005. The purpose of the IHR is to ensure maximum security against the international spread of diseases, with minimum interference with world travel and commerce. A copy of the current IHR and supporting information can be found on the WHO website (www.who.int/csr/ihr/en).

In addition to reporting public health events of international concern, the United

States must also inform the public about health requirements for entering other countries, such as the necessity of being vaccinated against yellow fever. Some countries require all travelers to have an International Certificate of Vaccination or Prophylaxis (ICVP) documenting yellow fever vaccine administration as a condition for entry, while other countries require vaccination against yellow fever only if travelers arrive from a country where the yellow fever virus is known to circulate. The Yellow Book and the CDC Travelers' Health website aim to communicate these requirements under the IHR (2005). Although this publication includes the most current available information, requirements can change. Current information must be accessed to ensure that these requirements are met; the CDC Travelers' Health website (www.cdc.gov/travel) may be checked for regularly updated information.

The Yellow Book is written primarily for clinicians, including physicians, nurses, and pharmacists. Others, such as people in the travel industry, multinational corporations, missionary and volunteer organizations, and individual travelers, can also find a wealth of information here.

This text is authored by subject-matter experts from within CDC and outside the agency. The guidelines presented in this book are evidence-based and supported by best practices. Internal text citations have not been included; however, a bibliography is included at the end of each section for those who would like to obtain more detailed information. The CDC Travelers' Health program and the CDC Foundation are pleased to partner with Oxford University Press, Inc., to publish the 2014 edition. In addition to the printed copy, a searchable, online version of the Yellow Book can be found on the CDC Travelers' Health website (www.cdc.gov/yellowbook).

NEW IN THIS EDITION

The Yellow Book reflects the ever-changing nature of travel medicine. Each new edition notes the changes in global disease distribution, vaccine and medication guidelines, and new developments in preventing travel health risks.

Some new sections in this edition include sections covering Travel Medicine Data Collection: GeoSentinel & Global TravEpiNet (later in this chapter) and Last-Minute Travelers (Chapter 8). In addition, sections such as *Escherichia coli*, Fascioliasis, and Salmonellosis (Nontyphoidal) have been added to the diseases covered in Chapter 3, while Cambodia: Angkor Wat, Thailand, and Vietnam have been added to the select destinations included in Chapter 4.

In addition to the country-specific yellow fever vaccine requirements and recommendations and malaria transmission information and prophylaxis recommendations, other country-specific vaccine recommendations have been added to the section located at the end of Chapter 3. This section is indicated by yellow-bordered edges.

Perspectives Editorial Sections

A continuing feature from previous editions is the incorporation of editorial sections entitled *Perspectives*. Some new *Perspectives* sections include Prioritizing for the Resource-Limited Traveler (Chapter 2), Terrorism (Chapter 2), and Malaria in Long-Term Travelers & Expatriates (Chapter 8). Although the body of evidence-based knowledge in the field of travel medicine is growing, there is recognition that the practice of this specialty involves not only science, but art as well. Thus, readers will notice a few sections that contain editorial discussions aiming to add depth and clinical perspective, as well as to discuss some controversies or differences in opinions and practice. *Perspectives* sections reflect the views and opinions of the authors and do not necessarily represent official CDC recommendations.

Historical Editorial Sections

Four new sections encompass the 2014 debut of a new category of historical editorial sections, entitled *For the Record*. Learning the background of certain clinical practices can give readers a better understanding of the health topic and prevention or treatment recommendations. Beyond the practical reasons, these sections are included because the editorial team thought they would be interesting for inquisitive readers.

CONTACT INFORMATION FOR CDC

Questions, comments, and suggestions for CDC Travelers' Health, including comments about this publication, may be made through the CDC-INFO contact center, toll-free at 800-CDC-INFO (800-232-4636) 8 AM to 8 PM Eastern (Monday–Friday, closed holidays) or by visiting www.cdc.gov and clicking on "Contact CDC-INFO" to submit your question through an online e-mail form.

Pre-Travel or Post-Travel Clinical Questions

Since CDC is not a medical facility, clinicians needing assistance with patients who are preparing for travel should consider referral to a travel clinic or a clinic listed on the International Society of Travel Medicine website (www.istm.org).

Clinicians with post-travel health questions regarding their patients may consider referral to a clinic listed on the ISTM website, the American Society of Tropical Medicine and Hygiene website (www.astmh.org), or a medical university with specialists in infectious diseases.

Malaria: Because of the clinical complexity of malaria, the CDC Malaria Branch offers clinicians assistance with the diagnosis or management of suspected cases of malaria. Clinicians can contact CDC's Malaria Branch telephone hotline during business hours at 770-488-7788 or toll-free at 855–856-4713. After hours and on weekends and holidays, a Malaria Branch clinician may be reached by calling 770-488-7100.

Other parasitic diseases: CDC has an online diagnostic assistance service, called DPDx, for laboratorians, pathologists, and other health professionals (see www.dpd.cdc.gov/dpdx/HTML/Contactus.htm). Additionally, clinicians may consult with CDC about evaluation and treatment of patients suspected to have a parasitic disease (404-718-4745; parasites@cdc.gov).

Yellow fever: Clinicians should contact their state or local health department or call 970-221-6400 for assistance with diagnostic testing for yellow fever infections and for questions about antibody response to vaccination.

CDC Emergency Operations Center: CDC maintains an Emergency Operations Center to assist local, state, and federal agencies (770-488-7100) 24 hours per day, 7 days per week. Assistance can also be given to health care providers with questions on emergency or urgent patient care. **Note:** this line is not intended for the general public.

All other questions for CDC may be directed to the CDC INFO contact center, toll-free at 800-CDC-INFO (800-232-4636) 8 AM to 8 PM Eastern (Monday–Friday, closed holidays) or cdcinfo@cdc.gov.

BIBLIOGRAPHY

1. United Nations World Tourism Organization. UNWTO World Tourism Barometer, Vol. 10 (September). Madrid: United Nations World Tourism Organization; 2012 [cited 2012 Sep 25]. Available from: http://dtxtq4w60xqpw.cloudfront.net/sites/all/files/pdf/unwto_barom12_05_sept_excerpt.pdf.

2. US Department of Commerce, Office of Travel and Tourism Industries. 2011 United States resident travel abroad. Washington, DC: US Department of Commerce; 2012 [cited 2012 Sep 25]. Available from: http://tinet.ita.doc.gov/outreachpages/download_data_table/2010_US_Travel_Abroad.pdf.

3. World Health Organization. International Health Regulations (2005). 2nd ed. Geneva: World Health Organization; 2008 [cited 2012 Sep 25]. Available from: http://www.who.int/ihr/9789241596664/en/index.html.

PLANNING FOR HEALTHY TRAVEL: RESPONSIBILITIES & RESOURCES

Kathryn E. Spruit-McGoff, C. Virginia Lee

International travel encompasses a wide array of activities, including business travel, sightseeing, adventure travel, international adoption, and visiting friends and relatives. The process of planning these trips involves relationships between the traveler, the clinicians, and the travel and tourism industry. This section outlines how these groups can work together to make travel safer, healthier, and more enjoyable.

RESPONSIBILITIES OF THE TRAVELER

Travelers need to understand the health risks that traveling internationally may pose and be actively involved in preparing for healthy travel. Unfortunately, studies have shown that most travelers from the United States and other countries do not seek pre-travel health advice.

Gathering Destination Information

Travelers should find out as many details as possible about their travel destinations, modes of travel, lodging, food, and activities during their trip. These details help the travel health provider tailor his or her advice in regard to immunizations, prophylaxis, and other health advice. Travelers can visit the CDC Travelers' Health website (www.cdc.gov/travel) for the latest health information for international destinations, which includes disease outbreaks, natural disasters, and other events with health-related concerns.

Seeking and Following Pre-Travel Health Advice

Obtaining pre-travel health care and advice from a clinician familiar with travel is an important step in preparing to travel internationally. Ideally, this visit should take place 4–6 weeks before travel, but even getting a consultation in the week before travel can be of value. The pre-travel visit includes a discussion of immunizations, prophylactic medications (such as antimalarial drugs),

and specific health advice for preventing and treating travelers' diarrhea and other illnesses the traveler may experience. Travelers who have chronic health issues or who take medications may also need to coordinate their pre-travel care with their regular doctors. CDC recommends that travelers prepare and carry a travel health kit (see Chapter 2, Travel Health Kits).

Avoiding Travel When Sick

Recently, more emphasis has been placed on advising people to avoid traveling while they are sick if they may have a communicable disease that can be spread easily to other people. Postponing or canceling a trip can be inconvenient and incur additional expenses, but these costs may be small compared with the public health costs of a disease outbreak, which may include a search for airline passengers who might have been exposed to the traveler's disease.

RESPONSIBILITIES OF THE CLINICIAN

Regardless of their specialty, most clinicians will encounter a traveling patient at some point in their practice. Clinicians, especially those in primary care, should know basic travel health information to determine the extent of health advice their patients should access before traveling, and be able to recognize common post-travel health symptoms and syndromes.

Incorporating Pre-Travel Care into One's Practice

At a minimum, clinicians can easily incorporate the topic of travel medicine into their practice by routinely asking patients if they are planning to travel internationally, particularly to a developing country. By doing so, clinicians can begin to raise awareness and emphasize the importance of a pre-travel consultation and the fact that international travel can pose special health risks. Inquiring in advance also allows time for the patient to receive comprehensive pre-travel care, either at the current visit or by scheduling a pre-travel consult before the planned trip. Additionally, patients who have more complex medical histories, or who need to see a specialist in travel medicine, would have time to adequately address any special needs. Clinicians should be particularly aware of people who were born in or may be visiting friends or relatives in developing countries. For more information on this population, refer to Chapter 8, Immigrants Returning Home to Visit Friends & Relatives (VFRs).

Before evaluating a traveler for a pre-travel consultation, the clinician should determine what level of information he or she is comfortable giving to the patient. Some clinicians may base their comfort level on aspects of trips, such as location, length, and type, on the complexity of the patient's medical history, or both. Common categories of service include the following:

- Referring all travelers to a travel clinic or a travel medicine specialist.
- Offering only basic pre-travel advice and common vaccinations for less complex situations, such as advising travelers who are going on a short vacation to a popular tourist destination, such as Mexico or the Caribbean.
- Providing complex pre-travel consultations and making a commitment to the practice of travel medicine.

Even if clinicians have decided to offer only pre-travel care for less complex situations and itineraries, they should take the time to give a comprehensive pre-travel consultation, incorporating vaccines, medications, and behavioral preventive recommendations. For more information, see Chapter 2, The Pre-Travel Consultation.

Clinicians who wish to provide pre-travel care in more complex consultations can extend their knowledge and expertise in several ways:

- Refer to Appendix A for additional information about the practice of travel medicine, professional resources, and certifications offered through professional organizations.

- As travel medicine is dynamic, clinicians who regularly advise travelers in pre-travel consultations need to maintain a current base of knowledge. Many different Internet resources and databases, although sometimes incomplete or in conflict with one another, are available for clinicians to use to keep abreast of the health issues in international travel (see Appendix B).
- In addition to general pre-travel consultations, some clinicians may also wish to become registered yellow fever vaccine providers. This process is initiated with one's state health department.

Incorporating Post-Travel Care into One's Practice

Recognizing common travel-related disease symptoms and syndromes is important in the primary care and emergency care settings, as these settings are usually where an ill returned traveler will initially seek medical care. When assessing a patient for a possible infectious disease, it is of paramount importance to remember to obtain a travel history. Patients with influenzalike symptoms may not remember to volunteer the fact that they have recently traveled to Africa, for example, and could have malaria, which is potentially life-threatening. Further information about post-travel medical care can be found in Chapter 5.

Additionally, clinicians should have a plan as to when they will refer a patient to a specialist and who that specialist would be, before the patient comes into the office seeking medical care. Patients needing more extensive post-travel care can be referred to a clinician in infectious diseases or clinical tropical medicine. The American Society of Tropical Medicine and Hygiene provides a listing of such clinicians on its website (www.astmh.org).

RESPONSIBILITIES OF THE TRAVEL AND TOURISM INDUSTRY

Customers often look to their travel agents to advise them on all aspects of their trip, including health risks and preventive actions they should take. Although the role of travel and tourism industry professionals is not to provide personal medical consultations, mentioning that health risks exist and referring travelers to a clinic or to the International

Society of Travel Medicine website (www. istm.org) are appropriate actions. In many cases, this may be the best opportunity to help someone who was not aware that pre-travel medical advice was important. The CDC Travelers' Health website can be consulted to give a general idea of the health risks the client may encounter on a given trip (www.cdc. gov/travel).

TRAVELERS' HEALTH WEBSITE FOR TRAVEL HEALTH ADVICE
Destination Pages
CDC's Travelers' Health website features destination-specific pages with information on current CDC assessments of disease risk and recommendations for healthy travel (wwwnc.cdc.gov/travel/destinations/list.

aspx). Destination pages contain information about endemic diseases and health risks with links to travel notices.

Travel Notices
Travel notices are a key feature of the website information. Notices are assigned different levels based on various factors relating to the disease, destination, and situation (see Box 1-1). Travel notices and more detailed information about the various levels of notices can be found at wwwnc.cdc.gov/travel/notices.htm.

The purpose of a travel notice is to inform and educate travelers and clinicians with health information and prevention recommendations regarding diseases, conditions, and disasters that they may encounter while abroad. Notices are destination-specific and

---

BOX 1-1. FACTORS THAT INFLUENCE TRAVEL NOTICE LEVELS

Disease Factors
- Case-fatality ratio
- Incubation period
- Period of communicability
- Susceptibility: resistance, risk, immunity, healthy carriers, vulnerable populations
- Transmission: airborne, vectorborne, waterborne, foodborne, bloodborne, multiple transmission routes
- Prevention: vaccine, prophylaxis, behaviors, efficacy of vaccine or drug
- Treatment: postexposure prophylaxis, medication, treatment failures, antibiotic resistance
- Sequelae: injury, disability

Destination Factors
- Occurrence: endemicity, past outbreaks
- Containment measures: public health infrastructure, political stability, access to potable water and sanitation, vector control methods, percent gross domestic product spent on health care, international interventions, ministry of health activities, importation
- Accessibility of medical care: clinics or hospitals in the area, internationally recognized clinics, availability of treatment or prophylaxis, available medical evacuation
- Frequency of visits by US travelers

Situation Factors
- New situation: appearance in a new area, expansion of an existing area, out of season, different population
- Scope: confirmed case count, probable case count, cases in health care staff or travelers, important event (even if small case numbers), population affected where event is occurring
- Quality of surveillance: credibility of surveillance, in-country CDC or World Health Organization staff, ministry of health reporting, public health surveillance systems
- Aftermath of disaster: people affected, water supply, environmental hazard, homelessness, risk of potential for illness and injury, diseases as a result of disaster, destruction of food and water sources, lack of medical supplies, environmental risks, risk of toxic spread

are usually posted for unexpected disease outbreaks or disasters. Travel notices also inform public health scientists to be aware of possible importation of disease into the United States.

CDC posts only confirmed events from official sources. Serious consideration is given to the impact, both positive and negative, before posting a notice. Notices are posted for the awareness and protection of travelers. Once posted, both outbreak and event notices are reviewed periodically (at least monthly) and updated or removed as indicated.

BIBLIOGRAPHY

1. Hamer DH, Connor BA. Travel health knowledge, attitudes and practices among United States travelers. J Travel Med. 2004 Jan–Feb;11(1):23–6.
2. Hatz CFR, Chen LH. Pre-travel consultation. In: Keystone JS, Freedman DO, Kozarsky PE, Connor BA, Nothdurft HD, editors. Travel Medicine. 3rd ed. Philadelphia: Saunders Elsevier; 2013. p. 31–6.
3. Keystone JS, Kozarsky PE, Freedman DO. Internet and computer-based resources for travel medicine practitioners. Clin Infect Dis. 2001 Mar 1;32(5):757–65.
4. Kozarsky PE, Keystone JS. Body of knowledge for the practice of travel medicine. J Travel Med. 2002 Mar–Apr;9(2):112–115.
5. MacDougall LA, Gyorkos TW, Leffondre K, Abrahamowicz M, Tessier D, Ward BJ, et al. Increasing referral of at-risk travelers to travel health clinics: evaluation of a health promotion intervention targeted to travel agents. J Travel Med. 2001 Sep–Oct;8(5):232–42.

TRAVEL EPIDEMIOLOGY
David O. Freedman

To prescribe optimal pre-travel advice, preventive measures, and education, travel health providers must be aware of the absolute and relative magnitude of the many travel-related health risks. Such knowledge allows travel health care providers to perform an epidemiologic and traveler-specific risk assessment so that these measures can be appropriately prioritized for each traveler. Travel-related health problems are self-reported by 22%–64% of travelers to the developing world; most of these problems are mild, self-limited illnesses such as diarrhea, respiratory infections, and skin disorders. Approximately 8% of the more than 50 million travelers to developing regions, or 4 million people, are ill enough to seek health care, either while abroad or upon returning home.

LIMITATIONS OF CURRENT EPIDEMIOLOGIC KNOWLEDGE
Knowledge of the precise risk for a specific disease in a specific location has proved elusive, despite several decades of interest and investigation. (For additional discussion, see Chapter 2, *Perspectives*: Risks Travelers Face.) A reasonably accurate estimate of the number of cases of a disease or infection in all travelers over a time period at a location is difficult to determine, as many will have returned to their home countries by the time the disease manifests symptoms. Similarly difficult to obtain is an exact denominator reflecting the total number of travelers to that location. An accurate numerator must be divided by an accurate denominator to calculate a true incidence rate or risk. Even this standard population-based approach assumes that past experience predicts future risk. In addition, disease risks are not stable over time, and current or real-time data are rarely available. Much of the frequently quoted numerical data regarding the incidence of infection in travelers are based on extrapolations of limited data, collected in limited samples of travelers anywhere from a few to >20 years ago. This knowledge base includes morbidity studies of various methodologic designs, each with its own set of strengths and weaknesses. These

studies have mostly examined a few key individual diseases in all travelers regardless of destination, profiles of disease occurrence at a few specific high-risk destinations, and disease occurrence in certain types of travelers with certain behaviors. Many have been single-clinic or single-destination studies that can lead to conclusions that are not generalizable to groups of travelers with different local, national, or cultural backgrounds.

INCIDENCE RATES AND ESTIMATES OF RISK

A compilation of best available incidence rate estimates, given the above limitations, is available and has been updated over the years (Figure 1-1). With the notable exception of malaria, the major preventable travel-related diseases are associated with relatively low risks, ranging from 1 in 100 for influenza to <1 in 100,000 for several diseases that often concern travelers. Hepatitis A may be taken as an example of a prototypical vaccine-preventable disease, with an estimated overall uncorrected incidence of approximately

1 in 5,000 travelers to the developing world. Thus, the odds against acquiring hepatitis A on a single short trip are greatly in the traveler's favor, as many travelers realize. Any considered vaccination should be presented in context as insurance against a relatively uncommon event, but one that may result in illness or other consequences.

For diseases with poor or fatal outcomes, such as meningococcal meningitis, rabies, or Japanese encephalitis, the context of less tolerance of even small risks needs to be communicated to travelers to help them make informed decisions about all available interventions. The incidence rates in Figure 1-1 reflect aggregate data and studies, and do not consider variations in risk behaviors, destination, season, duration of travel, or general style of travel. For many diseases, research into increased or decreased risk according to these variables is still in its infancy because of difficulties in tracking outcomes at remote destinations.

A more recent and novel approach to defining disease epidemiology in travelers has involved the use of collaborative networks of

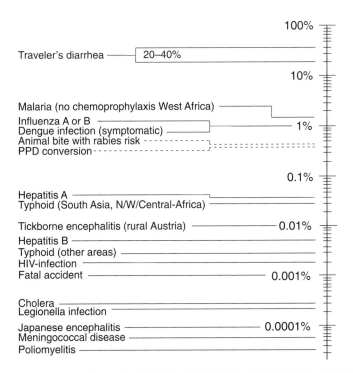

FIGURE 1-1. ESTIMATED INCIDENCE RATE PER MONTH OF INFECTIONS AND FATAL ACCIDENTS AMONG TRAVELERS IN DEVELOPING COUNTRIES, 2010[1]

[1]Unpublished; used with permission of Robert Steffen, Zurich, Switzerland.

specialized travel medicine clinics to collect and aggregate data on large samples of travelers (see the next section in this chapter, Travel Medicine Data Collection: GeoSentinel & Global TravEpiNet).

FUTURE CHALLENGES AND PRIORITIES FOR TRAVEL EPIDEMIOLOGY

Issues surrounding the relative merits of different methodologic approaches to defining travel-associated disease risk have recently been reviewed at length. In order to better characterize health risks and provide guidance to travelers, some epidemiologic priorities include the following:

- Obtaining travel-related data for many existing and potentially vaccine-preventable diseases. Current data are sparse, and incidence in local populations often may not reflect travelers' risk because of different risk behaviors, previous infection, or preexisting vaccination campaigns.

- Developing better surrogate markers for malaria exposure during travel to facilitate interventional studies for novel malaria chemoprophylaxis drugs or alternative dosing regimens. Such information is difficult to obtain because of the inability to perform placebo drug studies, given the life-threatening nature of the infection.
- Studying the effect of high-risk medical conditions or immunocompromising medications on travel outcomes.
- Improving understanding of the impact of host behavior related to different types of travel, such as tourism, business travel, travel to visit friends and relatives, missionary travel, and volunteer travel.
- Conducting research to gain more insight on exposure-related factors, such as urban vs rural travel, luxury vs rough travel, season of travel, and organized vs self-directed travel. Recent information on long-stay vs short-stay travel has been published.

BIBLIOGRAPHY

1. Chen LH, Wilson ME, Davis X, Loutan L, Schwartz E, Keystone J, et al. Illness in long-term travelers visiting GeoSentinel clinics. Emerg Infect Dis. 2009 Nov;15(11):1773–82.
2. Freedman DO, Weld LH, Kozarsky PE, Fisk T, Robins R, von Sonnenburg F, et al. Spectrum of disease and relation to place of exposure among ill returned travelers. N Engl J Med. 2006 Jan 12;354(2):119–30.
3. Hagmann S, Neugebauer R, Schwartz E, Perret C, Castelli F, Barnett ED, et al. Illness in children after international travel: analysis from the GeoSentinel Surveillance Network. Pediatrics. 2010 May;125(5):e1072–80.
4. Hill DR. Health problems in a large cohort of Americans traveling to developing countries. J Travel Med. 2000 Sep–Oct;7(5):259–66.
5. Jensenius M, Davis X, von Sonnenburg F, Schwartz E, Keystone JS, Leder K, et al. Multicenter GeoSentinel analysis of rickettsial diseases in international travelers, 1996–2008. Emerg Infect Dis. 2009 Nov;15(11):1791–8.
6. Leder K, Wilson ME, Freedman DO, Torresi J. A comparative analysis of methodological approaches used for estimating risk in travel medicine. J Travel Med. 2008 Jul–Aug;15(4):263–72.
7. Lederman ER, Weld LH, Elyazar IR, von Sonnenburg F, Loutan L, Schwartz E, et al. Dermatologic conditions of the ill returned traveler: an analysis from the GeoSentinel Surveillance Network. Int J Infect Dis. 2008 Nov;12(6):593–602.
8. Liese B, Mundt KA, Dell LD, Nagy L, Demure B. Medical insurance claims associated with international business travel. Occup Environ Med. 1997 Jul;54(7):499–503.
9. Mutsch M, Spicher VM, Gut C, Steffen R. Hepatitis A virus infections in travelers, 1988–2004. Clin Infect Dis. 2006 Feb 15;42(4):490–7.
10. Nicolls DJ, Weld LH, Schwartz E, Reed C, von Sonnenburg F, Freedman DO, et al. Characteristics of schistosomiasis in travelers reported to the GeoSentinel Surveillance Network 1997–2008. Am J Trop Med Hyg. 2008 Nov;79(5):729–34.
11. Peterson E, Chen LH, Schlagenhauf P, editors. Infectious Diseases: A Geographic Guide. Oxford, UK: Wiley-Blackwell; 2011.
12. Schwartz E, Weld LH, Wilder-Smith A, von Sonnenburg F, Keystone JS, Kain KC, et al. Seasonality, annual trends, and characteristics of dengue among ill returned travelers, 1997–2006. Emerg Infect Dis. 2008 Jul;14(7):1081–8.
13. Steffen R. Influenza in travelers: epidemiology, risk, prevention, and control issues. Curr Infect Dis Rep. 2010 May;12(3):181–5.
14. Steffen R, Amitirigala I, Mutsch M. Health risks among travelers—need for regular updates. J Travel Med. 2008 May–Jun;15(3):145–6.

15. Steffen R, deBernardis C, Banos A. Travel epidemiology—a global perspective. Int J Antimicrob Agents. 2003 Feb;21(2):89–95.
16. Steffen R, Rickenbach M, Wilhelm U, Helminger A, Schar M. Health problems after travel to developing countries. J Infect Dis. 1987 Jul;156(1):84–91.
17. Torresi J, Leder K. Defining infections in international travellers through the GeoSentinel Surveillance Network. Nat Rev Microbiol. 2009 Dec;7(12):895–901.
18. Whitty CJ, Mabey DC, Armstrong M, Wright SG, Chiodini PL. Presentation and outcome of 1107 cases of schistosomiasis from Africa diagnosed in a non-endemic country. Trans R Soc Trop Med Hyg. 2000 Sep–Oct;94(5):531–4.

1

TRAVEL MEDICINE DATA COLLECTION: GEOSENTINEL & GLOBAL TRAVEPINET

Regina C. LaRocque, David O. Freedman, Mark J. Sotir

During the past 2 decades, the knowledge base of travel medicine has been enhanced by medical provider networks designed to systematically collect data about travelers. This chapter discusses 2 of these networks, GeoSentinel Surveillance Network and Global TravEpiNet, both of which involve active participation of travel and tropical medicine clinics. Whereas GeoSentinel collects data from ill patients seen at clinics primarily during and after travel, Global TravEpiNet focuses on optimizing medical advice and care before travel.

GEOSENTINEL SURVEILLANCE NETWORK

GeoSentinel, a global surveillance system of travelers and migrants, operates under a cooperative agreement between the International Society of Travel Medicine and CDC and receives data from 54 travel and tropical medicine clinics on 6 continents. GeoSentinel conducts provider-based surveillance of travel-related illnesses and injuries to detect and respond to sentinel events, document ongoing disease trends, and provide a repository of data for analyses to improve epidemiologic expertise in the field of travel medicine. In addition, to facilitate communication and reporting of atypical and noteworthy events within the travel medicine community, GeoSentinel maintains a network membership of >200 travel medicine practitioners worldwide.

GeoSentinel clinics use a standard online data collection template to relate a specific diagnosis to a place and time of exposure. Exposure, if determined, can be at the country level or locally if ascertainable. Ancillary information submitted in real time to the central database includes country of residence, history of recent and previous travel, reason for travel, presenting signs and symptoms, pre-travel medical consult, and whether the patient is a classic traveler, an immigrant, or an expatriate. Records are segregated by clinical setting, which includes during or after travel and inpatient or outpatient. Specific diagnosis codes are used, and several codes are designated as "alarming diagnoses" to prompt more immediate attention.

GeoSentinel initiated data collection in 1997, and by the end of 2011 had generated >160,000 records on travelers seen at GeoSentinel site clinics. Of the patients with travel-related conditions reported by GeoSentinel clinics through the end of 2011, approximately 50% were seen after travel, 31% during travel, and 14% for illnesses related to their initial immigration travel. Among those seen after travel, 57% were leisure travelers; 14% were business travelers; 14% were missionaries, volunteer researchers, or aid workers; 12% were people visiting friends and relatives (VFR); and 2% were students. The most common destinations of returned travelers seen at GeoSentinel clinics were Mexico, Brazil, Egypt, Kenya, India, Thailand, and Indonesia.

GeoSentinel surveillance data have been used to report the spectrum of disease, document longitudinal disease trends, and detect sentinel events among traveling populations. Numerous reports using GeoSentinel data have been published; a list of publications, presentations, and citations can be found on the GeoSentinel website at www.istm.org/geosentinel/publicat.html. In 2006, a report was published describing spectrum of disease in 17,353 returning travelers from developing countries seen at GeoSentinel clinics and documenting both overall disease trends and regional disease occurrences. Additional studies using GeoSentinel data have been published, including reports focused on specific diseases such as dengue and malaria, animal-associated injuries, specific populations such as VFR travelers, destination-specific reports including the 2010 World Cup in South Africa and response to the 2010 Haiti earthquake, and outbreaks of leptospirosis and suspected sarcocystosis.

A continued focus of GeoSentinel will be to maintain systematic and timely data collection from sites, document trends and changes of illness patterns in travelers, and report new and unusual events in traveling populations. GeoSentinel will also seek to add new sites and expand its network membership. Further information on GeoSentinel can be found at www.istm.org/geosentinel/main.html.

GLOBAL TRAVEPINET

Global TravEpiNet was formed in 2009 to advance the pre-travel health care of US international travelers, particularly those at higher risk of travel-associated illness because of itinerary, purpose of travel, or existing medical conditions. Global TravEpiNet performs this work by systematically evaluating the health characteristics and pre-travel health care of travelers, developing evidence-based web tools for travelers and practitioners, and assessing the effect of pre-travel health interventions. As of September 2012, the Global TravEpiNet Consortium was composed of a network of 25 clinical sites across the United States, including primary care clinics, academic travel medicine practices, pharmacy-based practices, public health clinics, and occupational health clinics; many are registered to administer yellow fever vaccine.

Clinicians at Global TravEpiNet sites use a web tool to systematically collect data about the pre-travel health consultation. Data collected from the pre-travel consultation include demographics, travel itinerary, travel purpose, immunization history, vaccines administered, medication provided, and reasons for not administering a recommended vaccine. Data on >33,000 pre-travel consultations have been collected as of June 2012. More than 80% of travelers seen at Global TravEpiNet sites are visiting resource-poor destination countries. Africa is the most commonly visited region, and nearly a third of travelers visit multiple countries. Leisure (49%) is the most commonly reported purpose of travel, but business (15%), service work (15%), and VFR travelers (11%) are also common. Fifty-nine percent of travelers report an existing health condition before departure; 3% have an immune-suppressing condition of some type.

Patients declining recommended vaccines during the pre-travel consultation, particularly the influenza and rabies vaccines, have been identified as an area of concern within Global TravEpiNet. In particular, being a VFR traveler is an independent predictor of declining any recommended vaccine (OR, 1.45; 95% CI, 1.31–1.60). Global TravEpiNet is exploring the reasons that lead travelers to decline vaccines. Other areas of active research include determining the cost-effectiveness of the pre-travel consultation, evaluating specific traveling populations (such as VFR, pediatric, and immunocompromised travelers), and assessing the use of specific pre-travel interventions (such as yellow fever, Japanese encephalitis, and rabies vaccines).

Global TravEpiNet has identified that VFR travelers are less likely to seek timely pre-travel medical care and are more likely to decline recommended vaccines, even when they have sought medical advice. Because the Internet and primary care providers are common sources of health information for international travelers, especially VFR travelers, Global TravEpiNet has developed a number of web-based tools to optimize pre-travel health care for high-risk international travelers (Box 1-2). These publicly available web tools

BOX 1-2. PUBLICLY AVAILABLE TRAVEL RESOURCES FROM GLOBAL TRAVEPINET

- All resources are free, do not require registration, and can be accessed at www.healthful.travel.
- The **Travelers' Health Tool** encourages international travelers to seek pre-travel health advice and provides quick, itinerary-specific recommendations based on CDC guidelines.
- The **Healthcare Providers' Tool** guides clinicians through preparing a person for international travel and is up-to-date with CDC recommendations.

link directly to up-to-date recommendations from CDC. The Global TravEpiNet Consortium is also actively recruiting primary care and public health clinical sites that provide care to VFR and other high-risk travelers. More information on Global TravEpiNet, its web tools, and its membership can be found at www.healthful.travel.

BIBLIOGRAPHY

1. CDC. Notes from the field: acute muscular sarcocystosis among returning travelers—Tioman Island, Malaysia, 2011. MMWR Morb Mortal Wkly Rep. 2012 Jan 20;61(2):37–8.
2. CDC. Update: outbreak of acute febrile respiratory illness among college students—Acapulco, Mexico, March 2001. MMWR Morb Mortal Wkly Rep. 2001 May 11;50(18):359–60.
3. Esposito DH, Han PV, Kozarsky PE, Walker PF, Gkrania-Klotsas E, Barnett ED, et al. Characteristics and spectrum of disease among ill returned travelers from pre- and post-earthquake Haiti: The GeoSentinel experience. Am J Trop Med Hyg. 2012 Jan;86(1):23–8.
4. Freedman DO, Weld LH, Kozarsky PE, Fisk T, Robins R, von Sonnenburg F, et al. Spectrum of disease and relation to place of exposure among ill returned travelers. N Engl J Med. 2006 Jan 12;354(2):119–30.
5. Gautret P, Schwartz E, Shaw M, Soula G, Gazin P, Delmont J, et al. Animal-associated injuries and related diseases among returned travellers: a review of the GeoSentinel Surveillance Network. Vaccine. 2007 Mar 30;25(14):2656–63.
6. LaRocque RC, Rao SR, Lee J, Ansdell V, Yates JA, Schwartz BS, et al. Global TravEpiNet: a national consortium of clinics providing care to international travelers—analysis of demographic characteristics, travel destinations, and pretravel healthcare of high-risk US international travelers, 2009–2011. Clin Infect Dis. 2012 Feb 15;54(4):455–62.
7. LaRocque RC, Rao SR, Tsibris A, Lawton T, Barry MA, Marano N, et al. Pre-travel health advice-seeking behavior among US international travelers departing from Boston Logan International Airport. J Travel Med. 2010 Nov–Dec;17(6):387–91.
8. Leder K, Black J, O'Brien D, Greenwood Z, Kain KC, Schwartz E, et al. Malaria in travelers: a review of the GeoSentinel surveillance network. Clin Infect Dis. 2004 Oct 15;39(8):1104–12.
9. Leder K, Tong S, Weld L, Kain KC, Wilder-Smith A, von Sonnenburg F, et al. Illness in travelers visiting friends and relatives: a review of the GeoSentinel Surveillance Network. Clin Infect Dis. 2006 Nov 1;43(9):1185–93.
10. Mendelson M, Davis XM, Jensenius M, Keystone JS, von Sonnenburg F, Hale DC, et al. Health risks in travelers to South Africa: the GeoSentinel experience and implications for the 2010 FIFA World Cup. Am J Trop Med Hyg. 2010 Jun;82(6):991–5.
11. Schwartz E, Weld LH, Wilder-Smith A, von Sonnenburg F, Keystone JS, Kain KC, et al. Seasonality, annual trends, and characteristics of dengue among ill returned travelers, 1997–2006. Emerg Infect Dis. 2008 Jul;14(7):1081–8.

Perspectives

THE ROLE OF THE TRAVELER IN TRANSLOCATION OF DISEASE
Stephen M. Ostroff

Since humans began moving from one place to another, they have offered free passage to pathogens on themselves, in their belongings, or on their conveyances, and the consequences of such microbial hitchhiking have, at times, altered the course of history. Among the more notable examples are the great plagues that swept into Europe from Asia during the Middle Ages, the importation of smallpox to the Americas by European explorers, and the reverse movement of syphilis into Europe in those same returning explorers.

Although the movement of pathogens through travel is not a new phenomenon, today's increasing pace and scale of global human movement have enhanced the opportunities for disease spread. HIV infection, with symptoms that may be delayed for years, spread around the world less than a decade after it was recognized. In the 21st century, no place on the globe is more than a day from any other location, which gives even diseases with short incubation periods unprecedented opportunities for rapid spread. The following examples from the early part of this century illustrate the role travel plays in the translocation of infectious diseases. They also remind us that all travelers should take steps to prevent bringing more than luggage to their destinations.

INFLUENZA
Two new forms of influenza have recently emerged. One is avian influenza A (H5N1), which was first observed during a limited-scale outbreak in Hong Kong in 1997. After a brief hiatus, it reappeared in Vietnam in 2003 and has been in continuous circulation ever since. Even though H5N1 has primarily affected poultry, from 2003 through 2011, 578 human illnesses in 15 countries were reported, with an alarming case-fatality ratio of 59%. The countries with the most human disease (Indonesia, Vietnam, and Egypt) account for 80% of all cases and 78% of all deaths. All are tourist destinations, but no international travelers have become ill, largely because close contact with infected poultry is the primary risk factor for infection, and no sustained human-to-human transmission has been observed. However, movement of the virus between countries in goods carried by conveyances and animals has been documented.

In contrast, the rapid spread of influenza A (H1N1)pdm09 [pH1N1], which produced the first pandemic of the 21st century, was aided by infected travelers, both those who were symptomatic and those who were in the incubation stage. Although the virus was first identified in southern California in April 2009, human illnesses appeared weeks earlier in Mexico. Infected travelers who had visited Mexico were quickly detected in other parts of the world. An analysis of air traffic patterns found a very strong correlation between the volume of air travel from Mexico to a country and the likelihood pH1N1 was identified in

Perspectives sections are written as editorial discussions aiming to add depth and clinical perspective to the official recommendations contained in the book. The views and opinions expressed in this section are those of the author and do not necessarily represent the official position of CDC.

that location during the early stages of the pandemic. Aided by travel, this new virus rapidly found its way to dozens of countries after it was identified, resulting in a pandemic designation by the World Health Organization only 2 months later. This virus continues to circulate and has now become a seasonal influenza strain. The pH1N1 pandemic vividly demonstrates the potential for global dissemination of pathogens in a highly interconnected world.

SARS

The severe acute respiratory syndrome (SARS) epidemic of 2003 is another major example of the role of travel in the spread of infectious diseases in the 21st century. In February 2003, a professor from southern China, who was caring for patients with an unrecognized respiratory illness, traveled to a family wedding in Hong Kong while he was ill. His infection spread to 10 other travelers in his hotel, who then boarded airplanes to other parts of Asia, North America, and Europe, seeding a global epidemic of SARS that resulted in 8,098 cases and 774 deaths in 29 countries. Fortunately, characteristics of the virus, transmission dynamics of the disease, and aggressive public health measures contained the virus within months, but not before SARS produced widespread fear and economic and political turmoil. SARS had a major influence on the revisions to the International Health Regulations ratified in 2005.

CHILDHOOD VACCINE-PREVENTABLE DISEASES

Vaccination programs have substantially reduced the global prevalence of childhood infectious diseases. In the Western Hemisphere, indigenous measles transmission was declared eliminated in 2000, and diseases like mumps and rubella are at historical lows. Globally, poliomyelitis is on the verge of eradication, and endemic transmission of poliovirus is confined to only 3 countries. However, most vaccine-preventable diseases are highly transmissible and can easily spread in infected travelers. As one example, in recent years, transmission cycles were reestablished because poliovirus was imported into previously polio-free areas.

Measles

In the United States, clusters of measles continue to occur as a result of travel. These episodes have been precipitated by visitors from areas of the world where measles continues to circulate because of low vaccination coverage, susceptible US travelers going abroad, and overseas adoptees. These importations then ignite domestic outbreaks because of lower levels of population immunity in some communities, which is fueled largely by parents who elect not to vaccinate their children. In 2011, the United States reported 222 cases of measles, the largest number seen in 15 years. This number contrasts with a median of 56 cases reported per year from 2001 through 2008. Of the 2011 cases, 90% were definitely linked to importation (the remaining 10% were unknown), and 52 cases occurred in US residents exposed while abroad. The leading sources of importation were Europe (46%), Southeast Asia (26%), and the Western Pacific (15%), likely reflective of tourism patterns to and from areas with active measles transmission.

Mumps

Several recent large outbreaks of mumps in the United States are directly traceable to travel-related importation from Great Britain. A 2006 outbreak centered in Iowa, likely fueled by spring break travel, resulted in 6,584 mumps cases being reported across the country. A more recent outbreak that began in mid-2009, resulting in more than 2,000 cases in New York City and surrounding states, largely centered around an Orthodox Jewish community. This outbreak was started by a single traveler to Great Britain who returned to a summer camp in New York State. Mumps then spread to campers and staff, who carried it home to New York City and ignited sustained transmission for many months.

Polio

In 2002, only 6 countries had circulating indigenous wild-type poliovirus, but from 2002 through 2007, wild-type poliovirus spread to 27 previously disease-free countries in Africa and Asia through the movement of infected travelers. Northern Nigeria was the source of most of these illnesses, which reached all the way to Indonesia. Vaccination campaigns, guided by laboratory-based surveillance, largely disrupted transmission in these places, but travel continues to result in the spread of polio. In 2010, even as polio incidence decreased in Nigeria and India, 2 large outbreaks demonstrated the risk of introduction from poliovirus reservoirs. Spread of poliovirus into Tajikistan from India caused an outbreak of 458 cases and, subsequently, 18 cases in 2 other Central Asian republics and Russia. In central Africa, a large outbreak resulted after introduction of the virus from Angola, producing 441 cases in the Republic of Congo and an additional 104 cases in neighboring Democratic Republic of Congo. In 2011, cases of wild-type polio were identified in 16 countries, although only 1 recognized case occurred in India, which subsequently had no reported cases in more than a year. Although polio does not pose a threat to most travelers, it remains a serious concern for migrants, pilgrims, and people displaced by conflict; outbreaks heavily tax the public health resources of affected countries.

VECTORBORNE INFECTIONS

Several mosquito-transmitted diseases have expanded their range in the last decade. West Nile virus was introduced into New York City in 1999 and, in the next several years, spread throughout the Western Hemisphere, resulting in millions of human infections. The source and mode of introduction are unknown; although an infected traveler is a possibility, importation of infected birds or mosquitoes is considered more likely.

For 2 other major vectorborne infections (dengue and chikungunya), the role of travelers is clear. Neither of these viruses has an avian intermediary, and humans are amplifying hosts for both viruses, effectively moving these viruses from place to place. Dengue outbreaks are expanding in scale and scope, especially in Asia and South America. Since 2000, dengue virus has made incursions into the United States via infected travelers, producing outbreaks with local transmission in Texas, Hawaii (2001, 2011), and Florida (2009–2010, 2011). In Hawaii, for the first time since the 1940s, local dengue transmission was detected in 2001 when an outbreak in Maui resulted in 122 cases. The outbreak source was thought to be travelers from French Polynesia, which was experiencing an outbreak at the time. In 2010, an outbreak was identified in Oahu when 5 locally acquired dengue cases were linked to a sick traveler returning from the Philippines. In 2009, local dengue transmission was seen for the first time in Florida in 6 decades. This resulted in sustained local dengue transmission in 2009 and 2010; 93 cases of dengue were identified, principally among residents of the Florida Keys and tourists to the Florida Keys from other areas of the United States. Although dengue transmission appears to have subsided in the Florida Keys, in 2011 a total of 7 locally acquired infections were identified in 4 other Florida counties. The source of introduction of dengue virus to Florida is unknown, although many people from areas where dengue is endemic transit through the area.

Chikungunya virus was largely restricted to Africa and Asia until it began to appear on islands of the Indian Ocean in 2005, after an outbreak in Kenya in 2004. From there, it crossed to the Indian subcontinent in 2006, touching off major disease outbreaks, especially in southern India. Sizeable numbers of travelers to Indian Ocean tourist destinations and India have returned to Europe, North America, and Australia infected with chikungunya virus, and infected Indian nationals have also been seen in these locations. This has provided opportunities for local transmission of chikungunya virus to occur, including in northern Italy in 2007 and southeast France and south-central China in 2010. The source for translocation in Italy was a viremic traveler from India. A total of 205 locally acquired cases were acquired through infected *Aedes albopictus* mosquitoes, an invasive species that appeared in the area in the early 1990s. In contrast to West Nile in North America, chikungunya virus does not appear to have persisted in northern Italy. Many countries that have a viable vector for chikungunya virus remain at risk for importation and local transmission.

CHOLERA

In October 2010, cholera unexpectedly appeared in Haiti for the first time in recorded history. The cholera outbreak struck in the aftermath of the devastating January 2010 Haiti earthquake, which killed an estimated 316,000 people. The *Vibrio cholerae* strain (toxigenic serogroup O1, serotype Ogawa, biotype El Tor) responsible for the outbreak did not genetically resemble the Latin American outbreak strain that appeared in the 1990s or strains occasionally found along the coast of the Gulf of Mexico. Instead, it more closely resembled strains recently circulating in south Asia and Africa. A number of hypotheses were advanced regarding how the organism arrived in Haiti, including potential introduction by troops serving as part of the United Nations peacekeeping force housed upstream of the area where the first cases were recognized. Given Haiti's widespread poverty, poor sanitation, and population displacement in the aftermath of the earthquake, cholera spread rapidly. Shortly after it was recognized, cholera was causing thousands of cases throughout the country per week. As of April 2012, more than half a million cases had been recorded, with almost 300,000 hospitalizations and >7,000 deaths. Cholera subsequently spread to the Dominican Republic, which shares the island of Hispaniola, and Cuba. It also moved via travelers to and from Haiti to other countries, including the United States. Since these other locations have better sanitation infrastructure than Haiti, the risk of local spread of cholera is low. This outbreak provides a dramatic and unfortunate example of how disease can move from place to place with devastating consequences.

DRUG-RESISTANT PATHOGENS

Antimicrobial drug resistance among bacteria, viruses, fungi, and parasites is a growing problem. Travelers have frequently aided the spread of drug-resistant pathogens, including drug-resistant strains of *Neisseria gonorrhoeae*, methicillin-resistant *Staphylococcus aureus* (MRSA), and multidrug-resistant *Acinetobacter baumannii*. Highly drug-resistant strains of bacteria that are important causes

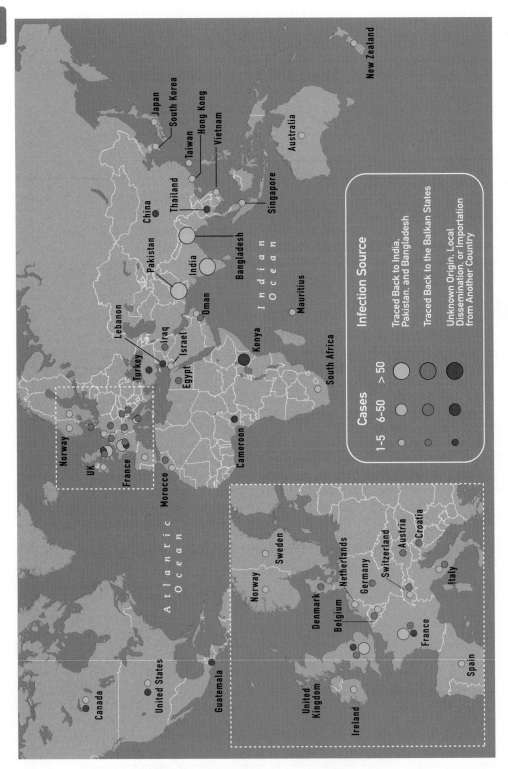

MAP 1-1. GLOBAL SPREAD OF NEW DELHI METALLO-β-LACTAMASE-PRODUCING *KLEBSIELLA PNEUMONIAE*, AS OF JUNE 2012[1]

[1] Adapted from Figure 4 in: Nordmann P, Naas T, Poirel L. Global spread of carbapenemase-producing Enterobacteriaceae. Emerg Infect Dis [serial on the Internet]. 2011 Oct [cited 2012 Sep 26]. Available from: http://dx.doi.org/10.3201/eid1710.110655. Additional data provided by Patrice Nordmann.

of health care–associated infection (HAI), for example, carbapenem-resistant Enterobacteriaceae (CRE), have emerged and been spread internationally via travelers. In 2006, HAI outbreaks due to CRE in Israel were linked to a strain common in the United States. More recently, a new and more transferrable drug-resistance mechanism responsible for CRE, known as the New Delhi metallo-β-lactamase-1 (NDM-1), was reported in 2009 in a Swedish citizen of Indian origin who developed medical problems requiring hospitalization while visiting India. After he returned to Sweden, the patient was again hospitalized, and strains of *Klebsiella pneumoniae* and *Escherichia coli* that produced NDM-1 were identified. In 2010, NDM-1 was identified in a series of 29 patients in Great Britain; at least 17 of the patients had traveled to the Indian subcontinent in the year before the diagnosis, and 14 of the 17 had been hospitalized during their visits. Similar findings in 3 patients were reported in the United States in 2010. Now, only a few years after the first case in Sweden, NDM-1 is being detected worldwide (Map 1-1), often first being seen in a patient who was previously hospitalized in the Indian subcontinent or the Balkans. This example shows how highly drug-resistant pathogens associated with health care can easily hitchhike from place to place. The growing phenomenon of medical tourism may further accelerate this trend.

DISEASE ASSOCIATED WITH GLOBAL GATHERINGS

The pilgrimage to Mecca is the world's largest annual event, drawing approximately 2 million Muslims from across the globe to Saudi Arabia. The history of the Hajj pilgrimage is an example of how diseases can spread to home countries of returning travelers after an international mass gathering. The intermingling and close contact offer ample opportunities for transmission of infectious diseases and rapid dissemination as pilgrims return home. In 2000, this occurred with *Neisseria meningitidis* serogroup W-135. Some vaccines used at that time did not cover this serogroup. After the event, 90 infections in returnees and their contacts were seen across Europe. In contrast, the number of infections in North America, where quadrivalent vaccine that covered W-135 was in use, was small. The outbreak strain of W-135 also quickly surfaced across areas of Africa, Asia, the Middle East, and the Indian Ocean, altering the epidemiologic patterns of meningococcal disease. As a result of this outbreak and similar cases in 2001, pilgrims to the Hajj are now required to be vaccinated with the quadrivalent vaccine.

These examples highlight the diversity of opportunities for microbial movement afforded by travel. No amount of vigilance is likely to eliminate such opportunities, especially since microbes can be silent travelers. However, all travelers should take precautions to prevent the spread of disease.

BIBLIOGRAPHY

1. CDC. Measles—United States, 2011. MMWR Morb Mortal Wkly Rep. 2012 Apr 20;61:253–7.
2. CDC. Resurgence of wild poliovirus type 1 transmission and consequences of importation—21 countries, 2002–2005. MMWR Morb Mortal Wkly Rep. 2006 Feb 17;55(6):145–50.
3. CDC. Update: mumps outbreak—New York and New Jersey, June 2009–January 2010.
   MMWR Morb Mortal Wkly Rep. 2010 Feb 12;59(5):125–9.
4. Chen LH, Wilson ME. The role of the traveler in emerging infections and magnitude of travel. Med Clin North Am. 2008 Nov;92(6):1409–32, xi.
5. Cleri DJ, Ricketti AJ, Vernaleo JR. Severe acute respiratory syndrome (SARS). Infect Dis Clin North Am. 2010 Mar;24(1):175–202.

6. Frerichs RR, Keim PS, Barrais R, Piarroux R. Nepalese origin of cholera epidemic in Haiti. Clin Microbiol Infect. 2012 Jun;18(6):E158–63.

7. Gushulak BD, MacPherson DW. Globalization of infectious diseases: the impact of migration. Clin Infect Dis. 2004 Jun 15;38(12):1742–8.

8. Khan K, Arino J, Hu W, Raposo P, Sears J, Calderon F, et al. Spread of a novel influenza A (H1N1) virus via global airline transportation. N Engl J Med. 2009 Jul 9;361(2):212–4.

9. Nordmann P, Naas T, Poirel L. Global spread of carbapenemase-producing Enterobacteriaceae. Emerg Infect Dis. 2011 Oct;17(10):1791–8.

10. Polgreen PM, Bohnett LC, Yang M, Pentella MA, Cavanaugh JE. A spatial analysis of the spread of mumps: the importance of college students and their spring-break-associated travel. Epidemiol Infect. 2010 Mar;138(3):434–41.

11. Reimer AR, Van Domselaar G, Stroika S, Walker M, Kent H, Tarr C, et al. Comparative genomics of *Vibrio cholerae* from Haiti, Asia, and Africa. Emerg Infect Dis. 2011 Nov;17(11):2113–21.

12. Rezza G, Nicoletti L, Angelini R, Romi R, Finarelli AC, Panning M, et al. Infection with chikungunya virus in Italy: an outbreak in a temperate region. Lancet. 2007 Dec 1;370(9602):1840–6.

13. Rogers BA, Aminzadeh Z, Hayashi Y, Paterson DL. Country-to-country transfer of patients and the risk of multi-resistant bacterial infection. Clin Infect Dis 2011;53:49–56.

14. Stoddard ST, Morrison AC, Vazquez-Prokopec GM, Paz Soldan V, Kochel TJ, Kitron U, et al. The role of human movement in the transmission of vector-borne pathogens. PLoS Negl Trop Dis. 2009;3(7):e481.

15. Taylor WR, Burhan E, Wertheim H, Soepandi PZ, Horby P, Fox A, et al. Avian influenza—a review for doctors in travel medicine. Travel Med Infect Dis. 2010 Jan;8(1):1–12.

16. Wilder-Smith A. Meningococcal disease: risk for international travellers and vaccine strategies. Travel Med Infect Dis. 2008 Jul;6(4):182–6.

17. Wilder-Smith A, Gubler DJ. Geographic expansion of dengue: the impact of international travel. Med Clin North Am. 2008 Nov;92(6):1377–90.

18. Wilson ME, Chen LH. NDM-1 and the role of travel in its dissemination. Curr Infect Dis Rep. 2012 Jun;14(3):213–26.

19. World Health Organization. Cumulative number of confirmed human cases of avian influenza A(H5N1) reported to WHO. Geneva: World Health Organization; 2012 [cited 2012 Sep 30]. Available from: http://www.who.int/influenza/human_animal_interface/H5N1_cumulative_table_archives/en/index.html.

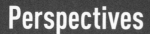

Perspectives

WHY GUIDELINES DIFFER
Alan J. Magill, David R. Shlim

INTRODUCTION

Numerous international, national, and professional organizations publish guidelines and recommendations that assist travel health providers in giving the best possible advice to prospective travelers. The CDC Yellow Book is one example of published recommendations. However, it is quickly apparent to both clinicians and patients that guidelines and recommendations differ, sometimes dramatically. Conflicting messages from authoritative sources may confuse patients and clinicians, and undermine the credibility of the source. It can be unsettling for patients to receive travel medicine advice, vaccines, and an antimalarial drug prescription from a provider, only to find that the recommendations conflict with what they have obtained from other sources, or even heard from other advisors. The skillful travel health provider will be able to help the traveler run this gauntlet of conflicting advice by knowing more about why guidelines differ.

HOW ARE GUIDELINES CREATED?

Most guidelines of interest to travel health providers and travelers focus on recommendations for immunizations, prophylactic medications, and self-treatment regimens (such as those for travelers' diarrhea). Guidelines come from many sources. A regulatory agency in each country must review and approve an application from the sponsor of a product in order for the product to be commercially distributed. Regulatory authorities review data from preli-censure clinical trials and also assess the manufacturing process. International organizations such as the World Health Organization (WHO) promote their own sets of guidelines. At national levels, agencies such as CDC make recommendations for the use of approved vaccines and medications for travelers. In addition, professional organizations may create consensus clinical practice guidelines based on published medical literature and expert opinion. Travel medicine–specific subscription services use experts to organize and present travel medicine recommendations for clinicians. However, these services can use information and sources that may not be fully validated by national and international authorities. Finally, vast quantities of unregulated opinions are published on the Internet. People new to travel medicine may not be aware of the decision-making process or the source information that results in formal recommendations from these organizations.

Regulatory Authorities

Countries typically have a national regulatory authority which acts as the government body that approves vaccines and drugs. In the United States, this is the

---

Food and Drug Administration (FDA). For the vaccines and medications commonly prescribed in a pre-travel consultation, providers are expected to use the products in accordance with the product label as approved by the FDA. The product label is a valuable source of information that is accurate at the time it is published. Manufacturers submit a detailed application that undergoes rigorous, multidisciplinary review. The approved product label reflects the information provided by the manufacturer in response to the requirements specified by a large body of regulatory law developed over many years. Since each country has different laws and requirements, approved products and their product labels may differ from country to country. This difference is then reflected in the national guidelines that relate to that product.

International Organizations

Travelers' health information is provided by WHO's publication, *International Travel and Health* (the "Green Book") and also in the WHO International Health Regulations 2005. Countries with less-developed or nonexistent regulatory agencies often default to the WHO guidelines, while more-developed countries with resources devoted to travelers' health may be aware of the WHO recommendations, but may not be able to reconcile WHO recommendations with their own country's recommendations in every situation.

US National Organizations

CDC provides recommendations for travel health and publishes those recommendations in this book. Subject-matter experts at CDC review information in their area of expertise and formulate recommendations. For vaccines, the Advisory Committee on Immunization Practices (ACIP) develops written recommendations for the administration of vaccines, including travelers' vaccines, to children and adults in the civilian population. Recommendations include age for vaccine administration, number of doses and dosing interval, and precautions and contraindications. ACIP, which is the only entity appointed by the federal government to make such recommendations, consists of 15 experts in fields associated with immunization who have been selected to provide advice and guidance to the US Department of Health and Human Services and CDC on the control of vaccine-preventable diseases (see Box 2-1).

Professional Organizations

Professional organizations often develop, write, and publish practice guidelines using committees of experts from their membership. These practice guidelines typically follow an evidence-based medicine approach that links recommendations to the strength and quality of the evidence as assessed by the committee members. The Infectious Disease Society of America has published a travel medicine practice guideline that many find useful. Practice guidelines, by their nature, are consensus documents.

Peer-Reviewed Medical Literature and Open Sources

As experience with a vaccine or a drug is acquired over the years, these results are often published in the peer-reviewed medical literature. In addition, people who use these products gain experience over time and develop their own opinions ("experience-based medicine"). The data that would be most useful in deciding how to use a vaccine or medication may not be available in published reports, so expert opinion attempts to interpret available information or provide background perspective.

WHY DO GUIDELINES DIFFER?

Guidelines in different countries and organizations may differ in substantial ways. Some of the reasons why guidelines differ include availability of products in different countries, a different cultural perception of risk, lack of evidence (or differing interpretations of the same evidence), and sometimes just honest differences in opinion among experts. Occasionally, public opinion may influence recommendations (for example, the widespread adverse publicity about mefloquine that was reported in the media).

Availability of Products

Travel health providers can only use the products that are available to them. Availability is determined by the regulatory approval status of the product and, to a lesser extent, the marketing and distribution plan of the manufacturer. Among the various vaccines and antimalarial drugs commercially available worldwide, the process for regulatory approvals varies greatly. For example, registering a new vaccine or antimalarial drug in the United States is a costly and rigorous process. If the market is insufficient to justify the expense of registration, then a commercial company may not seek registration in a particular country. The standards for licensure vary, and what may be sufficient for one regulatory authority may not suffice for another. For example, primaquine, an option for malaria chemoprophylaxis in the United States, is not registered or commercially available in Switzerland. Atovaquone-proguanil was available for malaria chemoprophylaxis in the United States before many other countries. On the other hand, an oral vaccine against cholera is approved for use and widely available in many countries, but is not approved by the FDA. Therefore, CDC and ACIP guidelines do not include any recommendations for the use of this vaccine.

Even when the same products are available, the recommendations for their use may differ. The capsular polysaccharide typhoid vaccine and the oral typhoid vaccine are examples. In the United States, a booster of the polysaccharide vaccine is recommended after 2 years, but in most European countries, a booster is recommended after 3 years. In the United States, a packet of 4 oral typhoid capsules is dispensed, whereas in Europe, 3 doses are considered adequate. The regulatory agencies may have reviewed the same data and drawn different conclusions, or they may have reviewed different data at separate times and reached different conclusions. Regulatory submissions to various agencies rarely are ready and occur at the same time; therefore, the data available for review by each agency may not be the same, for legitimate reasons.

Perception of Risk

People from varying backgrounds can view the same risk data and come to different conclusions as to the cost and benefit of preventing that risk. For example, national-level recommendations to prevent malaria while traveling to India vary widely. Germany does not recommend using standard prophylaxis for any travel to an Indian destination; standby emergency treatment (SBET or self-treatment) is the recommendation for identified risk destinations. The guidelines in the United Kingdom recommend only awareness and mosquito bite prevention for more than half the Indian subcontinent, including large cities and popular tourist destinations in the north and south, while recommending an individual risk assessment that is based on activities and types of travelers. Standard prophylaxis recommended in the UK guidelines is the combination of chloroquine plus proguanil (an option not available in the United States) for much of the middle of the subcontinent. However, CDC recommends malaria chemoprophylaxis for any Indian destination except for some mountainous areas of northern states above 2,000 m (6,561 ft). Is one of these guidelines better than the others? Not necessarily, as the recommendations may be based on the national experience with different types of travelers and the risk assessment approach of the organization formulating the national guidelines. For example, in 2010, CDC reported 216 malaria cases acquired in India by returning US travelers, the second highest absolute number of cases from any destination. However, when viewed as estimated relative case rates (the number of cases among US travelers attributable to each country divided by the estimated travel volume for US travelers to that country), countries in sub-Saharan Africa remain well above the median estimated risk, and India falls below the median estimated risk because of the much higher volume of travel to India. India reports active transmission in all provinces in the country. Based on the extremely large population of India, some of these provinces have high absolute numbers of cases but low case rates. Some countries base their recommendations on these relatively low case rates, but other countries believe that the high absolute numbers of cases result in large numbers of infective mosquitoes that can, in turn, infect travelers. In any case, travelers to India are likely to encounter diverse recommendations for malaria prevention on the Internet or from other travelers.

The best available data should always balance the risk of the intervention—and the costs—against the risk of the disease, so that the decision to recommend a vaccine or prophylactic medicine may be understood by the clinician and the traveler.

Lack of Evidence

In many cases, limited or no data are available to inform an evidence-based assessment. In this setting, travel health providers defer to expert opinion or an extrapolation from limited data in conjunction with expert opinion. In travel medicine, it is rare to have actual prospective numerator and denominator data on the risk of any vaccine-preventable diseases in travelers. For example, any data on the risk of hepatitis A in travelers would have to account for the immunization rate with hepatitis A vaccine. These data are rarely available, and therefore, we often rely on historical data that captured few actual cases.

CAN WE HARMONIZE GUIDELINES?

The complex nature of how we obtain, evaluate, and verify data, combined with the fundamental differences in risk perception, makes it likely that multiple, overlapping, and at times conflicting guidelines will continue to exist. However, given the international nature of travel medicine and the existence of the International Society of Travel Medicine, conflicting guidelines have decreased in the past decade. In one example of an effort to harmonize guidelines, from 2008 through 2010, WHO convened an international group of yellow fever and travel medicine experts to review available data on yellow fever virus transmission. The product of this collaboration was a country-specific list of yellow fever vaccine recommendations based on the geographic distribution of risk (see Chapter 3, Travel Vaccines & Malaria Information, by Country).

In summary, the role of the travel health provider is to become more sophisticated in his or her understanding of the various differences in guidelines, in interpreting this information, and in conveying it in an assured and comforting manner to travelers.

BIBLIOGRAPHY

1. CDC. Advisory Committee on Immunization Practices (ACIP). Atlanta: CDC; 2012 [cited 2012 Sep 25]. Available from: http://www.cdc.gov/vaccines/acip/index.html.

2. Chiodini P, Hill D, Lea G, Walker E, Whitty C, Bannister B. Guidelines for malaria prevention in travellers from the United Kingdom 2007. London: Health Protection Agency; 2007 [cited 2012 Sep 25]. Available from: http://www.hpa.org.uk/Publications/InfectiousDiseases/TravelHealth/0701Malariapreventionfortravellersfromthe UK.

3. Committee to Advise on Tropical Medicine and Travel. Canadian recommendations for the prevention and treatment of malaria among international travellers—2009. Can Commun Dis Rep. 2009 Jul;35 Suppl 1:1–82.

4. German Society for Tropical Medicine and International Health Association (DTG). [Recommendations for malaria prevention]. 2012 [cited 2012 Sep 25]. Available from: http://www.microsofttranslator.com/bv.aspx?from=de&to=en&a=http%3A%2F%2Fwww.dtg.org%2Fmalaria.html.

5. Hill DR, Ericsson CD, Pearson RD, Keystone JS, Freedman DO, Kozarsky PE, et al. The practice of travel medicine: guidelines by the Infectious Diseases Society of America. Clin Infect Dis. 2006 Dec 15;43(12):1499–1539.

6. World Health Organization. International Health Regulations (2005). Geneva: World Health Organization; 2008 [cited 2012 Sep 25]. Available from: http://www.who.int/ihr/9789241596664/en/index.html.

7. World Health Organization. International Travel and Health. Geneva: World Health Organization; 2012 [cited 2012 Sep 25]. Available from: http://www.who.int/ith/en/.

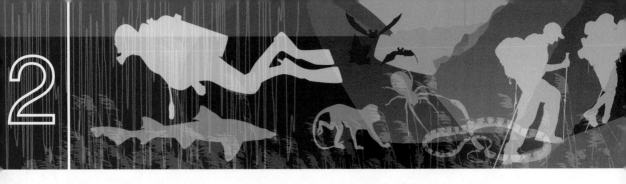

2

The Pre-Travel Consultation

THE PRE-TRAVEL CONSULTATION
Lin H. Chen

The pre-travel consultation offers a dedicated time to prepare travelers for the health concerns that might arise during their trips. The objectives of the pre-travel consultation are to assess the traveler's trip plans and determine potential health hazards; to educate the traveler regarding the anticipated risks and methods for prevention; to provide immunizations for vaccine-preventable diseases and medications for prophylaxis, self-treatment, or both; and to empower the traveler to manage his or her health throughout the trip.

QUALIFICATIONS FOR PROVIDING A PRE-TRAVEL CONSULTATION
Much evidence has accumulated relevant to travelers' health and forms the basis of pre-travel advice. Providers of pre-travel consultations should possess a general knowledge of the evidence base, understand disease epidemiology as well as routes of transmission and preventive measures, and be able to explore and discuss the risks clearly with travelers.

The outcome of a pre-travel consultation likely depends on the expertise and communication skills of the provider, as well as the health beliefs of the traveler. In-person counseling by trained staff can effectively deliver some messages, in particular with regard to

malaria risk and prevention. Familiarity with the traveler's destination, its culture, infrastructure, and disease patterns generates credibility for the advisor. An advisor with a passion for travel and personal travel experience may ably infuse vitality into the consultation and impart sound and memorable information.

Various disciplines of medicine provide pre-travel consultation, including primary care physicians, infectious diseases specialists, and travel medicine specialists. Primary care clinicians may have access to the traveler's medical history but may not have detailed knowledge of travel medicine. Travel medicine specialists have in-depth knowledge regarding immunizations, risks associated with specific destinations, and the implications of traveling with underlying conditions. Therefore, a comprehensive consultation with a travel medicine expert is indicated for any traveler with a complicated health history, special risks, or exotic or complicated itineraries.

COMPONENTS OF A PRE-TRAVEL CONSULTATION
Effective pre-travel consultations require attention to the health background of the traveler and incorporate the itinerary, trip

duration, travel style, and activities, all of which determine health risks (Table 2-1). Advice should be personalized, highlighting the likely exposures, and also reminding the traveler of ubiquitous risks such as injury, foodborne and waterborne infections, respiratory tract infections, and bloodborne and sexually transmitted infections. Written information is essential to supplement the oral advice and enable travelers to review the abundant instructions from their clinic visits. Balancing the cautions with an appreciation of the positive aspects of the journey leads to a more meaningful pre-travel consultation.

Assess Individual Risk

Many elements merit consideration in assessing a traveler's health risks. These factors can be incorporated into a paper intake form or electronic module to document the consultation (Table 2-1). Certain travelers may confront special risks. Recent hospitalization for serious problems may even lead the advisor to recommend delaying travel. Air travel is contraindicated for certain conditions. Other traveler characteristics that are associated with specific risks include travelers who are visiting friends or relatives, long-term travelers, travelers with chronic illnesses, immunocompromised travelers, pregnant travelers, and travelers with small children. More comprehensive discussion on advising travelers with specific needs is available in Chapter 8.

Manage Risk

Immunizations are a crucial component of pre-travel consultations, and the risk assessment forms the basis of recommendations for travel vaccines. At the same time, the pre-travel consultation presents an opportunity to update routine vaccines (Table 2-2).

The scope of pre-travel consultations includes preventive and self-treatment medications, such as malaria chemoprophylaxis, self-management of travelers' diarrhea, and prophylaxis or treatment for acute mountain sickness. Along with immunizations, prevention of malaria and travelers' diarrhea are key topics. If a traveler anticipates the need to treat motion sickness, jet lag, or severe allergic reactions, consider medications for self-management, such as motion sickness therapy, a sleep aid, and epinephrine. Prescribing multiple medications, particularly for travelers

already taking medications, warrants a review for possible drug interactions.

The pre-travel consultation also provides the ideal setting to review wellness strategies with travelers and to remind them of healthy practices during travel (Table 2-3). For travelers going to malaria-endemic countries, discuss malaria transmission, ways to reduce risk, and recommendations for chemoprophylaxis. Because of the frequent occurrence of travelers' diarrhea, advise travelers regarding food and water precautions and discuss a strategy to treat diarrhea if it occurs. Other topics to be explored are numerous and could be organized into a checklist, placing priority on the most serious and frequently encountered issues. General issues such as preventing injury and sunburn also deserve mention. Concise, written handouts can effectively summarize the salient issues.

Travelers with underlying health conditions require attention to their health issues as they relate to the destination and activities. For example, a traveler with a history of cardiac disease should carry medical reports, including a recent electrocardiogram. Asthma may flare in a traveler visiting a polluted city or from physical exertion during a hike; planning for treatment in case of asthma exacerbation can be lifesaving. Any allergies or serious medical conditions should be identified on a bracelet or a card to expedite medical care in emergency situations.

In addition to recognizing the traveler's characteristics, health background, and destination-specific risks, the exposures related to special activities also merit discussion. For example, river rafting in Africa could expose a traveler to schistosomiasis, and spelunking in Central America could put the traveler at risk of histoplasmosis.

Many medical issues that arise during travel can be self-managed. Therefore, travelers should be encouraged to carry a travel health kit with prescription and nonprescription medications. More detailed information for providers and travelers is given in Chapter 2, Travel Health Kits; Chapter 8, Travelers with Chronic Illnesses; Chapter 8, Humanitarian Aid Workers; and Appendix B.

Attention to the cost of recommended interventions may be critical. Some travelers may not be able to afford all of the indicated vaccines and medications, a situation

Table 2-1. Information necessary for a risk assessment during pre-travel consultations

Health Background

Past medical history	• Age • Sex • Underlying conditions • Allergies (especially any pertaining to vaccines, egg, or latex) • Medications
Special conditions	• Pregnancy • Breastfeeding • Disability or handicap • Immunocompromised • Older age • Psychiatric condition • Seizure disorder • Recent surgery • Recent cardiopulmonary event • Recent cerebrovascular event
Immunization history	• Routine vaccines • Travel vaccines
Prior travel experience	• Experience with malaria chemoprophylaxis • Experience with altitude • Illnesses related to prior travel

Trip Details

Itinerary	• Countries and specific regions, including order of countries if >1 country • Rural or urban
Timing	• Trip duration • Season of travel • Time to departure
Reason for travel	• Tourism • Business • Visiting friends and relatives (VFR) • Volunteer, missionary, or aid work • Research or education • Adventure • Pilgrimage • Adoption • Health care–seeking (medical tourism)
Travel style	• Independent travel or package tour • General hygiene standards at destination • Modes of transportation • Accommodations (such as tourist or luxury hotel, guest house, hostel or budget hotel, dormitory, local home or host family, or tent)
Special activities	• Disaster relief • High altitude or climbing • Diving • Cruise ship • Rafting • Cycling • Extreme sports

Table 2-2. Vaccines to update or consider during pre-travel consultations

VACCINE	TRAVEL-RELATED OCCURRENCES AND RECOMMENDATIONS
Routine Vaccines	
Haemophilus influenzae type b	No report of travel-related infection, although organism is ubiquitous.
Hepatitis B	Recommended for travelers visiting countries where HBsAg prevalence is ≥2% (see Map 3-4). Vaccination may be considered for all international travelers, regardless of destination, depending upon the traveler's behavioral risk as determined by the provider and traveler.
Human papillomavirus	No report of travel-acquired infection, although causal relationship is difficult to establish.
Influenza	Outbreaks have occurred on cruise ships, and 2009 influenza A(H1N1) illustrated the rapidity of spread via travel.
Measles, mumps, rubella	Infections are common in countries that do not immunize children routinely, including Europe. Outbreaks have occurred in the United States as a result of travel.
Meningococcal	Outbreaks occurred with Hajj pilgrimage, and the Kingdom of Saudi Arabia requires the quadrivalent vaccine for pilgrims.
Pneumococcal	Organism is ubiquitous and causal relationship to travel is difficult to establish.
Polio	Unimmunized or underimmunized travelers can acquire poliovirus, as occurred in a case reported in association with a stay with a host family in Latin America that had been declared polio-free.
Rotavirus	Common in developing countries, although not a common cause of travelers' diarrhea in adults. The vaccine is only recommended in young children.
Tetanus, diphtheria, pertussis	Rare cases of diphtheria have been attributed to travel. Pertussis has occurred in travelers, recently in adults whose immunity has waned.
Varicella	Infections are common in countries that do not immunize children routinely, as in most developing countries. Naturally occurring disease also occurs later in tropical countries.
Zoster	Travel (a form of stress) may trigger herpes zoster, but causal relationship is difficult to establish.

continued

TABLE 2-2. VACCINES TO UPDATE OR CONSIDER DURING PRE-TRAVEL CONSULTATIONS (continued)

Travel Vaccines

Cholera (not available in the United States)	Cases in travelers have occurred recently in association with travel to the Dominican Republic and Haiti.
Hepatitis A	Prevaccination incidence was 3–20 cases/1,000 person-months of travel, but recent surveillance indicated a decline to 3–11 cases/100,000 person-months of travel. Prevalence patterns of HAV infection may vary among regions within a country, and missing or obsolete data present a challenge. Some expert travel clinicians advise people traveling outside the United States to consider hepatitis A vaccination regardless of their country of destination.
Japanese encephalitis	Rare cases have occurred, estimated at <1 case/1 million travelers to endemic countries.
Rabies	Rabies preexposure immunization simplifies postexposure immunoprophylaxis.
Tickborne encephalitis (not available in the United States)	Cases have been identified in travelers with an estimated risk of 1/10,000 person-months in travelers. Endemic areas are expanding in Europe.
Typhoid	UK surveillance found the highest risk to be travel to India (6 cases/100,000 visits), Pakistan (9 cases/100,000 visits), and Bangladesh (21 cases/100,000 visits).
Yellow fever	Risk occurs mainly in defined areas of sub-Saharan Africa and the Amazon drainage of South America. Some countries require proof of vaccination for entry. For travelers visiting multiple countries, order of travel may make a difference in the requirements.

Abbreviation: HBsAg, hepatitis B surface antigen.

Table 2-3. Major topics for discussion during pre-travel consultations

Immunizations	• Review routine immunizations and those indicated for the specific itinerary.
Malaria chemoprophylaxis	• Determine if there is a risk of malaria. • Discuss personal protective measures. • Discuss risks and benefits of chemoprophylaxis, and recommended choices of chemoprophylaxis for the itinerary.

continued

TABLE 2-3. MAJOR TOPICS FOR DISCUSSION DURING PRE-TRAVEL CONSULTATIONS (continued)

Travelers' diarrhea	• Recommend strategies to minimize diarrhea. • Discuss antibiotics for self-treatment and adjunct medications such as loperamide.
Other vectorborne diseases	• Define risk of disease in specific itinerary and insect precautions needed.
Altitude illness	• Determine if the itinerary puts the traveler at risk of altitude illness. • Discuss preventive measures such as gradual ascent, adequate hydration, and medications to prevent and treat.
Other environmental hazards	• Caution the traveler to avoid contact with animals to reduce the potential for bites and scratches that can transmit rabies. • Advise to avoid walking barefoot as parasites can enter intact or damaged skin. • Advise to avoid wading or swimming in freshwater where there is risk for schistosomiasis or leptospirosis. • Remind travelers to apply sunscreen to skin exposed to the sun.
Personal safety	• Discuss precautions the traveler can take to minimize risks specific to the trip, such as traffic accidents, alcohol excess, personal assault, robbery, or drowning. • Provide information on travel health and medical evacuation insurance.
Sexual health and bloodborne pathogens	• Caution the traveler to avoid activities that can lead to sexually transmitted infections, unwanted pregnancy, or bloodborne infections. • Remind travelers to use condoms if they do have sex.

that requires prioritization of interventions. (See *Perspectives*: Prioritizing for the Resource-Limited Traveler section later in this chapter.)

Finally, a comprehensive pre-travel consultation should include providing the traveler with a record of immunizations administered.

BIBLIOGRAPHY

1. Angell SY, Behrens RH. Risk assessment and disease prevention in travelers visiting friends and relatives. Infect Dis Clin North Am. 2005 Mar;19(1):49–65.
2. Askling HH, Rombo L, Andersson Y, Martin S, Ekdahl K. Hepatitis A risk in travelers. J Travel Med. 2009 Jul–Aug;16(4):233–8.
3. CDC. Tick-borne encephalitis among US travelers to Europe and Asia—2000–2009. MMWR Morb Mortal Wkly Rep. 2010 Mar 26;59(11):335–8.
4. Chen LH, Hill DR. PIER Module: Travel immunizations. Philadelphia, PA: American College of Physicians [cited 2012 Feb 12]. Available from: http://pier.acponline.org/physicians/procedures/physpro272/ physpro272-wn.html (requires ACP membership for access).
5. Chen LH, Wilson ME, Davis X, Loutan L, Schwartz E, Keystone J, et al. Illness in long-term travelers visiting GeoSentinel clinics. Emerg Infect Dis. 2009 Nov;15(11):1773–82.
6. Christenson JC. Preparing families with children traveling to developing countries. Pediatr Ann. 2008 Dec;37(12):806–13.
7. DuPont HL, Ericsson CD, Farthing MJ, Gorbach S, Pickering LK, Rombo L, et al. Expert review of the evidence base for self-therapy of travelers' diarrhea. J Travel Med. 2009 May–Jun;16(3):161–71.

8. Freedman DO. Clinical practice. Malaria prevention in short-term travelers. N Engl J Med. 2008 Aug 7;359(6):603–12.

9. Freedman DO, Weld LH, Kozarsky PE, Fisk T, Robins R, von Sonnenburg F, et al. Spectrum of disease and relation to place of exposure among ill returned travelers. N Engl J Med. 2006 Jan 12;354(2):119–30.

10. Hartjes LB, Baumann LC, Henriques JB. Travel health risk perceptions and prevention behaviors of US study abroad students. J Travel Med. 2009 Sep–Oct;16(5):338–43.

11. Hatz CFR, Chen LH. Pre-travel consultation. In: Keystone JS, Freedman DO, Kozarsky PE, Connor BA, Nothdurft HD, editors. Travel Medicine. 3rd ed. Philadelphia: Saunders Elsevier; 2013. p. 31–6.

12. Hill DR, Ericsson CD, Pearson RD, Keystone JS, Freedman DO, Kozarsky PE, et al. The practice of travel medicine: guidelines by the Infectious Diseases Society of America. Clin Infect Dis. 2006 Dec 15;43(12):1499–539.

13. Hills SL, Griggs AC, Fischer M. Japanese encephalitis in travelers from non-endemic countries, 1973–2008. Am J Trop Med Hyg. 2010 May;82(5):930–6.

14. International Society of Travel Medicine. The body of knowledge for the practice of travel medicine. Atlanta: International Society of Travel Medicine; 2006 [cited 2012 Sep 18]. Available from: https://www.istm.org/WebForms/Members/MemberResources/Cert_Travhlth/Body.aspx.

15. LaRocque RC, Rao SR, Tsibris A, Lawton T, Barry MA, Marano N, et al. Pre-travel health advice-seeking behavior among US international travelers departing from Boston Logan International Airport. J Travel Med. 2010 Nov–Dec;17(6):387–91.

16. Mackell S. Traveler's diarrhea in the pediatric population: etiology and impact. Clin Infect Dis. 2005 Dec 1;41 Suppl 8:S547–52.

17. Mali S, Kachur SP, Arguin PM, Division of Parasitic Diseases and Malaria (CDC). Malaria surveillance—United States, 2010. MMWR Surveill Summ. 2012 Mar 2;61(2):1–17.

18. McCarthy AE, Mileno MD. Prevention and treatment of travel-related infections in compromised hosts. Curr Opin Infect Dis. 2006 Oct;19(5):450–5.

19. Patel TA, Armstrong M, Morris-Jones SD, Wright SG, Doherty T. Imported enteric fever: case series from the hospital for tropical diseases, London, United Kingdom. Am J Trop Med Hyg. 2010 Jun;82(6):1121–6.

20. Pitzurra R, Steffen R, Tschopp A, Mutsch M. Diarrhoea in a large prospective cohort of European travellers to resource-limited destinations. BMC Infect Dis. 2010;10:231.

21. Schlagenhauf P, Petersen E. Malaria chemoprophylaxis: strategies for risk groups. Clin Microbiol Rev. 2008 Jul;21(3):466–72.

22. Steffen R, Amitirigala I, Mutsch M. Health risks among travelers—need for regular updates. J Travel Med. 2008 May–Jun;15(3):145–6.

23. Talbot EA, Chen LH, Sanford C, McCarthy A, Leder K, Research Committee of the International Society of Travel Medicine. Travel medicine research priorities: establishing an evidence base. J Travel Med. 2010 Nov–Dec;17(6):410–5.

24. Toovey S, Moerman F, van Gompel A. Special infectious disease risks of expatriates and long-term travelers in tropical countries. Part II: infections other than malaria. J Travel Med. 2007 Jan–Feb;14(1):50–60.

25. World Health Organization. International travel and health. Geneva: World Health Organization; 2012 [cited 2012 Sep 25]. Available from: http://www.who.int/ith/en/.

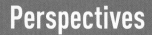

RISKS TRAVELERS FACE

David R. Shlim

Travel medicine is based on the concept of the reduction of risk. In the context of travel medicine, "risk" refers to the possibility of harm during the course of a planned trip. Some risks may be avoidable, and others may not. Vaccine-preventable diseases may be mostly avoidable, depending on the risk of the disease and the protective efficacy of the vaccine. Non-disease risks, such as motor vehicle accidents or drowning, account for a much higher percentage of deaths among travelers than infectious diseases.

For many years, travel medicine practitioners have felt that if they knew the statistics for a given risk, they could objectively advise travelers about that risk. However, it has become clear that the perception and tolerance of risk are subjective factors that must be considered when addressing risks of travel. Travel health providers may know statistics for a given risk, but whether the risk is considered high or low depends on the perception of the traveler or the travel medicine provider. For example, the risk of dying while trekking in Nepal is 15 deaths per 100,000 trekkers, but there is no objective way to determine whether this risk is high or low. When the manuscript that reported this risk of dying while trekking was peer-reviewed, one reviewer wrote, "You need to emphasize that these data show how dangerous trekking actually is." The other reviewer wrote, "You should make a point of stating that these data show how safe trekking is."

The subjective sense of risk is based on one's perception of risk ("15 per 100,000 means it's dangerous") and one's tolerance for risk ("it may be 15 per 100,000, but it's worth it"). This subjective sense of risk suffuses the field of travel medicine, but it is rarely discussed. Some travelers canceled travel plans to Asia because of their fear of H5N1 avian influenza, even though the actual risk to travelers was virtually zero. Other travelers plan to ascend Mount Everest, even though the risk of dying during an Everest climb is 1 in 40.

Regardless of the perception and tolerance of risk, the hazards associated with travel cannot be eliminated, just as the risks of staying home are not zero. Even the act of trying to prevent a risk—such as yellow fever—can lead to a fatal reaction to the vaccine in very rare cases. Therefore, the goal in travel and in travel medicine should be skillfully managing risk, rather than trying to eliminate risk. The pre-travel consultation is an opportunity to discuss risks and develop plans that minimize these risks. Each traveler may have individual concepts about the risks and benefits of vaccines, prophylaxis, and behavior modification.

Travelers should also consider the psychological and emotional aspects of foreign travel. Culture shock can occur on either end of a journey: on arrival when one encounters an entirely strange new world, and on return when one's

---

Perspectives sections are written as editorial discussions aiming to add depth and clinical perspective to the official recommendations contained in the book. The views and opinions expressed in this section are those of the author and do not necessarily represent the official position of CDC.

own world may temporarily appear unfamiliar. Travelers with underlying psychiatric conditions should be cautious when heading out to a stressful new environment, particularly if they are traveling alone.

Travel medicine providers should promote the understanding of the concept of commitment, the idea that certain parts of a journey cannot easily be reversed. A person trekking into a remote area may need to accept that rescue, if available at all, may be delayed for days. A person who has a myocardial infarction in a country with no advanced cardiac services may have a difficult time getting to definitive medical care. If the traveler has already contemplated these concerns and accepted them, it will be easier to deal with them if they come to pass.

Travel medicine practitioners should explore their own perception and tolerance of risk, so that they can help travelers find their individual comfort level when making decisions about destinations, activities, and prophylactic measures.

Perspectives

PRIORITIZING CARE FOR THE RESOURCE-LIMITED TRAVELER
Ilan Youngster, Elizabeth D. Barnett

Travelers seen in pre-travel clinic consultations often have financial constraints. Prioritizing immunizations and prophylactic medications should be part of an individualized assessment based not only on the travel profile and efficacy and safety of vaccines and medications, but also on associated costs. Travelers must often pay out of pocket for pre-travel care, as many health insurance plans do not cover travel immunizations and prophylaxis. Travelers with limited budgets tend to be at higher risk for acquiring travel-associated infections, as they often visit remote areas, stay in lower-grade accommodations, and are more likely to eat local street food. As an example, the estimated cost of a pre-travel consultation for a young backpacker planning a 4-week trip in West Africa will run as high as $1,400 for the initial consult and vaccinations, excluding malaria chemoprophylaxis. Clinicians need to understand travelers' financial constraints in order to provide realistic recommendations. Helping travelers with limited budgets decide how best to spend limited resources on travel vaccines and medications is one of the most challenging tasks of travel medicine specialists. The variety of insurance plans, number of travelers without adequate insurance coverage, and number of student and budget travelers vexes even the most savvy travel medicine clinics. This section provides guidance and strategies for prioritizing vaccine and medication choices for the busy practitioner.

VACCINES
Required Vaccines
Only 2 vaccines are categorically required for some travelers: meningococcal vaccine for pilgrims traveling to Mecca during the Hajj and yellow fever (see Chapter 3, Travel Vaccines & Malaria Information, by Country). If either of these is required for an itinerary, prioritize it since the traveler may be denied entry to the country without proof of vaccination.

Routine Vaccines
CDC recommends that all travelers should be up-to-date on routine vaccines before international travel, regardless of destination. Routine vaccines are generally associated with lower costs, as they are produced for mass administration as part of the scheduled national childhood and adult vaccination programs. The benefit of their administration extends beyond the travel period, and in many cases immunity for life is achieved. Moreover, many health insurance plans will reimburse the patient for the cost of their administration. If a traveler requires routine vaccines and cost is a limitation, he or she can explore opportunities for obtaining them in a health department or primary care setting, where cost may be lower than in a travel clinic. Prioritize the routine vaccines that protect against diseases for which the traveler is most likely to be at general risk. At this time, top priorities would be influenza vaccine and measles-containing vaccine.

Recommended Vaccines
The patient may have prior immunity to the disease for which immunization is being considered. In some settings, testing for antibody concentrations may be covered by insurance, while vaccines are not. Specifically, hepatitis A and B are vaccines important for travelers' health and should be considered for susceptible hosts. Testing for immunity to these infections may determine whether vaccination is warranted.

In recommending vaccines, a provider should consider the destination, the expected itinerary, seasonality, and baseline risk factors in the patient. Review the itinerary to determine the need for specific vaccines based on destination or purpose of travel: polio vaccine for travel to endemic countries, meningococcal vaccine for travel to the meningitis belt of sub-Saharan Africa or to an area where an outbreak is occurring, or hepatitis B vaccine for travelers likely to have blood and body fluid exposure (health care or humanitarian workers, for example).

Consider travel vaccines based on time until departure, risk at destination, effectiveness of vaccine, and likelihood of repeat travel. Hepatitis A vaccine will frequently be a good choice given the high efficacy, duration of immunity, and prevalence of risk. Parenteral typhoid vaccine may be less cost-effective for infrequent travelers (especially when departures are imminent and trip duration is short) because of the low efficacy, short duration of protection, and time needed for onset of effectiveness.

Educate about alternative ways to reduce risk; for example, avoiding animal bites, insect precautions, and food and water precautions. All travelers should practice these preventive behaviors, but they are critical for travelers who elect not to receive recommended vaccinations for financial reasons.

MALARIA CHEMOPROPHYLAXIS

Malaria chemoprophylaxis can also be a financial burden for the traveler. The risk of acquiring malaria in the affluent traveler staying in air-conditioned hotels and commuting in a rented car is much lower than that assumed by the young backpacker staying in a rural guesthouse or the traveler returning to his native land staying with friends or relatives. Tailoring advice to the traveler's financial needs in addition to his or her medical needs can improve compliance with prophylaxis and protect those who are at highest risk.

Every pre-travel consultation should include detailed advice about preventing mosquito bites (see Prevention against Mosquitoes, Ticks, & Other Insects & Arthropods later in this chapter). Malaria chemoprophylaxis, if needed, should be offered based on the risk profile of the traveler.

Costs associated with the different regimens vary widely. For example, based on current prices in the United States, a prophylactic treatment course for a 3-week trip to a malaria-endemic destination would be $30 for doxycycline, $45 for chloroquine, $80 for mefloquine, and $150 for atovaquone-proguanil (depending on health insurance and other factors). When cost is a primary consideration, doxycycline should be considered, although accompanied by detailed instructions about how to take this medication and information about potential adverse events and how to manage them. Atovaquone-proguanil cost may be equivalent with mefloquine for short trips, but mefloquine (or chloroquine, in the few regions where malaria remains susceptible) will be more cost-effective for longer trips. Travelers who raise the option of purchasing antimalarial drugs at their destination need to be advised about the risk of inappropriate and counterfeit medications (see *Perspectives*: Pharmaceutical Quality & Counterfeit Drugs later in this chapter).

PREVENTIVE BEHAVIORS

Budget travelers and those who cannot afford costly travel vaccines will continue to challenge travel medicine practitioners. Travelers who cannot afford all available vaccines will appreciate additional strategies to safeguard their health during travel. These strategies include information about safety and security and general information about sun protection, food hazards, and road traffic injury. Travelers can be reassured that this information addresses hazards that are, in fact, more common than many of the vaccine-preventable diseases and that the actions they take to avoid these hazards may, in the long run, be more beneficial than obtaining vaccines for diseases of low prevalence.

BIBLIOGRAPHY

1. Beutels P, Van Damme P, Piper Jenks N. Economic evaluation in travel medicine. In: DuPont HL, Steffen R, editors. Textbook of Travel Medicine and Health. 2nd ed. Hamilton, Ontario: Brian C Decker; 2001. p. 21–7.
2. Bryan JP. Cost considerations of malaria chemoprophylaxis including use of primaquine for primary or terminal chemoprophylaxis. Am J Trop Med Hyg. 2006 Sep;75(3):416–20.
3. Mangtani P, Roberts JA. Economic evaluations of travelers' vaccinations. In: Zuckerman JN, Jong EC, editors. Travelers' Vaccines. 2nd ed. Shelton, CT: People's Medical Publishing House; 2010. p. 553–67.
4. Steffen R, Connor BA. Vaccines in travel health: from risk assessment to priorities. J Travel Med. 2005 Jan-Feb;12(1):26–35.

GENERAL RECOMMENDATIONS FOR VACCINATION & IMMUNOPROPHYLAXIS

Andrew T. Kroger, Raymond A. Strikas

Recommendations for the use of vaccines and other biologic products (such as immune globulin [IG] products) in the United States are developed by the Advisory Committee on Immunization Practices (ACIP) and other groups, such as the American Academy of Pediatrics, the American Academy of Family Physicians, and the American College of Physicians. ACIP recommendations are based on scientific evidence of benefits (immunity to the disease) and risks (vaccine adverse reactions) and, where few or no data are available, on expert opinion. The recommendations include information on general immunization issues and the use of specific vaccines. Box 2-1 provides more information about ACIP. This section is based primarily on the ACIP General Recommendations on Immunization.

Evaluation of people before travel should include a review and provision of routine vaccines recommended based on age and other individual characteristics. Additionally, some routine vaccines are recommended at earlier ages for international travelers. For example, MMR (measles-mumps-rubella) vaccine is recommended for infants aged 6–11 months who travel abroad to protect them from measles. Recommendations for specific vaccines related to travel will depend on itinerary, duration of travel, and host factors. Vaccinations against diphtheria, tetanus, pertussis, measles, mumps, rubella, varicella, poliomyelitis, hepatitis A, hepatitis B, *Haemophilus influenzae* type b (Hib), rotavirus, human papillomavirus (HPV), and pneumococcal and meningococcal invasive disease are routinely administered in the United States, usually in childhood or adolescence. Influenza vaccine is routinely recommended for all people aged ≥6 months, each year. A dose of herpes zoster (shingles) vaccine is recommended for adults aged ≥60 years. If a person does not have a history of adequate protection against these diseases, immunizations appropriate to age and previous immunization status should be obtained, whether or not international travel is planned. A visit to a clinician for travel-related immunizations should be seen as an opportunity to bring an incompletely vaccinated person up-to-date on his or her routine vaccinations.

Both the child and adolescent vaccination schedules, and an adult vaccination schedule, are published annually in the *Morbidity and Mortality Weekly Report* (MMWR). Clinicians should obtain the most current schedules from the CDC Vaccines and Immunization

BOX 2-1. THE ADVISORY COMMITTEE ON IMMUNIZATION PRACTICES (ACIP)

In 1964, the Department of Health and Human Services chartered the Advisory Committee on Immunization Practices (ACIP) to provide guidance to CDC for making immunization policy. Guidance includes scheduling of vaccine doses, specific risk groups for whom vaccination is recommended, and vaccine contraindications and precautions.

The ACIP is composed of 15 voting members selected by the Secretary of Health and Human Services. ACIP chair, a consumer representative, and 13 members are balanced among various sectors, including academic immunology, medicine, and public health. In addition to the 15 voting members, the committee includes 8 ex officio members representing federal agencies and 26 nonvoting representatives of liaison organizations with broad responsibilities for vaccine development, administration of vaccines to various segments of the population, and operation of immunization programs. ACIP is subdivided into 4 permanent workgroups that address child/adolescent immunization schedules, adult immunization schedules, influenza vaccine, and general immunization issues. In addition to the 4 permanent workgroups, 7 additional workgroups focus on particular vaccines. Input into the development of immunization schedules is shared with professional organizations, including the American Academy of Pediatrics, American College of Physicians, American Academy of Family Physicians, American Congress of Obstetricians and Gynecologists, and American College of Nurse-Midwives.

ACIP workgroups are led by a member of ACIP who works in close collaboration with a CDC workgroup lead staff member. Members of the vaccine pharmaceutical industry may not serve as workgroup members. The workgroup develops consensus on various policy points, then the CDC workgroup lead writes specific content for presentation to the ACIP at large. When it is difficult to achieve consensus, options with plans are developed and presented to the ACIP at large for a vote.

The ACIP meets 3 times a year in a public meeting during which the various workgroups present content that has been developed and is ready for ACIP discussion or voting. Sometimes ACIP members are involved in academic vaccine research supported by the pharmaceutical industry. These members must state these conflicts and must recuse themselves from votes regarding vaccines manufactured by companies from which they receive support. The end result of various discussions and votes is an ACIP document published in CDC's *Morbidity and Mortality Weekly Report* (www.cdc.gov/mmwr), representing the official policy of the Department of Health and Human Services.

website (www.cdc.gov/vaccines/schedules). The text and many tables of this publication present recommendations for the use, number of doses, dose intervals, adverse reactions, precautions, and contraindications for vaccines and toxoids that may be indicated for travelers. Recommendations for travelers are not always the same as routine recommendations. For instance, most adults born after 1956 are recommended to receive 1 dose of MMR vaccine; however, international travelers of this age are recommended to receive 2 doses. One dose of MMR vaccine is also recommended for infants aged 6–11 months before they travel abroad. For specific vaccines and toxoids, additional details on background, adverse reactions, precautions, and contraindications, refer to the respective ACIP recommendations (http://www.cdc.gov/vaccines/acip/index.html).

SPACING OF IMMUNOBIOLOGICS
Simultaneous Administration

All commonly used vaccines can safely and effectively be given simultaneously (on the same day) at separate sites without impairing antibody responses or increasing rates of adverse reactions. This knowledge is particularly helpful for international travelers, for whom exposure to several infectious diseases might be imminent. Simultaneous administration of all indicated vaccines is encouraged for people who are the recommended age to receive these vaccines and for whom no contraindications exist. If not administered on the same day, an inactivated vaccine may be given at any time before or after a different inactivated vaccine or a live-virus vaccine.

The immune response to an injected or intranasal live-virus vaccine (such as MMR, varicella, yellow fever, or live attenuated influenza vaccine) might be impaired if administered within 28 days of another live-virus vaccine (within 30 days for yellow fever vaccine). Whenever possible, injected live-virus vaccines administered on different days should be given ≥28 days apart (≥30 days for yellow fever vaccine). If 2 injected or intranasal live-virus vaccines are not administered on the same day but <28 days apart (<30 days for yellow fever vaccine), the second vaccine should be readministered ≥28 days (≥30 days for yellow fever vaccine) after the second vaccine was administered.

Measles and other live-virus vaccines may interfere with the response to tuberculin skin testing and the interferon-γ release assay. Tuberculin skin testing, if otherwise indicated, can be done either on the day that live-virus vaccines are administered or 4–6 weeks later. Tuberculin skin testing is not a prerequisite for administration of any vaccine. Oral typhoid vaccine, a live attenuated bacterial vaccine, has not been associated with suppressing the response to tuberculosis testing.

Missed Doses and Boosters

All vaccines require a primary dose or series to ensure immunity, and some require periodic repeat, or booster, doses to maintain immunity. Travelers may forget to return to complete a series or for a booster at the specified time. Occasionally, the demand for a vaccine may exceed its supply, and providers may have difficulty obtaining vaccines. Information on vaccine shortages and recommendations can be found on the CDC Vaccines and Immunization website at www.cdc.gov/vaccines/vac-gen/shortages/default.htm.

In some cases, a scheduled dose of vaccine may not be given on time. If this occurs, the dose should be given at the next visit. Available data indicate that intervals between doses longer than those routinely recommended do not affect seroconversion rate or titer when the schedule is completed. Consequently, it is not necessary to restart the series or add doses of any vaccine because of an extended interval between doses. The only exception to this rule is oral typhoid vaccine in some circumstances. Some experts recommend repeating the series of oral typhoid vaccine if the 4-dose series is extended to more than 3 weeks. Information on revaccination (booster) doses of vaccines is listed in Table 2-4.

Table 2-4. Revaccination (booster) schedules

VACCINE	RECOMMENDATION
Hepatitis A	Booster doses not recommended for adults and children who have completed the primary series (2 doses) according to the routine schedule.[1]
Hepatitis B	Booster doses not recommended for adults and children who have completed the primary series (3 doses) according to the routine schedule.[1,2]
Influenza	1 annual dose (children aged 6 months to 9 years and certain incompletely vaccinated children should receive 2 doses separated by ≥4 weeks the first time that influenza vaccine is administered). Live attenuated influenza vaccine is approved only for healthy, nonpregnant people aged 2–49 years.
Japanese encephalitis (JE) (Vero cell formulation)	For people aged ≥17 years, if the primary series of Ixiaro was administered ≥1 year previously, a booster dose should be given before potential reexposure or if there is a continued risk for JE virus infection. There are no data on the use of Ixiaro as a booster dose after a primary series with JE-Vax. People who have received JE-Vax previously and require further vaccination against JE virus should receive a 2-dose primary series of Ixiaro. See the booster dose information in Chapter 3, Japanese Encephalitis.

continued

TABLE 2-4. REVACCINATION (BOOSTER) SCHEDULES (continued)

VACCINE	RECOMMENDATION
Measles, mumps, and rubella (MMR)	Two doses of MMR vaccine separated by ≥4 weeks or other evidence of immunity (such as serologic testing) are recommended for people born after 1956 who travel outside the United States. Revaccination is not recommended.
Meningococcal quadrivalent A, C, Y, W-135	Revaccination for people who received meningococcal polysaccharide vaccine or meningococcal conjugate vaccine, and who remain at increased risk for meningococcal disease (including some international travelers): Revaccination with meningococcal conjugate vaccine is recommended after 3 years for children who were previously vaccinated at ages 9 months to 6 years. Revaccination with meningococcal conjugate vaccine is recommended after 5 years for people who were previously vaccinated at ages 7–55 years, and every 5 years thereafter for people who are at continued risk.[3] Revaccination with meningococcal polysaccharide vaccine is recommended for adults >55 years who remain at increased risk 3–5 years after the last dose.
Pneumococcal (polysaccharide)	One-time revaccination 5 years after original dose for people with certain underlying medical conditions (such as asplenia) or people who were first vaccinated at <65 years of age.
Polio vaccine, inactivated (IPV)	For adults traveling to areas where poliomyelitis cases are still occurring, a single lifetime booster dose is recommended for those who have documentation of having completed a primary series.
Rabies preexposure vaccine	No serologic testing or boosters recommended for travelers. For people in high-risk groups (such as rabies laboratory workers), serologic testing and booster doses are recommended. See Table 3-15.
Rotavirus	Booster doses not recommended.
Tetanus, diphtheria, and acellular pertussis (Td, Tdap)	Tetanus and diphtheria booster dose is recommended every 10 years. A single dose of adolescent/adult formulation Td that includes acellular pertussis vaccine (Tdap) is recommended to replace 1 Td booster dose for people aged 11–64 years. Adults aged ≤65 years who have or who anticipate having close contact with an infant aged <12 months and who previously have not received Tdap should receive a single dose of Tdap to protect against pertussis and reduce the likelihood of transmission; all other adults aged ≥65 years who have not previously received Tdap may be given a single dose of Tdap instead of Td. See ACIP statement for details.
Typhoid intramuscular	Booster dose every 2 years for those who remain at continued risk.
Typhoid oral	Repeat series every 5 years for those who remain at continued risk.
Varicella	Revaccination is not recommended.
Yellow Fever	Repeat vaccination every 10 years for those who remain at risk.
Zoster	Revaccination is not recommended.

[1] A 3- or 4-dose series of combination hepatitis A-hepatitis B vaccine (HepA-HepB) is also available.
[2] Booster dosing may be appropriate for certain populations, such as hemodialysis patients.
[3] See: CDC. Updated recommendation from the Advisory Committee on Immunization Practices (ACIP) for revaccination of persons at prolonged increased risk for meningococcal disease. MMWR Morb Mortal Wkly Rep. 2009 Sep 25;58(37):1042–3.

Antibody-Containing Blood Products

Antibody-containing blood products, such as IG products, from the United States do not interfere with the immune response to yellow fever vaccine and are not believed to interfere with the response to live typhoid, live attenuated influenza, rotavirus, or zoster vaccines. When MMR and varicella vaccines are given shortly before, simultaneously with, or after an antibody-containing blood product, response to the vaccine can be diminished. The duration of inhibition of MMR and varicella vaccines is related to the dose of IG in the product. MMR or its components and varicella vaccines either should be administered ≥2 weeks before receipt of a blood product, or should be delayed 3–11 months after receipt of the blood product, depending on the vaccine (Table 2-5).

IG administration may become necessary for another indication after MMR or its individual components or varicella vaccines have been given. In such a situation, the IG may interfere with the immune response to the MMR or varicella vaccines. Vaccine virus replication and stimulation of immunity usually occur 2–3 weeks after vaccination. If the interval between administration of one of these vaccines and the subsequent administration of an IG preparation is ≥14 days, the vaccine need not be readministered. If the interval is <14 days, the vaccine should be readministered after the interval shown in Table 2-5, unless serologic testing indicates that antibodies have been produced.

If administration of IG becomes necessary, MMR or its components or varicella vaccines can be administered simultaneously with IG, with the recognition that vaccine-induced immunity can be compromised. The vaccine should be administered at a body site different from that chosen for the IG injection. Vaccination should be repeated after the interval noted in Table 2-5, unless serologic testing indicates antibodies have been produced.

When IG is given with the first dose of hepatitis A vaccine, the proportion of recipients who develop a protective level of antibody is not affected, but antibody concentrations are lower. Because the final concentrations of antibody are many times higher than those considered protective, this reduced immunogenicity is not expected to be clinically relevant.

IG preparations interact minimally with other inactivated vaccines and toxoids. Other inactivated vaccines may be given simultaneously, or at any time interval before or after an antibody-containing blood product is used. However, such vaccines should be administered at different sites from the IG.

VACCINATION OF PEOPLE WITH ACUTE ILLNESSES

Every opportunity should be taken to provide needed vaccinations. The decision to delay vaccination because of a current or recent acute illness depends on the severity of the symptoms and their cause. Although a moderate or severe acute illness is sufficient reason to postpone vaccination, minor illnesses (such as diarrhea, mild upper respiratory infection with or without low-grade fever, other low-grade febrile illness) are not contraindications to vaccination.

People with moderate or severe acute illness, with or without fever, should be vaccinated as soon as the condition improves. This precaution is to avoid superimposing adverse effects from the vaccine on underlying illness, or mistakenly attributing a manifestation of underlying illness to the vaccine. Antimicrobial therapy is not a contraindication to vaccination, with 3 exceptions:

- Antibacterial agents may interfere with the response to oral typhoid vaccine.
- Antiviral agents active against herpesviruses (such as acyclovir) may interfere with the response to varicella-containing vaccines.
- Antiviral agents active against influenza virus (such as zanamivir and oseltamivir) may interfere with the response to live attenuated influenza vaccine.

A physical examination or temperature measurement is not a prerequisite for vaccinating a person who appears to be in good health. Asking if a person is ill, postponing a vaccination for someone with moderate or severe acute illness, and vaccinating someone who does not have contraindications are appropriate procedures for clinic immunizations.

ALTERED IMMUNOCOMPETENCE

Altered immunocompetence is a general term that is often used interchangeably with the terms immunosuppression,

Table 2-5. Recommended intervals between administration of antibody-containing products and measles-containing vaccine or varicella-containing vaccine[1]

INDICATION	DOSE AND ROUTE	RECOMMENDED INTERVAL BEFORE MEASLES OR VARICELLA VACCINATION
Tetanus (TIG)	250 units (10 mg IgG/kg) IM	3 months
Hepatitis A (IG), duration of international travel <3-month stay ≥3-month stay	 0.02 mL/kg (3.3 mg IgG/kg) IM 0.06 mL/kg (10 mg IgG/kg) IM	 3 months 3 months
Hepatitis B prophylaxis (HBIG)	0.06 mL/kg (10 mg IgG/kg) IM	3 months
Rabies prophylaxis (HRIG)	20 IU/kg (22 mg IgG/kg) IM	4 months
Varicella prophylaxis (VZIG)	125 units/10 kg (60–200 mg IgG/kg) IM (maximum 625 units)	5 months

Measles prophylaxis (IG)
     Immunocompetent contact
     Immunocompromised contact
	
	0.25 mL/kg (40 mg IgG/kg) IM
	 0.50 mL/kg (80 mg IgG/kg) IM
		
		5 months
		 6 months

Botulism immune globulin, intravenous	1.5 mL/kg (75 mg IgG/kg) IV	6 months

Blood transfusion
     Red blood cells (RBCs), washed
     RBCs, adenine-saline added
     Packed RBCs (hematocrit 65%)[2]
     Whole blood (hematocrit 35%–50%)[2]
     Plasma/platelet products
	
	10 mL/kg (negligible IgG/kg) IV
	 10 mL/kg (10 mg IgG/kg) IV
	 10 mL/kg (60 mg IgG/kg) IV
	 10 mL/kg (80–100 mg IgG/kg) IV
	 10 mL/kg (160 mg IgG/kg) IV
		
		None
		 3 months
		 6 months
		 6 months
		 7 months

Cytomegalovirus prophylaxis (CMV IGIV)	150 mg/kg IV (maximum)	6 months
Respiratory syncytial virus (RSV) monoclonal antibody[3]	15 mg/kg IM	None

continued

TABLE 2-5. RECOMMENDED INTERVALS BETWEEN ADMINISTRATION OF ANTIBODY-CONTAINING PRODUCTS AND MEASLES-CONTAINING VACCINE OR VARICELLA-CONTAINING VACCINE[1] (continued)

INDICATION	DOSE AND ROUTE	RECOMMENDED INTERVAL BEFORE MEASLES OR VARICELLA VACCINATION
Intravenous immune globulin (IVIG)		
Replacement therapy	300–400 mg/kg IV	8 months
Immune thrombocytopenic purpura (ITP)	400 mg/kg IV	8 months
Postexposure varicella prophylaxis[4]	400 mg/kg IV	8 months
ITP	1 gm/kg IV	10 months
ITP or Kawasaki disease	1.6–2 gm/kg IV	11 months

Abbreviations: IG, immune globulin; IM, intramuscular; IV, intravenous.

[1] Adapted from Table 5, Kroger AT, Sumaya CV, Pickering LK, Atkinson WL. General recommendations on immunization: recommendations of the Advisory Committee on Immunization Practices (ACIP). MMWR Recomm Rep. 2011 Jan 28;60(RR-2):1–61. This table is not intended for determining the correct indications and dosage for the use of IG preparations. Unvaccinated people may not be fully protected against measles during the entire recommended interval, and additional doses of IG or measles vaccine may be indicated after measles exposure. Concentrations of measles antibody in an IG preparation can vary by manufacturer's lot. For example, more than a 4-fold variation in the amount of measles antibody titers has been demonstrated in different IG preparations. Rates of antibody clearance after receipt of an IG preparation can also vary. Recommended intervals are extrapolated from an estimated half-life of 30 days for passively acquired antibody and an observed interference with the immune response to measles vaccine for 5 months after a dose of 80 mg IgG/kg. Does not include zoster vaccine. Zoster vaccine may be given with antibody-containing products.

[2] Assumes a serum IgG concentration of 16 mg/mL.

[3] Contains only antibody to respiratory syncytial virus.

[4] IVIG is an alternative to VZIG for postexposure varicella prophylaxis. Both VZIG and IVIG should be administered within 96 hours of varicella exposure. Unlike VZIG, IVIG is a licensed product and in some situations might be obtained more quickly. For pregnant women who cannot obtain VZIG within 96 hours, monitoring for signs and symptoms of varicella disease and instituting treatment with acyclovir are an alternative to IVIG.

immunodeficiency, and a weakened immune system. It can be caused either by a disease (leukemia, HIV infection) or by drugs or other therapies (cancer chemotherapy, radiation therapy, prolonged high-dose corticosteroids). It can also include conditions such as asplenia and chronic renal disease.

Determination of altered immunocompetence is important because the incidence or severity of some vaccine-preventable diseases is higher in people with altered immunocompetence. Therefore, certain vaccines (such as inactivated influenza vaccine, pneumococcal vaccines) are recommended specifically for people with altered immunocompetence. Inactivated vaccine may be safely administered to a person with altered immunocompetence, although response to the vaccine may be suboptimal. The vaccine may need to be repeated after immune function has improved.

People with altered immunocompetence may be at increased risk for an adverse reaction after administration of live attenuated vaccines because of reduced ability to mount an effective immune response. Live vaccines should generally be deferred until immune function has improved. This is particularly important when planning to give yellow fever vaccine (see Chapter 3, Yellow Fever). For HIV-infected people with mild or moderate immunosuppression, MMR is recommended and varicella vaccine can be considered.

For an in-depth discussion, see Chapter 8, Immunocompromised Travelers.

VACCINATION SCHEDULING FOR LAST-MINUTE TRAVELERS

As noted, for people anticipating imminent travel, most vaccine products can be given during the same visit. Unless the vaccines given are booster doses of those typically given during childhood, vaccines may require a month or more to induce a sufficient immune response, depending on the vaccine and the number of doses in the series. Some vaccines require more than 1 dose for best protection. Recommended spacing should be maintained between doses (Table 2-6). Doses given at less than minimum intervals can lessen the antibody response. It is important to note that if a traveler needs yellow fever vaccination to meet a country requirement under the International Health Regulations, the yellow fever vaccine is not considered valid until 10 days after administration. Intervals between doses longer than those routinely recommended do not affect the immune response when the schedule is completed. Consequently, it is not necessary to restart the series or add doses of any vaccine because of an extended interval between doses.

Administration of a vaccine earlier than the recommended minimum age or at an interval shorter than the recommended minimum is discouraged. Table 2-6 lists the minimum age and minimum interval between doses for vaccines routinely recommended in the United States.

Because some travelers visit their health care providers at the last minute, studies have been performed to determine whether accelerated scheduling is adequate. This concern is primarily the case for hepatitis B vaccine or the combined hepatitis A and B vaccine. An accelerated schedule for combined hepatitis A and B vaccine has been approved by the Food and Drug Administration (FDA). It is unclear what level of protection any given traveler will have if he or she does not complete a full series of multidose vaccination.

ALLERGY TO VACCINE COMPONENTS

Vaccine components can cause allergic reactions in some recipients. These reactions can be local or systemic and can include anaphylaxis or anaphylactic-like responses. The vaccine components responsible can include the vaccine antigen, animal proteins, antibiotics, preservatives (such as thimerosal), or stabilizers (such as gelatin). The most common animal protein allergen is egg protein in vaccines prepared by using embryonated chicken eggs (influenza and yellow fever vaccines). Generally, people who can eat eggs or egg

products safely may receive these vaccines, while those with histories of anaphylactic allergy (swelling of the mouth and throat, difficulty breathing, hypotension, shock) to eggs or egg proteins ordinarily should not. Screening people by asking whether they can eat eggs without adverse effects is a reasonable way to identify those who might be at risk from receiving yellow fever and influenza vaccines. Protocols have been developed for testing and vaccinating people with anaphylactic reactions to egg ingestion. Recent studies have indicated that other components in vaccines in addition to egg proteins (such as gelatin) may cause allergic reactions, including anaphylaxis in rare instances.

Some vaccines contain a preservative or trace amounts of antibiotics to which people might be allergic. Providers administering the vaccines should carefully review the prescribing information before deciding if the rare person with such an allergy should receive the vaccine. No recommended vaccine contains penicillin or penicillin derivatives. Some vaccines (MMR and its individual component vaccines, inactivated polio vaccine [IPV], varicella, rabies) contain trace amounts of neomycin or other antibiotics; the amount is less than would normally be used for the skin test to determine hypersensitivity. However, people who have experienced anaphylactic reactions to this antibiotic generally should not receive these vaccines. Most often, neomycin allergy is a contact dermatitis—a manifestation of a delayed-type (cell-mediated) immune response rather than anaphylaxis. A history of delayed-type reactions to neomycin is not a contraindication to receiving these vaccines.

Thimerosal, an organic mercurial compound in use since the 1930s, has been added to certain immunobiologic products as a preservative. Thimerosal is present at preservative concentrations (trace quantities) in multidose vials of some brands of vaccine. Receiving thimerosal-containing vaccines has been postulated to lead to induction of allergy. However, there is limited scientific evidence for this assertion. Allergy to thimerosal usually consists of local delayed-type hypersensitivity reactions. Thimerosal elicits positive delayed-type hypersensitivity patch tests in 1%–18% of people tested, but these tests have limited or no clinical relevance. Most people do not experience reactions to

Table 2-6. Recommended and minimum ages and intervals between vaccine doses[1,2]

VACCINE AND DOSE NUMBER	RECOMMENDED AGE FOR THIS DOSE	MINIMUM AGE FOR THIS DOSE	MINIMUM INTERVAL TO NEXT DOSE[3]
Diphtheria and tetanus toxoids and acellular pertussis vaccine, pediatric (6 weeks through 6 years) (DTaP)-1[4]	2 months	6 weeks	4 weeks
DTaP-2	4 months	10 weeks	4 weeks
DTaP-3	6 months	14 weeks	6 months[5,6]
DTaP-4	15–18 months	12 months	6 months[5]
DTaP-5	4–6 years	4 years	NA
Haemophilus influenzae type b (Hib)-1[4,7]	2 months	6 weeks	4 weeks
Hib-2	4 months	10 weeks	4 weeks
Hib-3[8]	6 months	14 weeks	8 weeks
Hib-4	12–15 months	12 months	NA
Hepatitis A (HepA)-1	12–23 months	12 months	6 months[5]
HepA-2	≥18 months	18 months	NA
Hepatitis B (HepB)-1[4]	Birth	Birth	4 weeks
HepB-2	1–2 months	4 weeks	8 weeks
HepB-3[9]	6–18 months	24 weeks	NA
Herpes zoster[10]	≥60 years	60 years	NA
Human papillomavirus (HPV)-1[11]	11–12 years	9 years	4 weeks
HPV-2	2 months after dose 1	9 years, 4 weeks	12 weeks[12]

continued

TABLE 2-6. RECOMMENDED AND MINIMUM AGES AND INTERVALS BETWEEN VACCINE DOSES[1,2] (continued)

VACCINE AND DOSE NUMBER	RECOMMENDED AGE FOR THIS DOSE	MINIMUM AGE FOR THIS DOSE	MINIMUM INTERVAL TO NEXT DOSE[3]
HPV-3[12]	6 months after dose 1	9 years, 24 weeks	NA
Inactivated poliovirus (IPV)-1[4]	2 months	6 weeks	4 weeks
IPV-2	4 months	10 weeks	4 weeks
IPV-3	6–18 months	14 weeks	6 months
IPV-4[13]	4–6 years	4 years	NA
Influenza, inactivated[14]	≥6 months	6 months[15]	4 weeks
Influenza, live attenuated[14]	2–49 years	2 years	4 weeks
Japanese encephalitis, Vero cell (Ixiaro)-1[16]	≥17 years	≥17 years	28 days
Ixiaro-2	28 days after dose 1	≥17 years, 28 days	NA
Measles, mumps, and rubella (MMR)-1[17]	12–15 months	12 months	4 weeks
MMR-2[17]	4–6 years	13 months	NA
Meningococcal conjugate (MenACWY-1)[18]	11–12 years	9 months (Menactra) or 2 years (Menveo)	8 weeks[19]
MenACWY-2	16 years	11 months (Menactra) or 2 years, 8 weeks (Menveo)	NA
Meningococcal polysaccharide (MPSV4)-1[18]	NA	2 years	5 years
MPSV4–2	NA	7 years	NA
Pneumococcal conjugate (PCV)-1[7]	2 months	6 weeks	4 weeks

continued

TABLE 2-6. RECOMMENDED AND MINIMUM AGES AND INTERVALS BETWEEN VACCINE DOSES[1,2] (continued)

VACCINE AND DOSE NUMBER	RECOMMENDED AGE FOR THIS DOSE	MINIMUM AGE FOR THIS DOSE	MINIMUM INTERVAL TO NEXT DOSE[3]
PCV-2	4 months	10 weeks	4 weeks
PCV-3	6 months	14 weeks	8 weeks
PCV-4	12–15 months	12 months	NA
Pneumococcal polysaccharide (PPSV)-1	NA	2 years	5 years
PPSV-2[20]	NA	7 years	NA
Rabies-1 (preexposure)	See footnote 21	See footnote 21	7 days
Rabies-2	7 days after dose 1	7 days after dose 1	14 days
Rabies-3	21 days after dose 1	21 days after dose 1	NA
Rotavirus (RV)-1[22]	2 months	6 weeks	4 weeks
RV-2[22]	4 months	10 weeks	4 weeks
RV-3[22]	6 months	14 weeks	NA
Tetanus and reduced diphtheria toxoids (Td)	11–12 years	7 years	5 years
Tetanus toxoid, reduced diphtheria toxoid, and reduced acellular pertussis vaccine (Tdap)[23]	≥11 years	7 years	NA
Typhoid, inactivated (ViCPS)	≥2 years	≥2 years	NA
Typhoid, live attenuated (Ty21a)	≥6 years	≥6 years	See footnote 24
Varicella (Var)-1[17]	12–15 months	12 months	12 weeks[25]
Yellow fever	≥9 months[26]	≥9 months[26]	10 years

continued

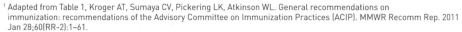

[1] Adapted from Table 1, Kroger AT, Sumaya CV, Pickering LK, Atkinson WL. General recommendations on immunization: recommendations of the Advisory Committee on Immunization Practices (ACIP). MMWR Recomm Rep. 2011 Jan 28;60(RR-2):1–61.

[2] Combination vaccines are available. Use of licensed combination vaccines is generally preferred over separate injections of their equivalent component vaccines (CDC. Combination vaccines for childhood immunization. MMWR Recomm Rep. 1999 May 14;48(RR-5):1–14.). When administering combination vaccines, the minimum age for administration is the oldest age for any of the individual components; the minimum interval between doses is equal to the largest interval of any of the individual components.

[3] See Table 2-4 for recommended revaccination (booster) schedules.

[4] Combination vaccines containing the HepB component are available (HepB-Hib, DTaP-HepB-IPV, HepA-HepB). These vaccines should not be administered to infants aged <6 weeks because of the other components (Hib, DTaP, IPV). HepA-HepB is not licensed for children aged <18 years in the United States.

[5] Calendar months.

[6] The minimum recommended interval between DTaP-3 and DTaP-4 is 6 months. However, DTaP-4 need not be repeated if administered ≥4 months after DTaP-3.

[7] For Hib and PCV, children receiving the first dose of vaccine at ≥7 months of age require fewer doses to complete the series (see the current childhood and adolescent immunization schedule at www.cdc.gov/vaccines).

[8] If PRP-OMP (Pedvax-Hib, Merck Vaccine Division) was administered at 2 and 4 months of age, a dose at 6 months of age is not indicated.

[9] HepB-3 should be administered ≥8 weeks after Hep B-2 and ≥16 weeks after Hep B-1; it should not be administered before age 24 weeks.

[10] Herpes zoster (shingles) vaccine is approved as a single dose for people aged ≥60 years.

[11] Bivalent HPV vaccine is approved for girls/women aged 10–25 years. It is recommended to prevent cervical and other anogenital cancers and precursors for girls/women aged 11–26 years. Quadrivalent HPV vaccine is approved for boys/men and girls/women aged 9–26 years. It is recommended to prevent cervical and other anogenital cancers, precursors, and genital warts for girls/women aged 11–26 years. It may be given to girls aged 9–10 years to prevent the same diseases, and to boys/men aged 9–26 years to prevent genital warts.

[12] The third dose of HPV should be administered ≥12 weeks after the second and ≥24 weeks after the first. Dose 3 need not be repeated if administered ≥16 weeks after dose 1.

[13] For people receiving an all-IPV or all-OPV series, if the third dose is given after the fourth birthday, a fourth dose is not needed.

[14] Two doses of influenza vaccine are recommended for children aged <9 years who are receiving the vaccine for the first time, and for certain incompletely vaccinated children (see reference 4). All others need only 1 dose annually. The doses of inactivated influenza vaccine are 0.25 mL for children aged 6–35 months and 0.5 mL for people aged ≥3 years.

[15] The minimum age for inactivated influenza vaccine varies by vaccine manufacturer. See package insert for vaccine-specific minimum ages.

[16] Ixiaro is approved by the Food and Drug Administration for people aged ≥17 years.

[17] Combination MMR-varicella can be used for children aged 12 months through 12 years. Also see footnote 25.

[18] Revaccination with meningococcal vaccine is recommended for people previously vaccinated who remain at high risk for meningococcal disease (see Table 2-4). MenACWY is preferred for revaccinating people aged 2–55 years (Bilukha OO, Rosenstein N. Prevention and control of meningococcal disease. Recommendations of the Advisory Committee on Immunization Practices (ACIP). MMWR Recomm Rep. 2005 May 27;54(RR-7):1–21.).

[19] Children aged 9–23 months who are vaccinated with Menactra (Sanofi Pasteur) should receive a 2-dose primary series administered 3 months apart (CDC. Recommendation of the Advisory Committee on Immunization Practices [ACIP] for use of quadrivalent meningococcal conjugate vaccine [MenACWY-D] among children aged 9 through 23 months at increased risk for invasive meningococcal disease. MMWR Morb Mortal Wkly Rep 2011: 60[40];1391–2.) People aged 2–55 years with persistent complement component deficiency (such as C5–C9, properdin, factor H, or factor D) and functional or anatomic asplenia and adolescents with human immunodeficiency virus (HIV) infection should receive a 2-dose primary series administered 2 months apart (CDC. Updated recommendations for use of meningococcal conjugate vaccines—Advisory Committee on Immunization Practices [ACIP], 2010. MMWR 2011;60[03]; 72–6).

[20] A second dose of PPSV is recommended for people aged ≥65 years who received a first dose at an age <65 years and at a 5-year minimum interval. A second dose is also recommended for people aged <65 years at highest risk for serious pneumococcal infection and those who are likely to have a rapid decline in pneumococcal antibody concentration (CDC. Prevention of pneumococcal disease: recommendations of the Advisory Committee on Immunization Practices [ACIP]. MMWR Recomm Rep. 1997 Apr 4;46(RR-8):1–24.).

[21] There is no minimum age for preexposure immunization for rabies (Manning SE, Rupprecht CE, Fishbein D, Hanlon CA, Lumlertdacha B, Guerra M, et al. Human rabies prevention—United States, 2008: recommendations of the Advisory Committee on Immunization Practices. MMWR Recomm Rep. 2008 May 23;57(RR-3):1–28.).

[22] The first dose of RV must be administered by 14 weeks and 6 days of age. The vaccine series should not be started at ≥15 weeks of age. The final dose in the series should be administered by age 8 months, 0 days. If Rotarix rotavirus vaccine is administered at 2 and 4 months of age, a dose at 6 months of age is not indicated.

[23] Only 1 dose of Tdap is recommended. Subsequent doses should be given as Td. Children aged 7–10 years who are not fully vaccinated against pertussis and for whom no contraindication to pertussis vaccine exists should receive a single dose of Tdap. If additional doses of tetanus and diphtheria toxoid-containing vaccines are needed, then children aged 7–10 years should be vaccinated according to catch-up guidance, with Tdap preferred as the first dose. Tdap vaccine, when indicated, should be administered regardless of the interval since the last dose of Td vaccine. For management of a tetanus-prone wound, the minimum interval after a previous dose of any tetanus-containing vaccine is 5 years.

[24] Oral typhoid vaccine is recommended to be administered 1 hour before a meal with a cold or lukewarm drink (temperature not to exceed body temperature—98.6°F [37°C]) on alternate days, for a total of 4 doses.

[25] The minimum interval from Var-1 to Var-2 for people beginning the series at ≥13 years of age is 4 weeks.

[26] Yellow fever vaccine may be administered to children aged <9 months in certain situations (Staples JE, Gershman M, Fischer M. Yellow fever vaccine: recommendations of the Advisory Committee on Immunization Practices [ACIP]. MMWR Recomm Rep. 2010 Jul 30;59(RR-7):1–27.).

thimerosal administered as a component of vaccines, even when patch or intradermal tests for thimerosal indicate hypersensitivity. A localized or delayed-type hypersensitivity reaction to thimerosal is not a contraindication to receipt of a vaccine that contains thimerosal.

Since mid-2001, vaccines routinely recommended for infants have been manufactured without thimerosal as a preservative. Additional information about thimerosal and the thimerosal content of vaccines is available on the FDA website (www.fda.gov/cber/vaccine/thimerosal.htm).

REPORTING ADVERSE EVENTS AFTER IMMUNIZATION

Modern vaccines are extremely safe and effective. Benefits and risks are associated with the use of all immunobiologics—no vaccine is completely effective or completely free of side effects. Adverse events after immunization have been reported with all vaccines, ranging from frequent, minor, local reactions to extremely rare, severe, systemic illness, such as that associated with yellow fever vaccine. Adverse events following specific vaccines and toxoids are discussed in detail in each ACIP statement. In the United States, clinicians are required by law to report selected adverse events occurring after vaccination with tetanus vaccine in any combination; pertussis in any combination; measles, mumps, or rubella, alone or in any combination; oral polio vaccine (OPV); IPV; hepatitis A; hepatitis B; varicella; Hib (conjugate); influenza; pneumococcal conjugate; rotavirus vaccines; HPV; and meningococcal vaccines (conjugate and polysaccharide). In addition, CDC strongly recommends that all vaccine adverse events be reported to the Vaccine Adverse Event Reporting System (VAERS), even if a causal relation to vaccination is not certain. VAERS reporting forms and information are available electronically at www.vaers.hhs.gov, or they may be requested by telephone: 800-822-7967 (toll-free). Clinicians are encouraged to report electronically at https://vaers.hhs.gov/esub/step1.

INJECTION ROUTE AND INJECTION SITE

Injectable vaccines are administered by intramuscular, intradermal, and subcutaneous routes. The method of administration of injectable vaccines depends in part on the presence of an adjuvant in some vaccines. The term *adjuvant* refers to a vaccine component distinct from the antigen, which enhances the immune response to the antigen. Vaccines containing an adjuvant (DTaP, DT, HPV, Td, Tdap, pneumococcal conjugate, Hib, hepatitis A, hepatitis B) should be injected into a muscle mass, because administration subcutaneously or intradermally can cause local irritation, induration, skin discoloration, inflammation, and granuloma formation.

Routes of administration are recommended by the manufacturer for each immunobiologic. Deviation from the recommended route of administration may reduce vaccine efficacy or increase local adverse reactions. Detailed recommendations on the route and site for all vaccines have been published in ACIP recommendations; a compiled list of these publications is available on the CDC website at www.cdc.gov/vaccines/pubs/ACIP-list.htm (also see Table C-1 in Appendix C).

BIBLIOGRAPHY

1. Ball LK, Ball R, Pratt RD. An assessment of thimerosal use in childhood vaccines. Pediatrics. 2001 May;107(5):1147–1154.

2. Bilukha OO, Rosenstein N. Prevention and control of meningococcal disease. Recommendations of the Advisory Committee on Immunization Practices (ACIP). MMWR Recomm Rep. 2005 May 27;54(RR-7):1–21.

3. CDC. Combination vaccines for childhood immunization. MMWR Recomm Rep. 1999 May 14;48(RR-5):1–14.

4. CDC. Prevention and control of influenza with vaccines: recommendations of the Advisory Committee on Immunization Practices (ACIP)—United States, 2012–13 influenza season. MMWR Morb Mortal Wkly Rep. 2012 Aug 17;61:613–8.

5. CDC. Updated recommendations for prevention of invasive pneumococcal disease among adults using the 23-valent pneumococcal polysaccharide vaccine (PPSV23). MMWR Morb Mortal Wkly Rep. 2010 Sep 3;59(34):1102–6.

6. CDC. Updated recommendations for use of meningococcal conjugate vaccines—Advisory Committee on Immunization Practices (ACIP), 2010. MMWR 2011;60(03):72–6.

7. CDC. Updated recommendations for use of tetanus toxoid, reduced diphtheria toxoid and acellular pertussis (Tdap) vaccine from the Advisory Committee on Immunization Practices, 2010. MMWR Morb Mortal Wkly Rep. 2011 Jan 14;60(1):13–5.

8. Kretsinger K, Broder KR, Cortese MM, Joyce MP, Ortega-Sanchez I, Lee GM, et al. Preventing tetanus, diphtheria, and pertussis among adults: use of tetanus toxoid, reduced diphtheria toxoid and acellular pertussis vaccine recommendations of the Advisory Committee on Immunization Practices (ACIP) and recommendation of ACIP, supported by the Healthcare Infection Control Practices Advisory Committee (HICPAC), for use of Tdap among health-care personnel. MMWR Recomm Rep. 2006 Dec 15;55(RR-17):1–37.

9. Kroger AT, Sumaya CV, Pickering LK, Atkinson WL. General recommendations on immunization: recommendations of the Advisory Committee on Immunization Practices (ACIP). MMWR Recomm Rep. 2011 Jan 28;60(RR-2):1–61.

10. Manning SE, Rupprecht CE, Fishbein D, Hanlon CA, Lumlertdacha B, Guerra M, et al. Human rabies prevention—United States, 2008: recommendations of the Advisory Committee on Immunization Practices. MMWR Recomm Rep. 2008 May 23;57(RR-3):1–28.

11. Nuorti JP, Whitney CG. Prevention of pneumococcal disease among infants and children—use of 13-valent pneumococcal conjugate vaccine and 23-valent pneumococcal polysaccharide vaccine: recommendations of the Advisory Committee on Immunization Practices (ACIP). MMWR Recomm Rep. 2010 Dec 10;59(RR-11):1–18.

12. Plotkin SA. Vaccines: correlates of vaccine-induced immunity. Clin Infect Dis. 2008 Aug 1;47(3):401–99.

13. Staples JE, Gershman M, Fischer M. Yellow fever vaccine: recommendations of the Advisory Committee on Immunization Practices (ACIP). MMWR Recomm Rep. 2010 Jul 30;59(RR-7):1–27.

14. Varricchio F, Iskander J, Destefano F, Ball R, Pless R, Braun MM, et al. Understanding vaccine safety information from the Vaccine Adverse Event Reporting System. Pediatr Infect Dis J. 2004 Apr;23(4):287–294.

15. Watson JC, Hadler SC, Dykewicz CA, Reef S, Phillips L. Measles, mumps, and rubella—vaccine use and strategies for elimination of measles, rubella, and congenital rubella syndrome and control of mumps: recommendations of the Advisory Committee on Immunization Practices (ACIP). MMWR Recomm Rep. 1998 May 22;47(RR-8):1–57.

16. Wood RA, Berger M, Dreskin SC, Setse R, Engler RJ, Dekker CL, et al. An algorithm for treatment of patients with hypersensitivity reactions after vaccines. Pediatrics. 2008 Sep;122(3):e771–7.

INTERACTIONS AMONG TRAVEL VACCINES & DRUGS

Ilan Youngster, Elizabeth D. Barnett

Vaccines and medications are prescribed frequently in pre-travel consultations, and potential interactions between vaccines and medications, including those already taken by the traveler, must be considered. Although a comprehensive list of interactions is beyond the scope of this section, some of the more serious interactions of commonly used travel-related vaccines and medications are discussed here.

INTERACTIONS BETWEEN VACCINES

In general, concomitant administration of multiple vaccines, including live attenuated immunizations, is safe and effective. Administering a live-virus vaccine within 4 weeks after administration of another live-virus vaccine can decrease immunogenicity to the second administered vaccine. This observation has given rise to the recommendation that live-virus vaccines should be administered the same day or ≥4 weeks apart. If the 4-week span is not achievable, the second vaccine may be administered sooner to afford some protection, but it should be readministered ≥4 weeks later if the traveler is at continued risk. A recent study examining concurrent administration of the yellow fever vaccine with the measles-mumps-rubella (MMR) vaccine in 12-month-old children showed slightly reduced immunogenicity to yellow fever and mumps components, compared with responses following separate vaccination with MMR and yellow fever vaccine 30 days apart. The clinical significance of this finding is uncertain at present.

INTERACTIONS BETWEEN TRAVEL VACCINES AND DRUGS
Oral Typhoid Vaccine

Live attenuated vaccines should generally be avoided in immunocompromised travelers, including those who are taking immunomodulators, calcineurin inhibitors, cytotoxic agents, antimetabolites, and high-dose steroids.

Antimicrobial agents may be active against the vaccine strain in the oral typhoid vaccine and may prevent an adequate immune response to the vaccine. Therefore, oral typhoid vaccine should not be given to people taking antibacterial agents. Vaccination with oral typhoid vaccine should be delayed for >72 hours after the administration of any such agent. Parenteral typhoid vaccine may be a more appropriate choice for these people.

Chloroquine and atovaquone-proguanil at doses used for malaria chemoprophylaxis may be given concurrently with the oral typhoid vaccine.

Rabies Vaccine

Concomitant use of chloroquine may reduce the antibody response to intradermal rabies vaccine administered for preexposure vaccination. The intramuscular route should be used for people taking chloroquine concurrently. (Currently, intradermal administration of rabies vaccine is not approved in the United States.)

INTERACTIONS BETWEEN ANTIMALARIALS AND SELECTED OTHER DRUGS

This section describes some of the more commonly encountered drug interactions. Any time a new medication is prescribed, clinicians should check for any interactions and inform the traveler of the potential risk.

Mefloquine

Mefloquine may interact with several categories of drugs, including other antimalarial drugs, drugs that alter cardiac conduction, and anticonvulsants. Mefloquine is associated with increased toxicities of the antimalarial drug lumefantrine (available in the United States in fixed combination to treat people with uncomplicated *Plasmodium falciparum* malaria), potentially causing fatal prolongation of the QTc interval. Lumefantrine should therefore be avoided or used with caution in patients taking mefloquine prophylaxis. Although no conclusive data are available with regard to coadministration of mefloquine and other drugs that may affect cardiac conduction, mefloquine should be used with caution or avoided in patients taking antiarrhythmic or β-blocking agents, calcium-channel blockers, antihistamines, H_1-blocking agents, tricyclic antidepressants, or phenothiazines. In general, mefloquine should also be avoided in travelers with a history of seizures. Mefloquine may also lower plasma levels of a number of anticonvulsants, such as valproic acid, carbamazepine, phenobarbital, and phenytoin; concurrent use of mefloquine with these agents should be avoided. Mefloquine can also lead to increased levels of calcineurin inhibitors and mTOR inhibitors (tacrolimus, cyclosporine A, and sirolimus) (see Table 8-2). Potent CYP3A4 inhibitors such as macrolides (clarithromycin, erythromycin), azole antifungals (ketoconazole, voriconazole, and itraconazole), and antiretroviral protease inhibitors may increase the levels of mefloquine, increasing the risk for QT prolongation. CYP3A4 inducers such as efavirenz, nevirapine, rifampin, and rifabutin may reduce plasma concentrations of mefloquine, and concurrent use should be avoided.

Chloroquine

Chloroquine may increase risk of prolonged QTc interval when given with other QT-prolonging agents (such as sotalol, amiodarone, and lumefantrine), and the combination should be avoided. Chloroquine inhibits CYP2D6; when given concomitantly with substrates of this enzyme (such as metoprolol, propranolol, fluoxetine, paroxetine, flecainide), increased monitoring for side effects may be warranted. Chloroquine absorption may be reduced by antacids or kaolin; ≥4 hours should elapse between doses of these medications. Concomitant use of cimetidine and chloroquine should be avoided, as cimetidine can inhibit the metabolism of chloroquine and may increase drug levels. CYP3A4 inhibitors such as ritonavir, ketoconazole, and erythromycin may also increase chloroquine levels, and concomitant use should be avoided. Chloroquine inhibits bioavailability of ampicillin, and 2 hours should elapse between doses. Chloroquine is also reported to decrease the bioavailability of ciprofloxacin and methotrexate. Chloroquine may increase digoxin levels; increased digoxin monitoring is warranted. Use of chloroquine could possibly also lead to increased levels of calcineurin inhibitors and should be used with caution.

Atovaquone-Proguanil

Tetracycline, rifampin, and rifabutin may reduce plasma concentrations of atovaquone and should not be used concurrently with atovaquone-proguanil. Metoclopramide may reduce bioavailability of atovaquone; unless no other antiemetics are available, this antiemetic should not be used to treat the vomiting that may accompany use of atovaquone at treatment doses. Atovaquone-proguanil should not be used with other medications that contain proguanil. Patients on anticoagulants may need to reduce their anticoagulant dose or monitor their prothrombin time more closely while taking atovaquone-proguanil, although coadministration of these drugs is not contraindicated. Atovaquone-proguanil may interact with antiretroviral protease inhibitors and efavirenz. Cimetidine and fluvoxamine interfere with the metabolism of proguanil and should therefore be avoided.

Doxycycline

Phenytoin, carbamazepine, and barbiturates may decrease the half-life of doxycycline. Patients on anticoagulants may need to reduce their anticoagulant dose while taking doxycycline because of its ability to depress plasma prothrombin activity. Absorption of tetracyclines may be impaired by bismuth subsalicylate, preparations containing iron, and antacids containing calcium, magnesium, or aluminum; these preparations should not be taken within 3 hours of taking doxycycline. Doxycycline may interfere with the bactericidal activity of penicillin, so these drugs, in general, should not be taken together. Doxycycline has no known interaction with antiretroviral agents, but concurrent use may lead to increased levels of calcineurin inhibitors and mTOR inhibitors (sirolimus).

INTERACTIONS WITH ANTIDIARRHEAL DRUGS

Fluoroquinolones

Increase in the international normalized ratio has been reported when levofloxacin and warfarin are used concurrently. Concurrent administration of ciprofloxacin and antacids that contain magnesium or aluminum hydroxide may reduce bioavailability of ciprofloxacin. Ciprofloxacin decreases clearance of theophylline and caffeine; theophylline levels should be monitored when ciprofloxacin is used concurrently. Ciprofloxacin and other fluoroquinolones should not be used with tizanidine. Sildenafil should not be used in patients on ciprofloxacin, as concomitant use is associated with increased rates of adverse effects. Fluoroquinolones have no known interaction with antiretroviral agents, but concurrent use may increase levels of calcineurin inhibitors and fluoroquinolone levels, and use should reflect renal function.

Azithromycin

Close monitoring for side effects of azithromycin is recommended when azithromycin is used with nelfinavir. Increased anticoagulant effects have been noted when azithromycin is used with warfarin; monitoring prothrombin time is recommended for people taking these drugs concomitantly. Additive QTc prolongation may occur when azithromycin is used with the antimalarial artemether, and concomitant therapy should be avoided. Drug interactions have been reported with macrolides and antiretroviral protease inhibitors, as well as efavirenz and nevirapine, and can increase risk of QTc prolongation. Concurrent use with macrolides may lead to increased levels of calcineurin inhibitors.

Rifaximin

No clinically significant drug interactions have been reported to date with rifaximin. Although the drug induces CYP3A4 enzymes, studies of concurrent administration of rifaximin with midazolam, and with a single dose of the oral contraceptive ethinylestradiol and norgestimate, did not show changes in the pharmacokinetics of these drugs.

INTERACTIONS WITH DRUGS USED FOR TRAVEL TO HIGH ALTITUDES

Acetazolamide

Acetazolamide produces alkaline urine that can increase the rate of excretion of barbiturates and salicylates and may potentiate salicylate toxicity, particularly if taking a high dose of aspirin. Decreased excretion of dextroamphetamine, anticholinergics, mecamylamine, ephedrine, mexiletine, or quinidine may also occur. Hypokalemia caused by corticosteroids may be potentiated by concurrent use of acetazolamide. Acetazolamide should not be given to patients taking the anticonvulsant topiramate, as concurrent use is associated with increased toxicity. Increased monitoring of cyclosporine, tacrolimus, and sirolimus is warranted if these drugs are given with acetazolamide. Concurrent administration of metformin and acetazolamide should be done with caution as there may be an additive risk for lactic acidosis.

Dexamethasone

Dexamethasone interacts with multiple classes of drugs. Using this drug to treat altitude illness may, however, be life-saving. Interactions may occur with dexamethasone and the following drugs and drug classes: macrolide antibiotics, anticholinesterases, anticoagulants, hypoglycemic agents, isoniazid, digitalis preparations, oral contraceptives, and phenytoin.

BIBLIOGRAPHY

1. Bouchaud O, Imbert P, Touze JE, Dodoo AN, Danis M, Legros F. Fatal cardiotoxicity related to halofantrine: a review based on a worldwide safety data base. Malar J. 2009;8:289.
2. CDC. Sudden death in a traveler following halofantrine administration—Togo, 2000. MMWR Morb Mortal Wkly Rep. 2001 Mar 9;50(9):169–70, 79.
3. Hoey LL, Lake KD. Does ciprofloxacin interact with cyclosporine? Ann Pharmacother. 1994 Jan;28(1):93–6.
4. Horowitz H, Carbonaro CA. Inhibition of the *Salmonella typhi* oral vaccine strain, Ty21a, by mefloquine and chloroquine. J Infect Dis. 1992 Dec;166(6):1462–4.
5. Keogh A, Esmore D, Spratt P, Savdie E, McCluskey P, Chang V. Acetazolamide and cyclosporine. Transplantation. 1988 Sep;46(3):478–9.
6. Kolawole JA, Mustapha A, Abdul-Aguye I, Ochekpe N, Taylor RB. Effects of cimetidine on the pharmacokinetics of proguanil in healthy subjects and in peptic ulcer patients. J Pharm Biomed Anal. 1999 Sep;20(5):737–43.
7. Kollaritsch H, Que JU, Kunz C, Wiedermann G, Herzog C, Cryz SJ Jr. Safety and immunogenicity of live oral cholera and typhoid vaccines administered alone or in combination with antimalarial drugs, oral polio vaccine, or yellow fever vaccine. J Infect Dis. 1997 Apr;175(4):871–5.
8. Nascimento Silva JR, Camacho LA, Siqueira MM, Freire Mde S, Castro YP, Maia Mde L, et al. Mutual interference on the immune response to yellow fever vaccine and a combined vaccine against measles, mumps and rubella. Vaccine. 2011 Aug 26;29(37):6327–34.
9. Pappaioanou M, Fishbein DB, Dreesen DW, Schwartz IK, Campbell GH, Sumner JW, et al. Antibody response to preexposure human diploid-cell rabies vaccine given concurrently with chloroquine. N Engl J Med. 1986 Jan 30;314(5):280–4.
10. Projean D, Baune B, Farinotti R, Flinois JP, Beaune P, Taburet AM, et al. In vitro metabolism of chloroquine: identification of CYP2C8, CYP3A4, and CYP2D6 as the main isoforms catalyzing N-desethylchloroquine formation. Drug Metab Dispos. 2003 Jun;31(6):748–54.
11. Ridtitid W, Wongnawa M, Mahatthanatrakul W, Raungsri N, Sunbhanich M. Ketoconazole increases plasma concentrations of antimalarial mefloquine in healthy human volunteers. J Clin Pharm Ther. 2005 Jun;30(3):285–90.

FEAR OF VACCINES
Paul Offit

Pre-travel consultations often provide the opportunity to update routine vaccinations for both children and adults. One of the first topics covered in such sessions is whether the traveler is immune to diseases such as measles and varicella. Unfortunately, in some circumstances, providers may be surprised to find that travelers have no interest in being vaccinated or in having their children vaccinated, whether for measles or other potentially life-threatening, travel-related infections, such as yellow fever.

Although travel-related vaccines may not have implications for community health, such as providing herd immunity, they can protect people against severe and occasionally fatal illness. For these vaccines, the discussion between clinicians and patients is one of weighing the risks and benefits of travel-related vaccines for particular destinations. Travelers are often at a higher risk of exposure to diseases for which routine vaccines provide protection, even when traveling to countries in Europe. For example, in 2011 the World Health Organization's European Region experienced a measles epidemic that affected >38,000 citizens, causing >10,000 hospitalizations and 10 deaths. The European measles outbreak belied a common belief that severe and occasionally fatal vaccine-preventable diseases are the province of the developing world.

Because so much is at stake, the travel health provider should educate all travelers, and especially parents, about the use of vaccines. Those providing travel health advice should familiarize themselves with the literature on the safety of both routine and travel-related vaccines, so they can address any concerns that their patients may have.

The history of the development of vaccination complacency and avoidance is a curious one. During the 1940s, parents in the United States did not hesitate to get the diphtheria, tetanus, and pertussis vaccines; they knew that diphtheria and pertussis were common killers of young children, and they had watched tetanus claim the lives of soldiers in World Wars I and II. During the 1950s, the polio vaccine was a godsend; everyone knew what poliovirus could do. During the 1960s, parents gladly accepted the measles, mumps, and rubella vaccines. They knew that measles caused thousands of hospitalizations and hundreds of deaths every year, mostly from pneumonia; that mumps was a common cause of deafness and a rare cause of sterility; and that rubella caused thousands of children to suffer severe birth defects of the eyes, ears, and heart.

The widespread use of vaccines caused a dramatic decrease—and in some cases a virtual elimination—of several diseases. Parents, no longer compelled by fear of the diseases around them, became complacent. Immunization rates plateaued. Now, the United States (as well as many European countries) finds itself in a situation where vaccine safety issues, real or imagined, are a primary concern. Parents confront a flood of misinformation from radio and television programs, magazine and newspaper articles, antivaccine blogs, YouTube, and Twitter. Vaccines—considered mankind's greatest lifesaver—are now feared by some to cause a variety of chronic diseases, including autism, diabetes, allergies, asthma, learning disabilities, multiple sclerosis, and attention deficit disorder. As a consequence, many parents are choosing not to immunize their children according to recommended schedules. Travel health providers must be aware of these issues and arm themselves with accurate information to properly educate their patients.

In addition to protecting the health of the vaccinee, vaccination safeguards the health of entire communities, both at home and possibly at travel destinations. Predictably, in communities with clusters of underimmunized children, the incidence of vaccine-preventable diseases has risen. More measles outbreaks occurred in the United States in 2011 than in any year since 1996, primarily due to the increase in imported measles cases. Pertussis outbreaks have swept the nation. *Haemophilus influenzae* type b meningitis has claimed the lives of several children in Minnesota and Pennsylvania, deaths that could have easily been avoided if parents had not feared vaccines more than the diseases they prevent. Some of these outbreaks have been linked to international travel to the United States.

So, where do we go from here? How do we again inspire people to vaccinate themselves and their children? One way would be to make parents aware of the impact of vaccine-preventable diseases and to provide the science that exonerates vaccines as a cause of chronic diseases in a manner that is compelling and easily understood. Some of this information is available from CDC (www.cdc.gov/vaccines/recs/acip/default.htm), the American Academy of Pediatrics (www.aap.org), the Immunization Action Coalition (www.immunize.org), the Vaccine Education Center at the Children's Hospital of Philadelphia (www.vaccine.chop.edu), Every Child By Two (www.ecbt.org), the National Network for Immunization Information (www.immunizationinfo.org), the Institute for Vaccine Safety at Johns Hopkins Hospital (www.vaccinesafety.edu), and Parents of Kids with Infectious Diseases (www.pkids.org), among other groups.

But is it enough? As providers whose job it is to protect people against vaccine-preventable diseases, travel-related or otherwise, we need to enhance our efforts to educate ourselves and our patients, so that we will not once again be compelled to vaccinate after witnessing the suffering, hospitalization, and death caused by vaccine-preventable diseases—an unwanted return to an earlier and darker phase in history.

BIBLIOGRAPHY

1. CDC. Increased transmission and outbreaks of measles—European region, 2011. MMWR Morb Mortal Wkly Rep. 2011 Dec 2;60(47):1605–10.
2. CDC. Invasive *Haemophilus influenzae* type B disease in five young children—Minnesota, 2008. MMWR Morb Mortal Wkly Rep. 2009 Jan 30;58(3):58–60.
3. CDC. Measles—United States, 2011. MMWR Morb Mortal Wkly Rep. 2012 Apr 20;61:253–7.
4. CDC. Pertussis outbreak in an Amish community—Kent County, Delaware, September 2004–February 2005. MMWR Morb Mortal Wkly Rep. 2006 Aug 4;55(30):817–21.
5. Centralized Information System for Infectious Diseases [database on the Internet]. WHO Regional Office for Europe. 2002 [cited 2012 Jul 31]. Available from: http://data.euro.who.int/cisid/?TabID=294730.
6. Chen RT, Mootrey G, DeStefano F. Safety of routine childhood vaccinations. An epidemiological review. Paediatr Drugs. 2000 Jul–Aug;2(4):273–90.

Self-Treatable Conditions

SELF-TREATABLE CONDITIONS

Alan J. Magill

Despite providers' best efforts, some travelers will become ill while traveling. Obtaining reliable and timely medical care during travel can be problematic in many destinations. As a result, prescribing certain medications in advance can empower the traveler to self-diagnose and treat common health problems. With some activities in remote settings, such as trekking, the only alternative to self-treatment would be no treatment. Pre-travel counseling may actually result in a more accurate self-diagnosis and treatment than relying on local medical care in some developing countries. In addition, the increasing awareness of substandard and counterfeit drugs in pharmacies in the developing world (as many as 50% of the drugs on the shelves) makes it more important for travelers to bring quality manufactured drugs with them from a reliable supplier in their own country (see *Perspectives:* Pharmaceutical Quality & Counterfeit Drugs later in this chapter).

Providing education and prescriptions is part of the pre-travel consultation. The key aspect of this strategy is to recognize the conditions for which the traveler may be at risk, given the travel itinerary, and to educate the traveler about the diagnosis and treatment of those particular conditions. The keys to successful self-treatment strategies are providing a simple disease or condition definition, providing one choice of treatment, and educating the traveler about the expected outcome of treatment. Using travelers' diarrhea as an example, a practitioner could provide the following advice:

- "Travelers' diarrhea" is the sudden onset of abnormally loose, frequent stools.
- The treatment is ciprofloxacin 500 mg, every 12 hours, for 1 day (2 doses).
- The traveler should feel better within 6–24 hours.

- If symptoms persist for 24–36 hours despite self-treatment, it may be necessary to seek medical attention.

To minimize the potential negative effects of a self-treatment strategy, the recommendations should follow a few key points:

- Drugs recommended must be safe, well tolerated, and effective for use as self-treatment.
- A drug's toxicity or potential for harm, if used incorrectly or in an overdose situation, should be minimal.
- Simple and clear directions are critical. Consider providing handouts describing how to use the drugs. Keeping the directions simple will increase the effectiveness of the strategy.

The following are some of the most common situations in which people would find self-treatment useful. The extent of self-treatment recommendations offered to the traveler should reflect the remoteness and difficulty of travel and the availability of reliable medical care at the particular destination. The recommended self-treatment options for each disease are provided in the designated section of the Yellow Book.

Travelers' diarrhea (TD) is perhaps the most frequent indication for self-treatment. The success of this strategy is based on the epidemiologic evidence that bacterial pathogens account for >90% of TD in short-term travelers. The recognition of antibiotic resistance for certain organisms in specific destinations has made the empiric choice of treatment somewhat more problematic in recent years (see the Travelers' Diarrhea section next in this chapter).

Altitude illness or acute mountain sickness (AMS) is a risk for travelers who ascend rapidly to altitudes >8,000 ft (2,440 m). Certain common travel destinations, such as Cuzco, Peru, or Lhasa, Tibet, involve flying to altitudes of 11,150 ft (3,400 m) or 12,000 ft (3,660 m), respectively. The symptoms of headache, anorexia, nausea, fatigue, lassitude, and poor sleep can largely be prevented or treated with acetazolamide (see the Altitude Illness section later in this chapter).

Jet lag affects almost everyone who crosses 3 or more time zones. There is no consensus on the optimal pharmacologic treatment or prevention of the symptoms of jet lag, but sleeping medication taken at the destination may help regularize sleep patterns (see the Jet Lag section later in this chapter).

Motion sickness can be a major deterrent to enjoyment for any susceptible person on a boat or a winding road. Premedication may help alleviate or ameliorate this bothersome syndrome (see the Motion Sickness section later in this chapter).

The self-treatment of suspected **respiratory infections** with empiric antibiotics is controversial. Almost all upper respiratory tract infections are initially caused by viruses. However, these viral infections, under the stress of travel, can lead to bacterial sinusitis, bronchitis, or pneumonia. Respiratory infections that last longer than a week without signs of improvement may require empiric antibiotics for recovery. Prolonged respiratory infections may have more of a negative effect on a trip than diarrheal disease (see the Respiratory Infections section later in this chapter).

Bacterial skin infections are not common among travelers, but when they occur, they can be particularly distressing. Bacterial abscesses or cellulitis can worsen rapidly and be very painful. If the traveler is in a remote area, or even more than a day's travel from medical care, the use of empiric antibiotic treatment can be beneficial (see Chapter 5, Skin and Soft Tissue Infections in Returned Travelers).

Urinary tract infections are common among many women, and carrying an antibiotic for empiric treatment of this condition may be valuable in many circumstances.

Vaginal yeast infections in women can be an annoying and debilitating problem. For women who know they are prone to infections, all sexually active women, and those who may be receiving antibiotics for other reasons, including doxycycline for malaria chemoprophylaxis, a self-treatment course of their preferred antifungal medication can be prescribed.

Occupational exposure to HIV is a particular risk to those participating in medical-related activities. Thousands of such people work in areas of sub-Saharan Africa, where the HIV prevalence may be higher than 15%–20%. A needlestick in this setting should prompt immediate wound care and the possible use of antiretroviral medications (see the Occupational Exposure to HIV section later in this chapter).

Malaria self-treatment is often referred to as standby emergency treatment (SBET). This strategy asks the traveler to use a therapeutic dose of a prescribed antimalarial drug when the traveler has a fever accompanied by systemic illness, and then proceed to reliable medical care within 24 hours. The goal is to prevent death or severe malaria. Since most travelers at risk of malaria should be advised to use prophylactic medication, this strategy is usually discouraged and reserved for a specific type of traveler under certain defined circumstances (see Chapter 3, Malaria).

TRAVELERS' DIARRHEA
Bradley A. Connor

DESCRIPTION
Travelers' diarrhea (TD) is the most predictable travel-related illness. Attack rates range from 30% to 70% of travelers, depending on the destination and season of travel. Traditionally, it was thought that TD could be prevented by following simple recommendations such as "boil it, cook it, peel, it, or forget

it," but studies have found that people who follow these rules may still become ill. Poor hygiene practice in local restaurants is likely the largest contributor to the risk for TD.

TD is a clinical syndrome that can result from a variety of intestinal pathogens. Bacterial pathogens are the predominant risk, thought to account for 80%–90% of TD. Intestinal viruses have been isolated in studies of TD, but they usually account for 5%–8% of illnesses, although improved diagnostics and their increased use for recognizing norovirus infections in travelers may change those percentages in the future. Protozoal pathogens are slower to manifest symptoms and collectively account for approximately 10% of diagnoses in longer-term travelers. What is commonly known as "food poisoning" involves the ingestion of preformed toxins in food. In this syndrome, vomiting and diarrhea may both be present, but symptoms usually resolve spontaneously within 12 hours.

INFECTIOUS AGENT

Bacteria are the most common cause of TD. Overall, the <u>most</u> common pathogen is enterotoxigenic *Escherichia coli*, followed by *Campylobacter jejuni*, *Shigella* spp., and *Salmonella* spp. Enteroadherent and other *E. coli* species are also common pathogens in bacterial diarrhea. There is increasing discussion of *Aeromonas* spp. and *Plesiomonas* spp. as potential causes of TD as well. Viral diarrhea can be caused by a number of pathogens, including norovirus, rotavirus, and astrovirus.

Etec
campy
shig
salm.

Giardia is the main protozoal pathogen found in TD. *Entamoeba histolytica* is a relatively uncommon pathogen in travelers. *Cryptosporidium* is also relatively uncommon. The risk for *Cyclospora* is highly geographic and seasonal: the most well-known risks are in Nepal, Peru, Haiti, and Guatemala. *Dientamoeba fragilis* is a low-grade but persistent pathogen that is occasionally diagnosed in travelers. The individual pathogens are each discussed in their own sections in Chapter 3, and persistent diarrhea in returned travelers is discussed in Chapter 5.

OCCURRENCE

The most important determinant of risk is travel destination, and there are regional differences in both the risk for and etiology of diarrhea. The world is generally divided into 3 grades of risk: low, intermediate, and high.

- Low-risk countries include the United States, Canada, Australia, New Zealand, Japan, and countries in Northern and Western Europe.
- Intermediate-risk countries include those in Eastern Europe, South Africa, and some of the Caribbean islands.
- High-risk areas include most of Asia, the Middle East, Africa, Mexico, and Central and South America.

RISK FOR TRAVELERS

TD occurs equally in male and female travelers and is more common in young adult travelers than in older travelers. In short-term travelers, bouts of TD do not appear to protect against future attacks, and >1 episode of TD may occur during a single trip. A cohort of expatriates residing in Kathmandu, Nepal, experienced an average of 3.2 episodes of TD per person in their first year. In more temperate regions, there may be seasonal variations in diarrhea risk. In south Asia, for example, much higher TD attack rates are reported during the hot months preceding the monsoon.

In environments where large numbers of people do not have access to plumbing or outhouses, the amount of stool contamination in the environment will be higher and more accessible to flies. Inadequate electrical capacity may lead to frequent blackouts or poorly functioning refrigeration, which can result in unsafe food storage and an increased risk for disease. Inadequate water supplies can lead to the absence of sinks for handwashing by restaurant staff, as well as direct contamination of foods, such as fruits and vegetables washed in contaminated water. Poor training in handling and preparation of food may lead to cross-contamination from meat, and inadequate disinfection of food preparation surfaces and utensils. In destinations in which effective food handling courses have been provided, the risk for TD has been demonstrated to decrease. However, some pathogens that cause TD, such as *Shigella sonnei*, are not unique to developing countries. The risk of TD is associated with the water, sanitation, and hygiene environment and practices in specific destinations, as well as the handling and preparation of food in restaurants in developed countries.

CLINICAL PRESENTATION

Bacterial diarrhea presents with the sudden onset of bothersome symptoms that can range from mild cramps and urgent loose stools to severe abdominal pain, fever, vomiting, and bloody diarrhea. Viral enteropathogens present in a similar fashion to bacterial pathogens, although with norovirus vomiting may be more prominent. Protozoal diarrhea, such as that caused by *Giardia intestinalis* or *E. histolytica*, generally has a more gradual onset of low-grade symptoms, with 2–5 loose stools per day. The incubation period of the pathogens can be a clue to the etiology of TD:

- Bacterial and viral pathogens have an incubation period of 6–48 hours.
- Protozoal pathogens generally have an incubation period of 1–2 weeks and rarely present in the first few weeks of travel. An exception can be *Cyclospora cayetanensis*, which can present quickly in areas of high risk.

Untreated bacterial diarrhea lasts 3–5 days. Viral diarrhea lasts 2–3 days. Protozoal diarrhea can persist for weeks to months without treatment. An acute bout of gastroenteritis can lead to persistent gastrointestinal symptoms, even in the absence of continued infection (see Chapter 5, Persistent Travelers' Diarrhea). Other postinfectious sequelae may include reactive arthritis and Guillain-Barré syndrome.

PREVENTION

For travelers to high-risk areas, several approaches may be recommended that can reduce, but never completely eliminate, the risk for TD. These include instruction regarding food and beverage selection, use of agents other than antimicrobial drugs for prophylaxis, and use of prophylactic antibiotics. Carrying small containers of alcohol-based hand sanitizers (containing ≥60% alcohol) may make it easier for travelers to clean their hands before eating. No vaccines are available for most pathogens that cause TD, but travelers should refer to the Hepatitis A and Typhoid & Paratyphoid Fever sections in Chapter 3 regarding vaccines that can prevent

other food- or waterborne infections to which travelers are prone.

Food and Beverage Selection

Care in selecting food and beverages for consumption helps to minimize the risk for acquiring TD. See the Food and Water Precautions section later in this chapter for CDC's detailed food and beverage recommendations. Although food and water precautions continue to be recommended, travelers may not always be able to adhere to the advice. Furthermore, many of the factors that ensure food safety, such as restaurant hygiene, are out of the traveler's control.

Nonantimicrobial Drugs for Prophylaxis

The primary agent studied for prevention of TD, other than antimicrobial drugs, is bismuth subsalicylate (BSS), which is the active ingredient in Pepto-Bismol. Studies from Mexico have shown this agent (taken daily as either 2 oz of liquid or 2 chewable tablets 4 times per day) reduces the incidence of TD by approximately 50%. BSS commonly causes blackening of the tongue and stool and may cause nausea, constipation, and rarely tinnitus. BSS should be avoided by travelers with aspirin allergy, renal insufficiency, and gout and by those taking anticoagulants, probenecid, or methotrexate. In travelers taking aspirin or salicylates for other reasons, the use of BSS may result in salicylate toxicity. BSS is not generally recommended for children aged <12 years; however, some clinicians use it off-label with caution in certain circumstances. Caution should be taken in administering BSS to children with viral infections, such as varicella or influenza, because of the risk for Reye syndrome. BSS is not recommended for children aged <3 years. Studies have not established the safety of BSS use for periods >3 weeks. Because of the number of tablets that need to be carried and the 4 times per day dosing, BSS is not commonly used as prophylaxis for TD.

The use of probiotics, such as *Lactobacillus* GG and *Saccharomyces boulardii*, has been studied in the prevention of TD in small numbers of people. Results are inconclusive, partially because standardized preparations of these bacteria are not reliably available. Some people report beneficial outcomes using bovine colostrum as a daily prophylaxis agent for TD. However, commercially sold preparations of bovine colostrum are marketed as dietary supplements that are not Food and Drug Administration (FDA) approved for medical indications. Because no data from rigorous clinical trials demonstrate efficacy in controlled trials, there is insufficient information to recommend the use of bovine colostrum to prevent TD.

Prophylactic Antibiotics

Prophylactic antibiotics are effective in the prevention of TD. Controlled studies have shown that diarrhea attack rates are reduced by 90% or more by the use of antibiotics. The prophylactic antibiotic of choice has changed over the past few decades as resistance patterns have evolved. Agents such as trimethoprim-sulfamethoxazole and doxycycline are no longer considered effective antimicrobial agents against enteric bacterial pathogens. The fluoroquinolones have been the most effective antibiotics for the prophylaxis and treatment of bacterial TD pathogens, but increasing resistance to these agents, mainly among *Campylobacter* species, may limit their benefit in the future. A nonabsorbable antibiotic, rifaximin, is being investigated but is not currently approved by the FDA for its potential use in TD prophylaxis. In one study, rifaximin reduced the risk for TD in travelers to Mexico by 77%.

At this time, prophylactic antibiotics should not be recommended for most travelers. Prophylactic antibiotics afford no protection against nonbacterial pathogens and can remove normally protective microflora from the bowel, rendering a traveler more susceptible to infection with resistant bacterial pathogens. Additionally, the use of antibiotics may be associated with allergic or adverse reactions in a certain percentage of travelers and may potentially contribute to drug resistance. The use of prophylactic antibiotics should be weighed against the result of using prompt, early self-treatment with antibiotics when TD occurs, which can limit the duration of illness to 6–24 hours in most cases. Prophylactic antibiotics may be considered for short-term travelers who are high-risk hosts (such as those who are immunosuppressed) or who are taking critical trips during which even a short bout of diarrhea could affect the trip.

TREATMENT

Antibiotics are the principal element in the treatment of TD and are effective in cases caused by bacterial pathogens that are susceptible to the particular antibiotic prescribed. Adjunctive agents used for symptomatic control may also be recommended. (See also the Self-Treatable Conditions section earlier in this chapter.)

Antibiotics

As bacterial causes of TD far outnumber other microbial causes, empiric treatment with an antibiotic directed at enteric bacterial pathogens remains the best therapy for TD. The benefit of treating TD with antibiotics has been proven in numerous studies. The effectiveness of a particular antimicrobial depends on the etiologic agent and its antibiotic sensitivity. Both as empiric therapy or for treatment of a specific bacterial pathogen, first-line antibiotics include those of the fluoroquinolone class, such as ciprofloxacin or levofloxacin. Increasing microbial resistance to the fluoroquinolones, especially among *Campylobacter* isolates, may limit their usefulness in some destinations, such as Thailand, where *Campylobacter* is prevalent. Increasing cases of fluoroquinolone resistance have been reported from other destinations and in other bacterial pathogens, including *Shigella* and *Salmonella*. A potential alternative to the fluoroquinolones in these situations is azithromycin. Rifaximin has been approved to treat TD caused by noninvasive strains of *E. coli*. However, since it is often difficult for travelers to distinguish between invasive and noninvasive diarrhea, and since they would have to carry a back-up drug in the event of invasive diarrhea, the overall usefulness of rifaximin as empiric self-treatment remains to be determined.

Single-dose or 1-day therapy for TD with a fluoroquinolone is well established, both by clinical trials and clinical experience. The best regimen for azithromycin treatment is not yet established. One study used a single dose of 1,000 mg, but side effects (mainly nausea) may limit the acceptability of this large dose. Azithromycin, 500 mg per day for 1–3 days, appears to be effective in most cases of TD.

Antimotility Agents

Antimotility agents provide symptomatic relief and serve as useful adjuncts to antibiotic therapy in TD. Synthetic opiates, such as loperamide and diphenoxylate, can reduce bowel movement frequency and enable travelers to ride on an airplane or bus while awaiting the effects of antibiotics. Loperamide appears to have antisecretory properties as well. The safety of loperamide when used along with an antibiotic has been well established, even in cases of invasive pathogens. Antimotility agents are not generally recommended for patients with bloody diarrhea or those who have diarrhea and fever. Loperamide can be used in children, and liquid formulations are available. In practice, however, these drugs are rarely given to small children (aged <6 years).

Oral Rehydration Therapy

Fluids and electrolytes are lost in cases of TD, and replenishment is important, especially in young children or adults with chronic medical illness. In adult travelers who are otherwise healthy, severe dehydration resulting from TD is unusual unless vomiting is prolonged. Nonetheless, replacement of fluid losses remains an adjunct to other therapy and helps the traveler feel better more quickly. Travelers should remember to use only beverages that are sealed, treated with chlorine, boiled, or are otherwise known to be purified. For severe fluid loss, replacement is best accomplished with oral rehydration solution (ORS), prepared from packaged oral rehydration salts, such as those provided by the World Health Organization, which are widely available at stores and pharmacies in most developing countries. ORS is prepared by adding 1 packet to the indicated volume of boiled or treated water—generally 1 liter. Travelers may find most ORS formulations to be relatively unpalatable, due to their saltiness. In less severe cases, rehydration can be maintained with any palatable liquid (including sports drinks), although overly sweet drinks, such as many sodas, can cause osmotic diarrhea if consumed in quantity.

Treatment of TD Caused by Protozoa

The most common parasitic cause of TD is *G. intestinalis*, and treatment options include metronidazole, tinidazole, and nitazoxanide (see Chapter 3, Giardiasis). Although cryptosporidiosis is usually a self-limited illness in immunocompetent people, nitazoxanide can be considered as a treatment option. Cyclosporiasis is treated with trimethoprim-sulfamethoxazole. Treatment of amebiasis is with metronidazole or tinidazole, followed by treatment with a luminal agent such as iodoquinol or paromomycin.

Treatment for Children

Children who accompany their parents on trips to high-risk destinations may be expected to have TD as well. There is no reason to withhold antibiotics from children who contract TD. In older children and teenagers, treatment recommendations for TD follow those for adults, with possible adjustments in the dose of medication. Macrolides such as azithromycin are considered first-line antibiotic therapy in children, although some experts now use short-course fluoroquinolone therapy (despite its not being FDA-approved for this indication in children) for travelers aged <18 years. Rifaximin is approved for use in children aged ≥12 years.

Infants and younger children with TD are at higher risk for developing dehydration, which is best prevented by the early use of ORS. Breastfed infants should continue to nurse on demand, and bottle-fed infants can continue to drink their formula. Older infants and children may eat a regular diet, depending on the level of their appetite while they are ill. Infants in diapers are at risk for developing a painful, eczematous rash on their buttocks in response to the liquid stool. Hydrocortisone cream will quickly improve this rash. More information about diarrhea and dehydration is discussed in Chapter 7, Traveling Safely with Infants and Children.

BIBLIOGRAPHY

1. Adachi JA, Jiang ZD, Mathewson JJ, Verenkar MP, Thompson S, Martinez-Sandoval F, et al. Enteroaggregative *Escherichia coli* as a major etiologic agent in traveler's diarrhea in 3 regions of the world. Clin Infect Dis. 2001 Jun 15;32(12):1706–9.

2. Black RE. Epidemiology of travelers' diarrhea and relative importance of various pathogens. Rev Infect Dis. 1990 Jan–Feb;12 Suppl 1:S73–9.

3. Connor BA. Sequelae of traveler's diarrhea: focus on postinfectious irritable bowel syndrome. Clin Infect Dis. 2005 Dec 1;41 Suppl 8:S577–86.

4. DuPont HL, Ericsson CD. Prevention and treatment of traveler's diarrhea. N Engl J Med. 1993 Jun 24;328(25):1821–7.

5. Greenwood Z, Black J, Weld L, O'Brien D, Leder K, Von Sonnenburg F, et al. Gastrointestinal infection among international travelers globally. J Travel Med. 2008 Jul–Aug;15(4):221–8.

6. Kendall ME, Crim S, Fullerton K, Han PV, Cronquist AB, Shiferaw B, et al. Travel-associated enteric infections diagnosed after return to the United States, Foodborne Diseases Active Surveillance Network (FoodNet), 2004–2009. Clin Infect Dis. 2012 Jun;54 Suppl 5:S480–7.

7. Shah N, DuPont HL, Ramsey DJ. Global etiology of travelers' diarrhea: systematic review from 1973 to the present. Am J Trop Med Hyg. 2009 Apr;80(4):609–14.

8. Shlim DR. Update in traveler's diarrhea. Infect Dis Clin North Am. 2005 Mar;19(1):137–49.

9. Swaminathan A, Torresi J, Schlagenhauf P, Thursky K, Wilder-Smith A, Connor BA, et al. A global study of pathogens and host risk factors associated with infectious gastrointestinal disease in returned international travellers. J Infect. 2009 Jul;59(1):19–27.

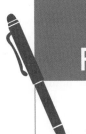

For the Record

A HISTORY OF THE DEFINITION & MANAGEMENT OF TRAVELERS' DIARRHEA

Herbert L. DuPont

BACKGROUND

Travelers' diarrhea (TD) is defined as the passage of ≥3 unformed stools per day plus ≥1 associated enteric symptoms, such as abdominal pain or cramps, occurring in a traveler after arrival, usually in a resource-limited destination. Many colorful terms have been used for the condition according to the places where diarrhea commonly occurred, such as Aztec Two-Step, Delhi Belly, Hong Kong Dog, Montezuma's Revenge, and the Pharaoh's Curse.

While it was known for centuries that diarrhea and dysentery complicated armed conflicts in international settings, it wasn't until the 1940s that diarrhea was closely correlated with international travel and relocation in tropical regions. In the 1950s, B. H. Kean from Cornell University increased awareness of the problem by studying travelers and students from the United States in Mexico. The field mushroomed in later years, when groups studied international students and travelers, expatriates, and military populations. The history of TD can be viewed in 3 time blocks.

PHASE 1. THE 1950S THROUGH THE 1960S—QUANTITATION OF THE PROBLEM AND SUCCESSFUL CHEMOPROPHYLAXIS

Kean and Waters studied the risk of TD among students and travelers to Mexico and demonstrated successful disease prevention with antibiotic chemoprophylaxis, which provided the first evidence that bacterial pathogens were responsible for most illness. Chemoprophylaxis was used in a little more than one-third of US visitors to Mexico in the 1950s and 1960s and was used by the

US, Australian, and British athletes competing in the Olympics in Mexico City in 1968.

PHASE 2. THE 1970S THROUGH THE 1990S—EPIDEMIOLOGY, ETIOLOGY, AND THERAPY

Clinical and epidemiologic features of TD were described. Microbiologic studies were carried out to determine the etiology of the illness, beginning with a study published in 1970 describing a single strain of *Escherichia coli* as the cause of TD in British troops stationed in Aden on the Red Sea. The next year, 2 strains of *E. coli* isolated from American soldiers with diarrhea acquired in Vietnam were shown to be enterotoxigenic in animals and adult volunteers, and 4 years later enterotoxigenic *E. coli* (ETEC) was found in most cases of TD among US students studying in a language school in Mexico.

The first clear evidence that antibiotics were effective in treating TD was in 1981 when trimethoprim-sulfamethoxazole (TMP-SMX) was shown to reduce the duration of the illness in a group of travelers with TD caused by different etiologies. Placebo-controlled clinical trials then demonstrated the value of fluoroquinolones in treating TD. Regions of the tropical and semitropical world were studied, allowing scientists to categorize areas according to risk that international visitors would face of acquiring TD.

Although prophylactic antibiotics were used by international travelers at the time, in 1985 chemoprophylaxis with systemic antibiotics was strongly discouraged because of concerns about adverse drug events and development of drug resistance. The Consensus Development Panel favored self-treatment with short-course (single-dose or 3 days) antibiotics.

PHASE 3. 2000 AND BEYOND—ANTIBIOTIC RESISTANCE AND CHRONIC COMPLICATIONS

During this phase, the fluoroquinolones, particularly ciprofloxacin, became the mainstay of therapy for TD. The poorly absorbed (<0.4%) rifamycin antibiotic, rifaximin, was found to be as effective as ciprofloxacin for the most common TD syndrome, watery diarrhea. After more than a decade of use of fluoroquinolones for a variety of infectious disease conditions, resistance to this class of drugs has become more common among some bacterial causes of TD, particularly *Campylobacter jejuni*. The emergence of resistance encouraged the wider use of azithromycin, either single-dose or 3-day courses, to treat TD.

Chemoprophylaxis was once more examined with bismuth subsalicylate or rifaximin, both of which appeared to have a more acceptable safety profile and fewer concerns about resistance compared with the absorbed antibiotics. Currently, there are no general recommendations for this approach.

With the knowledge that bacterial diarrhea may be associated with the development of postinfectious irritable bowel syndrome and that bacterial enteropathogens caused most cases of TD, studies of travelers were undertaken. These small studies found that 5%–10% of people developed new-onset irritable bowel syndrome after experiencing TD in Mexico or Asia, although in most of these people, no bacterial pathogen was identified. Studies are needed to further analyze this possible association and to develop and analyze methods of prevention, which could include early therapy (with passage of the first unformed stool), antibiotic chemoprophylaxis, or a vaccine.

BIBLIOGRAPHY

1. DuPont HL, Ericsson CD, Farthing MJ, Gorbach S, Pickering LK, Rombo L, et al. Expert review of the evidence base for prevention of travelers' diarrhea. J Travel Med. 2009 May–Jun;16(3):149–60.

2. DuPont HL, Formal SB, Hornick RB, Snyder MJ, Libonati JP, Sheahan DG, et al. Pathogenesis of *Escherichia coli* diarrhea. N Engl J Med. 1971 Jul 1;285(1):1–9.

3. DuPont HL, Jiang ZD, Ericsson CD, Adachi JA, Mathewson JJ, DuPont MW, et al. Rifaximin versus ciprofloxacin for the treatment of traveler's diarrhea: a randomized, double-blind clinical trial. Clin Infect Dis. 2001 Dec 1;33(11):1807–15.

4. DuPont HL, Reves RR, Galindo E, Sullivan PS, Wood LV, Mendiola JG. Treatment of travelers' diarrhea with trimethoprim/sulfamethoxazole and with trimethoprim alone. N Engl J Med. 1982 Sep 30;307(14):841–4.

5. Gorbach SL, Edelman R. Travelers' diarrhea: National Institutes of Health Consensus Development Conference. Bethesda, Maryland, January 28–30, 1985. Rev Infect Dis. 1986 May–Jun;8 Suppl 2:S109–233.

6. Gorbach SL, Kean BH, Evans DG, Evans DJ, Jr., Bessudo D. Travelers' diarrhea and toxigenic *Escherichia coli*. N Engl J Med. 1975 May 1;292(18):933–6.

7. Kean BH, Waters SR. The diarrhea of travelers. III. Drug prophylaxis in Mexico. N Engl J Med. 1959 Jul 9;261(2):71–4.

8. Kuschner RA, Trofa AF, Thomas RJ, Hoge CW, Pitarangsi C, Amato S, et al. Use of azithromycin for the treatment of *Campylobacter enteritis* in travelers to Thailand, an area where ciprofloxacin resistance is prevalent. Clin Infect Dis. 1995 Sep;21(3):536–41.

9. Okhuysen PC, Jiang ZD, Carlin L, Forbes C, DuPont HL. Post-diarrhea chronic intestinal symptoms and irritable bowel syndrome in North American travelers to Mexico. Am J Gastroenterol. 2004 Sep;99(9):1774–8.

10. Ouyang-Latimer J, Jafri S, VanTassel A, Jiang ZD, Gurleen K, Rodriguez S, et al. In vitro antimicrobial susceptibility of bacterial enteropathogens isolated from international travelers to Mexico, Guatemala, and India from 2006 to 2008. Antimicrob Agents Chemother. 2011 Feb;55(2):874–8.

11. Owen JR. Diarrhoea at the Olympics. Br Med J. 1968 Dec 7;4(5631):645.

12. Petruccelli BP, Murphy GS, Sanchez JL, Walz S, DeFraites R, Gelnett J, et al. Treatment of traveler's diarrhea with ciprofloxacin and loperamide. J Infect Dis. 1992 Mar;165(3):557–60.

13. Rowe B, Taylor J, Bettelheim KA. An investigation of traveller's diarrhoea. Lancet. 1970 Jan 3;1(7636):1–5.

14. Steffen R. Epidemiologic studies of travelers' diarrhea, severe gastrointestinal infections, and cholera. Rev Infect Dis. 1986 May–Jun;8 Suppl 2:S122–30.

15. Steffen R, van der Linde F, Gyr K, Schar M. Epidemiology of diarrhea in travelers. JAMA. 1983 Mar 4;249(9):1176–80.

16. Stermer E, Lubezky A, Potasman I, Paster E, Lavy A. Is traveler's diarrhea a significant risk factor for the development of irritable bowel syndrome? A prospective study. Clin Infect Dis. 2006 Oct 1;43(7):898–901.

17. Tribble DR, Sanders JW, Pang LW, Mason C, Pitarangsi C, Baqar S, et al. Traveler's diarrhea in Thailand: randomized, double-blind trial comparing single-dose and 3-day azithromycin-based regimens with a 3-day levofloxacin regimen. Clin Infect Dis. 2007 Feb 1;44(3):338–46.

18. Wistrom J, Jertborn M, Hedstrom SA, Alestig K, Englund G, Jellheden B, et al. Short-term self-treatment of travellers' diarrhoea with norfloxacin: a placebo-controlled study. J Antimicrob Chemother. 1989 Jun;23(6):905–13.

ALTITUDE ILLNESS

Peter H. Hackett, David R. Shlim

OVERVIEW

The stresses of the high-altitude environment include cold, low humidity, increased ultraviolet radiation, and decreased air pressure, all of which can cause problems for travelers. The primary concern, however, is hypoxia. At 10,000 ft (3,000 m), for example, the inspired PO_2 is only 69% of sea-level value. The degree of hypoxic stress depends on altitude, rate of ascent, and duration of exposure. Sleeping at high altitude produces the most hypoxia; day trips to high altitude with return to low altitude are much less stressful on the body. Typical high-altitude destinations include Cuzco, Peru (11,150 ft; 3,400 m), La Paz, Bolivia (12,400 ft; 3,780 m), Lhasa, Tibet (12,000 ft; 3,660 m), Everest Base Camp in Nepal (17,598 ft; 5,364 m), and Kilimanjaro in Tanzania (19,341 ft; 5,895 m).

The human body adjusts very well to moderate hypoxia, but requires time to do so (Box 2-2). The process of acute acclimatization to high altitude takes 3–5 days; therefore, acclimatizing for a few days at 8,000–9,000 ft (2,500–2,750 m) before proceeding to a higher altitude is ideal. Acclimatization prevents altitude illness, improves sleep, and increases comfort and well-being, although exercise performance will always be reduced compared with low altitude. Increase in ventilation is the most important factor in acute acclimatization; therefore, respiratory depressants must be avoided. Increased red-cell production does not play a role in acute acclimatization.

RISK FOR TRAVELERS

Inadequate acclimatization may lead to altitude illness in any traveler going to 8,000 ft (2,500 m) or higher. Susceptibility and resistance to altitude illness are genetic traits, and no simple screening tests are available to predict risk. Risk is not affected by training or physical fitness. Children are equally susceptible as adults; people aged >50 years have slightly lower risk. How a traveler has responded to high altitude previously is the most reliable guide for future trips, but is not infallible. However, given certain baseline susceptibility, risk is largely influenced by rate of ascent and exertion (see Table 2-7). Determining an itinerary that will avoid any occurrence of altitude illness is difficult because of variations in individual susceptibility, as well as in starting points and terrain. The goal for the traveler may not be to avoid all symptoms of altitude illness but to ensure that any illness remains mild.

CLINICAL PRESENTATION

Altitude illness is divided into 3 syndromes: acute mountain sickness (AMS), high-altitude cerebral edema (HACE), and high-altitude pulmonary edema (HAPE).

BOX 2-2. TIPS FOR ACCLIMATIZATION

- Ascend gradually, if possible. Try not to go directly from low altitude to >9,000 ft (2,750 m) sleeping altitude in 1 day. Once at >9,000 ft (2,750 m), move sleeping altitude no higher than 1,600 ft (500 m) per day, and plan an extra day for acclimatization every 3,300 ft (1,000 m).
- Consider using acetazolamide to speed acclimatization, if abrupt ascent is unavoidable.
- Avoid alcohol for the first 48 hours.
- Participate in only mild exercise for the first 48 hours.
- Having a high-altitude exposure at >9,000 ft (2,750 m) for 2 nights or more, within 30 days before the trip, is useful.

Table 2-7. Risk categories for acute mountain sickness

RISK CATEGORY	DESCRIPTION	PROPHYLAXIS RECOMMENDATIONS
Low	• People with no prior history of altitude illness and ascending to <9,000 ft (2,750 m) • People taking >2 days to arrive at 8,000–9,000 ft (2,500–2,750 m), with subsequent increases in sleeping elevation <1,600 ft (500 m) per day, and an extra day for acclimatization every 3,200 ft (1,000 m)	Acetazolamide prophylaxis generally not indicated.
Moderate	• People with prior history of AMS and ascending to 8,000–9,000 ft (2,500–2,750 m) in 1 day • No history of AMS and ascending to >9,000 ft (2,750 m) in 1 day • All people ascending >1,600 ft (500 m) per day (increase in sleeping elevation) at altitudes >9,000 ft (2,750 m), but with an extra day for acclimatization every 3,200 ft (1,000 m)	Acetazolamide prophylaxis would be beneficial and should be considered.
High	• History of AMS and ascending to >9,000 ft (2,750 m) in 1 day • All people with a prior history of HACE or HAPE • All people ascending to >11,400 ft (3,500 m) in 1 day • All people ascending >1,600 ft (500 m) per day (increase in sleeping elevation) >9,000 ft (2,750 m), without extra days for acclimatization • Very rapid ascents (such as <7-day ascents of Mount Kilimanjaro)	Acetazolamide prophylaxis strongly recommended.

Abbreviations: AMS, acute mountain sickness; HACE, high-altitude cerebral edema; HAPE, high-altitude pulmonary edema.

Acute Mountain Sickness

AMS is the most common form of altitude illness, affecting, for example, 25% of all visitors sleeping above 8,000 ft (2,500 m) in Colorado. Symptoms are those of an alcohol hangover: headache is the cardinal symptom, sometimes accompanied by fatigue, loss of appetite, nausea, and occasionally vomiting. Headache onset is usually 2–12 hours after arrival at a higher altitude and often during or after the first night. Preverbal children may develop loss of appetite, irritability, and pallor. AMS generally resolves with 24–72 hours of acclimatization.

High-Altitude Cerebral Edema

HACE is a severe progression of AMS and is rare; it is most often associated with HAPE. In addition to AMS symptoms, lethargy becomes profound, with drowsiness, confusion, and ataxia on tandem gait test. A person with

HACE requires immediate descent; death from HACE can ensue within 24 hours of developing ataxia if the person fails to descend.

High-Altitude Pulmonary Edema

HAPE can occur by itself or in conjunction with AMS and HACE; the incidence is 1 per 10,000 skiers in Colorado and up to 1 per 100 climbers at >14,000 ft (4,300 m). Initial symptoms are increased breathlessness with exertion, and eventually increased breathlessness at rest, associated with weakness and cough. Oxygen or descent is life-saving. HAPE can be more rapidly fatal than HACE.

Preexisting Medical Problems

Travelers with medical conditions, such as heart failure, myocardial ischemia (angina), sickle cell disease, or any form of pulmonary insufficiency, should be advised to consult a physician familiar with high-altitude medical issues before undertaking high-altitude travel. The risk for new ischemic heart disease in previously healthy travelers does not appear to be increased at high altitudes. People with diabetes can travel safely to high altitudes, but they must be accustomed to exercise and carefully monitor their blood glucose. In travelers with type 1 diabetes, diabetic ketoacidosis may be triggered by altitude illness and may be more difficult to treat in those on acetazolamide. Not all glucose meters read accurately at high altitudes.

Most people do not have visual problems at high altitudes. However, at very high altitudes some people who have had radial keratotomy may develop acute farsightedness and be unable to climb by themselves. LASIK and other newer procedures may produce only minor visual disturbances at high altitudes.

There are no studies or case reports of harm to a fetus if the mother travels briefly to high altitudes during pregnancy. However, it may be prudent to recommend that pregnant women do not stay at sleeping altitudes >12,000 ft (3,700 m), if possible. The dangers of having a pregnancy complication in remote, mountainous terrain should also be discussed.

DIAGNOSIS AND TREATMENT
Acute Mountain Sickness/High-Altitude Cerebral Edema

The differential diagnosis of AMS/HACE includes dehydration, exhaustion, hypoglycemia, hypothermia, or hyponatremia. Focal neurologic symptoms, or seizures, are rare in HACE and should lead to suspicion of an intracranial lesion or seizure disorder. Patients with AMS can descend ≥1,000 ft (300 m), and symptoms will rapidly abate. Alternatively, supplemental oxygen at 2 L per minute will relieve headache quickly and resolve AMS over hours, but it is rarely available. People with AMS can also safely remain at their current altitude and treat symptoms with nonopiate analgesics and antiemetics, such as ondansetron. They may also take acetazolamide, which speeds acclimatization and effectively treats AMS, but is better for prophylaxis than treatment. Dexamethasone is more effective than acetazolamide at rapidly relieving the symptoms of moderate to severe AMS. **If symptoms are getting worse while the traveler is resting at the same altitude, he or she must descend.**

HACE is a continuation of AMS and is diagnosed when neurologic findings, particularly ataxia, confusion, or altered mental status, are present. HACE may also occur in the presence of HAPE. People developing HACE in populated areas with access to medical care can be treated at altitude with supplemental oxygen and dexamethasone. In remote areas, descent should be initiated in any person suspected of having HACE. If descent is not feasible because of logistical issues, supplemental oxygen or a portable hyperbaric chamber should be used, if available.

High-Altitude Pulmonary Edema

Although the progression of decreased exercise tolerance, increased breathlessness, and breathlessness at rest is almost always recognizable as HAPE, the differential diagnosis includes pneumonia, bronchospasm, myocardial infarction, or pulmonary embolism. Descent in this situation is urgent and mandatory, and should be accomplished with as little exertion as is feasible for the patient. If descent is not immediately possible, supplemental oxygen or a portable hyperbaric chamber should be used. Patients with mild HAPE who have access to oxygen (at a hospital or high-altitude medical clinic, for example) may not need to descend to lower elevation and can be treated with oxygen at the current elevation. In the field setting, where resources are limited and there is a lower margin for error, nifedipine can be used as an adjunct to descent, oxygen, or portable hyperbaric therapy. A phosphodiesterase inhibitor may be used if nifedipine is not available, but concurrent use of multiple pulmonary vasodilators is not recommended.

Medications

In addition to the discussion below, recommendations for the usage and dosing of medications to prevent and treat altitude illness are outlined in Table 2-8. (See also the Self-Treatable Conditions section earlier in this chapter.)

Acetazolamide

Acetazolamide prevents AMS when taken before ascent and can speed recovery if taken after symptoms have developed. The drug works by acidifying the blood, which causes an increase in respiration and thus aids acclimatization. An effective adult dose that minimizes the common side effects of increased

Table 2-8. Recommended medication doses to prevent and treat altitude illness

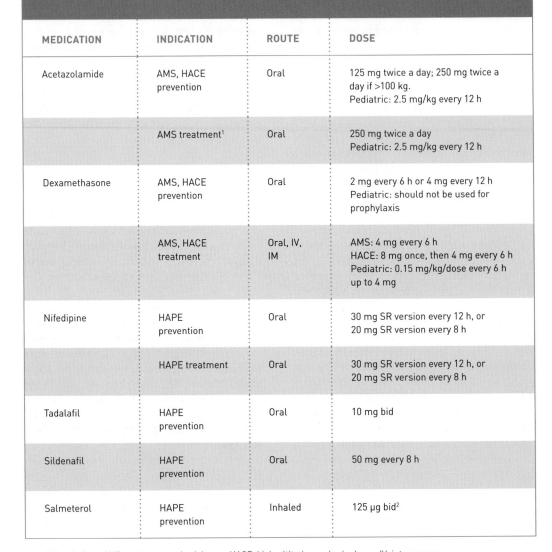

MEDICATION	INDICATION	ROUTE	DOSE
Acetazolamide	AMS, HACE prevention	Oral	125 mg twice a day; 250 mg twice a day if >100 kg. Pediatric: 2.5 mg/kg every 12 h
	AMS treatment[1]	Oral	250 mg twice a day Pediatric: 2.5 mg/kg every 12 h
Dexamethasone	AMS, HACE prevention	Oral	2 mg every 6 h or 4 mg every 12 h Pediatric: should not be used for prophylaxis
	AMS, HACE treatment	Oral, IV, IM	AMS: 4 mg every 6 h HACE: 8 mg once, then 4 mg every 6 h Pediatric: 0.15 mg/kg/dose every 6 h up to 4 mg
Nifedipine	HAPE prevention	Oral	30 mg SR version every 12 h, or 20 mg SR version every 8 h
	HAPE treatment	Oral	30 mg SR version every 12 h, or 20 mg SR version every 8 h
Tadalafil	HAPE prevention	Oral	10 mg bid
Sildenafil	HAPE prevention	Oral	50 mg every 8 h
Salmeterol	HAPE prevention	Inhaled	125 µg bid[2]

Abbreviations: AMS, acute mountain sickness; HACE, high-altitude cerebral edema; IV, intravenous; IM, intramuscular; HAPE, high-altitude pulmonary edema; SR, sustained release.
[1] Acetazolamide can also be used at this dose as an *adjunct* to dexamethasone in HACE treatment, but dexamethasone remains the primary treatment for that disorder.
[2] Should not be used as monotherapy and should only be used in conjunction with oral medications.

urination and paresthesias of the fingers and toes is 125 mg every 12 hours, beginning the day before ascent and continuing the first 2 days at altitude, or longer if ascent continues. Allergic reactions to acetazolamide are uncommon. As a nonantimicrobial sulfonamide, it does not cross-react with antimicrobial sulfonamides. However, it is best avoided by people with history of anaphylaxis to any sulfa. People with history of severe penicillin allergy have occasionally had allergic reactions to acetazolamide. The pediatric dose is 5 mg/kg/day in divided doses, up to 125 mg twice a day.

Dexamethasone
Dexamethasone is effective for preventing and treating AMS and HACE, and perhaps HAPE as well. Unlike acetazolamide, if the

drug is discontinued at altitude before acclimatization, rebound can occur. Acetazolamide is preferable to prevent AMS while ascending, with dexamethasone reserved for treatment, as an adjunct to descent. The adult dose is 4 mg every 6 hours. An increasing trend is to use dexamethasone for "summit day" on high peaks such as Kilimanjaro and Aconcagua, to prevent abrupt altitude illness.

Nifedipine

Nifedipine prevents HAPE and ameliorates it as well. For prevention, it is generally reserved for people who are particularly susceptible to the condition. The adult dose for prevention or treatment is 30 mg of extended release every 12 hours, or 20 mg every 8 hours.

Other Medications

Phosphodiesterase-5 inhibitors can also selectively lower pulmonary artery pressure, with less effect on systemic blood pressure. Tadalafil, 10 mg twice a day, during ascent can prevent HAPE and is being studied for treatment. When taken before ascent, gingko biloba, 100–120 mg twice a day, was shown to reduce AMS in adults in some trials, but it was not effective in others, probably due to variation in ingredients. Ibuprofen 600 mg every 8 hours was recently found to help prevent AMS, although it was not as effective as acetazolamide. However, it is nonprescription, inexpensive, and well tolerated.

PREVENTION OF SEVERE ALTITUDE ILLNESS OR DEATH

The main point of instructing travelers about altitude illness is not to eliminate the possibility, but to prevent death or evacuation due to altitude illness. Since the onset of symptoms and the clinical course are sufficiently slow and predictable, there is no reason for someone to die from altitude illness, unless trapped by weather or geography in a situation in which descent is impossible. Three rules can prevent death or serious consequences from altitude illness:

- Know the early symptoms of altitude illness, and be willing to acknowledge when they are present.
- Never ascend to sleep at a higher altitude when experiencing symptoms of altitude illness, no matter how minor they seem.
- Descend if the symptoms become worse while resting at the same altitude.

For trekking groups and expeditions going into remote high-altitude areas, where descent to a lower altitude could be problematic, a pressurization bag (such as the Gamow bag) can be beneficial. A foot pump produces an increased pressure of 2 lb/in^2, mimicking a descent of 5,000–6,000 ft (1,500–1,800 m), depending on the starting altitude. The total packed weight of bag and pump is about 14 lb (6.5 kg).

BIBLIOGRAPHY

1. Hackett P. High altitude and common medical conditions. In: Hornbein TF, Schoene RB, editors. High Altitude: an Exploration of Human Adaptation. New York: Marcel Dekker; 2001. p. 839–85.
2. Hackett PH, Roach RC. High altitude cerebral edema. High Alt Med Biol. 2004 Summer;5(2):136–46.
3. Hackett PH, Roach RC. High-altitude illness. N Engl J Med. 2001 Jul 12;345(2):107–14.
4. Hackett PH, Roach RC. High-altitude medicine and physiology. In: Auerbach PS, editor. Wilderness Medicine. 6th ed. Philadelphia: Mosby Elsevier; 2012. p. 2–33.
5. Johnson TS, Rock PB, Fulco CS, Trad LA, Spark RF, Maher JT. Prevention of acute mountain sickness by dexamethasone. N Engl J Med. 1984 Mar 15;310(11):683–6.
6. Luks AM, McIntosh SE, Grissom CK, Auerbach PS, Rodway GW, Schoene RB, et al. Wilderness Medical Society consensus guidelines for the prevention and treatment of acute altitude illness. Wilderness Environ Med. 2010 Jun;21(2):146–55.
7. Luks AM, Swenson ER. Medication and dosage considerations in the prophylaxis and treatment of high-altitude illness. Chest. 2008 Mar;133(3):744–55.
8. Maggiorini M, Brunner-La Rocca HP, Peth S, Fischler M, Bohm T, Bernheim A, et al. Both tadalafil and dexamethasone may reduce the incidence of high-altitude pulmonary edema: a randomized trial. Ann Intern Med. 2006 Oct 3;145(7):497–506.
9. Pollard A, Murdoch D. The High Altitude Medicine Handbook. 3rd ed. Abingdon, UK: Radcliffe Medical Press; 2003.
10. Pollard AJ, Niermeyer S, Barry P, Bartsch P, Berghold F, Bishop RA, et al. Children at high altitude: an international consensus statement by an ad hoc committee of the International Society for Mountain

Medicine, March 12, 2001. High Alt Med Biol. 2001 Fall;2(3):389–403.

11. Strom BL, Schinnar R, Apter AJ, Margolis DJ, Lautenbach E, Hennessy S, et al. Absence of cross-reactivity between sulfonamide antibiotics and sulfonamide nonantibiotics. N Engl J Med. 2003 Oct 23;349(17):1628–35.

12. van Patot MC, Leadbetter G 3rd, Keyes LE, Maakestad KM, Olson S, Hackett PH. Prophylactic low-dose acetazolamide reduces the incidence and severity of acute mountain sickness. High Alt Med Biol. 2008 Winter;9(4):289–93.

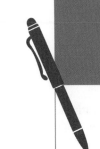

For the Record

A HISTORY OF THE DEFINITION & MANAGEMENT OF ALTITUDE ILLNESS
David R. Shlim

As explorers began to challenge the higher parts of the Earth, first in Europe in 1786 with the ascent of Mont Blanc and later in Asia and South America, the high-altitude environment occasionally proved unexpectedly fatal. Deaths in otherwise healthy young men were attributed to "heart failure" or "pneumonia," and a specific syndrome associated with rapid ascent was not suspected. The first detailed clinical descriptions of high-altitude pulmonary edema (HAPE) and high-altitude cerebral edema (HACE) were published in 1913 by Thomas Ravenhill, based on his work with high-altitude miners in Chile. Scottish physiologist A. M. Kellas also provided detailed descriptions of "mountain sickness" in papers that were a prelude to the British attempts on Mount Everest in the 1920s.

These early descriptions were overlooked until the syndromes of altitude illness were rediscovered in the early 1960s. Herbert Hultgren, a Stanford cardiologist, documented HAPE in the Andes in 1959. A year later, Charles Houston, a physician and mountain climber noted for an epic attempt on K2 in 1953, documented a case of pulmonary edema in a healthy 21-year-old backcountry skier in Aspen, Colorado, in which a cardiac cause was definitively ruled out. The first modern description of HACE is credited to Fitch in 1964. Originally, the spectrum of altitude illness was thought to include 3 syndromes: acute mountain sickness (AMS), along with HAPE and HACE. In recent times, however, AMS is understood to represent early HACE, although the term is still used. All the syndromes are classified under the term "altitude illness."

China, having annexed Tibet in the 1950s, invaded a remote corner of northern India in 1962 at altitudes of 15,000–18,000 feet. Chinese troops, attacking from the Tibetan plateau, had no problems with the altitude, but the Indian troops transported rapidly to those heights experienced considerable rates of altitude illness. The Indian physician treating these troops, Inder Singh, reported on almost 2,000 cases of altitude illness during the brief war. One of his key observations was that the severity of illness was not related to the altitude at which the symptoms began. Illness could be just as severe at 11,000 feet as at 18,000 feet. His insightful 1969 paper in the *New England Journal of Medicine* is well worth reading today.

The advent of high-altitude trekking in Nepal in the late 1960s and early 1970s opened up a new group of people—nonmountaineers—to the risk of altitude illness. The trekking route to Mount Everest involves walking on trails that range in altitude from 5,000–18,000 feet (1,525–5,500 m). The technical ease encouraged trekkers to ascend faster than they could acclimatize, and an estimated 5–10 people per year died of altitude illness in the Everest region in the early 1970s. In 1974, Dr. Peter Hackett trekked to Mount Everest and stayed to run an aid post at 14,000 feet on the way to Everest Base Camp. He remained in Nepal for 18 months and brought back detailed correlations between the risk of altitude illness and the rate of ascent.

At that time, trekkers had the choice of walking over several high passes on the way to Everest Base Camp, starting from close to Kathmandu, or flying into Lukla, an airstrip located at 9,000 feet. The trekkers who walked experienced altitude illness at a rate of 42%, while those who flew were ill at a rate of 60%. Dr. Hackett recommended 2 extra acclimatization days in the upper portions of the trek, which decreased the rate of altitude illness to <40%. His recommendations are still the basis of the itineraries for trekking to Everest Base Camp, even though the rate of altitude illness on this schedule remains approximately 35%.

In addition to trekkers walking into high-altitude destinations, travelers increasingly fly to a number of cities where they risk altitude illness, including Cuzco, Peru (11,150 ft, 3,400 m); Lhasa, Tibet (12,000 ft, 3,660 m); and La Paz, Bolivia (12,400 ft, 3,780 m). Tourists who fly from a low altitude to any of these destinations should consider taking acetazolamide to help prevent altitude illness.

In the 1930s, the antibiotic sulphanilamide was noted to cause metabolic acidosis and compensatory hyperventilation, an effect later attributed to inhibition of renal carbonic anhydrase. Another sulfonamide, acetazolamide, was a more potent carbonic anhydrase inhibitor. Inducing healthy people to breathe more was postulated to improve acclimatization to altitude, and in an article published in 1968, acetazolamide was shown to prevent altitude illness. To this day, acetazolamide remains the best drug to prevent altitude illness.

Because of variations in individual susceptibility and the modern tendency to take short trips that do not permit gradual acclimatization, altitude illness will continue to occur in travelers. However, there is no longer any reason why high-altitude sojourners should die of altitude illness. Education on acclimatization, recognition of symptoms, and appropriate response can ensure that an otherwise inconvenient and uncomfortable illness does not turn into a tragedy.

BIBLIOGRAPHY

1. Forwand SA, Landowne M, Follansbee JN, Hansen JE. Effect of acetazolamide on acute mountain sickness. N Engl J Med. 1968 Oct 17;279(16):839–45.
2. Hackett PH, Rennie D, Levine HD. The incidence, importance, and prophylaxis of acute mountain sickness. Lancet. 1976 Nov 27;2(7996):1149–55.
3. Singh I, Khanna PK, Srivastava MC, Lal M, Roy SB, Subramanyam CS. Acute mountain sickness. N Engl J Med. 1969 Jan 23;280(4):175–84.
4. Swenson ER. Carbonic anhydrase inhibitors and ventilation: a complex interplay of stimulation and suppression. Eur Res J. 1998 Dec;12(6):1242–7.
5. West JB. High life: a history of high-altitude physiology and medicine. New York: Oxford University Press; 1998.

[Handwritten at top of page: East → shift sleep 1-2 hrs earlier few days befr; West → "later"]

JET LAG
Lisa Libassi, Emad A. Yanni

OVERVIEW
Jet lag is a temporary sleep disorder among air travelers who rapidly travel across ≥3 time zones. Jet lag occurs as a result of the slow adjustment of the body clock to the destination time. Consequently, the daily rhythms and the internal drive for sleep and wakefulness are out of synchronization with the new environment.

The intrinsic body clock resides in the suprachiasmatic nuclei at the base of the hypothalamus, which contains melatonin receptors. Melatonin is manufactured in the pineal gland from tryptophan, and its synthesis and release are stimulated by darkness and suppressed by light; consequently, the secretion of melatonin is responsible for setting our sleep-wake cycle. The body clock is adjusted to the solar day by rhythmic cues in the environment, mainly the light–dark cycle, and the rhythmic secretion of melatonin. Exercise is also believed to exert an effect on the body clock, although with a somewhat weaker effect than other cues.

RISK FOR TRAVELERS
Eastward travel is associated with difficulty falling asleep at the destination bedtime and difficulty arising in the morning. Westward travel is associated with early evening sleepiness and predawn awakening at the travel destination. Travelers flying within the same time zone typically experience the fewest problems, such as nonspecific travel fatigue. Crossing more time zones or traveling eastward generally increases the time required for adaptation. After eastward flights, jet lag lasts for the number of days roughly equal to two-thirds the number of time zones crossed; after westward flights, the number of days is roughly half the number of time zones.

[Handwritten in left margin: east or many time zone difficult]

Individual responses to crossing time zones and ability to adapt to a new time zone vary. Increased age may contribute to a longer recovery period. The intensity and duration of jet lag are related to the number of time zones crossed, the direction of travel, the ability to sleep while traveling, the availability and intensity of local circadian time cues at the destination, and individual differences in phase tolerance.

CLINICAL PRESENTATION
Jet-lagged travelers may experience the following symptoms:

- Poor sleep, including delayed sleep onset (after eastward flight), early awakening (after westward flight), and fractionated sleep (after flights in either direction)
- Poor performance in physical and mental tasks during the new daytime
- Negative subjective changes such as fatigue, headache, irritability, stress, inability to concentrate, and depression
- Gastrointestinal disturbances and decreased interest in and enjoyment of meals

PREVENTION
Travelers can minimize jet lag by doing the following before travel:

- Exercise, eat a healthful diet, and get plenty of rest.
- Begin to reset the body clock by shifting the timing of sleep to 1–2 hours later for a few days before traveling westward and shifting the timing of sleep to 1–2 hours earlier for a few days before traveling eastward. It can also be helpful to shift mealtimes to hours that coincide with these changes.
- Seek exposure to bright light in the evening if traveling westward, in the morning if traveling eastward (although it requires high motivation and strict compliance with the prescribed light–dark schedules).
- Break up a long journey with a stopover, if possible.

Travelers should do the following during travel:

- Avoid large meals, alcohol, and caffeine.

- Drink plenty of water to remain hydrated.
- Move around on the plane to promote mental and physical acuity, as well as protect against deep vein thrombosis.
- Wear comfortable shoes and clothing.
- Sleep, if possible, during long flights.

Travelers should do the following on arrival at the destination:

- Avoid situations requiring critical decision making, such as important meetings, for the first day after arrival.
- Adapt to the local schedule as soon as possible.
- Depending on the number of time zones crossed, people with diabetes may need to adjust their insulin schedule during travel and on arrival at their destination. Providers should work with their patients to arrange schedule changes before travel.
- Optimize exposure to sunlight after arrival from either direction. Exposure to bright light in the morning moves the stage of circadian rhythm forward, while exposure to light in the evening delays the stage and encourages later sleep.
- Eat meals appropriate to the local time, drink plenty of water, and avoid excess caffeine or alcohol. Eat a balanced diet, including carbohydrates.
- Take short naps (20–30 minutes) to increase energy but not undermine nighttime sleep.

The use of the nutritional supplement melatonin is controversial for preventing jet lag. Some clinicians advocate the use of 0.5–5.0 mg of melatonin during the first few days of travel, and data suggest its efficacy. However, its production is not regulated by the Food and Drug Administration, and contaminants have been found in commercially available products. Current information also does not support the use of special diets to ameliorate jet lag.

TREATMENT

The 2008 American Academy of Sleep Medicine recommendations include the following:

- Remain on home time if the travel period is 2 days or less.
- Promote sleep with hypnotic medication, although the effects of hypnotics on daytime symptoms of jet lag have not been well studied.
- Nonaddictive sedative hypnotics (nonbenzodiazepines), such as zolpidem, have been shown in some studies to promote longer periods of high-quality sleep. If a benzodiazepine is preferred, a short-acting one, such as temazepam, is recommended to minimize oversedation the following day. Because alcohol intake is often high during international travel, the risk of interaction with hypnotics should be emphasized with patients.
- If necessary, promote daytime alertness with a stimulant such as caffeine in limited quantities. Avoid caffeine after midday.
- Take short naps (20–30 minutes), shower, and spend time in the afternoon sun.

(See also the Self-Treatable Conditions section earlier in this chapter.)

BIBLIOGRAPHY

1. Barion A, Zee PC. A clinical approach to circadian rhythm sleep disorders. Sleep Med. 2007 Sep;8(6):566–77.
2. Daurat A, Benoit O, Buguet A. Effects of zopiclone on the rest/activity rhythm after a westward flight across five time zones. Psychopharmacology (Berl). 2000 Apr;149(3):241–5.
3. Dubocovich ML, Markowska M. Functional MT1 and MT2 melatonin receptors in mammals. Endocrine. 2005 Jul;27(2):101–10.
4. Erren TC, Falaturi P, Morfeld P, Knauth P, Reiter RJ, Piekarski C. Shift work and cancer: the evidence and the challenge. Deutsches Arzteblatt international. 2010 Sep;107(38):657–62.
5. Herxheimer A. Jet lag. Clin Evid. 2005 Jun(13):2178–83.
6. Jamieson AO, Zammit GK, Rosenberg RS, Davis JR, Walsh JK. Zolpidem reduces the sleep disturbance of jet lag. Sleep Med. 2001 Sep;2(5):423–30.
7. Reid KJ, Chang AM, Zee PC. Circadian rhythm sleep disorders. Med Clin North Am. 2004 May;88(3):631–51, viii.
8. Reilly T, Waterhouse J, Edwards B. Jet lag and air travel: implications for performance. Clin Sports Med. 2005 Apr;24(2):367–80, xii.
9. Sack RL. Clinical practice. Jet lag. N Engl J Med. 2010 Feb 4;362(5):440–7.
10. Sack RL, Auckley D, Auger RR, Carskadon MA, Wright KP Jr, Vitiello MV, et al. Circadian rhythm

sleep disorders: part I, basic principles, shift work and jet lag disorders. An American Academy of Sleep Medicine review. Sleep. 2007 Nov 1;30(11):1460–83.

11. Waterhouse J, Edwards B, Nevill A, Atkinson G, Reilly T, Davies P, et al. Do subjective symptoms predict our perception of jet-lag? Ergonomics. 2000 Oct;43(10):1514–27.

12. Waterhouse J, Reilly T, Atkinson G, Edwards B. Jet lag: trends and coping strategies. Lancet. 2007 Mar 31;369(9567):1117–29.

MOTION SICKNESS
Emily W. Lankau

RISK FOR TRAVELERS

All people can develop motion sickness if given sufficient stimulus. However, people may vary in their susceptibility. Risk factors include:

- Age—children aged 2–12 years are especially susceptible, but infants and toddlers are generally immune.
- Sex—women are more likely to have motion sickness, especially when pregnant, menstruating, or on hormones.

- Migraines—people who get migraine headaches are more prone to motion sickness, especially during a migraine.
- Medication—some prescriptions can worsen the nausea of motion sickness (Table 2-9).

TREATMENT

Habituation to motion can be effective and has few long-term adverse side effects; however, as a method for controlling motion sickness, this can be a time-consuming and unpleasant approach. Many patients will

Table 2-9. Medications that may increase nausea

MEDICATION CLASS	EXAMPLES
Antibiotics	Azithromycin, metronidazole, erythromycin, trimethoprim-sulfamethoxazole
Antiparasitics	Albendazole, thiabendazole, iodoquinol, chloroquine, mefloquine
Estrogens	Oral contraceptives, estradiol
Cardiovascular	Digoxin, levodopa
Narcotic analgesics	Codeine, morphine, meperidine
Nonsteroidal analgesics	Ibuprofen, naproxen, indomethacin
Antidepressants	Fluoxetine, paroxetine, sertraline
Asthma medication	Aminophylline
Bisphosphonates	Alendronate sodium, ibandronate sodium, risedronate sodium

prefer medication. A primary side effect of most efficacious medications used for motion sickness is drowsiness, along with other drug-specific side effects. Some medications may interfere with or delay habituation. Because gastric stasis can occur with motion sickness, parenteral delivery may be advantageous.

Antihistamines are the most frequently used and widely available medications for motion sickness. Nonsedating ones appear to be less effective. Antihistamines commonly used for motion sickness include cinnarizine (not currently available in the United States), cyclizine, dimenhydrinate, meclizine, and promethazine (oral and suppository). Other common medications used to treat motion sickness are scopolamine (hyoscine, oral and transdermal), antidopaminergic drugs (such as prochlorperazine), metoclopramide, sympathomimetics, and benzodiazepines. Clinical trials have not shown efficacy for ondansetron in the prevention of nausea associated with motion sickness.

When recommending any of these medications to travelers, providers should make sure that patients understand the risks and benefits, possible undesirable side effects, and potential drug interactions. Some travelers may need to try the medication before travel to see what effect it has. (See also the Self-Treatable Conditions section earlier in this chapter.)

Medications in Children

For children aged 2–12 years, dimenhydrinate (Dramamine), 1–1.5 mg/kg per dose, or diphenhydramine (Benadryl), 0.5–1 mg/kg per dose up to 25 mg, can be given 1 hour before travel and every 6 hours during the trip. Because some children have paradoxical agitation with these medicines, a test dose should be given at home before departure. Antihistamines are not approved by the Food and Drug Administration to treat motion sickness in children. Caregivers should be reminded to always ask a physician, pharmacist, or other clinician if they have any questions about how to use or dose antihistamines in children before they administer the medication. Oversedation of young children with antihistamines can be life-threatening.

Scopolamine can cause dangerous adverse effects in children and should not be used; prochlorperazine and metoclopramide should be used with caution in children.

Medications in Pregnancy

Drugs with the most safety data regarding the treatment of the nausea of pregnancy are the logical first choice. Alphabetical scoring of the safety of medications in pregnancy may not be helpful, and clinicians should review the actual safety data or call the patient's obstetric provider for suggestions. Web-based information may be found at the websites www.Motherisk.org and www.Reprotox.org.

PREVENTION

Nonpharmacologic interventions to prevent or treat motion sickness include:

- Being aware of and avoiding situations that tend to trigger symptoms.
- Optimizing position to reduce motion or motion perception—for example, driving a vehicle instead of riding in it, sitting in the front seat of a car or bus, or sitting over the wing of an aircraft. Cabin location on a cruise ship does not appear to influence the likelihood of motion sickness.
- Reducing sensory input—lying prone, shutting eyes, or looking at the horizon.
- Maintaining hydration by drinking water, eating small meals frequently, and limiting alcoholic and caffeinated beverages.
- Adding distractions—listening to music or using aromatherapy scents such as mint or lavender. Flavored lozenges may also help, in particular ginger-flavored. Lozenges may also function as distractions or, in the case of ginger, may hasten gastric emptying.
- Using acupressure or magnets is advocated by some to prevent or treat nausea, although scientific data on efficacy of these interventions for preventing motion sickness are equivocal.

BIBLIOGRAPHY

1. Gahlinger PM. Cabin location and the likelihood of motion sickness in cruise ship passengers. J Travel Med. 2000 May–Jun;7(3):120–4.
2. Murdin L, Golding J, Bronstein A. Managing motion sickness. BMJ. 2011;343:d7430.
3. Priesol AJ. Motion Sickness. Deschler DG, editor. Waltham MA: UpToDate; 2012.
4. Takeda N, Morita M, Horii A, Nishiike S, Kitahara T, Uno A. Neural mechanisms of motion sickness. J Med Invest. 2001 Feb;48(1–2):44–59.

RESPIRATORY INFECTIONS

Regina C. LaRocque, Edward T. Ryan

OVERVIEW

Respiratory infection is a leading cause of seeking medical care in returning travelers and has been reported to occur in up to 20% of all travelers, which is almost as common as travelers' diarrhea. Upper respiratory infection is more common than lower respiratory infection. In general, the types of respiratory infections that affect travelers are similar to those in nontravelers, and exotic causes are rare.

INFECTIOUS AGENT

Viral pathogens are the most common cause of respiratory infection in travelers; causative agents include rhinovirus, respiratory syncytial virus, influenza virus, parainfluenza virus, human metapneumovirus, adenovirus, and coronavirus. Bacterial pathogens are less common and include *Streptococcus pneumoniae*, *Mycoplasma pneumoniae*, *Haemophilus influenzae*, and *Chlamydophila pneumoniae*. *Coxiella burnetii* and *Legionella pneumophila* can also cause outbreaks of respiratory illness. Respiratory infection due to viral pathogens may lead to bacterial sinusitis, bronchitis, or pneumonia.

RISK FOR TRAVELERS

Reported outbreaks are usually associated with common exposure in hotels and cruise ships or among tour groups. A few pathogens have been associated with outbreaks in travelers, including influenza virus, *L. pneumophila*, and *Histoplasma capsulatum*. The peak influenza season in the temperate Northern Hemisphere is December through February. In the temperate Southern Hemisphere, the peak influenza season is June through August. Travelers to tropical zones are at risk all year. Exposure to an infected person from another hemisphere, such as on a cruise ship or package tour, can lead to an outbreak of influenza at any time or place.

Air-pressure changes during ascent and descent of aircraft can facilitate the development of sinusitis and otitis media. Intermingling of large numbers of people in airports, travel hubs, transport vehicles, cruise ships, and hotels can also facilitate transmission of respiratory pathogens. Direct airborne transmission aboard aircraft is unusual because of frequent air recirculation and filtration, although influenza, tuberculosis, and other diseases have resulted from transmission in modern aircraft. Transmission of infection may occur between passengers who are seated near one another, usually through direct contact or droplets.

The air quality at many travel destinations may not be optimal, and exposure to sulfur dioxide, nitrogen dioxide, carbon monoxide, ozone, and particulate matter is associated with a number of health risks, including respiratory tract inflammation, exacerbations of asthma and chronic obstructive pulmonary disease, impaired lung function, bronchitis, and pneumonia. Certain travelers have a higher risk for respiratory tract infection, including children, the elderly, and people with comorbid pulmonary conditions, such as asthma and chronic obstructive pulmonary disease (COPD).

The risk for tuberculosis among travelers is low (see Chapter 3, Tuberculosis).

DIAGNOSIS

Identifying a specific etiologic agent, especially in the absence of pneumonia or serious disease, is not always clinically necessary. If indicated, the following methods of diagnosis can be used:

- Molecular methods are available to detect a number of respiratory viruses, including influenza virus, parainfluenza virus, adenovirus, human metapneumovirus, and respiratory syncytial virus, and for certain nonviral pathogens.
- Rapid tests are also available to detect some pathogens such as respiratory syncytial virus, influenza virus, *L. pneumophila*, and group A *Streptococcus*.
- Microbiologic culturing of sputum and blood, although insensitive, can help identify a causative respiratory pathogen.

CLINICAL PRESENTATION

Most respiratory tract infections, especially those of the upper respiratory tract, are mild and not incapacitating. Upper respiratory tract infections often cause rhinorrhea or pharyngitis. Lower respiratory tract infections, particularly pneumonia, can be more severe. Lower respiratory tract infections are more likely to cause fever, dyspnea, or chest pain than upper respiratory tract infections. Cough is often present in either upper or lower tract infections. People with influenza commonly have acute onset of fever, myalgia, headache, and cough. Pulmonary embolism should be considered in the differential diagnosis of travelers who present with dyspnea, cough, or pleurisy and fever, especially those who have recently been on long car or plane rides.

TREATMENT

Affected travelers are usually managed similarly to nontravelers, although travelers with progressive or severe illness should be evaluated for illnesses specific to their travel destinations and exposure history. Most respiratory infections are due to viruses, are mild, and do not require specific treatment or antibiotics. Self-treatment with antibiotics during travel can be considered for higher-risk travelers with symptoms of lower respiratory tract infection. A respiratory-spectrum fluoroquinolone such as levofloxacin or a macrolide such as azithromycin may be prescribed to the traveler for this purpose before travel. (See also the Self-Treatable Conditions section earlier in this chapter.)

The rate of influenza among travelers is not known. The difficulty in self-diagnosing influenza makes it problematic to decide whether to prescribe travelers a neuraminidase inhibitor for self-treatment. This practice should probably be limited to travelers with a specific underlying condition that may predispose them to severe influenza.

Specific situations that may require medical intervention include the following:

- Pharyngitis without rhinorrhea, cough, or other symptoms that may indicate infection with group A *Streptococcus*.
- Sudden onset of cough, chest pain, and fever that may indicate pneumonia (or pulmonary embolism), resulting in a situation where the traveler may be sick enough to seek medical care right away.
- Travelers with underlying medical conditions, such as asthma, pulmonary disease, or heart disease, who may need to seek medical care earlier than otherwise healthy travelers.

PREVENTION

Vaccines are available to prevent a number of respiratory diseases, including influenza, S. *pneumoniae* infection, H. *influenzae* type B infection (in young children), pertussis, diphtheria, varicella, and measles. Unless contraindicated, travelers should be vaccinated against influenza and be up-to-date on other routine immunizations. Preventing respiratory illness while traveling may not be possible, but common-sense preventive measures include the following:

- Minimizing close contact with people who are coughing and sneezing.
- Frequent handwashing, either with soap and water or alcohol-based hand sanitizers (containing ≥60% alcohol) when soap and water are not available.
- Using a vasoconstricting nasal spray immediately before air travel, if the traveler has a preexisting eustachian tube dysfunction, may help lessen the likelihood of otitis or barotrauma.

BIBLIOGRAPHY

1. Camps M, Vilella A, Marcos MA, Letang E, Muñoz J, Salvado E, et al. Incidence of respiratory viruses among travelers with a febrile syndrome returning from tropical and subtropical areas. J Med Virol. 2008 Apr;80(4):711–5.
2. Cobelens FG, van Deutekom H, Draayer-Jansen IW, Schepp-Beelen AC, van Gerven PJ, van Kessel RP, et al. Risk of infection with *Mycobacterium tuberculosis* in travellers to areas of high tuberculosis endemicity. Lancet. 2000 Aug 5;356(9228):461–5.
3. Foxwell AR, Roberts L, Lokuge K, Kelly PM. Transmission of influenza on international flights, May 2009. Emerg Infect Dis. 2011 Jul;17(7):1188–94.
4. Freedman DO, Weld LH, Kozarsky PE, Fisk T, Robins R, von Sonnenburg F, et al. Spectrum of disease and

relation to place of exposure among ill returned travelers. N Engl J Med. 2006 Jan 12;354(2):119–30.

5. Jauréguiberry S, Boutolleau D, Grandsire E, Kofman T, Deback C, Aït-Arkoub Z, et al. Clinical and microbiological evaluation of travel-associated respiratory tract infections in travelers returning from countries affected by pandemic A(H1N1) 2009 influenza. J Travel Med. 2012 Jan–Feb;19(1):22–7.

6. Leder K, Newman D. Respiratory infections during air travel. Intern Med J. 2005 Jan;35(1):50–5.

7. Leder K, Sundararajan V, Weld L, Pandey P, Brown G, Torresi J. Respiratory tract infections in travelers: a

review of the GeoSentinel surveillance network. Clin Infect Dis. 2003 Feb 15;36(4):399–406.

8. Luna LK, Panning M, Grywna K, Pfefferle S, Drosten C. Spectrum of viruses and atypical bacteria in intercontinental air travelers with symptoms of acute respiratory infection. J Infect Dis. 2007 Mar 1;195(5):675–9.

9. Medina-Ramon M, Zanobetti A, Schwartz J. The effect of ozone and PM10 on hospital admissions for pneumonia and chronic obstructive pulmonary disease: a national multicity study. Am J Epidemiol. 2006 Mar 15;163(6):579–88.

OCCUPATIONAL EXPOSURE TO HIV

Henry M. Wu, V. Ramana Dhara, Alan G. Czarkowski

RISK FOR HEALTH CARE WORKERS TRAVELING OUTSIDE THE UNITED STATES

The risk of occupational exposure to HIV is most closely related to the activities and duties of the health care worker, but the geographic location and practice setting can also affect the risk of exposure and the quality of postexposure care. Many factors can increase the risk of HIV infection due to occupational exposure in developing countries:

- Less stringent safety regulations or standards
- Unfamiliar practice conditions and equipment
- Limited availability of personal protective equipment or safety-engineered devices
- Increased prevalence of injection therapy and unsafe infection practices in many countries
- Challenging practice conditions that might result in barriers to Standard Precaution adherence (such as natural disasters or conflict zones)
- Performing unfamiliar medical procedures
- High prevalence of HIV infection (diagnosed and undiagnosed)
- Limited access to HIV treatment, resulting in high viral titers in source patients
- Limited resources for postexposure evaluation and treatment

Situations that put the health care worker at risk for HIV exposure can also expose the person to hepatitis B, hepatitis C, and other bloodborne pathogens that are endemic to the region visited.

TRANSMISSION

HIV may be transmitted occupationally to health care workers who are exposed to blood and other potentially infectious bodily fluids via percutaneous injury or splash exposures to mucous membranes or nonintact skin. Unfamiliar practice environments can put the health care worker at increased risk of exposure. In addition to blood, cerebrospinal fluid, synovial fluid, pericardial fluid, pleural fluid, peritoneal fluid, amniotic fluid, semen, and vaginal secretions are considered potentially infectious. Saliva, urine, sputum, nasal secretions, tears, feces, vomitus, and sweat are not considered infectious for HIV unless they are visibly bloody. Typically, exposures occur as a result of percutaneous exposure to contaminated sharps, including needles, lancets, scalpels, and broken glass (from capillary or test tubes). Skin exposures to potentially infectious bodily fluids are only considered to be at risk for HIV infection if there is evidence of compromised skin integrity (for example, dermatitis, abrasion, or open wound).

EPIDEMIOLOGY

The global number of HIV infections among health care workers attributable to sharps injuries has been estimated to be 1,000 cases (range, 200–5,000) per year. The risk of HIV transmission after a percutaneous exposure to HIV-infected blood is estimated to be approximately 0.3%, and after a mucous membrane exposure, approximately 0.09%. The risk of infection after percutaneous exposures is considered increased with exposure to larger blood volumes (visible blood on the injuring device, hollow-bore needles, deeper injuries, or procedures that involved direct cannulation of an artery or vein). Higher circulating viral load in the source patient is also thought to increase the risk of transmission, and evidence of this can include elevated plasma viral load (if the patient has been recently tested) or advanced stages of illness. The risk of HIV transmission after nonintact skin exposures has not been quantified but is thought to be less than the risk after mucous membrane exposure.

PREVENTION

People working internationally who will be engaging in occupational health care activities should consistently follow standard precautions to reduce the risk of occupational exposure to HIV and other bloodborne pathogens. Standard precautions include the use of personal protective equipment such as gloves, gowns, aprons, surgical masks, and protective eyewear. Additional information about occupational health and safety standards for bloodborne pathogens can be found at http://www.osha.gov/SLTC/bloodbornepathogens/index.html.

In addition, clinicians working internationally should:

- Ensure they are properly trained for all anticipated procedures, considering the locally available equipment.
- Maintain strict safety standards, even if local standards are less stringent.
- Ensure they are immune to hepatitis B and up-to-date on routine vaccinations before departure.
- Consider bringing their own protective equipment or safety-engineered medical devices if they are unsure of availability at their destination.
- Assess the local availability of reliable (or consider bringing) postexposure prophylaxis (PEP) for HIV. The choice of PEP regimen should be based on the most recent

guidelines for PEP and expert consultation (see Postexposure Prophylaxis, below).

POSTEXPOSURE MANAGEMENT

Health care workers who may have been occupationally exposed to HIV should immediately perform the following steps:

- Wash the exposed area with soap and water thoroughly. If mucous membrane exposure has occurred, flush the area with copious amounts of water or saline.
- If possible, assess the HIV status of the source. Rapid HIV testing is preferred. If the source's rapid HIV antibody test result is positive, assume that it is a true positive. Exposures originating from source patients who test HIV-negative are considered not to have HIV transmission risk, unless they have clinical evidence of primary HIV infection or HIV-related disease.
- Baseline HIV testing of the exposed health care worker should be performed at the time of the exposure. Before travel, health care workers should assess if reliable HIV testing is routinely available at the destination and, if it is not available, baseline testing before departure might be considered to provide supportive evidence in the event of a trip-related infection.
- Seek qualified medical evaluation as soon as possible to guide decisions on postexposure treatment and testing.
- Contact the National Clinicians' Postexposure Prophylaxis Hotline (PEPline) toll-free at 888-448-4911 (24 hours per day, 7 days per week) for assistance in assessing risk and advice on managing occupational exposures to HIV and other bloodborne pathogens (http://www.nccc.ucsf.edu/about_nccc/pepline). If the toll-free number is not accessible when calling from another country, the main administrative line for the National HIV/AIDS Clinicians' Consultation Center is 415-206-8700.
- Consider beginning PEP for HIV (see below).

Postexposure Prophylaxis

A number of medication combinations are available for PEP. Since these regimens have known toxicities and may change with updated guidelines, refer to MMWR's Updated US Public Health Service Guidelines for the Management of Occupational Exposures to

HIV and Recommendations for Postexposure Prophylaxis (http://aidsinfo.nih.gov/content-files/HealthCareOccupExpoGL.pdf) and seek expert consultation (either with local experts or through the PEPline) for more information about PEP recommendations. Specific regimens should be determined by clinicians familiar with the medications and the health care worker's medical history. Interactions exist between many antiretroviral medications and other medications. Expert consultants might also consider the possibility that the health care worker was exposed to a drug-resistant HIV strain (for example, if the source patient was treatment-experienced or the local prevalence of resistance is high).

If the exposed person chooses to initiate PEP, he or she must do so as soon as possible. PEP can be stopped if new information changes the assessment; however, waiting to start PEP until all information (HIV test results or the source patient's medical history) is gathered can decrease its efficacy.

Consider other potential infectious disease exposures from the source material, including hepatitis B virus or hepatitis C virus, and manage as appropriate.

Postexposure Testing and Counseling

People with occupational exposure to HIV should receive standard HIV testing as soon as possible after exposure as a baseline, with follow-up testing at 6 weeks, 3 months, and 6 months. Extended HIV follow-up testing for up to 12 months is recommended for those who become infected with HCV after exposure to a source coinfected with HIV and HCV. Postexposure counseling and medical evaluation should be provided, whether or not the exposed person receives PEP. The US embassy or consulate can assist in finding quality medical care.

Exposed health care workers should be advised to use precautions (abstinence from sexual contact or strict use of barrier protection with sexual activities, avoidance of blood or tissue donations, breastfeeding, or pregnancy) to prevent secondary transmission, especially during the first 6–12 weeks after exposure. When PEP is initiated, exposed health care workers should be counseled regarding drug toxicities, drug interactions, and the importance of adherence to PEP regimens. Drug side effects have historically been a common reason for PEP discontinuation, so monitoring for symptoms and proper management is essential. The emotional consequences of occupational exposures can be substantial and might be further exacerbated by stressors already present in the work environment. Psychological counseling should be considered an essential part of the management of exposures.

BIBLIOGRAPHY

1. Bell DM. Occupational risk of human immunodeficiency virus infection in healthcare workers: an overview. Am J Med. 1997 May 19;102(5B):9–15.
2. Canadian Centre for Occupation Health and Safety. Needlestick injuries. 2005 [cited 2012 May 28]. Available from: http://www.ccohs.ca/oshanswers/diseases/needlestick_injuries.html.
3. CDC. NIOSH alert: preventing needlestick injuries in health care settings. Cincinnati: National Institute for Occupational Safety and Health; 1999 [cited 2012 May 28]. Available from: http://www.cdc.gov/niosh/docs/2000-108/.
4. CDC. Notice to readers: updated information regarding antiretroviral agents used as HIV postexposure prophylaxis for occupational HIV exposure. MMWR Recomm Rep. 2007 Dec 14;56(49):1291–2.
5. CDC. Updated US Public Health Service guidelines for the management of occupational exposures to HBV, HCV, and HIV and recommendations for postexposure prophylaxis. MMWR Recomm Rep. 2001 Jun 29;50(RR-11):1–52.
6. Clinical and Laboratory Standards Institute. M29-A3 protection of laboratory workers from occupationally acquired infections: approved guideline. 3rd ed. 2005.
7. Gerberding JL. Clinical practice. Occupational exposure to HIV in health care settings. N Engl J Med. 2003 Feb 27;348(9):826–33.
8. Henderson DK. Management of needlestick injuries: a house officer who has a needlestick. JAMA. 2012 Jan 4;307(1):75–84.
9. International Healthcare Worker Safety Center. EPINet: Exposure Prevention Information Network. Charlottesville, VA: University of Virginia; 2010 [cited 2012 May 28]. Available from: http://www.healthsystem.virginia.edu/pub/epinet.
10. Mohan S, Sarfaty S, Hamer DH. Human immunodeficiency virus postexposure prophylaxis for medical trainees on international rotations. J Travel Med. 2010 Jul–Aug;17(4):264–8.
11. National HIV/AIDS Clinicians' Consultation Center. PEPline: the national clinicians' post-exposure

prophylaxis hotline. San Francisco: University of California, San Francisco; 2010 [cited 2012 May 28]. Available from: http://www.nccc.ucsf.edu/about_nccc/pepline/.

12. Occupational Safety and Health Administration. Regulations (standards—29 CFR): bloodborne pathogens–1910.1030. Washington, DC: Occupational Safety and Health Administration [cited 2012 Sep 18]. Available from: http://www.osha.gov/pls/oshaweb/owadisp.show_document?p_table=STANDARDS&p_id=10051.

13. Panlilio AL, Cardo DM, Grohskopf LA, Heneine W, Ross CS. Updated US Public Health Service guidelines for the management of occupational exposures to HIV and recommendations for postexposure prophylaxis. MMWR Recomm Rep. 2005 Sep 30;54(RR-9):1–17.

14. Prüss-Üstün A, Rapiti E, Hutin Y. Estimation of the global burden of disease attributable to

contaminated sharps injuries among health-care workers. Am J Ind Med. 2005 Dec;48(6):482–90.

15. Sagoe-Moses C, Pearson RD, Perry J, Jagger J. Risks to health care workers in developing countries. N Engl J Med. 2001 Aug 16;345(7):538–41.

16. Simonsen L, Kane A, Lloyd J, Zaffran M, Kane M. Unsafe injections in the developing world and transmission of bloodborne pathogens: a review. Bull World Health Organ. 1999;77(10):789–800.

17. Uslan DZ, Virk A. Postexposure chemoprophylaxis for occupational exposure to human immunodeficiency virus in traveling health care workers. J Travel Med. 2005 Jan–Feb;12(1):14–8.

18. Young TN, Arens FJ, Kennedy GE, Laurie JW, Rutherford G. Antiretroviral post-exposure prophylaxis (PEP) for occupational HIV exposure. Cochrane Database Syst Rev. 2007(1):CD002835.

Counseling & Advice for Travelers

FOOD & WATER PRECAUTIONS

John C. Watson, Michele C. Hlavsa, Patricia M. Griffin

Contaminated food and water often pose a risk for travelers. Among the infectious diseases that travelers can acquire from contaminated food and water are *Escherichia coli* infections, shigellosis or bacillary dysentery, giardiasis, cryptosporidiosis, norovirus infection, hepatitis A, and salmonelloses, including typhoid fever. Contaminated food and water can also pose a risk of cholera and a variety of conditions caused by protozoan and helminthic parasites. Many of the infectious diseases associated with contaminated food and water are caused by pathogens transmitted via the fecal-oral route. Drinking, inhaling, or touching contaminated water, including natural saltwater or freshwater or the water in inadequately treated swimming pools, interactive fountains, or hot tubs and spas can transmit these and other pathogens that can cause diarrhea, vomiting, or infection of the ears, eyes, skin, or the respiratory or nervous system (see Chapter 3 for specific infectious diseases).

FOOD

To avoid illness, travelers should be advised to select food with care. All raw food is subject to contamination. Raw or undercooked meat, fish, and shellfish can carry various intestinal pathogens. Particularly in areas where hygiene and sanitation are inadequate, travelers should be advised to avoid salads, uncooked vegetables, unpasteurized fruit juices, and unpasteurized milk and milk products, such as cheese and yogurt. Travelers should be advised to eat only food that is fully cooked and served hot and fruit that has been washed in clean water and then peeled by the traveler. Raw fruits that are eaten unpeeled (such as strawberries) or cut should be avoided, and fruits that are eaten peeled (such as bananas) should be peeled by the person who eats them. Always refrigerate perishable cooked food within 2 hours (1 hour at temperatures >90°F (32°C). Cooked food that has been stored should be thoroughly reheated before serving. These recommendations also apply to eggs, which should be thoroughly cooked, whether they are served alone or used in sauces. Consumption of food and beverages obtained from street vendors has been associated with an increased risk of illness.

Travelers should wash their hands with soap and water before eating, after using the bathroom or changing diapers, after caring for someone who is ill, and after direct contact with preschool-age children, animals, or feces. If soap and water are not available, use an alcohol-based hand sanitizer (with ≥60% alcohol).

The safest way to feed an infant aged <6 months is to breastfeed exclusively. If the infant is fed formula prepared from commercial powder, the powder should be reconstituted with hot water at a temperature of ≥158°F (≥70°C). This precaution will kill most pathogens with which the infant formula may have been contaminated during manufacturing or through handling after opening. To ensure that the water is hot enough (≥158°F; ≥70°C), travelers should prepare formula within 30 minutes after boiling the water for ≥1 minute (see the Water Disinfection for Travelers section later in this chapter). The prepared formula should be cooled to a safe temperature for feeding (for example, by placing in an ice bath that does not touch the nipple) and used within 2 hours of preparation. Bottles and nipples should be washed and then sterilized (in boiling water or in an electric sterilizer). Travelers may wish to pack enough formula for their trip, because manufacturing standards vary widely around the world.

Travelers should be advised not to bring perishable seafood from high-risk areas back to the United States. Cholera has occurred in people who ate crab that had been brought into the United States from Latin America by travelers. Moreover, travelers should not assume that food and water aboard commercial aircraft are safe, because food and water may be obtained in the country of departure, where hygiene and sanitation may be inadequate.

WATER

Drinking Water and Other Beverages

In many parts of the world, particularly where water treatment, sanitation, and hygiene are inadequate, tap water may contain disease-causing contaminants, including viruses, bacteria, and parasites. As a result, tap water in some places may be unsafe for drinking, preparing food and beverages, making ice, cooking, and brushing teeth. Contaminated tap water, including droplets and aerosols, may also cause illness if inadvertently swallowed or inhaled, as can occur during showering or bathing. Infants, young children, pregnant women, the elderly, and people whose immune systems are compromised because of AIDS, chemotherapy, or transplant medications may be especially susceptible to illness from some contaminants (such as *Cryptosporidium* and *Legionella*).

Travelers should avoid drinking or otherwise ingesting tap water unless they are reasonably certain it is not contaminated. Many people choose to disinfect or filter their water when traveling to destinations where safe tap water may not be available (see the Water Disinfection for Travelers section later in this chapter). Water contaminated with fuels or toxic chemicals, however, will not be made safe by boiling or disinfection; travelers should use a different source of water if they suspect this type of contamination.

In areas where tap water may be contaminated, commercially bottled water from an unopened, factory-sealed container or water that has been adequately disinfected should be used for brushing teeth and other oral hygiene.

Beverages made with boiled water and served steaming hot (such as tea and coffee) are generally safe to drink. When served in unopened, factory-sealed cans or bottles, carbonated beverages, commercially prepared fruit drinks, water, alcoholic beverages, and pasteurized drinks generally can be considered safe. Because water on the outside of cans and bottles may be contaminated, they should be wiped clean and dried before opening or drinking directly from the container.

Beverages that may not be safe for consumption include fountain drinks, fruit drinks made with tap water, iced tea, and iced coffee. Because ice may be made from contaminated water, travelers in areas with unsafe tap water should request that beverages be served without ice.

Recreational Water

Pathogens that cause gastrointestinal, respiratory, skin, ear, eye, and neurologic illnesses can be transmitted by contaminated water during swimming, wading, or participating in other activities in saltwater or freshwater or the water in inadequately treated pools, interactive fountains, or hot tubs and spas. Water contaminated by sewage, animal waste, wastewater runoff, or human feces from swimmers can appear clear and clean but still contain disease-causing pathogens or chemicals. Ingesting even small amounts of such water can cause illness. Pathogens, such as *Cryptosporidium*, can survive for days even in well-maintained pools and interactive fountains. Travelers should avoid ingesting any water in which they are swimming, wading, or participating in other recreational activities. They also should not swim when they have open cuts, abrasions, or other wounds that could serve as entry points for pathogens. To protect other swimmers, children and adults with diarrhea should *not* enter the water to avoid contaminating it.

Maintaining proper chlorine or bromine and pH levels is necessary to prevent transmission of most infectious pathogens in water in pools and interactive fountains. Travelers should avoid pools and interactive fountains if the water is cloudy. Additional pool user tips can be found at www.cdc.gov/healthywater/pdf/swimming/resources/pool-user-tips-factsheet.pdf.

Maintaining proper chlorine or bromine levels in hot tubs and spas may be especially difficult, because the high water temperature depletes their concentration. *Pseudomonas*, which can cause "hot tub rash" and "swimmer's ear," and *Legionella* (see Chapter 3, Legionellosis) can multiply in hot tubs and spas in which chlorine or bromine levels are not properly maintained. Travelers should avoid hot tubs and spas where bather limits are not enforced or where the water is visibly cloudy. Travelers can purchase and use test strips to check chlorine or bromine and pH levels before entering the water. Additional tips can be found at www.cdc.gov/healthywater/pdf/swimming/resources/hot-tub-user-tips-factsheet.pdf. Travelers at increased risk for legionellosis, such as the elderly or those with immunocompromising conditions such as cancer or diabetes, may choose to avoid high-risk areas such whirlpool spas (see Chapter 3, Legionellosis).

To protect their health in oceans, lakes, and rivers, travelers should not swim or wade 1) in water that may be contaminated with sewage or human or animal feces; 2) near storm drains; 3) after heavy rainfall; 4) in freshwater streams, canals, and lakes in schistosomiasis-endemic areas of the Caribbean, South America, Africa, and Asia (see Chapter 3, Schistosomiasis); 5) in water that may be contaminated with urine from animals infected with *Leptospira* (see Chapter 3, Leptospirosis); or 6) in warm seawater when they have cuts, abrasions, or other wounds. To help prevent a rare but fatal infection caused by *Naegleria fowleri* (www.cdc.gov/parasites/naegleria), a parasite found in warm freshwater around the world, travelers should avoid digging in or stirring up the sediment and should prevent water from entering the nose by holding the nose shut or wearing a nose clip when swimming, diving, or participating in similar activities in warm freshwater (including lakes, rivers, ponds, hot springs, or locations with water warmed by discharge from power plants and industrial complexes), especially during periods of high water temperature and low water levels.

BIBLIOGRAPHY

1. Backer H. Water disinfection for international and wilderness travelers. Clin Infect Dis. 2002 Feb 1;34(3):355–64.

2. Cartwright R, Colbourne J. Cryptosporidiosis and hotel swimming pools—a multifaceted challenge. Water Science and Technology: Water Supply. 2002;2(3):47–54.

3. CDC. Drinking water: camping, hiking, travel. Atlanta: CDC; 2012 [cited 2012 Sep 18]. Available from: http://www.cdc.gov/healthywater/drinking/travel/index.html.

4. CDC. For swimmers and hot tub users. Atlanta: CDC; 2012 [cited 2012 Sep 18]. Available from: http://

www.cdc.gov/healthywater/swimming/pools/for-swimmers-hot-tub-users.html.

5. CDC. Healthy swimming/recreational water. Atlanta: CDC; 2012 [cited 2012 Sep 18]. Available from: http://www.cdc.gov/healthywater/swimming/index.html.

6. CDC. Legionellosis resource site. Atlanta: CDC; 2012 [cited 2012 Sep 18]. Available from: http://www.cdc.gov/legionella/.

7. CDC. *Naegleria fowleri*—Primary amebic meningoencephalitis (PAM). Atlanta: CDC; 2012

[cited 2012 Sep 18]. Available from: http://www.cdc.gov/parasites/naegleria/.

8. CDC. *Vibrio vulnificus*. Atlanta: CDC; 2009 [cited 2012 Sep 18]. Available from: http://www.cdc.gov/nczved/divisions/dfbmd/diseases/vibriov/.

9. Eberhart-Phillips J, Besser RE, Tormey MP, Koo D, Feikin D, Araneta MR, et al. An outbreak of cholera from food served on an international aircraft. Epidemiol Infect. 1996 Feb;116(1):9–13.

10. Finelli L, Swerdlow D, Mertz K, Ragazzoni H, Spitalny K. Outbreak of cholera associated with crab brought from an area with epidemic disease. J Infect Dis. 1992 Dec;166(6):1433–5.

Perspectives

PREVENTION OF TRAVELERS' DIARRHEA—IT'S NOT ONLY WHAT YOU EAT & DRINK
David R. Shlim

Travel health providers in the 1980s seemed certain that travelers' diarrhea (TD) could be avoided by observing sensible food precautions. A consensus statement published in 1985 concluded, "Data indicate that meticulous attention to food and beverage preparation can decrease the likelihood of developing TD." The experts in the consensus group had 7 studies available to them at that time. In retrospect, it is surprising to note that 6 of the studies concluded that there was no relationship between recommended food and water precautions and the likelihood of developing TD. The seventh article showed a small correlation between eating "mistakes" and the likelihood of developing TD in the first 3 days of a journey.

Overall, the risk of acquiring TD in many countries has not decreased in the >50 years since the syndrome was first characterized in Mexico, despite decades of messages urging travelers to follow food and water precautions. The earliest study that addressed the question of food and water precautions was published in 1973; it concluded that "drinking bottled liquids, and avoiding salads, raw vegetables, and unpeeled fruits failed to prevent illness." In a study of returning travelers from Mexico and Peru published in 1978, in which >70% of travelers reported TD, the author noted that "avoidance of tap water, uncooked foods, and ice cubes did not make a difference in the outcome." In a famous study in 1983, a survey of >10,000 travelers worldwide found not only that observing food and water precautions failed to prevent TD, but also that people who claimed that they exercised more caution were at increased risk of acquiring TD: "Diarrhea seemed to occur more frequently the more a person tried to elude it!" Although careful travelers are unlikely to have more diarrhea than careless eaters, the authors were not able to confirm what seemed logical—that careful travelers will have *less* diarrhea.

Perspectives sections are written as editorial discussions aiming to add depth and clinical perspective to the official recommendations contained in the book. The views and opinions expressed in this section are those of the author and do not necessarily represent the official position of CDC.

Although these studies do not appear to support the traditional guidance, travelers should not abandon common sense in regard to being careful with food and water. However, the question remains as to why travelers do not measurably decrease their risk of diarrhea even when trying to be scrupulous with food and water precautions.

Since the 1980s, studies have suggested that *where* travelers eat makes more difference than *what* they eat. At least 3 studies have shown that people who eat in restaurants have a significantly higher risk of TD than expatriates who eat in their own homes. Investigation into the state of restaurant hygiene in several developing countries has demonstrated that many basic health precautions are violated. Some restaurants fail to provide sinks for employees to wash their hands after going to the toilet. Cutting boards may not be washed between cutting raw meat and peeling and cutting vegetables. Foods are cooked, but then may be left to sit at ambient temperatures for extended periods of time because of a paucity of refrigerator space or power cuts. Windows may not be screened to keep out flies. Defrosting meat can sit on a refrigerator shelf and drip juices on cooked foods. In tourist destinations where these restaurant violations were corrected, the rate of TD among the tourists visiting those sites decreased substantially.

How should this information be used in the pre-travel consultation? A few rules have been proven to help. Food that is served hot is almost always safe to eat. However, eating local foods is for some a major activity associated with travel, and travelers who eat only food that is cooked and "steaming," may feel as if they are missing an essential part of the travel experience. Foods that are cooked earlier in the day and sit out for long periods of time, such as on a buffet, can be unsafe. Dry foods such as cakes, cookies, and bread are usually safe. Beverages that come in factory-sealed containers are safe. All carbonated beverages that come in sealed bottles or cans should be safe because of their high acidity.

Because the risk of TD is not 100% avoidable by utilizing eating strategies, travelers should always be counseled on self-diagnosis and treatment strategies. Future reductions in the rate of TD are more likely to be attributable to improved restaurant hygiene in developing countries than strategies applied by travelers themselves. Expatriates can control food preparation in their own kitchens, but poor restaurant hygiene in developing countries will continue to pose a risk for a high percentage of travelers.

BIBLIOGRAPHY

1. Ashley DV, Walters C, Dockery-Brown C, McNab A, Ashley DE. Interventions to prevent and control food-borne diseases associated with a reduction in traveler's diarrhea in tourists to Jamaica. J Travel Med. 2004 Nov–Dec;11(6):364–7.
2. Blaser MJ. Environmental interventions for the prevention of travelers' diarrhea. Rev Infect Dis. 1986 May–Jun;8 Suppl 2:S142–50.
3. Ericsson CD, Pickering LK, Sullivan P, DuPont HL. The role of location of food consumption in the prevention of travelers' diarrhea in Mexico. Gastroenterology. 1980 Nov;79(5 Pt 1):812–6.
4. NIH Consensus Development Conference. Travelers' diarrhea. JAMA. 1985 May 10;253(18):2700–4.
5. Shlim DR. Looking for evidence that personal hygiene precautions prevent traveler's diarrhea. Clin Infect Dis. 2005 Dec 1;41 Suppl 8:S531–5.
6. Shlim DR. Update in traveler's diarrhea. Infect Dis Clin North Am. 2005 Mar;19(1):137–49.
7. Tjoa WS, DuPont HL, Sullivan P, Pickering LK, Holguin AH, Olarte J, et al. Location of food consumption and travelers' diarrhea. Am J Epidemiol. 1977 Jul;106(1):61–6.

WATER DISINFECTION FOR TRAVELERS
Howard D. Backer

RISK FOR TRAVELERS

Waterborne disease is a risk for international travelers who visit countries that have poor hygiene and inadequate sanitation, and for wilderness visitors who rely on surface water in any country, including the United States. The list of potential waterborne pathogens is extensive and includes bacteria, viruses, protozoa, and parasitic helminths. Most of the organisms that can cause travelers' diarrhea can be waterborne. Where treated tap water is available, most travelers' intestinal infections are probably transmitted by food, but aging or inadequate water treatment infrastructure may not effectively disinfect water during distribution. Where untreated surface or well water is used and there is no sanitation infrastructure, the risk of waterborne infection is high. Microorganisms with small infectious doses (such as *Giardia*, *Cryptosporidium*, *Shigella*, *Escherichia coli* O157:H7, and norovirus) can even cause illness through recreational water exposure, via inadvertent water ingestion.

Bottled water has become the convenient solution for most travelers, but in some places it may not be superior to tap water. Moreover, the plastic bottles create an ecological problem, since most developing countries do not recycle plastic bottles. All international travelers, especially long-term travelers or expatriates, should become familiar with and use simple methods to ensure safe drinking water. Table 2-10 compares benefits and limitations of different methods.

FIELD TECHNIQUES FOR WATER TREATMENT
Heat

Common intestinal pathogens are readily inactivated by heat. Microorganisms are killed in a shorter time at higher temperatures, whereas temperatures as low as 140°F (60°C) are effective with a longer contact time. Pasteurization uses this principle to kill foodborne enteric pathogens and spoiling organisms at temperatures between 140°F (60°C)

and 158°F (70°C), well below the boiling point of water (212°F [100°C]).

Although boiling is not necessary to kill common intestinal pathogens, it is the only easily recognizable end point that does not require a thermometer. All organisms except bacterial spores, which are rarely waterborne enteric pathogens, are killed in seconds at boiling temperature. In addition, the time required to heat the water from 60°C to boiling works toward heat disinfection. Although any water that is brought to a boil should be adequately disinfected, to allow for a margin of safety, boil for 1 minute. Although the boiling point decreases with altitude, it is still above temperatures required to inactivate enteric pathogens at typical travel and trekking elevations. To conserve fuel, the same results can be obtained by bringing water to a boil and then turning off the stove but keeping the container covered for several minutes.

If no other means of water treatment is available, a potential alternative to boiling is to use tap water that is too hot to touch, which is probably at a temperature between 131°F (55°C) and 140°F (60°C). This temperature may be adequate to kill pathogens if the water has been kept hot in the tank for some time. Travelers with access to electricity can bring a small electric heating coil or a lightweight beverage warmer to boil water.

Filtration and Clarification

Portable hand-pump or gravity-drip filters with various designs and types of filter media are commercially available to international travelers. Filter pore size is the primary determinant of a filter's effectiveness, but microorganisms also adhere to filter media by electrochemical reactions. Microfilters with "absolute" pore sizes of 0.1–0.4 μm are usually effective to remove cysts and bacteria but may not adequately remove viruses, which are a major concern in water with high levels of fecal contamination (Table 2-11). Filters that claim Environmental Protection Agency (EPA) designation of water "purifier" undergo

Table 2-10. Comparison of water disinfection techniques

TECHNIQUE	ADVANTAGES	DISADVANTAGES
Heat	• Does not impart additional taste or color • Single step that inactivates all enteric pathogens • Efficacy is not compromised by contaminants or particles in the water as for halogenation and filtration	• Does not improve taste, smell, or appearance of water • Fuel sources may be scarce, expensive, or unavailable • Does not prevent recontamination during storage
Filtration	• Simple to operate • Requires no holding time for treatment • Large choice of commercial product designs • Adds no unpleasant taste and often improves taste and appearance of water • Can be combined with halogens to remove or kill all pathogenic waterborne microbes	• Adds bulk and weight to baggage • Many do not reliably remove viruses • Channeling of water or high pressure can force microorganisms through the filter • More expensive than chemical treatment • Eventually clogs from suspended particulate matter and may require some field maintenance or repair • Does not prevent recontamination during storage
Halogens (chlorine, iodine)	• Inexpensive and widely available in liquid or tablet form • Taste can be removed by simple techniques • Flexible dosing • Equally easy to treat large and small volumes • Will preserve microbiologic quality of stored water	• Impart taste and odor to water • Flexibility requires understanding of principles • Iodine is physiologically active, with potential adverse effects • Not readily effective against *Cryptosporidium* oocysts • Efficacy decreases with low water temperature and decreasing water clarity • Corrosive and stain clothing
Chlorine dioxide	• Low doses have no taste or color • Simple to use and available in liquid or tablet form • More potent than equivalent doses of chlorine • Effective against all waterborne pathogens	• Volatile and sensitive to sunlight: do not expose tablets to air and use generated solutions rapidly • No persistent residual concentration, so does not prevent recontamination during storage
Ultraviolet (UV)	• Imparts no taste • Portable devices now available • Effective against all waterborne pathogens • Extra doses of UV can be used for added assurance and with no side effects • Solar UV exposure (SODIS) also provides moderate benefit	• Requires clear water • Does not improve taste or appearance of water • Relatively expensive (except solar) • Requires batteries or power source • Difficult to know if devices are delivering required UV doses • No persistent residual concentration, so does not prevent recontamination during storage

Table 2-11. Microorganism size and susceptibility to filtration

ORGANISM	AVERAGE SIZE (μm)	MAXIMUM RECOMMENDED FILTER RATING (μm ABSOLUTE)
Viruses	0.03	Not specified (optimally 0.01, ultrafiltration)
Enteric bacteria (*Escherichia coli*)	0.5 × 3.0–8.0	0.2–0.4 (microfiltration)
Cryptosporidium oocyst	4–6	1 (microfiltration)
Giardia cyst	6.0–10.0 × 8.0–15.0	3.0–5.0 (microfiltration)
Nematode eggs	30 × 60	Not specified; any microfilter
Schistosome larvae	50 × 100	Not specified; any microfilter

company-sponsored testing that has demonstrated removal of 10^6 bacteria, 10^4 (9,999 of 10,000) viruses, and 10^3 *Cryptosporidium* oocysts or *Giardia* cysts. (EPA does not independently test the validity of these claims.)

One new portable filter design includes hollow fiber technology, which is a cluster of tiny tubules with variable pore sizes that can remove virus-size particles. Reverse-osmosis filters achieve ultrafiltration levels that can remove microbiologic contamination and desalinate water. The high price and slow output of small hand-pump reverse-osmosis units prohibit use by land-based travelers; however, they are important survival aids for ocean voyagers.

Filters made from ceramic clay or simple sand and gravel (biosand) filters can be successfully used for households in developing countries or improvised in remote or austere situations when nothing else is available.

Coagulation-flocculation (CF) removes suspended particles that cause a cloudy appearance and bad taste and do not settle by gravity; this process removes many but not all microorganisms. CF is easily applied in the field. Alum, an aluminum salt that is widely used in food, cosmetic, and medical applications, or one of several other substances, is added to the water and stirred. The clumped particulates that form are allowed to settle, then poured through a coffee filter or fine cloth to remove the sediment. Tablets or packets of powder that combine flocculent and hypochlorite disinfection are available (products include Chlor-floc and PUR Purifier of Water [Proctor and Gamble—for humanitarian use, not sold commercially]).

Granular-activated carbon (GAC) purifies water by adsorbing organic and inorganic chemicals and most heavy metals, thereby improving odor, taste, and safety. GAC is a common component of household and field filters. It may trap but does not kill organisms. In field water treatment, GAC is best used after chemical disinfection to remove disinfection byproducts and the taste of iodine and chlorine (see Halogens below).

Chemical Disinfection
Halogens
The most common chemical water disinfectants are chlorine and iodine (halogens). Worldwide, chemical disinfection with chlorine is the most commonly used method for improving and maintaining the microbiologic

quality of drinking water. Sodium hypochlorite, the active ingredient in common household bleach, is the primary disinfectant promoted by CDC and the World Health Organization Safe Water System at a 1.5% concentration for household use in the developing world. Other chlorine-containing compounds, such as calcium hypochlorite and sodium dichloroisocyanurate, available in granular or tablet formulation, are also effective for household water treatment.

Given adequate concentrations and length of exposure (contact time), chlorine and iodine have similar activity and are effective against bacteria and viruses (www.cdc.gov/safewater/effectiveness-on-pathogens.html). *Giardia* cysts are more resistant to halogens; however, field-level concentrations, as well as the dosing and concentrations of halogen products, are targeted to the cysts, although the contact time recommended is longer. Also, because many factors in the field are uncontrolled, extending the contact time adds a margin of safety. However, some common waterborne parasites, such as *Cryptosporidium*, are poorly inactivated by halogen disinfection at practical concentrations, even with extended contact times. Therefore, chemical disinfection should be supplemented with adequate filtration to remove these microorganisms from drinking water. Cloudy water contains substances that will neutralize disinfectant, so it will require higher concentrations or contact times or, preferably, clarification through settling, CF, or filtration before disinfectant is added. Tablets that combine flocculent and disinfectant are available.

Both chlorine and iodine are available in liquid and tablet form. Because iodine has physiologic activity, WHO recommends limiting iodine water disinfection to a few weeks of emergency use. Iodine use is not recommended for people with unstable thyroid disease or known iodine allergy. Iodine should not be used by pregnant women because of the potential effect on the fetal thyroid.

The taste of halogens in water can be improved by several means:

- Reduce concentration and increase contact time proportionately.

- After the required contact time, run water through a filter that contains activated carbon.
- After the required contact time, add a 25-mg tablet of vitamin C (or a "tiny pinch" of powdered ascorbic acid), which reduces the disinfectant to tasteless and colorless forms of chloride or iodide.

Iodine Resins

Iodine resins transfer iodine to microorganisms that come into contact with the resin, but leave little iodine dissolved in the water. The resins have been incorporated into many different filter designs available for field use. Most contain a 1-µm cyst filter, which should effectively remove protozoan cysts. Few models are sold in the United States because of inconsistent test results, but some models are still available for international use.

Salt (Sodium Chloride) Electrolysis

Passing a current through a simple brine salt solution generates oxidants, including hypochlorite, which can be used to disinfect microbes. This technique has been engineered into a pocket-sized, battery-powered product.

Chlorine Dioxide

Chlorine dioxide (ClO_2) can kill most waterborne pathogens, including *Cryptosporidium* oocysts, at practical doses and contact times. Tablets and liquid formulations are available to generate chlorine dioxide in the field for small-quantity water treatment.

Ultraviolet (UV) Light

Extensive data show that UV light can kill bacteria, viruses, and *Cryptosporidium* oocysts in water. The effect depends on UV dose and exposure time, and requires clear water because suspended particles can shield microorganisms from UV rays. These units have limited effectiveness in water with high levels of suspended solids and turbidity. They also have no disinfection residual. Portable battery-operated units that deliver a metered, timed dose of UV are an effective way to disinfect small quantities of clear water in the field.

Solar Irradiation and Heating

UV irradiation by sunlight in the UVA range can substantially improve the microbiologic quality of water and may be used in austere emergency situations. Recent work has confirmed the efficacy and optimal procedures of the solar disinfection (SODIS) technique. Transparent bottles (such as clear plastic PET beverage bottles), preferably lying on a reflective surface, are exposed to sunlight for a minimum of 6 hours. UV and thermal inactivation are synergistic for solar disinfection of drinking water. Use of a simple reflector or solar cooker can achieve temperatures of 149°F (65°C), which will pasteurize the water after 4 hours. Solar disinfection is not effective on turbid water. If the headlines in a newspaper cannot be read through the bottle of water, then the water must be clarified before solar irradiation is used. Under cloudy conditions, water must be placed in the sun for 2 consecutive days.

Silver and Other Products

Silver ion has bactericidal effects in low doses and some attractive features, including absence of color, taste, and odor. The use of silver as a drinking water disinfectant is popular in Europe, but it is not approved for this purpose in the United States, because silver concentration in water is strongly affected by adsorption onto the surface of the container, and there has been limited testing on viruses and cysts. In the United States, silver is approved for maintaining microbiologic quality of stored water. Several other common products, including hydrogen peroxide, citrus juice, and potassium permanganate, have antibacterial effects in water and are marketed in commercial products for travelers. None have sufficient data to recommend them for primary water disinfection in the field.

THE PREFERRED TECHNIQUE

Table 2-12 summarizes field water disinfection techniques. The optimal technique for a person or group depends on personal preference, size of the group, water source, and the style of travel. Boiling is the most reliable single-step treatment, but certain filters, UV, and chlorine dioxide are also effective in most situations. Optimal treatment of highly contaminated or cloudy water may require CF followed by chemical disinfection. On long-distance, oceangoing boats where water must be desalinated during the voyage, only reverse-osmosis membrane filters are adequate.

Table 2-12. Summary of field water disinfection techniques

	BACTERIA	VIRUSES	*GIARDIA/* AMEBAS	CRYPTOSPORIDIA	NEMATODES/ CERCARIAE
Heat	+	+	+	+	+
Filtration	+	+/−[1]	+	+	+
Halogens	+	+	+[2]	−	+/−[3]
Chlorine dioxide and photocatalytic	+	+	+	+	+/−[3]

[1] Most filters make no claims for viruses. Reverse osmosis is effective. Virus removal is based on company claims of electrostatic attraction between viruses and filter media.
[2] Require higher concentrations and contact time.
[3] Eggs are not very susceptible to halogens but risk of waterborne transmission is very low.

BIBLIOGRAPHY

1. Backer H. Field water disinfection. In: Auerbach PS, editor. Wilderness medicine. 6th ed. Philadelphia: Elsevier Mosby; 2012. p. 1324–59.

2. Backer H, Hollowell J. Use of iodine for water disinfection: iodine toxicity and maximum recommended dose. Environ Health Perspect. 2000 Aug;108(8):679–84.

3. CDC. Safe water systems for the developing world: a handbook for implementing household-based water treatment and safe storage projects. Atlanta: CDC; 2001.

4. Center for Affordable Water and Sanitation Technology. Biosand filter. Alberta, Canada: Center for Affordable Water and Sanitation Technology; 2012 [cited 2012 Mar 18]. Available from: http://www.cawst.org/en/resources/biosand-filter.

5. Clasen T, Roberts I, Rabie T, Schmidt W, Cairncross S. Interventions to improve water quality for preventing diarrhoea (review). Cochrane Database Syst Rev [Internet]. 2009 (3). Available from: http://onlinelibrary.wiley.com/doi/10.1002/14651858.CD004794.pub2/full.

6. Departments of the Army, Navy, and Air Force. TB MED 577 Technical bulletin: sanitary control and surveillance of field water supplies. Washington, DC: US Army Medical Department; 2010 [cited 2012 Sep 18]. Available from: http://armypubs.army.mil/med/DR_pubs/dr_a/pdf/tbmed577.pdf.

7. Groh CD, MacPherson DW, Groves DJ. Effect of heat on the sterilization of artificially contaminated water. J Travel Med. 1996 Mar 1;3(1):11–3.

8. Joyce TM, McGuigan KG, Elmore-Meegan M, Conroy RM. Inactivation of fecal bacteria in drinking water by solar heating. Appl Environ Microbiol. 1996 Feb;62(2):399–402.

9. Korich DG, Mead JR, Madore MS, Sinclair NA, Sterling CR. Effects of ozone, chlorine dioxide, chlorine, and monochloramine on *Cryptosporidium parvum* oocyst viability. Appl Environ Microbiol. 1990 May;56(5):1423–8.

10. Lantagne DS. Sodium hypochlorite dosage for household and emergency water treatment. Journal of American Water Works Association. 2008;100(8):106–19.

11. McGuigan KG, Joyce TM, Conroy RM, Gillespie JB, Elmore-Meegan M. Solar disinfection of drinking water contained in transparent plastic bottles: characterizing the bacterial inactivation process. J Appl Microbiol. 1998 Jun;84(6):1138–48.

12. Sobsey MD, Stauber CE, Casanova LM, Brown JM, Elliott MA. Point of use household drinking water filtration: A practical, effective solution for providing sustained access to safe drinking water in the developing world. Environ Sci Technol. 2008 Jun 15;42(12):4261–7.

13. Swiss Federal Institute of Aquatic Science and Technology. SODIS method. Dübendorf, Switzerland: Swiss Federal Institute of Aquatic Science and Technology; 2012 [cited 2012 Mar 3]. Available from: http://www.sodis.ch/methode/index_EN.

FOOD POISONING FROM MARINE TOXINS
Vernon E. Ansdell

Seafood poisoning from marine toxins is an underrecognized hazard for travelers, particularly in the tropics and subtropics. Furthermore, the risk is increasing because of factors such as climate change, coral reef damage, and spread of toxic algal blooms.

CIGUATERA FISH POISONING

Ciguatera fish poisoning occurs after eating reef fish contaminated with toxins such as ciguatoxin or maitotoxin. These potent toxins originate from small marine organisms (dinoflagellates) that grow on and around coral reefs. Dinoflagellates are ingested by herbivorous fish. The toxins are then concentrated as they pass up the food chain to large carnivorous fish (usually >6 lb, 2.7 kg) and finally to humans. Toxins are concentrated in fish liver, intestinals, roe, and head.

Gambierdiscus toxicus, which produces ciguatoxin, may proliferate on dead coral reefs more quickly than other dinoflagellates. The risk of ciguatera is likely to increase as more coral reefs die because of climate change, ocean acidification, construction, and nutrient runoff.

Risk for Travelers
More than 50,000 cases of ciguatera poisoning occur globally every year. The incidence

in travelers to highly endemic areas has been estimated as high as 3 per 100. Ciguatera is widespread in tropical and subtropical waters, usually between the latitudes of 35°N and 35°S; it is particularly common in the Pacific and Indian Oceans and the Caribbean Sea. The incidence and geographic distribution of ciguatera poisoning are increasing. Newly recognized areas of risk include the Canary Islands, the eastern Mediterranean, and the western Gulf of Mexico.

Fish that are most likely to cause ciguatera poisoning are carnivorous reef fish, including barracuda, grouper, moray eel, amberjack, sea bass, or sturgeon. Omnivorous and herbivorous fish such as parrot fish, surgeonfish, and red snapper can also be a risk.

Clinical Presentation

Typical ciguatera poisoning results in a gastrointestinal illness and may also cause neurologic symptoms. Although very rare, cardiovascular collapse may result. The first symptoms usually appear 1–3 hours after eating contaminated fish and include nausea, vomiting, diarrhea, and abdominal pain.

Neurologic symptoms usually appear 3–72 hours after the meal and include paresthesias, pain in the teeth or the sensation that the teeth are loose, itching, metallic taste, blurred vision, or even transient blindness. Cold allodynia (dysesthesia when touching cold water or objects) is characteristic, though there can be acute sensitivity to both hot and cold. Neurologic symptoms usually last a few days to several weeks.

Chronic neuropsychiatric symptoms resembling chronic fatigue syndrome may be disabling, last several months or longer, and include malaise, depression, headaches, myalgias, and fatigue. Cardiac manifestations include bradycardia, other arrhythmias, and hypotension.

The overall death rate from ciguatera poisoning is approximately 0.1% but varies according to the toxin dose and availability of medical care to deal with complications. The diagnosis of ciguatera poisoning is based on the clinical signs and symptoms and a history of eating fish that are known to carry ciguatera toxin. Commercial kits to test for ciguatera in fish are unreliable; however, reliable fish testing can be done by the US Food and Drug Administration (FDA). There is no easily available clinical test for ciguatera in humans.

Prevention

Travelers can take the following precautions to prevent ciguatera fish poisoning:

- Avoid or limit consumption of the reef fish listed above.
- Never eat high-risk fish such as barracuda or moray eel.
- Avoid the parts of the fish that concentrate ciguatera toxin: liver, intestines, roe, and head.

Remember that ciguatera toxins do not affect the texture, taste, or smell of fish, and they are not destroyed by gastric acid, cooking, smoking, freezing, canning, salting, or pickling.

Treatment

There is no specific antidote for ciguatoxin or maitotoxin. Treatment is generally for specific symptoms and includes supportive care. Intravenous mannitol has been reported to reduce the severity and duration of neurologic symptoms, particularly if given within 48 hours of the appearance of symptoms.

SCOMBROID

Scombroid, one of the most common fish poisonings, occurs worldwide in both temperate and tropical waters. The illness occurs after eating improperly refrigerated or preserved fish containing high levels of histamine, and often resembles a moderate to severe allergic reaction.

Fish typically associated with scombroid have naturally high levels of histidine in the flesh and include tuna, mackerel, mahimahi (dolphin fish), sardine, anchovy, herring, bluefish, amberjack, and marlin. Histidine is converted to histamine by bacterial overgrowth in fish that has been improperly stored after capture. Histamine and other scombrotoxins are resistant to cooking, smoking, canning, or freezing.

Clinical Presentation

Symptoms of scombroid poisoning resemble an acute allergic reaction and usually appear 10–60 minutes after eating contaminated fish. They include flushing of the face and upper body (resembling sunburn), severe headache, palpitations, itching, blurred vision, abdominal cramps, and diarrhea. Untreated, symptoms usually resolve within 12 hours. Rarely, there may be respiratory compromise, malignant arrhythmias, and hypotension requiring hospitalization. Diagnosis is usually clinical. A clustering of cases helps exclude the possibility of fish allergy.

Prevention

Fish contaminated with histamine may have a peppery, sharp, salty, or "bubbly" feel but may also look, smell, and taste normal. The key to prevention is to make sure that the fish is properly iced, refrigerated, or immediately frozen after it is caught (<38°F, <3.3°C). Cooking, smoking, canning, or freezing will not destroy histamine in contaminated fish.

Treatment

Scombroid poisoning usually responds well to antihistamines (H_1-receptor blockers, although H_2-receptor blockers may also be of benefit).

SHELLFISH POISONING

Several forms of shellfish poisoning may occur after ingesting filter-feeding bivalve mollusks (such as mussels, oysters, clams, scallops, and cockles) that contain potent toxins. The toxins originate in small marine organisms (dinoflagellates or diatoms) that are ingested and concentrated by shellfish.

Risk for Travelers

Contaminated shellfish may be found in temperate and tropical waters, typically during or after dinoflagellate blooms called harmful algal blooms (HABs). One example of a HAB is the Florida red tide caused by *Karenia brevis*.

Clinical Presentation

Poisoning results in gastrointestinal and neurologic illness of varying severity. Symptoms typically appear 30–60 minutes after ingesting toxic shellfish but can be delayed for several hours. Diagnosis is usually one of exclusion and is usually made clinically in patients who recently ate shellfish.

Paralytic Shellfish Poisoning

This is the most common and most severe form of shellfish poisoning. Symptoms usually appear 30–60 minutes after eating toxic

shellfish and include numbness and tingling of the face, lips, tongue, arms, and legs. There may be headache, nausea, vomiting, and diarrhea. Severe cases are associated with ingestion of large doses of toxin and clinical features such as ataxia, dysphagia, mental status changes, flaccid paralysis, and respiratory failure. The case-fatality ratio averages 6% and is dependent on the availability of modern medical care, including mechanical ventilation. The death rate may be particularly high in children.

Neurotoxic Shellfish Poisoning

Neurotoxic shellfish poisoning usually presents as gastroenteritis accompanied by minor neurologic symptoms, resembling mild ciguatera poisoning or mild paralytic shellfish poisoning. Inhalation of aerosolized toxin in the sea spray associated with a Florida red tide (*Karenia brevis* bloom) can induce bronchoconstriction and may cause acute, temporary respiratory discomfort in healthy people. People with asthma may experience more severe and prolonged effects.

Diarrheic Shellfish Poisoning

This produces chills, nausea, vomiting, abdominal cramps, and diarrhea. No deaths have been reported.

Amnesic Shellfish Poisoning

This is a rare form of shellfish poisoning that has been reported to produce gastroenteritis and neurologic symptoms that may be severe. There are little data on this type of poisoning.

Prevention

Shellfish poisoning can be prevented by avoiding potentially contaminated bivalve mollusks. This is particularly important in areas during or shortly after algal blooms, which may be locally referred to as "red tides," "brown tides," etc. Travelers to developing countries should avoid eating all shellfish, because they carry a high risk of viral and bacterial infections. Marine shellfish toxins cannot be destroyed by cooking or freezing.

Treatment

Treatment is symptomatic and supportive. Severe cases of paralytic shellfish poisoning may require mechanical ventilation.

BIBLIOGRAPHY

1. Ansdell V. Food-borne illness. In: Keystone JS, Freedman DO, Kozarsky PE, Connor BA, Nothdurft HD, editors. Travel Medicine. 3rd ed. Philadelphia: Saunders Elsevier; 2013. p. 425–32.

2. Backer L, Fleming L, Rowan A, Baden D. Epidemiology and public health of human illnesses associated with harmful marine algae. In: Hallegraeff GM, Anderson DM, Cembella A, editors. Manual on Harmful Marine Microalgae. Paris: UNESCO; 2003. p. 723–49.

3. Hungerford JM. Scombroid poisoning: a review. Toxicon. 2010 Aug 15;56(2):231–43.

4. Isbister GK, Kiernan MC. Neurotoxic marine poisoning. Lancet Neurol. 2005 Apr;4(4):219–28.

5. Palafox NA, Buenoconsejo-Lum LE. Ciguatera fish poisoning: review of clinical manifestations. J Toxicol Toxin Rev. 2001;20(2):141–60.

6. Schnorf H, Taurarii M, Cundy T. Ciguatera fish poisoning: a double-blind randomized trial of mannitol therapy. Neurology. 2002 Mar 26;58(6):873–80.

7. Sobel J, Painter J. Illnesses caused by marine toxins. Clin Infect Dis. 2005 Nov 1;41(9):1290–6.

8. Stewart I, Lewis RJ, Eaglesham GK, Graham GC, Poole S, Craig SB. Emerging tropical diseases in Australia. Part 2. Ciguatera fish poisoning. Ann Trop Med Parasitol. 2010 Oct;104(7):557–71.

PROTECTION AGAINST MOSQUITOES, TICKS, & OTHER INSECTS & ARTHROPODS

Roger S. Nasci, Emily Zielinski-Gutierrez, Robert A. Wirtz, William G. Brogdon

Vaccines or chemoprophylactic drugs are available to protect against some vectorborne diseases such as yellow fever and malaria; however, travel health practitioners should advise travelers to use repellents and other general protective measures against biting arthropods. The effectiveness of malaria chemoprophylaxis is variable, depending on patterns of drug resistance, bioavailability, and compliance with medication, and no similar preventive measures exist for other mosquitoborne diseases such as dengue, chikungunya, or West Nile virus.

The Environmental Protection Agency (EPA) regulates repellent products in the United States. CDC recommends that consumers use repellent products that have been registered by EPA. EPA registration indicates the materials have been reviewed and approved for both efficacy and human safety when applied according to the instructions on the label.

GENERAL PROTECTIVE MEASURES

Avoid outbreaks. To the extent possible, travelers should avoid known foci of epidemic disease transmission. The CDC website provides updates on regional disease transmission patterns and outbreaks (www.cdc.gov/travel).

Be aware of peak exposure times and places. Exposure to arthropod bites may be reduced if travelers modify their patterns or locations of activity. Although mosquitoes may bite at any time of day, peak biting activity for vectors of some diseases (such as dengue and chikungunya) is during daylight hours. Vectors of other diseases (such as malaria) are most active in twilight periods (dawn and dusk) or in the evening after dark. Avoiding the outdoors or taking preventive actions (such as using repellent) during peak biting hours may reduce risk. Place also matters; ticks and chiggers are often found in grasses and other vegetated areas. Local health officials or guides may be able to point out areas with increased arthropod activity.

Wear appropriate clothing. Travelers can minimize areas of exposed skin by wearing long-sleeved shirts, long pants, boots, and hats. Tucking in shirts, tucking pants into socks, and wearing closed shoes instead of sandals may reduce risk. Repellents or insecticides, such as permethrin, can be applied to clothing and gear for added protection. (Additional information on clothing is below.)

Check for ticks. Travelers should inspect themselves and their clothing for ticks during outdoor activity and at the end of the day. Prompt removal of attached ticks can prevent some infections. Showering within 2 hours of being in a tick-infested area reduces the risk of some tickborne diseases.

Bed nets. When accommodations are not adequately screened or air conditioned, bed nets are essential in providing protection and reducing discomfort caused by biting insects. If bed nets do not reach the floor, they should be tucked under mattresses. Bed nets are most effective when they are treated with a pyrethroid insecticide. Pretreated, long-lasting bed nets can be purchased before traveling, or nets can be treated after purchase. Effective, treated nets may also be available in destination countries. Nets treated with a pyrethroid insecticide will be effective for several months if they are not washed. Long-lasting pretreated nets may be effective for much longer.

Insecticides and spatial repellents. More spatial repellent products are becoming commercially available. These products, containing active ingredients such as metofluthrin and allethrin, augment aerosol insecticide sprays, vaporizing mats, and mosquito coils that have been available for some time. Such products can help to clear rooms or areas of mosquitoes (spray aerosols) or repel mosquitoes from a circumscribed area (coils, spatial repellents).

Although many of these products appear to have repellent or insecticidal activity under particular conditions, they have not yet been adequately evaluated in peer-reviewed studies for their efficacy in preventing vectorborne disease. Travelers should supplement the use of these products with repellent on skin or clothing and using bed nets in areas where vectorborne diseases are a risk or biting arthropods are noted. Since some products available internationally may contain pesticides that are not registered in the United States, it may be preferable for travelers to bring their own. Insecticides and repellent products should always be used with caution, avoiding direct inhalation of spray or smoke.

Optimum protection can be provided by applying the repellents described in the following sections to clothing and to exposed skin (Box 2-3).

REPELLENTS FOR USE ON SKIN AND CLOTHING

CDC has evaluated information published in peer-reviewed scientific literature and data available from EPA to identify several types of EPA-registered products that provide repellent activity sufficient to help people reduce the bites of disease-carrying mosquitoes. Products containing the following active ingredients typically provide reasonably long-lasting protection:

- **DEET** (chemical name: N,N-diethyl-m-toluamide or N,N-diethyl-3-methyl-benzamide). Products containing DEET include, but are

---

BOX 2-3. MAXIMIZING PROTECTION FROM MOSQUITOES

To optimize protection against mosquitoes and reduce the risk of mosquito-transmitted diseases:
- Wear a long-sleeved shirt, long pants, and socks.
- Treat clothing with permethrin or purchase pretreated clothing.
  - > Permethrin-treated clothing will retain repellent activity through multiple washes.
  - > Repellents used on skin can also be applied to clothing but provide shorter duration of protection (same duration as on skin) and must be reapplied after laundering.
- Apply lotion, liquid, or spray repellent to exposed skin.
- Ensure adequate protection during times of day when mosquitoes are most active.
  - > Dengue, yellow fever, West Nile, and chikungunya vector mosquitoes bite mainly from dawn to dusk.
  - > Malaria and Japanese encephalitis vector mosquitoes bite mainly from dusk to dawn.
- Use common sense. Reapply repellents as protection wanes and mosquitoes start to bite.

not limited to, Off!, Cutter, Sawyer, and Ultrathon.

- **Picaridin** (KBR 3023 [Bayrepel] and icaridin outside the United States; chemical name: 2-(2-hydroxyethyl)-1-piperidinecarboxylic acid 1-methylpropyl ester). Products containing picaridin include, but are not limited to, Cutter Advanced, Skin So Soft Bug Guard Plus, and Autan (outside the United States).
- **Oil of lemon eucalyptus (OLE)** or **PMD** (chemical name: para-menthane-3,8-diol), the synthesized version of OLE. Products containing OLE and PMD include, but are not limited to, Repel and Off! Botanicals. This recommendation refers to EPA-registered repellent products containing the active ingredient OLE (or PMD). "Pure" oil of lemon eucalyptus (essential oil not formulated as a repellent) is not recommended; it has not undergone similar, validated testing for safety and efficacy, is not registered with EPA as an insect repellent, and is not covered by this recommendation.
- **IR3535** (chemical name: 3-[N-butyl-N-acetyl]-aminopropionic acid, ethyl ester). Products containing IR3535 include, but are not limited to, Skin So Soft Bug Guard Plus Expedition and SkinSmart.

EPA characterizes the active ingredients DEET and picaridin as "conventional repellents" and OLE, PMD, and IR3535 as "biopesticide repellents," which are either derived from or are synthetic versions of natural materials.

Repellent Efficacy

Published data indicate that repellent efficacy and duration of protection vary considerably among products and among mosquito species. Product efficacy and duration of protection are also markedly affected by ambient temperature, level of activity, amount of perspiration, exposure to water, abrasive removal, and other factors. In general, higher concentrations of active ingredient provide longer duration of protection, regardless of the active ingredient. Products with <10% active ingredient may offer only limited protection, often 1–2 hours. Products that offer sustained-release or controlled-release (microencapsulated) formulations, even with lower active ingredient concentrations, may provide longer protection times. Studies suggest that concentrations of

DEET above approximately 50% do not offer a marked increase in protection time against mosquitoes; DEET efficacy tends to plateau at a concentration of approximately 50%. CDC recommends using products with ≥20% DEET on exposed skin to reduce biting by ticks that may spread disease.

Recommendations are based on peer-reviewed journal articles and scientific studies and data submitted to regulatory agencies. People may experience some variation in protection from different products. Regardless of what product is used, if travelers start to get insect bites they should reapply the repellent according to the label instructions, try a different product, or, if possible, leave the area with biting insects.

Ideally, repellents should be purchased before traveling and can be found online or in hardware stores, drug stores, and supermarkets. A wide variety of repellents can be found in camping, sporting goods, and military surplus stores. When purchasing repellents overseas, look for the active ingredients specified above on the product labels; some names of products available internationally have been specified in the list above.

Repellents and Sunscreen

Repellents that are applied according to label instructions may be used with sunscreen with no reduction in repellent activity; however, limited data show a one-third decrease in the sun protection factor (SPF) of sunscreens when DEET-containing insect repellents are used after a sunscreen is applied. Products that combine sunscreen and repellent are not recommended, because sunscreen may need to be reapplied more often and in larger amounts than needed for the repellent component to provide protection from biting insects. In general, the recommendation is to use separate products, applying sunscreen first and then applying the repellent. Due to the decrease in SPF when using a DEET-containing insect repellent after applying sunscreen, travelers may need to reapply the sunscreen and repellent more frequently.

Repellents and Insecticides for Use on Clothing

Clothing, hats, shoes, bed nets, jackets, and camping gear can be treated with permethrin for added protection. Products such as Permanone and Sawyer permethrin are registered with EPA specifically for use by consumers to treat clothing and gear. Alternatively, clothing pretreated with permethrin is commercially available, marketed to consumers in the United States as Insect Shield or BugsAway.

Permethrin is a highly effective insecticide-acaricide and repellent. Permethrin-treated clothing repels and kills ticks, chiggers, mosquitoes, and other biting and nuisance arthropods. Clothing and other items must be treated 24–48 hours in advance of travel to allow them to dry. As with all pesticides, follow the label instructions when using permethrin clothing treatments.

Permethrin-treated materials retain repellency or insecticidal activity after repeated laundering but should be retreated, as described on the product label, to provide continued protection. Clothing that is treated before purchase is labeled for efficacy through 70 launderings. Clothing treated with the other repellent products described above (such as DEET) provides protection from biting arthropods but will not last through washing and will require more frequent reapplications.

Precautions when Using Insect Repellents

Travelers should take the following precautions:

- Apply repellents only to exposed skin or clothing, as directed on the product label. Do not apply repellents under clothing.
- Never use repellents over cuts, wounds, or irritated skin.
- When using sprays, do not spray directly on face—spray on hands first and then apply to face. Do not apply repellents to eyes or mouth, and apply sparingly around ears.
- Wash hands after application to avoid accidental exposure to eyes or ingestion.
- Children should not handle repellents. Instead, adults should apply repellents to their own hands first, and then gently spread on the child's exposed skin. Avoid applying directly to children's hands.
- Use just enough repellent to cover exposed skin or clothing. Heavy application and saturation are generally unnecessary for effectiveness. If biting insects do not respond to a thin film of repellent, apply a bit more.
- After returning indoors, wash repellent-treated skin with soap and water or bathe.

This is particularly important when repellents are used repeatedly in a day or on consecutive days.

- Wash treated clothing before wearing it again. This precaution may vary with different repellents—check the product label.

If a traveler experiences a rash or other reaction, such as itching or swelling, from an insect repellent, the repellent should be washed off with mild soap and water and its use discontinued. If a severe reaction has occurred, a local poison-control center should be called for further guidance, if feasible. Travelers seeking health care because of the repellent should take the repellent to the doctor's office and show the doctor. Permethrin should *never* be applied to skin but only to clothing, bed nets, or other fabrics as directed on the product label.

Children and Pregnant Women

Most repellents can be used on children aged >2 months. Protect infants aged <2 months from mosquitoes by using an infant carrier draped with mosquito netting with an elastic edge for a tight fit. Products containing OLE specify that they should not be used on children aged <3 years. Other than the safety tips listed above, EPA does not recommend any additional precautions for using registered repellents on children or on pregnant or lactating women.

Useful Links

- Choosing an Insect Repellent (EPA): www.epa.gov/pesticides/insect/choose.htm
- Using Insect Repellents Safely (EPA): http://epa.gov/pesticides/insect/safe.htm
- Insect Repellent Use and Safety (CDC): www.cdc.gov/ncidod/dvbid/westnile/qa/insect_repellent.htm
- National Pesticide Information Center—Choosing and Using Insect Repellents: http://npic.orst.edu/ingred/ptype/repel.html

BEDBUGS

There has been a recent resurgence in bedbug infestations worldwide, particularly in developed countries. Although bedbugs do not transmit diseases, their bites may be a nuisance. Travelers can take measures to avoid bedbug bites and avoid transporting them in luggage and clothing (Box 2-4).

BOX 2-4. BEDBUGS AND INTERNATIONAL TRAVEL

A recent resurgence in bedbug infestations worldwide, particularly in developed countries, is thought to be related to the increase in international travel, pest control strategy changes in travel lodgings, and insecticide resistance. Bedbug infestations have been increasingly reported in hotels, theaters, and any locations where people congregate, even in the workplace, dormitories, and schools. Bedbugs may be transported in luggage and on clothing. Transport of personal belongings in contaminated transport vehicles is another means of spread of these insects.

Bedbugs are small, flat insects that are reddish-brown in color, wingless, and range from 1 to 7 mm in length. While bedbugs have not been shown to transmit disease, their bites can produce strong allergic reactions and considerable emotional stress.

Protective Measures against Bedbugs

Travelers should be encouraged to take the following precautions to avoid or reduce their exposure to bedbugs:

- Inspect the premises of hotels or other sleeping locations for bedbugs on mattresses, box springs, bedding, and furniture, particularly built-in furniture with the bed, desk, and closets as a continuous structural unit. Travelers who observe evidence of bedbug activity—whether it be the bugs themselves or physical signs such as blood-spotting on linens—should seek alternative lodging.
- Keep suitcases closed when they are not in use and try to keep them off the floor.
- Remove clothing and personal items (such as toiletry bags and shaving kits) from the suitcase only when they are in use.
- Carefully inspect clothing and personal items before returning them to the suitcase.
- Keep in mind that bedbug eggs and nymphs are very small and can be easily overlooked.

Prevention is by far the most effective and inexpensive way to protect oneself from these pests. The costs of ridding a personal residence of these insects are considerable, and efforts at control are often not immediately successful even when conducted by professionals.

BIBLIOGRAPHY

1. Barnard DR, Bernier UR, Posey KH, Xue RD. Repellency of IR3535, KBR3023, para-menthane-3,8-diol, and DEET to black salt marsh mosquitoes (Diptera: Culicidae) in the Everglades National Park. J Med Entomol. 2002 Nov;39(6):895–9.
2. Barnard DR, Xue RD. Laboratory evaluation of mosquito repellents against *Aedes albopictus*, *Culex nigripalpus*, and *Ochlerotatus triseriatus* (Diptera: Culicidae). J Med Entomol. 2004 Jul;41(4):726–30.
3. Centers for Disease Control and Prevention, Environmental Protection Agency. Joint statement on bed bug control in the United States from the US Centers for Disease Control and Prevention (CDC) and the US Environmental Protection Agency (EPA). Atlanta: US Department of Health and Human Services; 2010 [updated 2011 Feb 17; cited 2012 Sep 18]. Available from: http://www. cdc.gov/nceh/ehs/publications/bed_bugs_cdc-epa_ statement.htm.
4. Fradin MS, Day JF. Comparative efficacy of insect repellents against mosquito bites. N Engl J Med. 2002 Jul 4;347(1):13–8.
5. Montemarano AD, Gupta RK, Burge JR, Klein K. Insect repellents and the efficacy of sunscreens. Lancet. 1997 Jun 7;349(9066):1670–1.
6. Murphy ME, Montemarano AD, Debboun M, Gupta R. The effect of sunscreen on the efficacy of insect repellent: a clinical trial. J Am Acad Dermatol. 2000 Aug;43(2 Pt 1):219–22.
7. Thavara U, Tawatsin A, Chompoosri J, Suwonkerd W, Chansang UR, Asavadachanukorn P. Laboratory and field evaluations of the insect repellent 3535 (ethyl butylacetylaminopropionate) and DEET against mosquito vectors in Thailand. J Am Mosq Control Assoc. 2001 Sep;17(3):190–5.

SUNBURN
Vernon E. Ansdell, Amy K. Reisenauer

OVERVIEW

Increased exposure to UV radiation occurs near the equator, during summer months, at high elevation, and between 10 AM and 4 PM. Reflection from the snow, sand, and water increases exposure, a particularly important consideration for snow skiing, beach activities, swimming, and sailing. In addition, several common medications may cause photosensitivity reactions in travelers:

- Acetazolamide
- Amiodarone
- Antibiotics (fluoroquinolones, sulfonamides, and tetracyclines, especially demeclocycline and doxycycline)
- Furosemide
- Nonsteroidal anti-inflammatory drugs
- Phenothiazines
- Sulfonylureas
- Thiazide diuretics
- Voriconazole

Medical conditions such as connective tissue diseases, polymorphous light eruption, rosacea, and vitiligo can increase sun sensitivity, and alcohol consumption can lead to behavioral changes that increase the risk of sunburn.

Both UVA rays (320–400 nm) and UVB rays (290–320 nm) are carcinogenic. UVA rays are present throughout the day and can pass through window glass. UVA rays cause premature aging of the skin and are primarily responsible for drug-related phototoxicity and photoallergic reactions. UVB rays are most intense from 10 AM to 4 PM, are blocked by window glass, and are most responsible for sunburn. Serious burns are painful, and the skin may be red, tender, swollen, and blistered. These sunburns may be accompanied by fever, headache, itching, and malaise. Cumulative overexposure to the sun leads to premature aging of the skin, including wrinkling and age spots and an increased risk for skin cancer, including basal cell carcinoma, squamous cell carcinoma, and melanoma.

Repeated exposure to sunlight can also result in ocular pterygium formation, cataracts, and macular degeneration.

PREVENTION
Sun Avoidance

Sun exposure is the most preventable risk factor for skin cancer, including melanoma. Staying indoors or seeking shade between 10 AM and 4 PM is very important in limiting exposure to UV rays, particularly UVB rays. Be aware that sunburn and sun damage can occur even on cloudy days and even when one sits under an umbrella or in the shade. Sunburn can occur after as little as 10–15 minutes of unprotected sun exposure in a fair-skinned person. Tanning beds and sun lamps are also carcinogenic and should be avoided.

Protective Clothing

Wide-brimmed hats, long sleeves, and long pants protect against UV rays. Tightly woven clothing and darker fabrics provide additional protection. High-UPF (ultraviolet protection factor >30) clothing is recommended for travelers at increased risk of sunburn or with a history of skin cancer. This type of clothing contains colorless compounds, fluorescent brighteners, or treated resins that absorb UV rays. A laundry additive, such as the product SunGuard, can be used to add UV protection to clothing. Sunglasses that provide 100% protection against UV radiation are strongly recommended.

Sunscreens

Sun protection factor (SPF) defines the extra protection against UVB rays that a person receives by using a sunscreen. For example, if a person using SPF 15 sunscreen normally acquires a sunburn in 20 minutes without protection, the benefit will be 20×15 minutes (300 minutes; 5 hours) extra protection with sunscreen. SPF does not refer to protection against UVA rays.

Physical sunscreens contain titanium dioxide or zinc oxide, inorganic molecules that are confined to the stratum corneum and reflect and scatter both visible and UV light. They are effective, broad-spectrum sunscreens that protect against both UVA and UVB radiation. With the advent of nanotechnology, these products no longer cause an opaque white film on the skin and have become cosmetically acceptable for widespread use. They are recommended for people who burn easily or who take medications that may cause photosensitivity reactions.

Chemical sunscreens absorb rather than reflect UV radiation. A combination of chemical agents is recommended to provide broad-spectrum protection against UVA and UVB rays. Although the Food and Drug Administration recommends using sunscreen with ≥15 SPF, the American Academy of Dermatology recommends using sunscreen with ≥30 SPF. A debate exists as to the value of additional protection provided by sunscreens with SPFs >15. In a controlled environment, the marginal protection provided by these high-SPF sunscreens is only 2%–4%. However, since most people underapply sunscreen, the higher-SPF sunscreens may have a margin of safety and give the user at least an SPF 15 level of protection. Travelers should consider the following key points regarding sunscreens:

- Choose a sunscreen with ≥15 SPF to ensure adequate UVB protection.
- For UVA protection, look for the following active ingredients: zinc oxide, titanium dioxide, avobenzone, ecamsule, oxybenzone, dioxybenzone, or sulisobenzone.
- Use products that contain both UVA and UVB protection.
- Select a waterproof or water-resistant product. Waterproof sunscreens confer approximately 80 minutes of protection in the water, and water-resistant products offer 40 minutes of protection.
- Apply to dry skin 15 minutes before exposure to the sun.
- At least 1 oz (2 tablespoons or enough to fill a shot glass) of sunscreen is needed to cover the exposed areas of the body. Most people only apply 25%–50% of the recommended amount of sunscreen, which decreases the achieved SPF.

- Apply to all exposed areas, especially the ears, scalp, back of the neck, tops of the feet, and backs of the hands.
- Reapply every 2 hours and after sweating, swimming, or towel-drying (even on cloudy days).
- Use a lip balm or lipstick with ≥15 SPF.
- The Food and Drug Administration requires that all sunscreens retain their original strength for at least 3 years. Always check the expiration date and discard all expired product.
- Sunscreens should be applied to the skin before insect repellents. (Note: DEET-containing insect repellents may decrease the SPF of sunscreens by one-third. Sunscreens may increase absorption of DEET through the skin.)
- Avoid products that contain both sunscreens and insect repellents, because sunscreen may need to be reapplied more often and in larger amounts than the repellent.

TREATMENT

Travelers with sunburn should maintain hydration and stay in a cool, shaded, or indoor environment. Topical and oral nonsteroidal anti-inflammatory drugs decrease erythema if used before or soon after exposure to UVB rays and may relieve symptoms such as headache, fever, and local pain. The pain of sunburn is usually most intense 6–48 hours after sun exposure, and skin usually peels 4–7 days later. Topical steroids are of limited benefit, and systemic steroids appear to be ineffective in alleviating the pain. Cool compresses, colloidal oatmeal baths, moisturizing creams, and topical aloe vera gel may relieve symptoms. Oral diphenhydramine may relieve pruritus. If blisters occur, they should be left intact to promote faster healing. Open erosions should be coated with petrolatum jelly and covered with sterile gauze to decrease the risk of infection. If infection occurs, oral antibiotics may be necessary. In severe cases of sunburn, dehydration and hypovolemia may occur, presenting with severely inflamed or reddened skin, disorientation, dizziness or fainting, nausea, chills, high fever, and headache. Hospitalization for intravenous rehydration and narcotic analgesics for pain relief may be required in these extreme cases.

BIBLIOGRAPHY

1. Diffey BL, Grice J. The influence of sunscreen type on photoprotection. Br J Dermatol. 1997 Jul;137(1):103–5.

2. Gu X, Wang T, Collins DM, Kasichayanula S, Burczynski FJ. In vitro evaluation of concurrent use of commercially available insect repellent and sunscreen preparations. Br J Dermatol. 2005 Jun;152(6):1263–7.

3. Han A, Maibach HI. Management of acute sunburn. Am J Clin Dermatol. 2004;5(1):39–47.

4. Krakowski AC, Kaplan LA. Exposure to radiation from the sun. In: Auerbach PS, editor. Wilderness Medicine. 6th ed. Philadelphia: Mosby Elsevier; 2012. p. 294–313.

5. McLean DI, Gallagher R. Sunscreens. Use and misuse. Dermatol Clin. 1998 Apr;16(2):219–26.

6. Murphy ME, Montemarano AD, Debboun M, Gupta R. The effect of sunscreen on the efficacy of insect repellent: a clinical trial. J Am Acad Dermatol. 2000 Aug;43(2 Pt 1):219–22.

7. Wang SQ, Stanfield JW, Osterwalder U. In vitro assessments of UVA protection by popular sunscreens available in the United States. J Am Acad Dermatol. 2008 Dec;59(6):934–42.

8. Wang SQ, Tooley IR. Photoprotection in the era of nanotechnology. Seminars in cutaneous medicine and surgery. 2011 Dec;30(4):210–3.

PROBLEMS WITH HEAT & COLD
Howard D. Backer, David R. Shlim

OVERVIEW

International travelers encounter environments that may include extremes of climate to which the traveler is not accustomed. Exposure to heat and cold can result in serious injury or death. Travelers should investigate climate extremes that they will face during their journey and prepare with proper clothing, knowledge, and equipment.

PROBLEMS ASSOCIATED WITH A HOT CLIMATE
Risk for Travelers

Many of the most popular travel destinations are tropical or desert areas. Travelers who sit on the beach or by the pool and do only short walking tours incur minimal risk of heat illness. Those who do strenuous hiking, biking, or work in the heat are at risk, especially travelers coming from cool or temperate climates who are not in good physical condition and are not acclimatized to the heat.

Clinical Presentations
Physiology of Heat Injuries

Tolerance to heat depends largely on physiologic factors, unlike cold environments where adaptive behaviors are more important. The major means of heat dissipation are radiation while at rest and evaporation of sweat during exercise, both of which become minimal with air temperatures above 95°F (35°C) and high humidity.

The major organs involved in temperature regulation are the skin, where sweating and heat exchange take place, and the cardiovascular system, which must increase blood flow to shunt heat from the core to the surface, while meeting the metabolic demands of exercise. Cardiovascular status and conditioning are the major physiologic variables affecting the response to heat stress at all ages. In addition to environmental conditions and intensity of exercise, dehydration is the most important predisposing factor in heat illness. Dehydration also reduces exercise performance, decreases time to exhaustion, and increases internal heat load; temperature and heart rate increase in direct proportion to the level of dehydration. Sweat is a hypotonic fluid containing sodium and chloride. Sweat rates commonly reach 1 L per hour and may exceed this level, which may result in substantial fluid and sodium loss.

Minor Heat Disorders

Heat cramps are painful muscle contractions following exercise in heat. They begin an hour or more after stopping exercise, most often involving heavily used muscles in the calves, thighs, and abdomen. Rest and passive stretching of the muscle, supplemented by fluids and salt, will rapidly relieve symptoms. Water with a salty snack is sufficient; an oral salt solution, as in rehydration solutions, can be made by adding one-fourth to one-half teaspoon of table salt (or 2 1-g salt tablets) to 1 L of water. To improve taste, add a few teaspoons of sugar and/or orange juice or lemon juice.

Heat syncope is sudden fainting in heat that occurs in unacclimatized people while standing in the heat or after 15–20 minutes of exercise. Consciousness rapidly returns to normal when the patient is supine. Rest, relief from heat, and oral fluids are sufficient treatment.

Heat edema is mild swelling of the hands and feet, more frequent in women during the first few days of heat exposure. It resolves spontaneously and should not be treated with diuretics, which may delay heat acclimatization and cause dehydration.

Prickly heat (such as miliaria or heat rash) manifests as small, red, itchy lesions on the skin caused by obstruction of the sweat ducts. It is best prevented by wearing light, loose clothing and avoiding heavy, continuous sweating.

Major Heat Disorders
Heat exhaustion
Most people who experience acute collapse or other symptoms associated with exercise in the heat are suffering from heat exhaustion, simply defined as the inability to continue exertion in the heat. The presumed cause of heat exhaustion is loss of fluid and electrolytes, but there are no objective markers to define the syndrome, which is a spectrum ranging from minor complaints to a vague boundary shared with heat stroke. Transient mental changes, such as irritability, confusion, or irrational behavior may be present, but major neurologic signs, such as seizures or coma, indicate heat stroke or hyponatremia. Body temperature may be normal or mildly elevated.

Most cases can be treated with supine rest in the shade or other cool place, and oral water or fluids containing glucose and salt. Spontaneous cooling occurs, and patients recover within hours without progression to more serious illness. An oral solution for treating heat exhaustion can be made by adding one-fourth to one-half teaspoon of table salt (or 2 1-g salt tablets) to 1 L of water plus 4–6 teaspoons of sugar. To further improve taste, add one-quarter cup of orange juice or 2 teaspoons of lemon juice. Commercial sports-electrolyte drinks or water with snacks are also effective. Plain water plus salty snacks may be more palatable and equally effective. Subacute heat exhaustion may develop over several days and is often misdiagnosed as "summer flu" because of findings of weakness, fatigue, headache, dizziness, anorexia, nausea, vomiting, and diarrhea. Treatment is as described for acute heat exhaustion.

Exercise-associated hyponatremia
Hyponatremia (low sodium [salt] levels in the blood) occurs in both endurance athletes and recreational hikers, due to loss of sodium through sweating and replacement of fluids with excessive amounts of plain water.

In the field setting, altered mental status with normal body temperature and a history of large volumes of water intake suggest hyponatremia. The vague and nonspecific symptoms are the same as those described for hyponatremia in other settings (for example, anorexia, nausea, emesis, headache, muscle weakness, lethargy, confusion, and seizures). Symptoms of heat exhaustion and early hyponatremia are similar. Hyponatremia can be distinguished by persistent alteration of mental status without elevated temperature. Delay in onset of major neurologic symptoms (confusion, seizures, or coma) or deterioration after cessation of exercise and heat exposure point to hyponatremia.

The recommendation of forcing fluid during prolonged exercise and the attitude that "you can't drink too much" are major contributors to exercise-associated hyponatremia. Prevention includes drinking as one desires to relieve thirst and to maintain urine output. During prolonged exercise or heat exposure, supplemental sodium should be taken. Most sports-electrolyte drinks do not contain sufficient amounts of sodium to prevent hyponatremia; however, salt tablets often cause nausea and vomiting. For hikers, food is the most efficient vehicle for salt replacement. Trail snacks should include salty foods (such as trail mix, crackers, pretzels, and jerky) and not just sweets.

Heat stroke

Heat stroke is an extreme medical emergency requiring aggressive cooling measures and hospitalization for support. Damage is related to duration, as well as peak elevation of body temperature. Heat stroke is the only form of heat illness in which the mechanisms for thermal homeostasis have failed. As a result of uncontrolled fever and circulatory collapse, organ damage can occur in the brain, liver, kidneys, and heart. The onset of heat stroke may be acute (exertional heat stroke), which can affect healthy people who are exercising in the heat, or gradual (nonexertional heat stroke, also referred to as classic or epidemic), which occurs from passive heat exposure in those with chronic illness.

Early symptoms are similar to those of heat exhaustion, with confusion or change in personality, loss of coordination, dizziness, headache, and nausea that progress to severe symptoms. A presumptive diagnosis of heat stroke is made in the field when people have elevation of body temperature (hyperpyrexia) and marked alteration of mental status, including delirium, convulsions, and coma. Body temperatures in excess of 106°F (41°C) can be observed; even without a thermometer, people will feel hot to the touch. If a thermometer is available, a rectal temperature is the safest and most reliable way to check the temperature of someone who may have heat stroke.

In the field, immediately institute cooling measures by one of several simple methods:

- Use evaporative cooling by maximizing skin exposure, spraying tepid water on the skin, and maintaining air movement over the body by fanning.
- Apply ice or cold packs to the neck, axillas, and groin. Vigorously massage the skin to prevent constriction of blood vessels and try to avoid shivering, which will increase body temperature.
- Immerse the person in cool water, such as a nearby pool or natural body of water. (Always attend and hold the person while in the water.)

Unless the recovery is rapid, the person should be evacuated to a hospital. If that is not possible, encourage rehydration for those able to take oral fluids, and monitor closely for several hours for temperature swings. Delayed complications in the first 24–48 hours may include liver or kidney damage and bleeding.

Prevention of Heat Disorders
Heat Acclimatization
Heat acclimatization is a process of physiologic adaptation to a hot environment that occurs in both residents and visitors. The result of acclimatization is an increase in sweating with less salt content, and decreased energy expenditure with lower rise in body temperature for a given workload. Only partial adaptation occurs by passive exposure to heat. Full acclimatization, especially cardiovascular response, requires 1–2 hours of exercise in the heat each day. Most acclimatization changes occur within 10 days, provided a suitable amount of exercise is taken each day in the heat. After this time, only increased physical fitness will result in further exercise tolerance. Decay of acclimatization occurs within days to weeks if there is no heat exposure.

Physical Conditioning and Acclimatization
Higher levels of physical fitness improve exercise tolerance and capacity in heat, but not as much as acclimatization. If possible, travelers should acclimatize before leaving by exercising ≥1 hour daily in the heat. If this is not possible before departing, exercise during the first week of travel in a hot climate should be limited in intensity and duration. It is a good idea to conform to the local practice in most hot regions and avoid strenuous activity during the hottest part of the day.

Clothing
Clothing should be lightweight, loose, and light-colored to allow maximum air circulation for evaporation yet give protection from the sun. A wide-brimmed hat markedly reduces radiant heat exposure.

Fluid and Electrolyte Replacement
During exertion, fluid intake improves performance and decreases the likelihood of illness. Reliance on thirst alone is not sufficient to prevent dehydration, bearing in

mind the potential danger of hyponatremia. During mild to moderate exertion, electrolyte replacement offers no advantage over plain water. However, for those exercising many hours in heat, salt replacement is recommended. Eating salty snacks or lightly salting mealtime food or fluids is the most efficient way to replace salt losses. Salt tablets, when swallowed whole, may cause gastrointestinal irritation and vomiting, but 2 tablets can be dissolved in 1 L of water. Urine volume and color are readily available means to monitor fluid needs.

PROBLEMS ASSOCIATED WITH A COLD CLIMATE
Risk for Travelers

Travelers do not have to be in an arctic or high-altitude environment to encounter problems with the cold. Humidity, rain, and wind can produce hypothermia even with temperatures around 50°F (10°C). Reports of severe hypothermia in international travelers are rare. Many high-altitude destinations are not wilderness areas, and villages offer an escape from extreme weather. In Nepal, trekkers almost never experience hypothermia, except in the rare instance in which they get lost in a storm. Even in a temperate climate, a traveler in a small boat that overturns in very cold water can rapidly become hypothermic.

Clinical Presentations
Hypothermia

Hypothermia can be defined, in general terms, as having a core body temperature below 95°F (35°C). When people are faced with an environment in which they cannot keep warm, they first feel chilled, then begin to shiver, and eventually stop shivering as their metabolic reserves are exhausted. At that point, body temperature continues to decrease, depending on the ambient temperatures. As the core temperature falls, neurologic functioning decreases until almost all hypothermic people with a core temperature of 86°F (30°C) or lower are comatose. The record low core body temperature in an adult who survived is 56°F (13°C). Travelers headed to a cold climate should be encouraged to ask questions and research clothing and equipment. Modern clothing, gloves, and particularly footwear have greatly decreased the chances of suffering cold injury in extreme climates. Cold injuries occur more often after accidents, such as avalanches or unexpected nights outside, than during normal recreational activities.

Travelers who will be engaging in recreational activities or working around cold water face a different sort of risk. Immersion hypothermia can render a person unable to swim or keep floating in <15 minutes. In these cases, a personal flotation device is critical, as is knowledge about self-rescue and righting a capsized boat.

The other medical conditions associated with cold affect mainly the skin and the extremities. These can be divided into nonfreezing cold injuries and freezing injuries (frostbite).

Nonfreezing Cold Injury

The nonfreezing cold injuries are trench foot, pernio (chilblains), and cold urticaria. **Trench foot** (immersion foot) is caused by prolonged immersion of the feet in cold water (32°F–59°F, 0°C–15°C). The damage is mainly to nerves and blood vessels, and the result is pain that is aggravated by heat and a dependent position of the limb. Severe cases can take months to resolve. Unlike the treatment for frostbite, immersion foot should not be rapidly rewarmed, which can make the damage much worse.

Pernio are localized, inflammatory lesions that occur mainly on the hands of susceptible people. They can occur with exposure to only moderately cold weather. The bluish-red lesions are thought to be caused by prolonged, cold-induced vasoconstriction. As with trench foot, rapid rewarming should be avoided, as it makes the pain worse. Nifedipine may be an effective treatment.

Cold urticaria involves the formation of localized or general wheals and itching after exposure to cold. It is not the absolute temperature that induces this form of urticaria but the rate of change of temperature in the skin.

Freezing Cold Injury
Categories of frostbite

Frostbite is the term that is used to describe tissue damage from direct freezing of the skin. Modern equipment and clothing have decreased the risk of frostbite resulting from adventure tourism, and frostbite occurs mainly during an accident, severe unexpected weather, or as a result of poor planning.

Once frostbite injury has occurred, little can be done to reverse the changes. Therefore, taking great care to prevent frostbite is crucial. Frostbite is usually graded like burns. First-degree frostbite involves reddening of the skin without deeper damage. The prognosis for complete healing is virtually 100%. Second-degree frostbite involves blister formation. Blisters filled with clear fluid have a better prognosis than blood-tinged blisters. Third-degree frostbite represents full-thickness injury to the skin and possibly the underlying tissues. No blister forms, the skin darkens over time and may turn black, and if the tissue is completely devascularized, amputation will be necessary.

Management of frostbite

Frostbitten skin is numb and appears whitish or waxy. The generally accepted method for treating a frozen digit or limb is through rapid rewarming in water heated to 104°F–108°F (40°C–42°C). The frozen area should be completely immersed in the warm water. A thermometer is needed to ensure the water is kept at the correct temperature. Rewarming can be associated with severe pain, and analgesics can be given if needed. Once the area is rewarmed, it must be safeguarded against freezing again. It is thought to be better to keep digits frozen a little longer and rapidly rewarm them, than to allow them to thaw out slowly or to thaw and refreeze. A cycle of freeze-thaw-refreeze is devastating to tissue and leads more directly to the need for amputation.

Once the area has rewarmed, it can be examined. If blisters are present, note whether they extend to the end of the digit.

Proximal blisters usually mean that the tissue distal to the blister has suffered full-thickness damage. Treatment consists of avoiding further mechanical trauma to the area and preventing infection. Reasonable field treatment consists of washing the area thoroughly with a disinfectant such as povidone-iodine, putting dressings between the toes or fingers to prevent maceration, using fluffs (expanded gauze sponges) for padding, and covering with a roller gauze bandage. These dressings can safely be left on for up to 3 days at a time. By leaving the dressings on longer, the traveler can preserve what may be limited supplies of bandages. Prophylactic antibiotics are not needed in most situations.

In the rare situation in which a foreign traveler suffers frostbite and can be evacuated to an advanced medical setting within 24 hours, there may be a role for thrombolytics, such as prostacyclin and recombinant tissue plasminogen activator. If you are managing frostbite in the first 24 hours, you should consult someone with expertise in frostbite as soon as possible. The risks and benefits of using these drugs should be carefully considered in each patient. Beyond 24 hours after thawing, these interventions are probably not beneficial.

Once the patient has reached a definitive medical setting, there should be no rush to do surgery. The usual time from injury to surgery is 4–5 weeks. Technetium (Tc)-99 scintigraphy and magnetic resonance imaging can be used to help define the extent of the damage. Once the delineation between dead tissue and viable becomes clear, surgery that preserves the remaining digits can be planned.

BIBLIOGRAPHY

1. Armstrong LE, Casa DJ, Millard-Stafford M, Moran DS, Pyne SW, Roberts WO. American College of Sports Medicine position stand. Exertional heat illness during training and competition. Med Sci Sports Exerc. 2007 Mar;39(3):556–72.

2. Cauchy E, Cheguillaume B, Chetaille E. A controlled trial of a prostacyclin and rt-PA in the treatment of severe frostbite. N Engl J Med. 2011 Jan 13;364(2):189–90.

3. Epstein Y, Moran DS. Extremes of temperature and hydration. In: Keystone JS, Freedman DO, Kozarsky PE, Connor BA, Nothdurft HD, editors. Travel Medicine.

3rd ed. Philadelphia: Saunders Elsevier; 2013. p. 381–90.

4. Freer L, Imray CHE. Frostbite. In: Auerbach PS, editor. Wilderness Medicine. 6th ed. Philadelphia: Mosby Elsevier; 2012. p. 181–201.

5. O'Brien KK, Leon LR, Kenefick RW. Clinical management of heat-related illnesses. In: Auerbach PS, editor. Wilderness Medicine. 6th ed. Philadelphia: Mosby Elsevier; 2012. p. 232–8.

6. Rogers IR, Hew-Butler T. Exercise-associated hyponatremia: overzealous fluid consumption. Wilderness Environ Med. 2009 Summer;20(2):139–43.

INJURIES & SAFETY

David A. Sleet, Douglas R. Roehler, Michael F. Ballesteros

OVERVIEW

According to the World Health Organization (WHO), injuries are among the leading causes of death and disability in the world, and they are the leading cause of preventable death in travelers. Among travelers, data show that injuries are one of the leading causes for consulting a physician, for hospitalization, for repatriation, and for death. Worldwide, among people aged 5–29 years, injuries account for 7 of the 15 leading causes of death. US citizens abroad are 10 times more likely to die as the result of an injury than from an infectious disease; injuries cause 23% of deaths of US citizens while abroad, compared with only 2% caused by infectious diseases. Contributing to the injury toll while traveling are exposure to unfamiliar and perhaps risky environments, differences in language and communications, less stringent product safety and vehicle standards, unfamiliar rules and regulations, a carefree holiday or vacation spirit leading to more risk-taking behavior, and overreliance on travel and tour operators to protect one's safety and security.

From 2009 through 2011, an estimated 2,773 US citizens died from nonnatural causes, such as injuries and violence, while in foreign countries (excluding deaths occurring in the wars in Iraq and Afghanistan). Motor vehicle crashes—not crime or terrorism—are the number 1 killer of healthy US citizens living, working, or traveling in foreign countries. From 2009 through 2011, road traffic crashes accounted for 27% of deaths to US citizens abroad. Other common causes of death included homicides (22%), suicides (14%), and drowning (12%) (Figure 2-1). Other less common but serious injuries are related to natural disasters, aviation accidents, drugs, terrorism, falls, burns, and poisoning.

If a traveler is seriously injured, emergency care may not be available or acceptable by US standards. Trauma centers capable of providing optimal care for serious injuries are uncommon outside urban areas in many foreign destinations.

Although men are more likely than women to die from injuries while abroad, acquaintance rape and sexual assault are special risks to female travelers. Travelers should be aware of the increased risk of certain injuries while traveling or residing abroad, particularly in low- and middle-income countries (LMICs) and be prepared to take preventive steps. Injuries are the primary reason for US citizens abroad to be transported back to the United States by air medical transport.

ROAD TRAFFIC INJURIES

Globally, an estimated 3,500 people are killed each day, including 720 children, in road traffic crashes involving cars, buses, motorcycles, bicycles, trucks, and pedestrians. Annually, 1.3 million are killed and 20–50 million are injured in traffic crashes—a number likely to double by 2030. More than 90% of these casualties (and 96% of child injury deaths) occur in LMICs. Table 2-13 lists the countries with the highest death rates from road traffic crashes.

International efforts to combat road deaths command a tiny fraction of the resources deployed to fight diseases such as malaria and tuberculosis, yet the burden of road traffic injuries is comparable. In response to this crisis, in March 2010 the 64th General Assembly of the United Nations described the global road safety crisis as "a major public health problem" and proclaimed 2011–2020 as "The Decade of Action for Road Safety." On April 19, 2012, the United Nations General Assembly adopted a new resolution (A/66/L.43) to improve global road safety by implementing plans for the decade, setting ambitious targets, and monitoring global road traffic fatalities.

According to Department of State data, road traffic crashes are the leading cause of injury deaths to US citizens while abroad (Figure 2-1). Recent estimates show that 743 US citizens were killed in road traffic crashes from 2009 through 2011. Approximately 16% of these road traffic deaths involved motorcycles, and 7% involved pedestrians. A study from Bermuda reported that the rate of

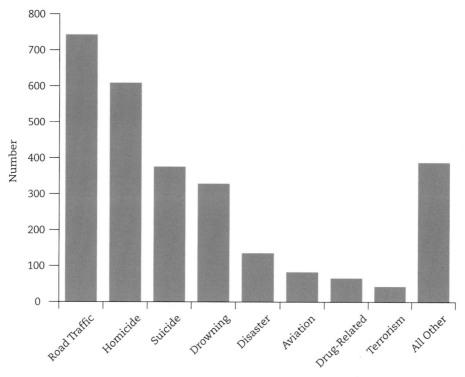

FIGURE 2-1. LEADING CAUSES OF INJURY DEATH FOR US CITIZENS IN FOREIGN COUNTRIES, 2009–2011[1,2]

[1] Data from US Department of State. Death of US citizens abroad by non-natural causes. Washington, DC: US Department of State; 2012. Available from: http://travel.state.gov/law/family_issues/death/death_600.html.
[2] Excludes deaths of US citizens fighting wars in Afghanistan or Iraq.

motorbike injuries is much higher in tourists than in the local population, and the rate is highest in people aged 50–59 years. Motor vehicle rentals in Bermuda and some other small Caribbean islands are typically limited to motorbikes for tourists, possibly contributing to the higher rates of motorbike injuries. Loss of vehicular control, unfamiliar equipment, and inexperience with motorized 2-wheelers contributed to crashes and injuries, even at speeds <30 miles per hour.

Road traffic crashes are common among foreign travelers for a number of reasons: lack of familiarity with the roads, driving on the opposite side of the road, lack of seat belt use, the influence of alcohol, poorly made or maintained vehicles, travel fatigue, poor road surfaces without shoulders, unprotected curves and cliffs, and poor visibility due to lack of adequate lighting. In many LMICs, unsafe roads and vehicles and an inadequate transportation infrastructure contribute to the traffic injury problem. In many of these countries, motor vehicles often share the road with vulnerable road users, such as

pedestrians, bicyclists, and motorcycle users. The mix of traffic involving cars, buses, taxis, rickshaws, large trucks, and even animals (on one road or in a single travel lane) increases the risk for crashes and injuries.

Millions of US citizens travel to Mexico each year, and >150,000 people cross the US–Mexico border daily. Travelers should be particularly cautious in Mexico; from 2009 through 2011, 27% of all deaths of US citizens abroad occurred in Mexico, where >220 lost their lives in motor vehicle crashes, and another 299 were victims of homicide.

Traffic death rates in 20 countries most frequented by US citizens are listed in Table 2-14. Strategies to reduce the risk of traffic injury are shown in Table 2-15. The Association for International Road Travel (www.asirt.org) and Make Roads Safe (www.makeroadssafe.org) have useful safety information for international travelers, including road safety checklists and country-specific driving risks. The Department of State has safety information useful to international travelers, including road safety and security

Table 2-13. Ranking of the countries with the 20 highest estimated traffic death rates
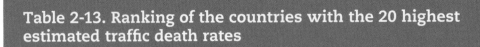

COUNTRY	REPORTED NUMBER OF TRAFFIC DEATHS[1,2]	ESTIMATED TRAFFIC DEATH RATE PER 100,000 POPULATION PER YEAR[1,2]
Eritrea	81	48.4
Cook Islands (New Zealand)	6	45.0
Egypt	15,983	41.6
Libya	2,138	40.5
Afghanistan	1,179	39.0
Iraq	1,932	38.1
Angola	2,358	37.7
Niger	570	37.7
United Arab Emirates	1,056	37.1
The Gambia	54	36.6
Iran	22,918	35.8
Mauritania	262	35.5
Ethiopia	2,441	35.0
Sudan	2,227	34.7
Mozambique	1,952	34.7
Tunisia	1,497	34.5
Kenya	3,760	34.4
Guinea-Bissau	512	34.4
Tanzania	2,595	34.3
Chad	814	34.3

[1] Data from World Health Organization. Global Status Report on Road Safety: Time for Action. Geneva: WHO; 2009. Available from: http://whqlibdoc.who.int/publications/2009/9789241563840_eng.pdf.
[2] Deaths reported in the local population in 2006 or 2007. For comparison, the number of reported traffic deaths in the United States in 2007 was 42,642, with an estimated traffic death rate of 13.9 per 100,000 population.

Table 2-14. Estimated traffic death rates in the 20 countries most frequently traveled by US citizens

COUNTRY[1,2]	REPORTED NUMBER OF TRAFFIC DEATHS[3,4]	ESTIMATED TRAFFIC DEATH RATE PER 100,000 POPULATION PER YEAR[3,4]
Mexico	22,103	20.7
The Philippines	1,185	20.0
Dominican Republic	1,838	17.3
India	105,725	16.8
China	96,611	16.5
Costa Rica	688	15.4
South Korea	6,166	12.8
Jamaica	350	12.3
Colombia	5,409	11.7
Italy	5,669	9.6
Spain	4,104	9.3
Canada	2,889	8.8
Ireland	365	8.5
France	4,620	7.5
Germany	4,949	6.0
Israel	398	5.7
United Kingdom	3,298	5.4
Japan	6,639	5.0
Switzerland	370	4.9
The Netherlands	791	4.8

[1] Hong Kong, Aruba, and Taiwan excluded due to incomplete data.
[2] Data from the US Department of Commerce. 2011 United States resident travel abroad. Washington, DC: US Department of Commerce; 2011. Available from: http://tinet.ita.doc.gov/outreachpages/download_data_table/2011_US_Travel_Abroad.pdf.
[3] World Health Organization. Global Status Report on Road Safety: Time for Action. Geneva: WHO; 2009. Available from: http://whqlibdoc.who.int/publications/2009/9789241563840_eng.pdf.
[4] Deaths reported in the local population in 2006 or 2007. For comparison, the number of reported traffic deaths in the United States in 2007 was 42,642, with an estimated traffic death rate of 13.9 per 100,000 population.

Table 2-15. Recommended strategies to reduce injuries while abroad

MECHANISM OR TYPE OF INJURY	PREVENTION STRATEGIES
Road Traffic Crashes	
Seat belts and child safety seats	Always use safety belts and child safety seats. Rent vehicles with seat belts; when possible, ride in taxis with seat belts and sit in the rear seat; bring child safety seats and booster seats from home for children to ride properly restrained.
Driving hazards	When possible, avoid driving at night in low- and middle-income countries; always pay close attention to the correct side of the road when driving in countries that drive on the left.
Country-specific driving hazards	Check the Association for Safe International Road Travel website for driving hazards or risks by country (www.asirt.org).
Motorcycles, motor bikes, and bicycles	Always wear helmets (bring a helmet from home, if needed). When possible, avoid driving or riding on motorcycles or motorbikes, including motorcycle and motorbike taxis. Traveling overseas is a bad time to learn to drive a motorcycle or motorbike.
Alcohol-impaired driving	Alcohol increases the risk for all causes of injury. Do not drive after consuming alcohol, and avoid riding with someone who has been drinking.
Cellular telephones	Do not use a cellular telephone or text while driving. Many countries have enacted laws banning cellular telephone use while driving, and some countries have made using any kind of telephone, including hands-free, illegal while driving.
Taxis or hired drivers	Ride only in marked taxis, and try to ride in those that have safety belts accessible. Hire drivers familiar with the area.
Bus travel	Avoid riding in overcrowded, overweight, or top-heavy buses or minivans.
Pedestrians	Be alert when crossing streets, especially in countries where motorists drive on the left side of the road. Walk with a companion or someone from the host country.
Other Tips	
Airplane travel	Avoid using local, unscheduled aircraft. If possible, fly on larger planes (>30 seats), in good weather, during the daylight hours, and with experienced pilots. Children <2 years should sit in a child safety seat, not on a parent's lap. Whenever possible, parents should travel with a safety seat for use before, during, and after a plane ride.

continued

TABLE 2-15. RECOMMENDED STRATEGIES TO REDUCE INJURIES WHILE ABROAD (continued)

MECHANISM OR TYPE OF INJURY	PREVENTION STRATEGIES
Drowning	Avoid swimming alone or in unfamiliar waters. Wear life jackets while boating or during water recreation activities.
Burns	Reside below the sixth floor to maximize rescue in case of a fire. Bring your own smoke alarm.
Violence	
Country-specific	The Department of State provides useful safety information for international travelers. Read the consular information sheets, travel warnings, and any public announcements for country-specific personal security risks and safety tips (www.travel.state.gov).
Assault	When in low- and middle-income countries or high-poverty areas, avoid traveling at night in unfamiliar environments. Use alcohol in moderation, and do not travel alone. If confronted, give up all valuables, and do not resist attackers.

alerts, international driving permits, and travel insurance (www.travel.state.gov).

Before flying with children, parents and caregivers should check to make sure that their child restraint system is approved for use on an aircraft. This approval should be printed on the system's information label or on the device itself. The Federal Aviation Administration (FAA) recommends that a child weighing <20 pounds use a rear-facing child restraint system. A forward-facing child safety seat should be used for children weighing 20–40 pounds. FAA has also approved a harness-type device for children weighing 22–44 pounds.

WATER AND AQUATIC INJURIES

Drowning accounts for 2% of all deaths of US citizens abroad. Although risk factors have not been clearly defined, these deaths are most likely related to unfamiliarity with local water currents and conditions, inability to swim, and the absence of lifeguards on duty. Rip currents can be especially dangerous, as are sea animals such as urchins, jellyfish, coral, and sea lice. Alcohol also contributes to drowning and boating mishaps.

Drowning was the leading cause of injury death to US citizens visiting countries where water recreation is a major activity, such as Fiji, The Bahamas, Jamaica, and Costa Rica. Young men are particularly at risk of head and spinal cord injuries from diving into shallow water, and alcohol is a factor in some cases.

Boating can be a hazard, especially if boaters are unfamiliar with the boat, do not know proper boating etiquette or rules for watercraft navigation, or are new to the water environment in a foreign country. Many boating fatalities result from inexperience or failure to wear lifejackets.

Scuba diving is a frequent pursuit of travelers in coastal destinations. The death rate among all divers worldwide is thought to be 15–20 deaths per 100,000 divers per year. Travelers should either be experienced divers or dive with a reliable dive shop and instructors. See the Scuba Diving section later in this chapter for more a more detailed discussion about diving risks and preventive measures.

OTHER UNINTENTIONAL INJURIES

From 2009 through 2011, aviation incidents, drug-related incidents, and deaths classified as "other unintentional injuries" accounted for 18% of all injury deaths to US citizens abroad (Figure 2-1). This figure includes 120

Americans who died as a result of the January 12, 2010, Haiti earthquake. Fires can be a substantial risk in LMICs where building codes do not exist or are not enforced, there are no smoke alarms, there is no emergency access to 9-1-1 services, and the fire department's focus is on putting out fires rather than on fire prevention or victim rescue.

Travel by local, lightweight aircraft in many countries can be risky. From 2009 through 2011, an estimated 83 US citizens abroad were killed in aircraft crashes. Travel on unscheduled flights, in small aircraft, at night, in inclement weather, and with inexperienced pilots carries the highest risk.

Travel health providers, vendors of travel services, and travelers themselves should consider the following:

- Travelers should consider purchasing special travel health and medical evacuation insurance if their destinations include countries where there may not be access to good medical care (see the Travel Insurance, Travel Health Insurance, & Medical Evacuation Insurance section later in this chapter).
- Because trauma care is poor in many countries, victims of injuries and violence can die before reaching a hospital, and there may be no coordinated ambulance service available. In remote areas, medical assistance and modern drugs may be unavailable, and travel to the nearest medical facility can take a long time.
- Adventure activities, such as mountain climbing, skydiving, whitewater rafting, dune-buggying, and kayaking, are popular with travelers. The lack of rapid emergency trauma response, inadequate trauma care in remote locations, and sudden, unexpected weather changes that compromise safety and hamper rescue efforts, can delay access to care.
- Travelers should avoid using local, unscheduled, small aircraft. If available, choose larger aircraft (>30 seats), as they have most likely undergone more strict and regular safety inspections. Larger aircraft also provide more protection in the event of a crash. For country-specific airline crash events, see www.airsafe.com.
- When traveling by air with young children, consider bringing a child safety seat approved for use on an aircraft.

- To prevent fire-related injuries, travelers should select accommodations no higher than the sixth floor. (Fire ladders generally cannot reach higher than the sixth floor.) Hotels should be checked for smoke alarms and preferably sprinkler systems. Travelers may want to bring their own smoke alarm. Two escape routes from buildings should always be identified. Crawling low under smoke and covering one's mouth with a wet cloth are helpful in escaping a fire. Families should agree on a meeting place outside the building in case a fire erupts.
- Improperly vented heating devices may cause poisoning from carbon monoxide. Carbon monoxide at the back of boats near the engine can be especially dangerous. Travelers may want to carry a personal detector that can sound an alert in the presence of this lethal gas.
- Travelers should consider learning basic first aid and CPR before travel overseas with another person. Travelers should bring a travel health kit, which should be customized to the anticipated itinerary and activities (see the Travel Health Kits section later in this chapter).

VIOLENCE-RELATED INJURIES

Violence is a leading worldwide public health problem and a growing concern of US citizens traveling, working, or residing abroad. Each year, >1.6 million people lose their lives to violence, and only one-fifth are casualties of armed conflicts. Rates of violent deaths in LMICs are >3 times those in higher-income countries, although there are variations within countries.

Homicide is the second-leading cause of injury death among US citizens abroad; it accounted for >600 deaths from 2009 through 2011 (Figure 2-1). For some LMICs, such as the Dominican Republic, Honduras, Mexico, and the Philippines, homicide was the leading cause of injury death for US citizens, accounting for 41% of all US citizen injury deaths in those 4 countries.

Travelers to foreign countries are viewed by many criminals as wealthy, naïve targets, who are inexperienced, unfamiliar with the culture, and inept at seeking assistance once victimized. Traveling in high-poverty areas or regions of civil unrest, using alcohol or drugs, and traveling in unfamiliar environments at night increase the likelihood that a traveler will be the victim of violence.

To avoid violence while abroad, travelers should limit travel at night, travel with a companion, and vary routine travel habits. Travelers abroad should not wear expensive clothing or accessories. Criminals are less likely to victimize upper floors of buildings, so travelers should avoid accommodations on the ground floor and avoid rooms immediately next to the stairs. Travelers should lock all doors and windows and may even consider carrying and using a door intruder alarm and a rubber doorstop that can be used as a supplemental lock. If confronted, travelers should give up all valuables and not resist attackers. Victims of a crime overseas should contact the nearest US embassy, consulate, or consular agency for assistance.

Suicide is the third-leading cause of injury death to US citizens abroad (13%). For longer-term travelers (such as missionaries and volunteers), social isolation and substance abuse, particularly in the face of living in areas of poverty and rigid gender roles, may increase the risk of depression and suicide. See the Mental Health & Travel section later in this chapter for more detailed information.

BIBLIOGRAPHY

1. ASIRT.org [Internet]. Rockville, MD: Association for Safe International Road Travel; c2002–12 [cited 2012 Sep 18]. Available from: www.asirt.org.

2. Balaban V, Sleet D. Prevention of injuries to children traveling. In: Kamat D, Fischer P, editors. Textbook of Child Global Health. Elk Grove Village, IL: American Academy of Pediatrics; 2011.

3. Ball DJ, Machin N. Foreign travel and the risk of harm. Int J Inj Contr Saf Promot. 2006 Jun;13(2):107–15.

4. Carey MJ, Aitken ME. Motorbike injuries in Bermuda: a risk for tourists. Ann Emerg Med. 1996 Oct;28(4):424–9.

5. Cortes LM, Hargarten SW, Hennes HM. Recommendations for water safety and drowning prevention for travelers. J Travel Med. 2006 Jan–Feb;13(1):21–34.

6. Death of US citizens abroad by non-natural causes [database on the Internet]. US Department of State. c2002– [cited 2012 Sep 18]. Available from: http://travel.state.gov/law/family_issues/death/death_600.html.

7. FIA Foundation for the Automobile and Society. Make roads safe report: a decade of action for road safety. FIA Foundation for the Automobile and Society; 2009 [cited 2012 Sep 18]. Available from: http://www.fiafoundation.org/publications/Pages/PublicationHome.aspx.

8. Guse CE, Cortes LM, Hargarten SW, Hennes HM. Fatal injuries of US citizens abroad. J Travel Med. 2007 Sep–Oct;14(5):279–87.

9. Krug EG, Mercy JA, Dahlberg LL, Zwi AB. The world report on violence and health. Lancet. 2002 Oct 5;360(9339):1083–8.

10. Lawson CJ, Dykewicz CA, Molinari NA, Lipman H, Alvarado-Ramy F. Deaths in international travelers arriving in the United States, July 1, 2005 to June 30, 2008. J Travel Med. 2012 Mar–Apr;19(2):96–103.

11. Leggat PA, Fischer PR. Accidents and repatriation. Travel Med Infect Dis. 2006 May–Jul;4(3–4):135–46.

12. Li G, Pressley JC, Qiang Y, Grabowski JG, Baker SP, Rebok GW. Geographic region, weather, pilot age, and air carrier crashes: a case-control study. Aviat Space Environ Med. 2009 Apr;80(4):386–90.

13. McInnes RJ, Williamson LM, Morrison A. Unintentional injury during foreign travel: a review. J Travel Med. 2002 Nov–Dec;9(6):297–307.

14. Patel D. Occupational travel. Occup Med. 2011 Jan;61(1):6–18.

15. Peden M, Scurfield R, Sleet D, Mohan D, Hyder AA, Jarawan E, et al. World report on road traffic injury prevention. Geneva: World Health Organization; 2004.

16. Tonellato DJ, Guse CE, Hargarten SW. Injury deaths of US citizens abroad: new data source, old travel problem. J Travel Med. 2009 Sep-Oct;16(5):304–10.

17. US Department of Commerce. 2008 United States resident travel abroad. Washington, DC: US Department of Commerce; 2010 [cited 2012 Sep 18]. Available from: http://tinet.ita.doc.gov/outreachpages/download_data_table/2008_US_Travel_Abroad.pdf.

18. US Department of State. Tips for traveling abroad. Washington, DC: US Department of State; 2012 [cited 2012 Sep 18]. Available from: http://www.travel.state.gov/travel/tips/tips_1232.html.

19. World Health Organization. Mobile phone use: a growing problem of driver distraction. Geneva: World Health Organization; 2011 [cited 2012 Sep 18]. Available from: http://www.who.int/violence_injury_prevention/publications/road_traffic/distracted_driving_en.pdf.

Perspectives

TERRORISM
Ashika Devi Bhan, Ali S. Khan

The explosion on Pan Am Flight 103 over Lockerbie in 1988. The 1997 Luxor massacre in Egypt. The 2002 Bali nightclub bombing. The Madrid train attacks of 2004, and the London Underground explosions the following year. The Mumbai Taj hotel attack in 2008. Even though such events are rare, terrorist attacks arouse a great deal of concern among travelers. They also demonstrate that travelers can become victims of terrorism, either directed against the country in which they are traveling or specifically targeted against foreigners in the country. In the latter case, travelers' risk is based on their apparent country of origin and may be higher than the overall risk in the country they are visiting. In either circumstance, the unpredictable nature of terrorism has become an unfortunate part of the travel and tourism landscape.

From October 2002 through December 2011, 289 American citizens abroad died as a result of terrorist action (about 4% of nonnatural deaths). In 2010 alone, >11,500 terrorist attacks were reported in 72 countries, injuring approximately 50,000 people and killing 13,200. US citizens were among the victims: 15 were killed and 9 were injured in 2010. More than 75% of these terrorist incidents took place in South Asia and the Near East.

Although these data may alarm potential travelers, it is important to keep the threat of terrorism in perspective. An estimated 28.5 million US residents traveled abroad in 2010, and the leading cause of death of US citizens in foreign countries is not crime or terrorism but motor vehicle crashes. From 2009 through 2011, road traffic crashes accounted for 27% of US citizen deaths abroad due to injuries, followed by homicide (22%) and drowning (12%). When the adverse events that can happen during travel are ranked by likelihood, terrorism is near the bottom of a very long list.

Although unlikely, when terrorism does occur, the aftermath can be devastating, and travelers can take measures to reduce their risk of either being a target or becoming caught in the crossfire. The first and perhaps best protection is to avoid travel to areas with a persistent record of terrorist incidents. Some countries consistently rank among the most dangerous for American travelers. The Department of State (www.state.gov) maintains travel warnings, issues security alerts, and updates reports on global terrorism and countries to avoid.

The Department of State provides additional information about terrorism that can be useful for citizens abroad. Travelers are advised that terrorists may use tactics such as bombings, suicide operations, shootings, assassinations, kidnappings, hijackings, and the use of chemical, biological, radiologic, or nuclear materials. The weapons they use may be conventional or unconventional. Their targets can be both official and private interests, including residential areas, business offices, hotels, restaurants, clubs, markets, schools, places of worship, public areas, high-profile sporting events, and other tourist destinations where travelers gather. Terrorists are also likely to attack public transportation systems and other tourist infrastructure. Many have targeted or attempted to attack not only aviation but also subways, rail systems, and maritime transportation.

Travelers can minimize their risk of being a victim of terrorism abroad by taking a number of common-sense precautions. The following guidelines can be used by any traveler but may be especially important for those who are visiting a high-risk destination:

Before departing:

- Safety begins before leaving home. The Department of State encourages travelers to enroll in the Smart Traveler Enrollment Program, a free service provided by the US government to citizens who are traveling to (or living in) a foreign country. This program provides up-to-date safety and security announcements and makes it easier for the embassy to contact enrollees in an emergency.
- Obtain as much country-specific information as possible from the Department of State, travel agencies, and passport offices. Learn about products and services offering travel assistance.
- Schedule direct flights and fly to safer cities, if possible. Avoid stops in high-risk airports or areas.
- Keep luggage to a minimum—overburdened travelers are easy targets. Carry on as little as possible. If luggage is checked, hide luggage tags that include personal information such as name, address, or company name.
- Leave behind a folder of important information, such as copies of important papers, legal documents, financial records, itineraries, and instructions in case of an incident.
- When packing, choose clothing that does not single you out as a tourist (such as T-shirts emblazoned with the flag or logos of the traveler's local sports team). Try to blend in with the locals.

Upon arrival:

- Minimize time spent in publicly accessible areas of the airport, which are less protected. Move quickly from the check-in counter to secured areas. Leave the airport as soon as possible.
- Keep an eye out for and avoid abandoned packages, briefcases, and other suspicious items; report them to airport authorities.
- Register with the US embassy or consulate. Keep a card containing their phone number, along with other emergency numbers.
- Take only well-marked modes of local transportation. For taxis, check the driver's name and license. Rent a car (similar to local models) from an established company.
- Know where the nearest emergency exits are.

While touring the country:

- Keep a low profile, particularly in areas frequented by foreign tourists. Dress and act so that you avoid attention. Remain as anonymous as possible.
- Do not give out your name, company, or position to strangers. Be cautious about what you say to strangers or what others may overhear. Do not discuss travel plans with those without a need to know.

- Exercise caution in public transportation systems and other tourist infrastructure, such as subways, train stations, elevators, marketplaces, and festivals.
- When renting a car, check for loose wires or suspicious activity around it. Drive with the windows closed.
- Avoid public demonstrations and other civil disturbances.
- Avoid situations in which anti-American sentiments may be expressed.
- Do not display items that may be offensive to local customs or culture. These vary by location but may include political documents, religious items, pornography, or liquor.
- Avoid patterns and routines that provide an easy target. Vary the time and route of regular outings if you are in a location for an extended period. Be wary of people observing your comings and goings.
- Look out for unattended packages or bags in public places and other crowded areas. Be cautious of unexpected packages. Report any suspicious activity to local police. Many terrorist attacks are foiled by the vigilance of ordinary people.
- Be aware of the location of safe havens such as police stations, hotels, and hospitals. Devise a plan of action to be used if an incident occurs.
- Do not invite strangers into your hotel room or meet at unfamiliar or remote locations.
- Regularly check travel advice and information for the country being visited. Watch and read daily news reports about the region.

These strategies incorporate the same defensive alertness and good judgment that people should use to keep safe from crime at home or abroad. Awareness (not paranoia) is key—taking precautions to be aware of surroundings and adopting protective measures. Although the odds are in favor of a safe trip, travelers can and do become victims of terrorism. The possibility of terrorist threats should not take away from the adventure and joys of travel, but the wise traveler will weigh the risks, plan ahead, and take safety measures to ensure peace of mind during the journey.

BIBLIOGRAPHY

1. Death of US citizens abroad by non-natural causes [database on the Internet]. US Department of State. c2002– [cited 2012 Sep 18]. Available from: http://travel.state.gov/law/family_issues/death/death_600.html.

2. US Department of Commerce, International Trade Administration. Profile of US resident travelers visiting overseas destinations: 2010 outbound. Washington, DC: US Department of Commerce; 2011 [cited 2012 Sep 18]. Available from: http://tinet.ita.doc.gov/outreachpages/download_data_table/2010_Outbound_Profile.pdf.

3. US Department of State. A safe trip abroad. Washington, DC: US Department of State; 2012 [cited 2012 Sep 18]. Available from: http://travel.state.gov/travel/tips/safety/safety_1747.html.

4. US Department of State. Tips for traveling abroad. Washington, DC: US Department of State; 2012 [cited 2012 Sep 18]. Available from: http://travel.state.gov/travel/tips/tips_1232.html#terrorism.

5. US Department of State. Worldwide Caution. Washington, DC: US Department of State; 2012 [cited 2012 Sep 18]. Available from: http://travel.state.gov/travel/cis_pa_tw/pa/pa_4787.html.

6. US Department of State, Office of the Coordinator for Counterterrorism. Country reports on terrorism 2010. Washington, DC: US Department of State; 2011 [cited 2012 Sep 19]. Available from: http://www.state.gov/documents/organization/170479.pdf.

ANIMAL-ASSOCIATED HAZARDS

Nina Marano, G. Gale Galland

HUMAN INTERACTION WITH ANIMALS: A RISK FACTOR FOR INJURY AND ILLNESS

Animals tend to avoid humans, but they can attack if they perceive threat, are protecting their young or territory, or are injured or ill. Although attacks by wild animals are more dramatic, attacks by domestic animals are far more common, and secondary infections of wounds may result in serious systemic disease. In addition, animals can transmit zoonotic infections such as rabies. Of the estimated 35,000–55,000 rabies deaths every year worldwide, >95% occur as a result of dog bites in the developing countries of Africa and Asia. A recent 10-year retrospective review of dog bites in Austria showed that 75% of the bites were preventable because the person had intentionally interacted with the dog.

BITE OR SCRATCH WOUNDS

Animal bites present a risk for rabies, tetanus, and other bacterial infections. Animals' saliva can be so heavily contaminated with bacteria that a bite may not even be necessary to cause infection if the animal licks a preexisting cut or scratch. Young children are more likely to be bitten by animals and to sustain more severe injuries from animal bites.

Prevention

Before departure, travelers should have a current tetanus vaccination or documentation of having received a booster vaccination within the previous 5–10 years. Travel health providers should assess a traveler's need for preexposure rabies immunization according to the guidelines in Table 3-15. While traveling, people should never try to pet, handle, or feed unfamiliar animals (whether domestic or wild, even in captive settings such as game ranches or wild animal petting zoos), particularly in areas where rabies is endemic. To mitigate the risk of exposure to rabies, dogs and other mammals should be avoided.

Management

In order to prevent infection, all wounds should be promptly cleaned with soap and water, and the wound promptly debrided, if necrotic tissue, dirt, or other foreign materials are present. These steps of wound care are especially important for tetanus- or rabies-prone wounds (see the Rabies and Tetanus sections in Chapter 3). Travelers who might have been exposed to rabies should contact a reliable health care provider as soon as possible for advice about rabies postexposure prophylaxis. Travelers who received their most recent tetanus toxoid–containing vaccine >5 years previously, or who have not received ≥3 doses of tetanus toxoid–containing vaccines, may require a dose of tetanus toxoid–containing vaccine (Tdap, Td, or DTaP) according to ACIP guidelines.

MONKEYS

Macaques are native to Asia and North Africa. Additionally, descendants of North African populations of Barbary macaques inhabit Gibraltar, the only place that wild populations of macaques are found in Europe. They are also housed in research facilities, zoos, and wildlife or amusement parks and are kept as pets in private homes throughout the world. Monkey bites occasionally occur in certain urban sites, such as temples in Nepal or India.

Macaque bites can transmit herpes B virus, a virus related to the herpes simplex viruses that cause oral and genital ulcers. Herpes B infection is rare in humans. The virus was discovered in 1933, and since that time approximately 50 human cases have been reported, with an 80% case-fatality ratio. No cases of herpes B infection have been reported in people exposed to monkeys in the wild. Most documented cases have resulted from occupational exposures. However, travelers to areas where macaques range freely should be aware of the potential risk. A monkey infected with herpes B may appear completely healthy.

Documented routes of human infection with herpes B virus include animal bites and scratches, exposure to infected tissue or body fluids from splashes, and in one instance, human-to-human transmission. Even minor scratches or bites should be considered potential exposures, because, experimentally, herpes B virus has been isolated from surfaces for up to 2 weeks after it was applied. The incubation period ranges from <1 week to 1 month or longer. Neurologic symptoms develop as the virus infects the central nervous system and may lead to ascending paralysis and respiratory failure. Increased public and clinician awareness about the risks associated with an injury from a macaque, improved first aid after exposure, the availability of better diagnostic tests, and improved antiviral therapeutics have decreased the case-fatality ratio to 20% in treated people. As a result, from 1987 through 2004 only 5 infections were fatal.

Although only macaque bites pose a herpes B virus threat, any monkey bite may pose a threat for rabies.

Prevention

Travelers should never attempt to feed, pet, or otherwise handle any monkeys.

Management

After a monkey bite or scratch, travelers should be advised to thoroughly clean the wound and seek medical care immediately to be evaluated for possible rabies and herpes B postexposure prophylaxis. Additional information and photos of macaques can be found at the website for the National B Virus Resource Center at the Georgia State University Viral Immunology Center (www2.gsu.edu/~wwwvir).

BATS

Bats can be found almost anywhere in the world except the polar regions and extreme deserts. Bats are reservoir hosts for viruses that can cross species barriers to infect humans and other domestic and wild mammals. Viral infections such as rabies and viral hemorrhagic fevers can be transmitted from bats to people. It is not possible to tell if a bat has rabies; however, any bat that is active by day, is found where bats are not usually seen (for example, indoors or outdoors in areas near humans), or is unable to fly is far more likely to be rabid. A recent example of an imported case of Marburg fever in a tourist who had visited a "python cave" in western Uganda illustrates the risk of acquiring diseases from contact with cave-dwelling bats. This same cave was the source of a fatal case of Marburg hemorrhagic fever in a Dutch tourist in 2008. Exposure to bats can occur during adventure activities, such as caving or spelunking, and can include bites, scratches, and mucosal or cutaneous exposure to bat saliva. Like any other wild animal, bats, whether sick or healthy, will bite in self-defense if handled.

Prevention

Bats should never be handled. Travelers should be discouraged from going into caves or mines that have large bat infestations. Depending on the country being visited, preexposure rabies vaccination may be recommended for people engaged in activities such as caving.

Management

If a bite occurs or if infectious material (such as saliva) from a bat gets into the eyes, nose, mouth, or a wound, the traveler should wash the affected area thoroughly and get medical advice immediately. Any suspected or documented bite or scratch from a bat anywhere in the world should be grounds for seeking postexposure rabies immunoprophylaxis.

People usually know when they have been bitten by a bat. However, bats have tiny teeth, and not all wounds may be apparent. Travelers should seek medical advice even in the absence of an obvious bite wound if they wake up to find a bat in the room or see a bat in the room of an unattended child.

RODENTS

Rodents carry a variety of viral, bacterial, and parasitic agents that may pose a threat to human health. Human exposure can occur directly by a bite or scratch, or indirectly by exposure to surfaces or water contaminated with urine or feces. Rodents should never be handled. Travelers should avoid places that have evidence of infestation with rodents and should avoid contact with rodent feces. Travelers should not eat or drink anything that is suspected to be contaminated by rodent feces or urine.

Management

Wild rodents are unlikely to have rabies; how-ever, each exposure needs to be evaluated as follows:

- If the bite was provoked (such as through feeding, petting, or playing with the animal) and the animal appeared healthy, the ani-mal was probably not rabid at the time of the bite. Most experts would not recommend postexposure prophylaxis in this situation.
- If the bite was unprovoked or the animal appeared unhealthy and is unavailable for testing, rabies postexposure prophylaxis should be considered.

Travelers who were exposed to rodents and who develop febrile illness shortly after returning home should be evaluated by a cli-nician. Depending on the history and symp-toms, diseases such as yersiniosis, plague, leptospirosis, hantavirus and rickettsial infec-tions, Lyme disease, tickborne encephalitis, poxvirus, and bartonellosis (all discussed in further detail in Chapter 3) should be included in the list of possible diagnoses.

SNAKES

Poisonous snakes are hazards in many loca-tions, although deaths from snakebites are rare. Snakebites usually occur in areas where dense human populations coexist with dense snake populations, such as Southeast Asia, sub-Saharan Africa, and tropical areas in the Americas.

Prevention

Common sense is the best precaution. Most snake bites result from startling, handling, or harassing snakes. Therefore, all snakes should be left alone. Travelers should be aware of their surroundings, especially at night and during warm weather when snakes tend to be more active. For extra precaution, when prac-tical, travelers should wear heavy, ankle-high or higher boots and long pants when walking outdoors in areas possibly inhabited by ven-omous snakes.

Management

Travelers should be advised to seek imme-diate medical attention any time a bite wound breaks the skin or when snake venom is ejected into their eyes or mucous membranes. Immobilization of the affected limb and application of a pressure bandage that does not restrict blood flow are recom-mended first aid measures while the victim is moved as quickly as possible to a medical facility. Incision of the bite site and tourni-quets that restrict blood flow to the affected limb are not recommended. Specific therapy for snakebites is controversial and should be left to the judgment of local emergency medi-cal personnel. Specific antivenoms are avail-able for some snakes in some areas, so trying to ascertain the species of snake that bit the victim may be critical.

INSECTS AND OTHER ARTHROPODS

Bites and stings from spiders and scorpions can be painful and can result in illness and death, particularly among infants and chil-dren. Other insects and arthropods, such as mosquitoes and ticks, can transmit infec-tions. See the Protection against Mosquitoes, Ticks, & Other Insects & Arthropods section earlier in this chapter.

MARINE ANIMALS

Most marine animals are generally harm-less unless threatened. Most injuries are the result of chance encounters or defensive maneuvers. Resulting wounds have many common characteristics: bacterial contami-nation, foreign bodies, and occasionally venom. Venomous injuries from marine fish and invertebrates are increasing with the popularity of surfing, scuba diving, and snor-keling. Most species responsible for human injuries, including stingrays, jellyfish, stone-fish, sea urchins, and scorpionfish, live in tropical coastal waters.

Prevention

Travelers should be advised to maintain vigi-lance while engaging in recreational water activities. Prevention is the best defense:

- Avoid contact. This may be difficult in con-ditions of poor visibility, rough water, cur-rents, and confined areas.
- Do not attempt to feed, handle, tease, or annoy marine animals.
- Wear protective clothing, such as protec-tive footwear.
- Make an effort to find out which animals may be encountered at the destination

and learn about their characteristics and habitats before engaging in recreational water activities.

Management

In case of injury, identifying the species involved can help determine the best course of treatment. Signs and symptoms may not appear for hours after contact, or the animal may not have been seen or recognized at the time of injury. In such cases treatment is based on the injury presentation. Symptoms of venomous injuries can range from mild swelling and redness at the site to more severe symptoms, such as difficulty breathing or swallowing, chest pain, or intense pain at the site of the sting, for which immediate medical treatment should be sought. Management will vary according to the severity of symptoms and can include medications, such as diphenhydramine, steroids, pain medication, and antibiotics.

BIRDS

Ill birds have been associated with cases of highly pathogenic avian influenza in humans. When traveling in an area where outbreaks of avian influenza have been reported, travelers should avoid contact with live poultry (such as chickens, ducks, geese, pigeons, turkeys, and quail) or any wild birds and should avoid settings where avian influenza A (H5N1)-infected poultry may be present, such as commercial or backyard poultry farms and live poultry markets. Travelers should not eat uncooked or undercooked poultry or poultry products, including dishes that contain uncooked eggs or poultry blood. Other pathogens from birds may infect humans through infected feces or by aerosol. These cause diseases such as histoplasmosis (see Chapter 3, Histoplasmosis), salmonellosis (see Chapter 3, Salmonellosis [Nontyphoidal]), psittacosis, and avian mycobacteriosis. Travelers should wash their hands if they come in contact with bird feces.

BIBLIOGRAPHY

1. Callahan M. Bites, stings and envenoming injuries. In: Keystone JS, Freedman DO, Kozarsky PE, Connor BA, Nothdurft HD, editors. Travel Medicine. 3rd ed. Philadelphia: Saunders Elsevier; 2013. p. 413–24.

2. CDC. Dog-bite-related fatalities—United States, 1995–1996. MMWR Morb Mortal Wkly Rep. 1997 May 30;46(21):463–7.

3. CDC. Nonfatal dog bite-related injuries treated in hospital emergency departments—United States, 2001. MMWR Morb Mortal Wkly Rep. 2003 Jul 4;52(26):605–10.

4. Cohen JI, Davenport DS, Stewart JA, Deitchman S, Hilliard JK, Chapman LE. Recommendations for prevention of and therapy for exposure to B virus (cercopithecine herpesvirus 1). Clin Infect Dis. 2002 Nov 15;35(10):1191–203.

5. Davis RF, Johnston GA, Sladden MJ. Recognition and management of common ectoparasitic diseases in travelers. Am J Clin Dermatol. 2009;10(1):1–8.

6. Diaz JH. The global epidemiology, syndromic classification, management, and prevention of spider bites. Am J Trop Med Hyg. 2004 Aug;71(2):239–50.

7. Feldman KA, Trent R, Jay MT. Epidemiology of hospitalizations resulting from dog bites in California, 1991–1998. Am J Public Health. 2004 Nov;94(11):1940–1.

8. Gibbons RV. Cryptogenic rabies, bats, and the question of aerosol transmission. Ann Emerg Med. 2002 May;39(5):528–36.

9. Gold BS, Dart RC, Barish RA. Bites of venomous snakes. N Engl J Med. 2002 Aug 1;347(5):347–56.

10. Huff JL, Barry PA. B-virus (cercopithecine herpesvirus 1) infection in humans and macaques: potential for zoonotic disease. Emerg Infect Dis. 2003 Feb;9(2):246–50.

11. Löe J, Röskaft E. Large carnivores and human safety: a review. Ambio. 2004 Aug;33(6):283–8.

12. Meerburg BG, Singleton GR, Kijlstra A. Rodent-borne diseases and their risks for public health. Crit Rev Microbiol. 2009;35(3):221–70.

13. Pan American Health Organization. Rabies. In: Acha PN, Szyfres B, editors. Zoonoses and Communicable Diseases Common to Man and Animals. 3rd ed. Washington, DC: Pan American Health Organization; 2003. p. 246–76.

14. Schalamon J, Ainoedhofer H, Singer G, Petnehazy T, Mayr J, Kiss K, et al. Analysis of dog bites in children who are younger than 17 years. Pediatrics. 2006 Mar;117(3):e374–9.

15. Warrell DA. Treatment of bites by adders and exotic venomous snakes. BMJ. 2005 Nov 26;331(7527):1244–7.

16. World Health Organization. WHO Expert Consultation on rabies. World Health Organ Tech Rep Ser. 2005;931:1–88.

NATURAL DISASTERS & ENVIRONMENTAL HAZARDS

Josephine Malilay, Dahna Batts, Armin Ansari, Charles W. Miller, Clive M. Brown

NATURAL DISASTERS

Travelers should be aware of the potential for natural phenomena such as hurricanes, floods, tsunamis, tornadoes, or earthquakes. Natural disasters can contribute to the transmission of some diseases, especially since water supplies and sewage systems may be disrupted; sanitation and hygiene may be compromised by population displacement and overcrowding; and normal public health services may be interrupted.

When arriving at a destination, travelers should be familiar with local risks for seismic, flood-related, landslide-related, tsunami-related, and other hazards, as well as warning systems, evacuation routes, and shelters in areas of high risk.

Disease Risks

The risk for infectious diseases among travelers to affected areas is minimal unless a disease is endemic in an area before the disaster, because transmission cannot take place unless the causative agent is present. Although typhoid can be endemic in developing countries, natural disasters have seldom led to epidemic levels of disease. Floods have been known to prompt outbreaks of leptospirosis and cholera in areas where the organism is found in water sources (see the Leptospirosis and Cholera sections in Chapter 3).

When water and sewage systems have been disrupted, safe water and food supplies are of great importance in preventing enteric disease transmission. If contamination is suspected, water should be boiled or disinfected (see the Water Disinfection for Travelers section earlier in this chapter). Travelers who are injured during a natural disaster should have a medical evaluation to determine what additional care may be required for wounds potentially contaminated with feces, soil, or saliva, or that have been exposed to fresh or sea water that may contain parasites or bacteria.

Tetanus booster status should always be kept current.

Various vaccine-preventable diseases have been eliminated or are near elimination in some developing countries. However, if someone who has the disease travels to the country, the disease could be reintroduced, leading to an outbreak. Therefore, it is very important that people traveling to offer relief or other services in countries affected by natural disasters be protected against such diseases or not be sick when entering a country.

Injuries

After a natural disaster, deaths are rarely due to infectious diseases. Rather they are most often due to blunt trauma, crush-related injuries, or drowning. Therefore, travelers should be aware of the risks for injury during and after a natural disaster. In floods, people should avoid driving through swiftly moving water. Travelers should exercise caution during clean-up, particularly when encountering downed power lines, water-affected electrical outlets, interrupted gas lines, and stray or frightened animals. During natural disasters, technological malfunctions may release hazardous materials (such as release of toxic chemicals from a point source displaced by strong winds, seismic motion, or rapidly moving water).

Environmental Risks

Natural disasters often lead to wide-ranging air pollution in large cities. For example, uncontrolled forest fires have caused widespread pollution over vast expanses. Natural or manmade disasters resulting in massive structural collapse or dust clouds can cause the release of chemical or biologic contaminants (such as asbestos or the arthrospores that lead to coccidioidomycosis). Health risks associated with these environmental occurrences have not been fully studied. Travelers with chronic pulmonary disease or who are immunocompromised may be more suscep-tible to adverse effects from these types of exposures.

Event-Specific Information

Typically, after natural disasters of a magni-tude that may affect travelers, current infor-mation about the disaster, as well as travel health information specific to those need-ing to travel to the affected area, is provided on the CDC website (www.cdc.gov/travel). Recommendations may include specific immunizations or cautions about unique hazards in the affected area.

ENVIRONMENTAL HAZARDS
Air

Air pollution may be found in large cities throughout the world; its sources are often attributed to automobile exhaust and indus-trial emissions and may be aggravated by cli-mate and geography. Specifically, particulate matter (PM), or particle pollution, consisting of fine particles 2.5 µm or smaller in diam-eter, may enter the lungs and cause serious health problems. Travelers should be aware that global long-term average PM2.5 concen-trations have been estimated to exceed the World Health Organization's Air Quality PM2.5 Interim Target-1 (35 µg/m^3 annual average) in eastern and central Asia and North Africa.

Although the harmful effects of air pol-lution are difficult to avoid when visiting some cities, limiting strenuous activity and not smoking can help. Any risk to healthy short-term travelers to such areas is probably small, but people with preexisting health conditions (such as asthma, chronic obstructive pulmo-nary disease, or heart disease) could be more susceptible. Avoiding dust clouds and areas of heavy dust or haze is wise.

Water

Rivers, lakes, and oceans may be contami-nated with organic or inorganic chemical compounds (such as heavy metals or other toxins); harmful algal blooms (cyanobacteria) that can be toxic both to fish and to people who eat the fish, or who swim or bathe in the water; and pathogens from human and ani-mal waste that may cause disease in swim-mers. Such hazards may not be immediately apparent in a body of water. Available drink-ing water may also be contaminated; see the

Water Disinfection for Travelers section ear-lier in this chapter for guidance on ensuring water is safe to drink.

Extensive water damage after major hurricanes and floods increases the likeli-hood of mold contamination in buildings. Travelers may visit flooded areas overseas as part of emergency, medical, or humanitar-ian missions. Mold is a more serious hazard for people with conditions such as impaired host defenses or mold allergies. To prevent exposure that could result in adverse health effects from disturbed mold, people should adhere to the following recommendations:

- Avoid areas where mold contamination is obvious.
- Use personal protective equipment (PPE), such as gloves, goggles, and a tight-fitting approved N-95 respirator. Travelers should take sufficient PPE with them, as these may be scarce in the countries visited.
- Keep hands, skin, and clothing clean and free from mold-contaminated dust.
- Review the CDC guidance, Mold Prevention Strategies and Possible Health Effects in the Aftermath of Hurricanes and Major Floods (www.cdc.gov/mmwr/preview/mmwrhtml/rr5508a1.htm), which provides recommen-dations for dealing with mold in these settings.

Radiation

Natural background radiation levels can vary substantially from region to region, but these natural variations are not a health concern for either the traveler or resident population. Travelers should be aware of regions known to have been contaminated with radioactive materials, such as the areas surrounding the Chernobyl nuclear power plant in Ukraine and the Fukushima Daiichi nuclear power plant in Japan.

The Chernobyl plant is located 100 km (62 miles) northwest of Kiev. This 1986 acci-dent contaminated regions in 3 republics—Ukraine, Belarus, and Russia—with the highest radioactive ground contamination within 30 km (19 miles) of Chernobyl.

The Fukushima Daiichi plant is located 240 km (150 miles) north of Tokyo. The area within a 20-km (32-mile) radius of the plant is restricted, and Japanese authorities also advised evacuation from locations farther away to the northwest of the plant. This incident occurred in 2011, and as Japanese authorities continue to clean the affected areas and monitor the situation, travel advisories may change. US travelers are advised to check the website of the US embassy in Tokyo for up-to-date information. There are no travel advisories for Tokyo or any city or region south of Tokyo. Travelers who choose to reside for >1 year within 80 km of the Fukushima Daiichi nuclear plant should consult with local authorities to receive guidance on expected levels of radiation and recommendations for reducing exposure to radiation. In addition, pregnant women, children, and the elderly should avoid residing within 30 km of the Fukushima Daiichi Nuclear Plant.

More than 450,000 travelers to the United States originate from Japan each month. During the height of the Fukushima releases, there was some concern about those travelers bringing contamination into the United States with them. Based on radiologic contamination screening at points of entry into the United States, 3 travelers arriving from Japan after the incident had low levels of contamination and were not considered to pose a health hazard to themselves or others.

In most countries, known areas of radioactive contamination are fenced or marked with signs. These areas should not be trespassed. Any traveler seeking long-term (more than a few months) residence near a known or suspected contaminated area should consult with staff of the nearest US embassy and inquire about any applicable advisories in that area regarding drinking water quality or purchase of meat, fruit, and vegetables from local farmers. Radiation emergencies are rare events. In case of such an emergency, however, travelers should follow instructions provided by local emergency and public health authorities. If such information is not forthcoming, US travelers should immediately seek advice from the nearest US embassy.

Natural disasters (such as floods) may also displace industrial or clinical radioactive sources. In all circumstances, travelers should exercise caution when they encounter unknown objects or equipment, especially if they bear the radioactive symbol. Travelers who encounter a questionable object should notify authorities.

BIBLIOGRAPHY

1. Ansari A. Radiation threats and your safety: a guide to preparation and response for professionals and community. Boca Raton, FL: Taylor & Francis/CRC Press; 2009.
2. Brandt M, Brown C, Burkhart J, Burton N, Cox-Ganser J, Damon S, et al. Mold prevention strategies and possible health effects in the aftermath of hurricanes and major floods. MMWR Recomm Rep. 2006 Jun 9;55(RR-8):1–27.
3. Eisenbud M, Gesell TF. Environmental Radioactivity: from Natural, Industrial, and Military Sources. 4th ed. San Diego: Academic Press; 1997.
4. Food and Drug Administration, Center for Devices and Radiological Health. Accidental radioactive contamination of human food and animal feeds: recommendations for state and local agencies. Rockville, MD: US Department of Health and Human Services; 1998 [cited 2012 Sept 18]. Available from: http://www.fda.gov/downloads/MedicalDevices/DeviceRegulationandGuidance/GuidanceDocuments/UCM094513.pdf.
5. National Council on Radiation Protection and Measurements. Ionizing radiation exposure of the population of the United States: recommendations of the National Council on Radiation Protection and Measurements. Bethesda, MD: National Council on Radiation Protection and Measurements; 2009 [cited 2012 Sep 18]. Available from: http://www.knovel.com/knovel2/Toc.jsp?BookID=2562.
6. Noji EK. The Public Health Consequences of Disasters. New York: Oxford University Press; 1997.
7. Nukushina J. Japanese earthquake victims are being exposed to high density of asbestos. We need protective masks desperately. Epidemiol Prev. 1995 Jun;19(63):226–7.
8. PAHO. Natural Disasters: Protecting the Public's Health. Washington, DC: PAHO Emergency Preparedness Program; 2000 [cited 2012 Sep 18]. Available from: http://www.paho.org/English/dd/ped/SP575.htm.
9. Schneider E, Hajjeh RA, Spiegel RA, Jibson RW, Harp EL, Marshall GA, et al. A coccidioidomycosis outbreak following the Northridge, Calif, earthquake. JAMA. 1997 Mar 19;277(11):904–8.
10. Scientific Committee on the Effects of Atomic Radiation. Annex J: exposure and effects of the Chernobyl accident. Sources and Effects of Ionizing Radiation. New York: United Nations; 2000. p. 451–556.

11. van Donkelaar A, Martin RV, Brauer M, Kahn R, Levy R, Verduzco C, et al. Global estimates of ambient fine particulate matter concentrations from satellite-based aerosol optical depth: development and application. Environ Health Perspect. 2010 Jun;118(6):847–55.

12. Watson JT, Gayer M, Connolly MA. Epidemics after natural disasters. Emerg Infect Dis. 2007 Jan;13(1):1–5.

13. Young S, Balluz L, Malilay J. Natural and technologic hazardous material releases during and after natural disasters: a review. Sci Total Environ. 2004 Apr 25;322(1–3):3–20.

SCUBA DIVING
Daniel A. Nord

OVERVIEW

An estimated 3 million people participate in recreational diving in the United States, and many travel to tropical areas of the world to dive. Traveling divers can face a variety of medical challenges, but because dive injuries are generally rare, few clinicians are trained in their diagnosis and treatment. Therefore, the recreational diver must be able to recognize the signs of injury and find qualified dive medicine help when needed.

PREPARING FOR DIVE TRAVEL

Planning for dive-related travel should take into account any recent changes in health, including injuries or surgery, and medication use. Respiratory disorders (such as asthma), disorders that affect higher function and consciousness (such as diabetes or seizures), psychological problems (such as anxiety), cardiovascular disease, and pregnancy raise special concerns about diving fitness.

DIVING DISORDERS
Barotrauma
Ear and sinus

Ear barotrauma is the most common injury in divers. On descent, failure to equalize pressure changes in the middle ear space creates a pressure gradient across the eardrum. This pressure change must be controlled through proper equalization techniques to avoid bleeding or fluid accumulation in the middle ear and avoid stretching or rupture of the eardrum and the membranes covering the windows of the inner ear. Symptoms of barotrauma include the following:

- pain
- tinnitus (ringing in the ears)
- vertigo (dizziness or sensation of spinning)
- sensation of fullness
- effusion (fluid accumulation in the ear)
- decreased hearing

Paranasal sinuses, because of their relatively narrow connecting passageways, are especially susceptible to barotrauma, generally on descent. With small changes in pressure (depth), symptoms are usually mild and subacute but can be exacerbated by continued diving. Larger pressure changes, especially with forceful attempts at equilibration (Valsalva maneuver), can be more injurious. Additional risk factors for ear and sinus barotrauma include the following:

- earplugs
- medications
- ear or sinus surgery
- nasal deformity
- disease

A diver who may have sustained ear or sinus barotrauma should discontinue diving and seek medical attention.

Pulmonary

A scuba diver must reduce the risk of lung overpressure problems by breathing normally and ascending slowly when breathing compressed gas. Overinflation of the lungs can result if a scuba diver ascends toward the surface without exhaling, which may happen, for example, when a novice diver panics. During ascent, compressed gas trapped in the lung increases in volume until the expansion exceeds the elastic limit of lung tissue, causing damage and allowing gas bubbles to escape into 1 or more of 3 possible locations:

- Gas entering the pleural space can cause lung collapse or pneumothorax.
- Gas entering the space around the heart, trachea, and esophagus (the mediastinum) causes mediastinal emphysema and frequently tracks under the skin (subcutaneous emphysema) or into the tissue around the larynx, sometimes precipitating a change in voice characteristics.
- Gas rupturing the alveolar walls can enter the pulmonary capillaries and pass via the pulmonary veins to the left side of the heart, where it is distributed according to relative blood flow, resulting in arterial gas embolism (AGE).

While mediastinal or subcutaneous emphysema usually resolves spontaneously, pneumothorax generally requires specific treatment to remove the air and reinflate the lung. AGE is a medical emergency, requiring intervention, which includes recompression treatment with hyperbaric oxygen.

Lung overinflation injuries from scuba diving can range from dramatic and life threatening to mild symptoms of chest pain and dyspnea. Although pulmonary barotrauma is relatively uncommon in divers, prompt medical evaluation is necessary, and evidence for this condition should always be considered in the presence of respiratory or neurologic symptoms following a dive.

Decompression Illness

Decompression illness (DCI) is an all-inclusive term that describes the dysbaric injuries (AGE) and decompression sickness (DCS). Because the 2 diseases are considered to result from separate causes, they are described here separately. However, from a clinical and practical standpoint, distinguishing between them in the field may be impossible and unnecessary, since the initial treatment is the same for both. Decompression illness can occur even in divers who have carefully followed the standard decompression tables and the principles of safe diving. Serious permanent injury may result from either AGE or DCS.

Arterial Gas Embolism

Gas entering the arterial blood through ruptured pulmonary vessels can distribute bubbles into the body tissues, including the heart and brain, where they disrupt circulation. AGE

may cause minimal neurologic symptoms, dramatic symptoms that require immediate attention, or death. Common signs and symptoms include the following:

- numbness
- weakness
- tingling
- dizziness
- blurred vision
- chest pain
- personality change
- paralysis or seizures
- loss of consciousness

In general, any scuba diver who surfaces unconscious or loses consciousness within 10 minutes after surfacing should be assumed to have AGE. Intervention with basic life support is indicated, including the administration of 100% oxygen, followed by rapid evacuation to a hyperbaric oxygen treatment facility.

Decompression Sickness

Breathing air under pressure causes excess inert gas (usually nitrogen) to dissolve in body tissues. The amount dissolved is proportional to and increases with depth and time. As the diver ascends to the surface, the excess dissolved gas must be cleared through respiration via the bloodstream. Depending on the amount dissolved and the rate of ascent, some gas can supersaturate tissues, where it separates from solution to form bubbles, interfering with blood flow and tissue oxygenation and causing the following signs and symptoms of DCS:

- joint aches or pain
- numbness or tingling
- mottling or marbling of skin
- coughing spasms or shortness of breath
- itching
- unusual fatigue
- dizziness
- weakness
- personality changes
- loss of bowel or bladder function
- staggering, loss of coordination, or tremors
- paralysis
- collapse or unconsciousness

FLYING AFTER DIVING

The risk of developing decompression sickness is increased when divers are exposed to increased altitude too soon after a dive. The cabin pressure of commercial aircraft may be the equivalent of 6,000–8,000 ft (1,829–2,438 m). Thus, divers should avoid flying or an altitude exposure >2,000 ft (610 m) for:

- ≥12 hours after surfacing from a single no-decompression dive
- ≥18 hours after repetitive dives or multiple days of diving
- substantially longer than 18 hours after dives where decompression stops were required

These recommended preflight surface intervals do not eliminate risk of DCS, and longer surface intervals will further reduce this risk.

PREVENTING DIVING DISORDERS

Recreational divers should dive conservatively and well within the no-decompression limits of their dive tables or computers. Risk factors for DCI are primarily dive depth, dive time, and rate of ascent. Additional factors such as repetitive dives, strenuous exercise, dives to depths >60 ft (18.3 m), altitude exposure soon after a dive, and certain physiological variables also increase risk. Divers should be cautioned to stay hydrated and rested and dive within the limits of their training. Diving is a skill that requires training and certification and should be done with a companion.

TREATMENT OF DIVING DISORDERS

Definitive treatment of DCI begins with early recognition of symptoms, followed by recompression with hyperbaric oxygen. A high concentration (100%) of supplemental oxygen is recommended. Surface-level oxygen given for first aid may relieve the signs and symptoms of decompression illness and should be administered as soon as possible. Divers are often dehydrated, either because of incidental causes, immersion, or DCI itself, which can cause capillary leakage. Administration of isotonic glucose-free intravenous fluid is recommended in most cases. Oral rehydration fluids may also be helpful, provided they can be safely administered (for example, if the diver is conscious). The definitive treatment of DCI is recompression and oxygen administration in a hyperbaric chamber.

Divers Alert Network (DAN) maintains 24-hour emergency consultation and evacuation assistance at 919-684-9111 (collect calls are accepted). DAN will help with managing the injured diver, help decide if recompression is needed, provide the location of the closest recompression facility, and help arrange patient transport. DAN can also be contacted for routine, nonemergency consultation by telephone at 919-684-2948, extension 222, or by accessing the DAN website (www.diversalertnetwork.org).

Travelers who plan to scuba dive may want to ascertain whether there are recompression facilities at their destination before embarking on their trip.

HAZARDOUS MARINE LIFE

The oceans and waterways are filled with creatures and, although some are capable of wounding and poisoning, most marine animals are generally harmless unless threatened. Most injuries are the result of chance encounters or defensive maneuvers. Resulting wounds have many common characteristics: bacterial contamination, foreign bodies, and occasionally venom. See the Animal-Associated Hazards section earlier in this chapter for prevention and injury management recommendations.

BIBLIOGRAPHY

1. Brubakk AO, Neuman TS, Bennett PB, Elliott DH. Bennett and Elliott's Physiology and Medicine of Diving. 5th ed. London: Saunders; 2003.
2. Dear G, Pollock N. DAN America Dive and Travel Medical Guide. 5th ed. Durham, NC: Divers Alert Network; 2009.
3. Moon RE. Treatment of decompression illness. In: Bove AA, Davis JC, editors. Bove and Davis' Diving Medicine. 4th ed. Philadelphia: WB Saunders; 2004. p. 195–223.
4. Neuman TS, Thom SR. Physiology and medicine of hyperbaric oxygen therapy. Philadelphia, PA: Saunders; 2008.
5. Sheffield P, Vann R. Flying after recreational diving, workshop proceedings of the Divers Alert Network 2002 May 2. Durham, NC: Divers Alert Network; 2004 [cited 2012 Sep 18]. Available from: http://www.diversalertnetwork.org/research/projects/fad/workshop/FADWorkshopProceedings.pdf.

MEDICAL TOURISM

C. Virginia Lee, Victor Balaban

OVERVIEW

"Medical tourism" is the term commonly used to describe people traveling outside their home country for medical treatment. Traditionally, international medical travel involved patients from less-developed countries traveling to a medical center in a developed country for treatment that was not available in their home country. In the United States, the term "medical tourism" generally refers to people traveling to less-developed countries for medical care. Medical tourism is a worldwide, multibillion-dollar phenomenon that is expected to grow substantially in the next 5–10 years. However, little reliable epidemiologic data on medical tourism exist. Studies using different definitions and methods have estimated there are 60,000–750,000 medical tourists annually from around the world.

The most common categories of procedures that people pursue during medical tourism trips are cosmetic surgery, dentistry, cardiology (cardiac surgery), and orthopedic surgery. Common destinations include Thailand, Mexico, Singapore, India, Malaysia, Cuba, Brazil, Argentina, and Costa Rica. The type of procedure and the destination need to be considered when reviewing the risk of travel for medical care.

Most medical tourists rely on private companies or "medical concierge" services to identify foreign health care facilities, and they pay for their care out of pocket. Some insurers and large employers have alliances with overseas hospitals to control health care costs, and several major medical schools in the United States have developed joint initiatives with overseas providers, such as the Harvard Medical School Dubai Center, the Johns Hopkins Singapore International Medical Center, and the Duke-National University of Singapore. Whether these joint ventures will increase the number of US citizens who go overseas for health care is unknown.

Travel health providers should advise prospective medical tourists to determine if health care facilities they are considering are accredited by the Joint Commission International (JCI). JCI is the international division of the Joint Commission Resources, a US-based, not-for-profit affiliate of the Joint Commission that certifies health care facilities in the United States. As of March 2012, JCI has accredited 368 international hospitals in 46 countries. These can be found at www.jointcommissioninternational.org/JCI-Accredited-Organizations. As more facilities are accredited, more providers will likely offer incentives for their patients to travel overseas for care.

PRE-TRAVEL ADVICE FOR MEDICAL TOURISTS

As discussed in Chapter 1, Planning for Healthy Travel: Responsibilities & Resources, patients who elect to travel for medical reasons should consult a travel health provider for advice tailored to individual health needs, preferably ≥4–6 weeks before travel. In addition to other considerations for healthy travel related to their destination, medical tourists should consider the risks associated with surgery and travel, either while being treated or while recovering from treatment. Air pressure in an aircraft is equivalent to the pressure at an altitude of about 6,000–8,000 ft (1,829–2,438 m). Patients should not travel for 10 days after chest or abdominal surgery to avoid risks associated with this change in pressure. Flying and surgery both increase the risk of the development of blood clots and the formation of pulmonary emboli. The American Society of Plastic Surgeons advises people who have had cosmetic procedures of the face, eyelids, or nose, or who have had laser treatments, to wait 7–10 days before flying. Patients are also advised to avoid "vacation" activities such as sunbathing, drinking alcohol, swimming, taking long tours, and engaging in strenuous activities or exercise after surgery. The Aerospace Medical Association has published medical guidelines for airline travel that provide useful information on the risks of travel with certain medical conditions (www.asma.org/asma/media/asma/Travel-Publications/paxguidelines.pdf).

TRANSPLANT TOURISM

One controversial form of medical tourism is "transplant tourism," which is travel for the purpose of receiving an organ purchased from an unrelated donor for transplant. An estimated 5%–10% of all kidney transplants in 2007 were from commercial living donors or vendors (although most of these were not transplant tourism). In 2004, the World Health Assembly Resolution 57.18 encouraged member countries to "take measures to protect the poorest and vulnerable groups from 'transplant tourism' and the sale of tissues and organs." A meeting in 2008 in Istanbul addressed the issue of transplant tourism and organ trafficking, which resulted in a call for these activities to be prohibited. In view of those events, the World Health Organization revised the Guiding Principles on Human Cell, Tissue and Organ Transplantation and released those revised principles in March 2009. A 2007 report on the international organ trade found that China, the Philippines, and Pakistan were the largest organ-exporting countries. Several studies have indicated potential problems that travelers and clinicians need to be aware of when considering transplantation overseas: the donor and

---

BOX 2-5. GUIDING PRINCIPLES ON MEDICAL TOURISM[1]

The American Medical Association advocates that employers, insurance companies, and other entities that facilitate or promote medical care outside the United States adhere to the following principles:

(a) Medical care outside the United States must be voluntary.

(b) Financial incentives to travel outside the United States for medical care should not limit the diagnostic and therapeutic alternatives that are offered to patients, or restrict treatment or referral options.

(c) Patients should be referred for medical care only to institutions that have been accredited by recognized international accrediting bodies (e.g., the Joint Commission International or the International Society for Quality in Health Care).

(d) Prior to travel, local follow-up care should be coordinated and financing should be arranged to ensure continuity of care when patients return from medical care outside the United States.

(e) Coverage for travel outside the United States for medical care must include the costs of necessary follow-up care upon return to the United States.

(f) Patients should be informed of their rights and legal recourse prior to agreeing to travel outside the United States for medical care.

(g) Access to physician licensing and outcome data, as well as facility accreditation and outcomes data, should be arranged for patients seeking medical care outside the United States.

(h) The transfer of patient medical records to and from facilities outside the United States should be consistent with Health Insurance Portability and Accountability Action (HIPAA) guidelines.

(i) Patients choosing to travel outside the United States for medical care should be provided with information about the potential risks of combining surgical procedures with long flights and vacation activities.

---

[1] From American Medical Association. New AMA guidelines on medical tourism. Chicago: AMA; 2008. Available from: http://www.ama-assn.org/ama1/pub/upload/mm/31/medicaltourism.pdf.

the procedures lacked documentation, most patients received fewer immunosuppressive drugs than is current practice in the United States, and most patients did not receive antibiotic prophylaxis. However, it is not clear if these issues are representative of the issues faced by all patients who travel for transplants.

GUIDELINES FOR TRAVELERS SEEKING MEDICAL CARE ABROAD

Several professional organizations have developed guidelines that include questions useful for travelers when discussing medical or dental care abroad, either with the facility providing the care or with the group facilitating the trip.

When considering a trip overseas for medical care, travelers should be aware of the guiding principles developed by the American Medical Association (Box 2-5). For cosmetic surgery, the American Society for Plastic Surgery (ASPS) developed a briefing paper that includes a patient safety checklist (Box 2-6). Similarly, the American Dental Association provides informational documents, including "Traveler's Guide to Safe Dental Care" through the Global Dental Safety Organization for Safety and Asepsis Procedures (Box 2-7). Although the dental guidelines were not developed for medical tourists, they provide useful information for travelers to consider when selecting a facility or planning a trip for medical or dental

---

BOX 2-6. PATIENT SAFETY CHECKLIST FOR COSMETIC SURGERY[1]

To help ensure optimal results and to limit risks and complications, the American Society for Plastic Surgery (ASPS) offers the following tips to anyone considering cosmetic surgery in the United States.

Do Your Homework: Research the procedure, the benefits, and the risks. Refer to www.plasticsurgery.org for the latest information on plastic surgery procedures.

Have Realistic Expectations: Ask your plastic surgeon questions about how the surgery will work for you: identify expectations and understand side effects and recovery time.

Be Informed: Talk to patients who have had your procedure so you know what to expect.

Require a Medical Evaluation: Consult with your plastic surgeon for an evaluation and discuss your full medical history to determine the most appropriate treatment.

Choose an ASPS Member Surgeon: Why? ASPS Member Surgeons are qualified, trained, properly certified, experienced in your procedure, and operate only in accredited facilities.

Ask Questions:

- Are you an ASPS Member Surgeon?
- Are you certified by the American Board of Plastic Surgery?
- Do you have hospital privileges to perform this procedure? If so, at which hospitals?
- How many procedures of this type have you performed?
- Am I a good candidate for this procedure? What will be expected of me to get optimal results?
- Where and how will you perform my procedure?
- Is the surgical facility accredited?
- What are the risks involved with my procedure?
- How long a recovery period can I expect, and what kind of help will I need during my recovery?
- Will I need to take time off work? If so, how long?
- How much will my procedure cost? Are financing options available?
- How are complications handled?

---

[1] Excerpt from American Society of Plastic Surgeons. Cosmetic surgery tourism briefing paper. Arlington Heights, IL: American Society of Plastic Surgeons; 2010. Available from: http://www.plasticsurgery.org/News-and-Resources/Briefing-Papers/Cosmetic-Surgery-Tourism.html.

BOX 2-7. PATIENT CHECKLIST FOR OBTAINING SAFE DENTAL CARE DURING INTERNATIONAL TRAVEL[1]

Before you leave:

- Visit your dentist for a check-up to reduce the chances you will have a dental emergency.
- See a health care provider to receive any needed vaccinations, medications, and advice related to your travel destination.

When seeking treatment for a dental emergency during your trip:

- Consult hotel staff or the American Embassy or consulate for assistance in finding a dentist.
- If possible, consider recommendations from Americans living in the area or from other trusted sources.

If the answers to any of the asterisked (*) items below are "No," you should have reservations about the office's infection control standards. If the answer to a two-star item (**) is "No," consider making a swift but gracious exit.

When making the appointment, ask:

- Do you use new gloves for each patient?*
- Do you use an autoclave (steam sterilizer) or dry heat oven to sterilize your instruments between patients?**
- Do you sterilize your handpieces (drills)?* (If not, do you disinfect them?)**
- Do you use new needles for each patient?**
- Is sterile (or boiled) water used for surgical procedures?** (In areas where drinking water is unsafe, the water also may cause illness if used for dental treatment.)

Upon arriving at the office, observe the following:

- Is the office clean and neat?
- Do staff wash their hands, with soap, between patients?**
- Do they wear gloves for all procedures?**
- Do they clean and disinfect or use disposable covers on surfaces touched during treatment?

[1] Excerpt from Organization for Safety and Asepsis Procedures. Traveler's guide to safe dental care. Annapolis, MD: Organization for Safety and Asepsis Procedures; 2001. Available from: http://www.osap.org/?page=TravelersGuide.

care. These 3 guides are targeted for specific groups; however, they provide an indication of the types of questions that people considering travel for medical care should discuss with their regular health care provider. In addition to these guidelines, the European Union is working to establish harmonized standards of care for professional services such as plastic or aesthetic surgery. These standards, released for comment in early 2012, will provide additional guidance for medical tourists in evaluating facilities and services.

BIBLIOGRAPHY

1. Aerospace Medical Association. Medical Guidelines for Airline Travel. 2nd ed. Alexandria, VA: Aerospace Medical Association; 2003.
2. American Medical Association. New AMA Guidelines on Medical Tourism. Chicago: AMA; 2008 [cited 2012 Sep 18]. Available from: http://www.ama-assn.org/ama1/pub/upload/mm/31/medicaltourism.pdf.
3. American Society of Plastic Surgeons. Cosmetic Surgery Tourism Briefing Paper. Arlington Heights: American Society of Plastic Surgeons; 2010 [cited 2012 Sep 18]. Available from: http://www.plasticsurgery.org/News-and-Resources/Briefing-Papers/Cosmetic-Surgery-Tourism.html.
4. Bookman MZ, Bookman KR. Medical Tourism in Developing Countries. New York: Palgrave MacMillan; 2007.

5. Budiani-Saberi DA, Delmonico FL. Organ trafficking and transplant tourism: a commentary on the global realities. Am J Transplant. 2008 May;8(5):925–9.

6. Ehrbeck T, Guevara C, Mango PD. Mapping the market for medical travel. McKinsey Quarterly. 2008(May).

7. Einhorn B, Arnst C. Outsourcing the patients: more US health insurers are slashing costs by sending policyholders overseas for pricey procedures. Businessweek News. 2008 Mar 13.

8. Galland Z. Medical tourism: the insurance debate: most insurers balk at covering medical procedures performed overseas, but some are exploring the option Businessweek News. 2008 Nov 9.

9. Gill J, Madhira BR, Gjertson D, Lipshutz G, Cecka JM, Pham PT, et al. Transplant tourism in the United States: a single-center experience. Clin J Am Soc Nephrol. 2008 Nov;3(6):1820–8.

10. Horowitz MD, Rosensweig JA, Jones CA. Medical tourism: globalization of the healthcare marketplace. MedGenMed. 2007;9(4):33.

11. JointCommissionInternational.org [Internet]. Oak Brook, IL: Joint Commission International; c2002–2011 [cited 2012 Sep 18]. Available from: http://www.jointcommissioninternational.org/.

12. Keckley PH, Underwood HR. Medical Tourism: Consumers in Search of Value. Washington, DC: Deloitte Center for Health Solutions; 2008.

13. Merion RM, Barnes AD, Lin M, Ashby VB, McBride V, Ortiz-Rios E, et al. Transplants in foreign countries among patients removed from the US transplant waiting list. Am J Transplant. 2008 Apr;8(4 Pt 2):988–96.

14. Organization for Safety and Asepsis Procedures. Traveler's guide to safe dental care. Annapolis, MD: Organization for Safety and Asepsis Procedures; 2001 [cited 2012 Sep 18]. Available from: http://www.osap.org/?page=TravelersGuide.

15. Reed CM. Medical tourism. Med Clin North Am. 2008 Nov;92(6):1433–46, xi.

16. Sajjad I, Baines LS, Patel P, Salifu MO, Jindal RM. Commercialization of kidney transplants: a systematic review of outcomes in recipients and donors. Am J Nephrol. 2008;28(5):744–54.

17. Sanford C, Merck. Air travel. Whitehouse Station, NJ: Merck Sharp & Dohme Corp; 2009 [cited 2012 Sep 18]. Available from: http://www.merck.com/mmpe/sec22/ch333/ch333b.html#CBBIEDEH.

18. Shimazono Y. The state of the international organ trade: a provisional picture based on integration of available information. Bull World Health Organ. 2007 Dec;85(12):955–962.

19. US Department of Commerce. 2008 United States resident travel abroad. Washington, DC: US Department of Commerce; 2008 [cited 2012 Sep 18]. Available from: http://tinet.ita.doc.gov/outreachpages/download_data_table/2008_US_Travel_Abroad.pdf.

20. US Department of Health and Human Services. 2007 annual report of the US Organ Procurement and Transplantation Network and the Scientific Registry of Transplant Recipients: transplant data 1997–2006. Rockville, MD: US Department of Health and Human Services; 2007 [cited 2012 Sep 18]. Available from: http://www.ustransplant.org/annual_reports/current/ar_archives.htm.

21. World Health Organization. Guiding principles on human organ transplantation. Geneva: World Health Organization; 2010 [cited 2012 Sep 18]. Available from: http://www.who.int/ethics/topics/transplantation_guiding_principles/en/index1.html.

22. World Health Organization. Human organ and tissue transplantation. Geneva: World Health Organization; 2009 [updated 2012 Sep 18]. Available from: http://apps.who.int/gb/ebwha/pdf_files/A62/A62_15-en.pdf.

DEEP VEIN THROMBOSIS & PULMONARY EMBOLISM

Nimia Reyes, Scott Grosse, Althea Grant

BACKGROUND

Deep vein thrombosis (DVT) is a condition in which a blood clot develops in the deep veins, most commonly in the lower extremities. A part of the clot can break off and travel to the lungs, causing a pulmonary embolism (PE), which can be life threatening. About 25% of calf vein DVTs, if left untreated, will extend to involve the proximal lower extremity veins (popliteal, femoral, or iliac veins); a proximal lower extremity DVT, if left untreated, has about a 50% risk of leading to a PE. Venous thromboembolism (VTE) is a term that includes both DVT and PE. Many cases are asymptomatic and resolve spontaneously. VTE is often recurrent, and long-term complications, such as postthrombotic syndrome after a DVT or chronic thromboembolic pulmonary hypertension after a PE, are frequent.

More than 300 million people travel on long-haul flights each year. An association between VTE and air travel was first reported in the early 1950s, and since then, long-haul air travel has become more common, leading to increased concerns about travel-related VTE.

PATHOGENESIS

Virchow's classic triad for thrombus formation is venous stasis, vessel wall damage, and the hypercoagulable state. Prolonged cramped sitting during long-distance travel interferes with venous flow in the legs and causes venous stasis. Seat-edge pressure on the popliteal area may contribute to vessel wall damage as well as venous stasis. Coagulation activation may result from an interaction between cabin conditions (such as hypobaric hypoxia) and individual risk factors for VTE. Studies of the pathophysiologic mechanisms for the increased risk of VTE after long-distance travel have not produced consistent results, but venous stasis appears to play a major role; other factors specific to air travel may increase coagulation activation, particularly in passengers with individual risk factors for VTE.

INCIDENCE

The annual incidence of VTE in the general population has been estimated at 0.1% but is higher in subpopulations with risk factors for VTE (Box 2-8). The actual incidence of travel-related VTE is difficult to determine, since there is no consensus on the definition of travel-related VTE, particularly in regards to duration of travel and time window after travel. Estimates of travel-related VTE incidence vary because of differences between studies in duration of travel, measured outcome, time window after the flight, and the populations studied.

In general, the overall incidence of travel-related VTE is low. Two studies reported that the absolute risk of VTE for flights >4 hours is 1 in 4,656 flights and 1 in 6,000 flights. People who travel on long-distance flights are generally healthier and therefore are at lower risk for VTE than the general population.

Five prospective studies that assessed the incidence of DVT among travelers at low to intermediate risk for VTE after travel >8 hours yielded an overall incidence of VTE of 0.5%, while the incidence of symptomatic VTE was 0.3%.

ASSOCIATION WITH TRAVEL

Numerous studies have examined the association between travel, particularly air travel, and VTE. However, these studies had differences in methods. Outcomes ranged from asymptomatic DVT to symptomatic DVT/PE to severe or fatal PE. Asymptomatic DVT is estimated to be 5- to 20-fold more common than symptomatic events. Definitions of long-distance travel ranged from flight duration >3 hours to >10 hours (most >4 hours). The time window until illness after the flight ranged from hours after landing to ≥8 weeks (most 4 weeks).

Published studies have yielded varying results; some studies found that long-distance travel increased the risk of VTE, and others either found no definitive evidence that it increased the risk of VTE or found that it increased the risk only if ≥1 additional risk factors were present. Most studies found long-distance air travel to be a weak risk factor for VTE, and most VTE occurred as asymptomatic DVT of uncertain clinical significance in passengers with additional preexisting risk factors.

Long-distance air travel may increase the risk of VTE by 2- to 4-fold. A similar increase in risk is also seen with other modes of travel, such as car, bus, or train, implying that the increase in risk is caused mainly by prolonged limited mobility rather than by the cabin environment. The risk is the same for economy-class and business-class travel. The risk increases with increasing travel duration and with preexisting risk factors. The risk decreases with time after air travel; most air travel–related VTE occurs within the first 1–2 weeks after the flight and returns to baseline by 8 weeks.

RISK FACTORS

Most travel-related VTE occurs in passengers with risk factors for VTE (Box 2-8). Some studies have shown that 75%–99.5% of those who developed travel-related VTE had ≥1 preexisting risk factor; one study showed that 20%

BOX 2-8. VENOUS THROMBOEMBOLISM (VTE) RISK FACTORS

General risk factors for VTE include the following:

- Older age (increasing risk after age 40)
- Obesity (BMI >30 kg/m²)
- Estrogen use (hormonal contraceptives or hormone replacement therapy)
- Pregnancy and the postpartum period
- Thrombophilia (such as factor V Leiden mutation or antiphospholipid syndrome) or a family history of VTE
- Previous VTE
- Active cancer
- Serious medical illness (such as congestive heart failure or inflammatory bowel disease)
- Recent surgery, hospitalization, or trauma
- Limited mobility
- Central venous catheterization

had ≥5 risk factors. For travelers without pre-existing risk factors, the risk of travel-related venous thromboembolism is low. However, a person may not be aware that he or she has a risk factor such as inherited thrombophilia. The combination of air travel with pre-existing individual risk factors may have a synergistic effect on the risk for VTE.

For air travelers, height appears to be an additional risk factor. Risk of travel-related VTE increases with height <1.6 m (5 feet, 3 inches). Unlike car seats, airline seats are higher and cannot be adjusted to a person's height; therefore, shorter passengers who travel by air may experience seat-edge pressure to the popliteal area. Risk of travel-related VTE also increases with height >1.9 m (6 ft, 3 in), possibly because taller passengers have less leg room.

CLINICAL PRESENTATION
Signs and symptoms of DVT/PE are nonspecific:

- Typical signs or symptoms of DVT in the extremities include pain or tenderness, swelling, increased warmth in the affected area, and redness or discoloration of the overlying skin.
- The most common signs or symptoms of acute PE include unexplained shortness of breath, pleuritic chest pain, cough or hemoptysis, and syncope.

DIAGNOSIS
Imaging studies are needed for diagnosis:

- Duplex ultrasonography is the standard imaging procedure for diagnosis of DVT. Contrast venography is the gold standard but is invasive and uses potentially harmful contrast material. Magnetic resonance venography imaging and computed axial tomography venography are less frequently used.
- Computed tomographic pulmonary angiography is the standard imaging procedure for diagnosis of PE. Ventilation-perfusion scan is the second-line imaging procedure. Pulmonary angiography is the gold standard but is invasive and uses potentially harmful contrast material. Magnetic resonance angiography can also be used.

PREVENTIVE MEASURES FOR LONG-DISTANCE TRAVELERS
The American College of Chest Physicians published the 9th edition of their Antithrombotic Therapy and Prevention of Thrombosis Evidence-Based Clinical Practice Guidelines in February 2012. Recommendations for long-distance travelers (considered grade 2C: weak recommendation, low- or very low-quality evidence) are the following:

1. For long-distance travelers at increased risk of VTE (Box 2-8), frequent ambulation, calf muscle exercise, and sitting in an aisle seat if feasible are suggested.
2. For long-distance travelers at increased risk of VTE (Box 2-8), use of properly fitted, below-knee graduated compression stockings (GCS)

providing 15–30 mm Hg of pressure at the ankle during travel is suggested. For all other long-distance travelers, use of GCS is not recommended.

3. For long-distance travelers, the use of aspirin or anticoagulants to prevent VTE is not recommended.

There is no evidence for an association between dehydration and travel-related VTE and no direct evidence that drinking plenty of nonalcoholic beverages to ensure adequate hydration or avoiding alcoholic beverages has a protective effect. Therefore, while maintaining hydration is reasonable and unlikely to cause harm, it cannot be strongly recommended specifically to prevent travel-related VTE.

There is evidence that immobility while flying is a risk for VTE and indirect evidence that maintaining mobility may prevent VTE. In view of the role of venous stasis in the pathogenesis of travel-related VTE, it would be reasonable to recommend frequent ambulation and calf muscle exercises for long-distance travelers.

Compared with aisle seats, window seats in one study were reported to increase the risk 2-fold, particularly in obese passengers, who had a 6-fold increase in risk. Aisle seats are reported to have a protective effect, compared with window or middle seats, probably because passengers are freer to move around.

GCS are indicated for long-distance travelers at increased risk. GCS appear to reduce asymptomatic DVT in travelers and are generally well tolerated.

Global use of anticoagulants for long-distance travel is not indicated. Pharmacologic prophylaxis for long-distance travelers at particularly high risk should be decided on an individual basis. In cases where the potential benefits of pharmacologic prophylaxis outweigh the possible adverse effects, anticoagulants rather than antiplatelet drugs are recommended.

RECOMMENDATIONS

1. General measures for long-distance travelers (Figure 2-2):
   a. Calf muscle exercises
   b. Frequent ambulation
   c. Aisle seating when feasible
2. Additional measures for long-distance travelers at increased risk of VTE:
   a. Properly fitted below-knee GCS
   b. Anticoagulant prophylaxis only in particularly high-risk cases where the potential benefits outweigh the risks

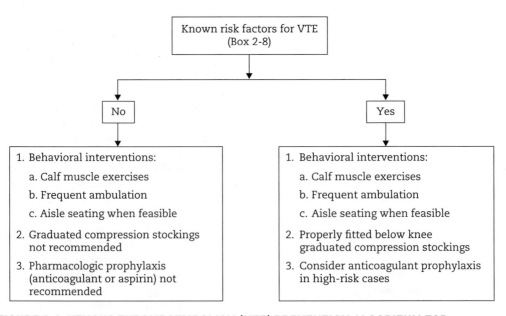

FIGURE 2-2. VENOUS THROMBOEMBOLISM (VTE) PREVENTION ALGORITHM FOR LONG-DISTANCE TRAVELERS

BIBLIOGRAPHY

1. Adi Y, Bayliss S, Rouse A, Taylor RS. The association between air travel and deep vein thrombosis: systematic review & meta-analysis. BMC cardiovascular disorders. 2004 May 19;4:7.

2. Arya R, Barnes JA, Hossain U, Patel RK, Cohen AT. Long-haul flights and deep vein thrombosis: a significant risk only when additional factors are also present. Br J Haematol. 2002 Mar;116(3):653–4.

3. Aryal KR, Al-Khaffaf H. Venous thromboembolic complications following air travel: what's the quantitative risk? A literature review. Eur J Vasc Endovasc Surg. 2006 Feb;31(2):187–99.

4. Bartholomew JR, Schaffer JL, McCormick GF. Air travel and venous thromboembolism: minimizing the risk. Cleve Clin J Med. 2011 Feb;78(2):111–20.

5. Belcaro G, Geroulakos G, Nicolaides AN, Myers KA, Winford M. Venous thromboembolism from air travel: the LONFLIT study. Angiology. 2001 Jun;52(6):369–74.

6. Cannegieter SC, Doggen CJ, van Houwelingen HC, Rosendaal FR. Travel-related venous thrombosis: results from a large population-based case control study (MEGA study). PLoS Med. 2006 Aug;3(8):e307.

7. Chandra D, Parisini E, Mozaffarian D. Meta-analysis: travel and risk for venous thromboembolism. Ann Intern Med. 2009 Aug 4;151(3):180–90.

8. Clarke M, Hopewell S, Juszczak E, Eisinga A, Kjeldstrom M. Compression stockings for preventing deep vein thrombosis in airline passengers. Cochrane Database Syst Rev. 2006(2):CD004002.

9. Eklof B, Maksimovic D, Caprini JA, Glase C. Air travel-related venous thromboembolism. Disease-a-month : DM. 2005 Feb–Mar;51(2–3):200–7.

10. Gavish I, Brenner B. Air travel and the risk of thromboembolism. Intern Emerg Med. 2011 Apr;6(2):113–6.

11. Kahn SR, Lim W, Dunn AS, Cushman M, Dentali F, Akl EA, et al. Prevention of VTE in nonsurgical patients: antithrombotic therapy and prevention of thrombosis, 9th ed: American College of Chest Physicians evidence-based clinical practice guidelines. Chest. 2012 Feb;141(2 Suppl):e195S–226S.

12. Kuipers S, Cannegieter SC, Middeldorp S, Robyn L, Buller HR, Rosendaal FR. The absolute risk of venous thrombosis after air travel: a cohort study of 8,755 employees of international organisations. PLoS Med. 2007 Sep;4(9):e290.

13. Kuipers S, Schreijer AJ, Cannegieter SC, Buller HR, Rosendaal FR, Middeldorp S. Travel and venous thrombosis: a systematic review. J Intern Med. 2007 Dec;262(6):615–34.

14. Martinelli I, Taioli E, Battaglioli T, Podda GM, Passamonti SM, Pedotti P, et al. Risk of venous thromboembolism after air travel: interaction with thrombophilia and oral contraceptives. Arch Intern Med. 2003 Dec 8–22;163(22):2771–4.

15. Paganin F, Bourde A, Yvin JL, Genin R, Guijarro JL, Bourdin A, et al. Venous thromboembolism in passengers following a 12-h flight: a case-control study. Aviat Space Environ Med. 2003 Dec;74(12):1277–80.

16. Schobersberger W, Schobersberger B, Partsch H. Travel-related thromboembolism: mechanisms and avoidance. Expert Rev Cardiovasc Ther. 2009 Dec;7(12):1559–67.

17. Schreijer AJ, Cannegieter SC, Caramella M, Meijers JC, Krediet RT, Simons RM, et al. Fluid loss does not explain coagulation activation during air travel. Thromb Haemost. 2008 Jun;99(6):1053–9.

18. Schreijer AJ, Cannegieter SC, Doggen CJ, Rosendaal FR. The effect of flight-related behaviour on the risk of venous thrombosis after air travel. Br J Haematol. 2009 Feb;144(3):425–9.

19. Toff WD, Jones CI, Ford I, Pearse RJ, Watson HG, Watt SJ, et al. Effect of hypobaric hypoxia, simulating conditions during long-haul air travel, on coagulation, fibrinolysis, platelet function, and endothelial activation. JAMA. 2006 May 17;295(19):2251–61.

20. Trujillo-Santos AJ, Jimenez-Puente A, Perea-Milla E. Association between long travel and venous thromboembolic disease: a systematic review and meta-analysis of case-control studies. Ann Hematol. 2008 Feb;87(2):79–86.

21. Watson HG, Baglin TP. Guidelines on travel-related venous thrombosis. Br J Haematol. 2011 Jan;152(1):31–4.

22. World Health Organization. WHO Research Into Global Hazards of Travel (WRIGHT) project: final report of phase I. Geneva: World Health Organization; 2007 [cited 2012 Apr 4]. Available from: http://www.who.int/cardiovascular_diseases/wright_project/phase1_report/en/index.html.

MENTAL HEALTH & TRAVEL

Thomas H. Valk

INTRODUCTION

International travel is stressful. Stressors vary to some extent with the type of travel, short-term travel likely offering the least stress and frequent travel and expatriation the most. Given the stressors of travel, preexisting psychiatric disorders can recur, and latent, undiagnosed problems can become apparent for the first time.

OCCURRENCE IN TRAVELERS

Incidence data based on population surveys of travelers are nonexistent. Data from clinical populations include the following:

- Patel et al. conducted a study of urgent repatriation of British diplomats and found that 11% of medical evacuations were "nonphysical," or psychological in nature. Using the authors' data, an overall incident rate of 0.34% for psychological evacuations occurred for their population. Of these, 41% were for some form of depression.
- Another study examined psychiatric evacuations over a 5-year period in the US Foreign Service population from 1982 through 1986. Using an unpublished estimate of the population served in this study, an overall incidence rate of 0.16% for psychiatric evacuations occurred. Of these, fully 50% were for substance abuse or affective disorder. Mania and hypomanic states accounted for 2.8% of these evacuations.
- Streltzer studied psychiatric emergencies in travelers to Hawaii and estimated a rate of 0.22% for tourists and 2.25% for transient travelers versus a rate of 1.25% for nontravelers. In order of decreasing frequency, diagnoses in this population were schizophrenia, alcohol abuse, anxiety reactions, and depression.

THE PRE-TRAVEL CONSULTATION AND MENTAL HEALTH EVALUATION

Any pre-travel consultation should include a mental health screening, especially for those planning extended travel or residence in a foreign country. Since travel medicine specialists rarely have mental health credentials, a full mental health inquiry with mental status examination and a psychiatric review of symptoms would not be practicable or productive. Rather, a brief inquiry aimed at eliciting previously diagnosed psychiatric disorders should be undertaken. To introduce this portion of the consultation and to elicit the most cooperation, the practitioner could enumerate the following facts:

- International travel is stressful for everyone and has been associated with the emergence or reemergence of mental health problems.
- The availability of culturally compatible mental health services varies widely.
- Laws regarding the use of illicit substances can be severe in some countries.

The practitioner can then ask about factors that might indicate a mental health problem:

- Any previously treated or diagnosed psychiatric disorders and the type of treatment involved (inpatient, outpatient, medications).
- Current treatment for any psychiatric disorders and their nature.
- Current or past use of illicit substances.
- Any diagnosis of substance use disorder, or suggestion from medical service providers, friends, or family that the traveler might be using alcohol or other substances to excess.
- Any immediate family history of serious mental health problems.

In general, any history of inpatient treatment, psychotic episode, violent or suicidal behavior, affective disorder (including mania, hypomania, or major depression), any treatment for substance use problems, and any current treatments would warrant further evaluation by a mental health professional, preferably one who has had some experience in problems relating to international travel. On occasion, the patient's mental status upon examination may be notably abnormal, which would also warrant a referral.

Other issues that may be encountered and should be addressed during the pre-travel consultation include the following:

- Customs regulations: Traveling through customs with medications for personal use can be problematic in countries where those medications are prohibited. It is always wise to carry them in their original containers, along with a letter from the prescribing physician indicating that the medications have been prescribed for medical reasons. Even with these precautions, problems may still occur at customs. Occasionally the country's embassy can be helpful prior to travel, but their advice may not be reliable. A health care provider in the destination country may be able to provide guidance about medication restrictions.
- Psychotropic medication refills: Obtaining these medications while living overseas can be problematic, as availability or even legality of the medication varies from country to country. Again, a check with the country's embassy may be helpful, as would a check with a reputable in-country pharmacy or health care provider.
- Measuring drug levels: Locating laboratory facilities for the determination of lithium levels or for other mood-stabilizing medications may be challenging and should be investigated prior to travel. High temperatures and increased sweating could lead to toxicity, even on the same dose.
- Mefloquine: In general, patients with mental health issues should not be prescribed mefloquine for malarial chemoprophylaxis because of its potential for neuropsychiatric side effects.
- Alcoholics Anonymous (AA) and Narcotics Anonymous (NA) meetings: Currently sober patients with substance use disorders should consider seeking out AA and NA meetings, depending upon their length of stay and stability of their sobriety.
- Sexual activity: An increase in sexual activity is often associated with international travel, along with casual and unprotected sex (see Chapter 3, *Perspectives:* Sex and Tourism). A frank discussion of sexual activity and its associated risks and precautions should be undertaken.
- Evacuation insurance: Travelers with mental health problems should consider travel health and medical evacuation insurance for emergencies when abroad.

POST-TRAVEL MENTAL HEALTH ISSUES

Travel health practitioners may be in a unique position to inquire about traumatic experiences a traveler might have had that may lead to posttraumatic stress disorder (PTSD). Travelers continuously exposed to high levels of stress, such as disaster relief workers, may experience a subclinical syndrome of PTSD.

If the traveler has had such an experience, clinicians should inquire about possible symptoms:

- Reexperiencing the event could include recurrent and intrusive recollections or distressing dreams of the event or feeling as if the event is happening again.
- Avoidance symptoms can include avoiding thoughts, feelings, activities, places, or people that lead to memories of the event.
- Arousal symptoms can include difficulty sleeping or concentrating, irritability, or an exaggerated startle response.

As symptoms may occur months or even years after an event, education about the possibility of having such symptoms in the future is worthwhile. If there is any doubt about a possible reaction to a traumatic event, referral to a psychiatrist is warranted.

BIBLIOGRAPHY

1. Benedek DM, Wynn GH. Clinical manual for management of PTSD. Arlington, VA: American Psychiatric Publishing, Inc.; 2011.
2. Liese B, Mundt KA, Dell LD, Nagy L, Demure B. Medical insurance claims associated with international business travel. Occup Environ Med. 1997 Jul;54(7):499–503.
3. Patel D, Easmon CJ, Dow C, Snashall DC, Seed PT. Medical repatriation of British diplomats resident overseas. J Travel Med. 2000 Mar–Apr;7(2):64–9.
4. Streltzer J. Psychiatric emergencies in travelers to Hawaii. Compr Psychiatry. 1979 Sep–Oct;20(5):463–8.
5. Valk TH. Psychiatric and psychosocial counseling of the international traveler and expatriate family. Shoreland's Travel Medicine Monthly. 1998;2(7):1, 3–5, 10.
6. Valk TH. Psychiatric medical evacuations within the Foreign Service. Foreign Serv Med Bull. 1988;268:9–11.

TRAVEL HEALTH KITS
Amanda Whatley Lee

OVERVIEW

Regardless of the destination, all international travelers should assemble and carry a travel health kit. The contents of a travel health kit should be tailored to the traveler's needs, type and length of travel, and destinations. Kits can be assembled at home or purchased at a local store, pharmacy, or online.

A travel health kit can help to ensure travelers have supplies they need to:

- Manage preexisting medical conditions and treat any exacerbations of these conditions
- Prevent illness related to traveling
- Take care of minor health problems as they occur

By bringing medications from home, travelers avoid having to purchase them at their destination. See *Perspectives*: Pharmaceutical Quality & Counterfeit Drugs later in this chapter for information about the risks associated with purchasing medications abroad. Even when the quality of medications is reliable, medications people are used to taking at home may be sold by different names or dosage units in other countries, presenting additional challenges.

TRAVELING WITH MEDICATIONS

All medications should be carried in their original containers with clear labels, so the contents are easily identified. The patient's name and dosing regimen should be on each container. Although many travelers prefer placing medications into small containers or packing them in daily-dose containers, officials at ports of entry may require proper identification of medications.

Travelers should carry copies of all prescriptions, including their generic names. For controlled substances and injectable medications, travelers should carry a note from the prescribing physician or from the travel clinic on letterhead stationery. Certain medications are not permitted in some countries. If there is a question about these restrictions, particularly regarding controlled substances, travelers should contact the embassy or consulate of the destination country.

A travel health kit is useful only when it is easily accessible. It should be carried with the traveler at all times (such as in a carry-on bag), although sharp objects must remain in checked luggage. Travelers should make sure that any liquid or gel-based items packed in the carry-on bags do not exceed the size limits. Exceptions are made for certain medical reasons; check the Transportation Security Administration for US outbound and inbound travel (toll-free at 855-787-2227 M–F 8 AM to 11 PM or at www.tsa.gov/travelers/airtravel/disabilityandmedicalneeds/index.shtm) and the embassy or consulate of the destination country for their restrictions.

SUPPLIES FOR PREEXISTING MEDICAL CONDITIONS

Travelers with preexisting medical conditions should carry enough medication for the duration of their trip and an extra supply, in case the trip is extended for any reason. If additional supplies or medications would be needed to manage exacerbations of existing medical conditions, these should be carried as well. The clinician managing a traveler's preexisting medical conditions should be consulted for the best plan of action (see Chapter 8, Travelers with Chronic Illnesses).

People with preexisting conditions, such as diabetes or allergies, should consider wearing an alert bracelet (such as those available from www.medicalert.org) and making sure this information is on a card in their wallet and with their other travel documents.

GENERAL TRAVEL HEALTH KIT SUPPLIES

Although the following is not a comprehensive list, basic items that should be considered for a travel health kit are listed below. See Chapters 7 and 8 for additional suggestions that may be useful in planning the contents of a kit for travelers with specific needs.

Medications

- Destination-related, if applicable:
  > Antimalarial medications
  > Medication to prevent or treat altitude illness
- Pain or fever (one or more of the following, or an alternative):
  > Acetaminophen
  > Aspirin
  > Ibuprofen
- Stomach upset or diarrhea:
  > Over-the-counter antidiarrheal medication (such as loperamide [Imodium] or bismuth subsalicylate [Pepto-Bismol])
  > Antibiotic for self-treatment of moderate to severe diarrhea
  > Packets of oral rehydration salts for dehydration
  > Mild laxative
  > Antacid
- Upper respiratory tract discomfort:
  > Antihistamine

  > Decongestant, alone or in combination with antihistamine
  > Cough suppressant or expectorant
  > Cough drops
- Anti-motion sickness medication
- Epinephrine auto-injectors* (such as an EpiPen 2-Pak), especially if history of severe allergic reaction or anaphylaxis; smaller-dose packages are available for children
- Any medications, prescription or over the counter, taken on a regular basis at home.
- Needles or syringes, if needed, such as for people with diabetes. Needles and syringes can be difficult to purchase in some locations, so take more than what is needed for the length of the trip. (These items will require a letter from the prescribing physician on letterhead stationery.)

Basic First Aid

- Disposable latex-free exam gloves (≥2 pairs)
- Adhesive bandages, multiple sizes
- Gauze
- Adhesive tape
- Elastic bandage wrap for sprains and strains
- Triangular bandage to wrap injuries and to make an arm or shoulder sling
- Antiseptic
- Cotton swabs
- Tweezers**
- Scissors**
- Antifungal and antibacterial spray or creams
- 1% hydrocortisone cream
- Anti-itch gel or cream for insect bites and stings
- Aloe gel for sunburns
- Moleskin or molefoam for blister prevention and treatment
- Saline eye drops
- Saline nose drops or spray
- Digital thermometer
- First aid quick reference card

Other Important Items

- Insect repellent (see the Protection against Mosquitoes, Ticks, & Other Insects & Arthropods section earlier in this chapter for recommended types)

---

*Note: Injectable epinephrine and antihistamines should always be carried on one's person, including during air, sea, and land travel, for immediate treatment of a severe allergic reaction. Travelers with a history of severe allergic reactions should consider bringing along a short course of oral steroid medication (prescription required from doctor) and antihistamines as additional treatment of a severe allergic reaction.

**Note: If traveling by air, travelers should pack these sharp items in checked baggage, since they could be confiscated by airport or airline security if packed in carry-on bags. Small bandage scissors with rounded tips may be available for purchase in certain stores or online.

- Sunscreen (≥15 SPF)
- Antibacterial hand wipes or an alcohol-based hand sanitizer, containing ≥60% alcohol
- Useful items in certain circumstances:
  - > Extra pair of contact lenses, prescription glasses, or both, for people who wear corrective lenses
  - > Mild hypnotic medication (such as zolpidem [Ambien]), other sleep aid, or antianxiety medication
  - > Latex condoms
  - > Water purification tablets
  - > Commercial suture or syringe kits to be used by a local clinician. (These items will require a letter from the prescribing physician on letterhead stationery.)

Contact Card

Travelers should carry a contact card with the street addresses, phone numbers, and e-mail addresses of the following:

- Family member or close contact remaining in the United States
- Place of lodging at the destination
- Health care provider(s) at home
- Medical insurance information
- Travel insurance, travel health insurance, and medical evacuation insurance information
- Area hospitals or clinics, including emergency services
- US embassy or consulate in the destination country or countries

See the Obtaining Health Care Abroad for the Ill Traveler section later in this chapter for information about how to locate local health care and embassy or consulate contacts.

Travelers should also leave a copy of this contact card with a family member or close contact who will remain in the United States, in case of an emergency.

COMMERCIAL MEDICAL KITS

Commercial medical kits are available for a wide range of circumstances, from basic first aid to advanced emergency life support. Many pharmacy, grocery, retail, and outdoor sporting goods stores sell their own basic first aid kits. Travelers who choose to purchase a health kit should review the contents of the kit carefully to ensure that it has everything needed. Additional items may be necessary and can be added to the purchased kit.

For more adventurous travelers, a number of companies produce advanced medical kits and will even customize kits based on specific travel needs. In addition, specialty kits are available for managing diabetes, dealing with dental emergencies, and handling aquatic environments. Below is a list of websites supplying a wide range of medical kits. There are many suppliers, and this list is not meant to be all-inclusive.

- American Red Cross: www.redcrossstore.org
- Adventure Medical Kits: www.adventure medicalkits.com
- Chinook Medical Gear: www.chinookmed. com
- International Medical Center: www.travel doc.com/products/kits.aspx
- Travel Medicine, Inc.: www.travmed.com
- Wilderness Medicine Outfitters: www.wil dernessmedicine.com

BIBLIOGRAPHY

1. Goodyer L. Travel medical kits. In: Keystone JS, Freedman DO, Kozarsky PE, Connor BA, Nothdurft HD, editors. Travel Medicine. 3rd ed. Philadelphia: Saunders Elsevier; 2013. p. 63–6.
2. Harper LA, Bettinger J, Dismukes R, Kozarsky PE. Evaluation of the Coca-Cola company travel health kit. J Travel Med. 2002 Sep–Oct; 9(5):244–6.
3. Rose SR, Keystone JS. Chapter 2, trip preparation. In: Rose SR, Keystone JS, editors. International Travel Health Guide. 14th ed. Northampton: Travel Medicine, Inc; 2008.

Perspectives

PHARMACEUTICAL QUALITY & COUNTERFEIT DRUGS
Michael D. Green

GENERAL INFORMATION
Counterfeit and substandard drugs are an international problem contributing to illness, death, toxicity, and drug resistance. A counterfeit drug is a compound that is not made by an authorized manufacturer but is presented to the consumer as if it were. Both the packaging and pill construction of counterfeit drugs are often virtually identical to the authentic medication. Substandard drugs are medicines made by a licensed manufacturer but fail to comply with pharmaceutical regulatory standards. These drugs may not contain the proper proportion of ingredients and are consequently less effective or may cause an adverse reaction. Regulatory agencies in the United States, such as the Food and Drug Administration (FDA), protect citizens from products that are inherently unsafe. In developing countries, regulatory controls are much less effective or even nonexistent, leading to conditions that allow proliferation of counterfeit and substandard drugs. Overall, global estimates of drug counterfeiting are ambiguous, depending on region, but proportions range from 1% of sales in developed countries to >10% in developing countries. In specific regions in Africa, Asia, and Latin America, chances of purchasing a counterfeit drug may be >30%.

Since counterfeit drugs are not made by the legitimate manufacturer and are produced under unlawful circumstances, toxic contaminants or lack of proper ingredients may result in serious harm. For example, the active pharmaceutical ingredient may be completely lacking, present in small quantities, or substituted by a less-effective compound. In addition, the wrong inactive ingredients (excipients) can contribute to poor drug dissolution and bioavailability. As a result, a patient may not respond to treatment or may have adverse reactions to unknown substituted or toxic ingredients.

Before international departure, travel health providers should alert travelers to the dangers of counterfeit and substandard drugs and provide suggestions on how to avoid them.

HOW TO AVOID COUNTERFEIT DRUGS WHEN TRAVELING
The best way to avoid counterfeit drugs is to reduce the need to purchase medications abroad. Anticipated amounts of medications for chronic conditions (such as hypertension, sinusitis, arthritis, and hay fever); medications for gastroenteritis (travelers' diarrhea); and prophylactic medications for infectious diseases (such as malaria) should all be purchased before traveling.

Before departure, travelers should do the following:

- Purchase all medicines needed for the trip in advance. Prescriptions written in the United States usually cannot be filled overseas, and over-the-counter medicines may not be available in many foreign countries. Checked baggage

Perspectives sections are written as editorial discussions aiming to add depth and clinical perspective to the official recommendations contained in the book. The views and opinions expressed in this section are those of the author and do not necessarily represent the official position of CDC.

can get lost; therefore, travelers should pack as much as possible in a carry-on bag and bring extra medicine in case of travel delays.

- Make sure medicines are in their original containers. If the drug is a prescription, the patient's name and dose regimen should be on the container.
- Bring the "patient prescription information" sheet. This sheet provides information on common generic and brand names, use, side effects, precautions, and drug interactions.

If travelers run out and require additional medications, they should take steps to ensure the medicines they buy are safe:

- Purchase medicines from a legitimate pharmacy. Patients should not buy from open markets, street vendors, or suspicious-looking pharmacies; they should request a receipt when making the purchase. The US embassy may be able to help find a legitimate pharmacy in the area.
- Do not buy medicines that are substantially cheaper than the typical price. Although generics are usually less expensive, many counterfeited brand names are sold at prices substantially below the normal price for that particular brand.
- Make sure the medicines are in their original packages or containers. If travelers receive medicines as loose tablets or capsules supplied in a plastic bag or envelope, they should ask the pharmacist to see the container from which the medicine was originally dispensed. The traveler should record the brand, batch number, and expiration date. Sometimes a wary consumer will prompt the seller into supplying quality medicine.
- Be familiar with medications. The size, shape, color, and taste of counterfeit medicines may be different from the authentic. Discoloration, splits, cracks, spots, and stickiness of the tablets or capsules are indications of a possible counterfeit. Travelers should keep examples of authentic medications to compare if they purchase the same brand.
- Be familiar with the packaging. Different color inks, poor-quality print or packaging material, and misspelled words are clues to counterfeit drugs. Travelers should keep an example of packaging for comparison, and observe the expiration date to make sure the medicine has not expired.

USEFUL WEBSITES

General Information about Counterfeit Drugs

- CDC: wwwnc.cdc.gov/travel/contentCounterfeitDrugs.aspx
- World Health Organization:
    > www.who.int/mediacentre/factsheets/fs275/en
    > www.who.int/medicines/services/counterfeit/overview/en
- Food and Drug Administration: www.fda.gov//Drugs/DrugSafety/ucm170314.htm
- US Pharmacopeia: www.usp.org/worldwide

Traveling and Customs Guidelines

Researching what travelers can pack and bring back into the United States, especially for travelers with disabilities and medical conditions, is helpful in preparing for travel.

- Transportation Security Administration: www.tsa.gov/travelers/airtravel/disabilityandmedicalneeds/index.shtm
- Customs and Border Protection: www.cbp.gov/xp/cgov/travel/clearing/restricted/medication_drugs.xml

Reporting Counterfeit Cases

- World Health Organization: www.who.int/medicines/services/counterfeit/report/en/

BIBLIOGRAPHY

1. Bate R, Jin GZ, Mathur A. Does price reveal poor-quality drugs? Evidence from 17 countries. J Health Econ. 2011 Dec;30(6):1150–63.
2. Nayyar GM, Breman JG, Newton PN, Herrington J. Poor-quality antimalarial drugs in southeast Asia and sub-Saharan Africa. Lancet Infect Dis. 2012 Jun;12(6):488–96.
3. Newton P, Fernandez F, Green M. Counterfeit and substandard antimalarial drugs. In: Schlagenhauf-Lawlor P, editor. Travelers' Malaria. 2nd ed. Hamilton, ON: BC Decker; 2008. p. 331–42.
4. Newton PN, Green MD, Fernandez FM, Day NP, White NJ. Counterfeit anti-infective drugs. Lancet Infect Dis. 2006 Sep;6(9):602–13.
5. World Health Organization. Medicines: counterfeit medicines [fact sheet no. 275]. Geneva: World Health Organization; 2012 [cited 2012 Sep 18]. Available from: http://www.who.int/mediacentre/factsheets/fs275/en/.

OBTAINING HEALTH CARE ABROAD FOR THE ILL TRAVELER

Theresa E. Sommers

INTRODUCTION

The quality and availability of proper medical care abroad may be variable. Before departure, travelers should consider how they would access adequate health care during their trip, should a medical problem arise. Many insurance plans provide coverage for emergency health care while abroad, but travelers should check with their carriers to confirm what coverage is offered and what requirements exist. At a minimum, travelers will need to provide copies of bills and invoices to initiate reimbursement. Travelers should also be aware that emergency health coverage does not usually cover emergency evacuation or the costs of altered itineraries. Travelers may purchase specific policies to cover these expenses (see below).

LOCATING ADEQUATE HEALTH CARE PROVIDERS AND FACILITIES ABROAD

Before going abroad, travelers should identify adequate health care providers and facilities at their destination. This is especially true for travelers with preexisting or complicated medical issues. Travelers who require regular dialysis need to arrange appointments at an adequate clinical site before arriving at their destination. Similarly, pregnant travelers should identify reliable health facilities before going abroad.

The following resources list health care providers and facilities around the world:

- The Department of State (www.usembassy.gov) can help travelers locate medical services and notify friends, family, or employer of an emergency.
- The International Society of Travel Medicine (ISTM) maintains a directory of health care professionals with expertise in travel medicine in almost 50 countries worldwide. Search these clinics at www.istm.org.
- The International Association for Medical Assistance to Travelers (IAMAT) maintains an international network of physicians, hospitals, and clinics that have agreed to provide care to members while abroad. Membership is free, although donations are suggested. Search for clinics at http://www.iamat.org/doctors_clinics.cfm.
- The Joint Commission International (JCI) aims to improve patient safety through accreditation and certification of health care facilities worldwide. Facilities that

are accredited through JCI demonstrate a standard level of quality. A list of these facilities can be found at http://www. jointcommissioninternational.org/JCI-Accredited-Organizations.

- Embassies and consulates in other countries, hotel doctors, and credit card companies (especially those with special privileges) may also provide information.
- Supplemental medical insurance plans acquired prior to travel will often enable access to local providers in many countries through a 24-hour emergency hotline.

For more information on medical insurance, see the next section in this chapter, Travel Insurance, Travel Health Insurance, & Medical Evacuation Insurance.

In addition to identifying quality health care, travelers, especially those with chronic or complicated medical issues, should know all the names of their chronic conditions and allergies, their blood type, and current medications (including generic names), ideally in the local language. Travelers should also wear medical identification jewelry (such as a MedicAlert bracelet), if appropriate.

AVOID TRAVEL WHEN SICK

Travelers should evaluate their health before travel to ensure that they are healthy enough for their itinerary and should avoid travel if they become ill before or during their trip. Some airlines check for visibly sick passengers in the waiting area and during boarding. If a passenger looks visibly ill, the airline may prohibit that person from boarding. Travelers may be reluctant to postpone or cancel a trip when ill because of their financial investment in a trip, among other factors.

Encouraging travelers, especially those with chronic or complicated health conditions, to purchase trip cancellation insurance, which will protect some or all of the investment in a trip, may increase compliance with this recommendation.

DRUGS AND OTHER PHARMACEUTICALS

The quality of drugs and medical products abroad cannot be guaranteed, as they may not meet US standards or could be counterfeit (see *Perspectives*: Pharmaceutical Quality & Counterfeit Drugs earlier in this chapter). To

minimize risks associated with substandard drugs and pharmaceuticals, travelers should:

- Bring with them all the medicines that they think they will need, including pain relievers and antidiarrheal medication.
- Use caution when buying medications abroad, especially those that do not require a prescription. In many developing countries, a variety of drugs can be purchased without a prescription.
- Insist that a new needle and syringe be used when receiving an injection. Travelers who know beforehand that they will require injections during their trip can bring their own injection supplies (see the Travel Health Kits section earlier in this chapter).
- Carry an epinephrine autoinjector, if needed, in carry-on luggage and include a letter from the prescribing physician that explains the allergy and a copy of the prescription.

BLOOD SAFETY

A medical emergency abroad, such as a motor vehicle accident or trauma, could result in need for a blood transfusion. Not all countries have accurate, reliable, and systematic screening of blood donations for infectious agents, which increases the risk of transfusion-related transmission of disease. Although it is difficult to ensure access to safe blood, there are a few measures travelers can take to increase their chances of having a safe blood transfusion in the event of a medical emergency:

- Avoid blood transfusions as much as possible, particularly in developing countries. Travelers should receive a blood transfusion only in life-or-death situations.
- If a blood transfusion is required, travelers should make every effort to ensure that the blood has been screened for transmissible diseases, including HIV. Although this is difficult to do at the point of service, travelers who plan ahead and locate medical services before traveling will increase their chances of obtaining higher-quality care abroad.
- Travelers may consider registering with agencies such as the Blood Care Foundation that attempt to rapidly deliver reliable

blood products to members while abroad (http://www.bloodcare.org.uk/blood_trans-fusion_abroad.html).

All travelers should consider being immunized against hepatitis B virus before travel, especially those who travel frequently to developing countries, those whose itinerary indicates spending a prolonged period in developing countries, and those whose activities (such as adventure travel) put them at higher risk for serious injury.

BIBLIOGRAPHY

1. Kolars JC. Rules of the road: a consumer's guide for travelers seeking health care in foreign lands. J Travel Med. 2002 Jul–Aug; 9(4):198–201.
2. World Health Organization. Blood safety [fact sheet no. 279]. Geneva: World Health Organization; 2011 [cited 2012 Sep 18]. Available from: http://www.who.int/worldblooddonorday/media/who_blood_safety_factsheet_2011.pdf.
3. World Health Organization. Medicines: spurious/falsely-labelled/ falsified/counterfeit (SFFC) medicines [fact sheet no. 275]. Geneva: World Health Organization; 2012 [cited 2012 Sep 18]. Available from: http://www.who.int/mediacentre/factsheets/fs275/en/.

TRAVEL INSURANCE, TRAVEL HEALTH INSURANCE, & MEDICAL EVACUATION INSURANCE

Theresa E. Sommers

INTRODUCTION

Severe illness or injury abroad may result in a financial burden on travelers. Although planning for every possible contingency is impossible, travelers can reduce the cost of a medical emergency by considering the purchase of 3 types of insurance for their trip: travel insurance, travel health insurance, and medical evacuation insurance. These insurance policies can be purchased before a trip to provide coverage in the event of an illness or injury and may be of particular importance to travelers with chronic medical conditions. Basic accident or travel insurance may even be required for travelers to certain destinations.

TRAVEL INSURANCE

Travel insurance protects the financial investment in a trip, including lost baggage and trip cancellation. Travelers may be more likely to avoid travel when sick if they know their financial investment in the trip is protected. Depending on the policy, this type of insurance may or may not cover medical expenses abroad, so travelers need to carefully research the coverage offered to determine if additional travel health and medical evacuation insurance is needed.

PAYING FOR HEALTH SERVICES ABROAD

Medical care abroad usually requires cash or credit card payment at the point of service, regardless of whether the traveler has insurance coverage in their home country. This could result in a large out-of-pocket expenditure of perhaps thousands of dollars. Additionally, the existence of nationalized health care services in a given destination does not ensure that nonresidents will be given full coverage. When paying out-of-pocket for care, travelers should obtain copies of all bills and receipts and, if necessary, contact a US consular officer, who can assist US citizens with transferring funds from the United States.

The possibility of these large out-of-pocket medical expenses makes a discussion of insurance options an important part of any pre-travel consultation. Although insurance should be a consideration for all travelers, it is particularly important for travelers who are planning to be outside the United States for an extended period of time, have underlying health conditions, or plan to participate in high-risk activities on their trip.

DOMESTIC HEALTH INSURANCE

Some health insurance carriers in the United States may provide coverage for emergencies that occur while traveling abroad. Travelers should carefully examine their coverage and planned itinerary to determine exactly which medical services, if any, will be covered abroad and the level of supplemental insurance needed. The following is a list of characteristics to consider:

- Exclusions for treating exacerbations of preexisting medical conditions
- The company's policy for "out-of-network" services
- Coverage for complications of pregnancy (or for a neonate, especially if the newborn requires intensive care)
- Exclusions for high-risk activities such as skydiving, scuba diving, and mountain climbing
- Exclusions regarding psychiatric emergencies or injuries related to terrorist attacks or acts of war
- Whether preauthorization is needed for treatment, hospital admission, or other services
- Whether a second opinion is required before obtaining emergency treatment
- Whether there is a 24-hour physician-backed support center

SUPPLEMENTAL TRAVEL HEALTH AND MEDICAL EVACUATION INSURANCE

Short-term supplemental policies that cover health care costs on a trip can be purchased, and are relatively inexpensive. Medical evacuation coverage may be purchased separately or in conjunction with travel health insurance. Domestic insurance policies may not cover medical evacuation from a resource-poor area to a hospital where definitive care can be obtained, which can cost more than $100,000. Frequent travelers may want to consider purchasing annual policies or even policies that will provide coverage for repatriation to one's home country.

Medical evacuation companies may have better resources and experience in some parts of the world than others; travelers may want to ask about a company's resources in a given area, especially if planning a trip to remote destinations. The traveler should scrutinize all policies carefully before purchase, looking for those that provide the following:

- Arrangements with hospitals to guarantee payments directly
- Assistance via a 24-hour physician-backed support center (critical for medical evacuation insurance)
- Emergency medical transport to facilities that are equivalent to those in the home country or to the home country itself
- Any specific medical services that may apply to their circumstances, such as coverage of high-risk activities

Even if an insurance provider is selected carefully, travelers should be aware that unexpected delays in care may still arise, especially in remote destinations. In special circumstances, travelers may be advised to postpone or cancel international trips if the health risks are too high.

FINDING AN INSURANCE PROVIDER

The following resources, although not all-inclusive, provide information about purchasing travel health and medical evacuation insurance:

- Department of State (www.travel.state.gov)
- International SOS (www.internationalsos.com)
- MEDEX (www.medexassist.com)
- International Association for Medical Assistance to Travelers (www.iamat.org)
- American Association of Retired Persons (www.aarp.org) (for information about Medicare supplement plans, see below)

SPECIAL CONSIDERATIONS FOR TRAVELERS WITH UNDERLYING MEDICAL CONDITIONS

Travelers with underlying medical conditions should take extra precautions in preparing for travel. These travelers should choose a medical assistance company that allows customers to store their medical history before departure, so it can be accessed from anywhere in the world. Travelers should carry a letter from their physician listing their medical conditions and current medications (including their generic names), written in the local language if possible. Those with cardiac disease should carry a copy (paper or electronic) of their most recent ECG. They should also pack all medications in their original bottles, checking beforehand with the destination's embassy to ensure that none are considered illegal narcotics in the destination country.

SPECIAL CONSIDERATIONS FOR MEDICARE BENEFICIARIES

The Social Security Medicare program does not provide coverage for medical costs outside the United States, except in limited circumstances. Some Medigap plans may provide limited coverage for emergency care abroad. As with all travelers, Medicare beneficiaries should examine their coverage carefully and supplement with additional travel health insurance as needed.

CHECKLIST FOR DISCUSSING INSURANCE WITH TRAVELERS

The following checklist can be used for guiding an insurance discussion during a pre-travel consultation. In short, travelers should:

- Consider travel, travel health, and medical evacuation insurance.
- Scrutinize their domestic health insurance policy to see what medical services may or may not be covered abroad.
- Locate medical services in areas that they plan to visit and carry this information with them on their trip.
- Carry copies of their insurance policy identity cards, including any supplemental insurance purchased for a trip, and insurance claim forms.
- Retain copies of all bills and receipts for medical care received abroad.

BIBLIOGRAPHY

1. American Association of Retired Persons, Education and Outreach. Overview of Medicare supplemental insurance. Washington, DC: American Association of Retired Persons; 2010 [cited 2012 Sep 18]. Available from: http://www.aarp.org/health/medicare-insurance/info-10-2008/overview_medicare_supplemental_insurance.html.
2. Centers for Medicare and Medicaid Services. Medicare coverage outside the United States. Baltimore: CMS; 2010 [cited 2012 Sep 18]. Available from: http://www.medicare.gov/Publications/Pubs/pdf/11037.pdf.
3. Leggat PA, Carne J, Kedjarune U. Travel insurance and health. J Travel Med. 1999 Dec;6(4):243–8.
4. Teichman PG, Donchin Y, Kot RJ. International aeromedical evacuation. N Engl J Med. 2007 Jan 18;356(3):262–70.
5. US Department of State. Medical insurance. Washington, DC: US Department of State; 2010 [cited 2012 Sep 18]. Available from: http://travel.state.gov/travel/cis_pa_tw/cis/cis_1470.html.

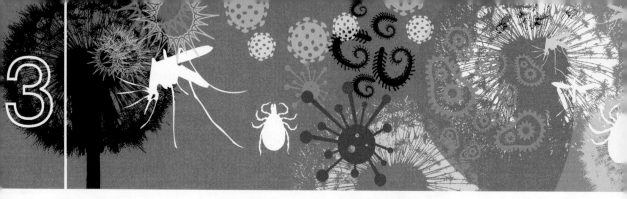

Infectious Diseases Related To Travel

AMEBIASIS

Sharon L. Roy

INFECTIOUS AGENT

The protozoan parasite *Entamoeba histolytica*.

TRANSMISSION

Fecal-oral route, either directly by person-to-person contact (such as by diaper-changing or sexual practices) or indirectly by eating or drinking fecally contaminated food or water.

EPIDEMIOLOGY

Distributed worldwide, particularly in the tropics; more common in areas of poor sanitation. Long-term travelers (duration >6 months) are significantly more likely than short-term travelers (duration <1 month) to develop *E. histolytica* infection. People at higher risk for severe disease are those who are pregnant, immunocompromised, or receiving corticosteroids; associations with diabetes and alcohol use have also been reported.

CLINICAL PRESENTATION

Most patients have a gradual illness onset days or weeks after infection. Symptoms include cramps, watery or bloody diarrhea, and weight loss and may last several weeks. Occasionally, the parasite may spread to other organs (extraintestinal amebiasis), most commonly the liver. Amebic liver abscesses may be asymptomatic, but most patients present with fever and right upper quadrant abdominal pain, usually in the absence of diarrhea.

DIAGNOSIS

Microscopy does not distinguish between *E. histolytica* (pathogenic), *E. dispar*, and *E. moshkovskii*. The latter 2 have historically been considered nonpathogenic, but new evidence suggests they might cause illness. More specific tests such as EIA or PCR are needed to confirm the diagnosis of *E. histolytica*. Additionally, serologic tests can help diagnose extraintestinal amebiasis.

TREATMENT

For symptomatic intestinal infection and extraintestinal disease, treatment with metronidazole or tinidazole should be followed by treatment with iodoquinol or paromomycin. Asymptomatic patients infected with *E. histolytica* should also be treated with iodoquinol or paromomycin, because they can infect others and because 4%–10% develop disease within a year if left untreated.

PREVENTION

Food and water precautions (see Chapter 2, Food & Water Precautions) and hand hygiene. Avoid fecal exposure during sexual activity.

CDC website: www.cdc.gov/parasites/amebiasis

BIBLIOGRAPHY

1. Bercu TE, Petri WA, Behm JW. Amebic colitis: new insights into pathogenesis and treatment. Curr Gastroenterol Rep. 2007 Oct;9(5):429–33.

2. Petri WA Jr, Singh U. Diagnosis and management of amebiasis. Clin Infect Dis. 1999 Nov;29(5):1117–25.

3. Stanley SL Jr. Amoebiasis. Lancet. 2003 Mar 22;361(9362):1025–34.

ANGIOSTRONGYLIASIS, NEUROLOGIC

Barbara L. Herwaldt

INFECTIOUS AGENT

Angiostrongylus cantonensis, rat lungworm, a nematode parasite.

TRANSMISSION

Various species of rats are the definitive hosts of the parasite, known as the rat lungworm. Rats are only able to infect snails and slugs, which are the intermediate hosts. Transmission to humans occurs by consuming infected snails or slugs or contaminated raw produce or vegetable juices. Infective larvae have also been found in freshwater shrimp, crabs, and frogs, considered transport (paratenic) hosts.

EPIDEMIOLOGY

Most described cases have occurred in Asia and the Pacific Basin (such as in parts of Thailand, Taiwan, mainland China, the Hawaiian Islands, and other Pacific Islands); however, cases have been reported in many areas of the world, including the Caribbean.

CLINICAL PRESENTATION

Incubation period is typically 1–3 weeks but ranges from 1 day to >6 weeks. *A. cantonensis* is considered the most common infectious cause of eosinophilic meningitis in humans. Common manifestations include headache, photophobia, stiff neck, nausea, vomiting, fatigue, and body aches. Abnormal skin sensations (such as tingling or painful feelings) are more common than in other types of meningitis. A low-grade fever might be noted. Symptoms are usually self-limited but may persist for weeks or months. Severe cases can be associated with paralysis, blindness, or death.

DIAGNOSIS

Typically presumptive, on the basis of clinical and epidemiologic criteria in people with otherwise unexplained eosinophilic meningitis.

TREATMENT

The larvae die spontaneously, and supportive care usually suffices. Clinicians may consult with CDC about evaluation and treatment of patients (404-718-4745; parasites@cdc.gov).

PREVENTION

Food and water precautions, particularly:

- Avoid eating raw or undercooked snails, slugs, and other possible hosts.
- Eat raw produce, such as lettuce, only if it has been thoroughly washed or treated with bleach. Such measures might provide some protection but may not eliminate the risk.
- Wear gloves (and wash hands) if snails or slugs are handled.

CDC website: www.cdc.gov/parasites/angio strongylus

BIBLIOGRAPHY

1. Hochberg NS, Blackburn BG, Park SY, Sejvar JJ, Effler PV, Herwaldt BL. Eosinophilic meningitis attributable to *Angiostrongylus cantonensis* infection in Hawaii: clinical characteristics and potential exposures. Am J Trop Med Hyg. 2011 Oct;85(4):685–90.

2. Wang QP, Lai DH, Zhu XQ, Chen XG, Lun ZR. Human angiostrongyliasis. Lancet Infect Dis. 2008 Oct;8(10):621–30.

ANTHRAX

Sean V. Shadomy, Chung K. Marston

INFECTIOUS AGENT

Aerobic, gram-positive, encapsulated, spore-forming, nonmotile, nonhemolytic, rod-shaped bacterium *Bacillus anthracis*.

TRANSMISSION

B. anthracis is primarily transmitted by direct contact with *B. anthracis*-infected animals or their carcasses or with contaminated products from infected animals, including meat, hides, wool, or items made with those products, such as drums or wool clothing.

Anthrax normally presents in 3 forms: cutaneous, gastrointestinal, and inhalation. Introduction of the spores through the skin can result in cutaneous anthrax; abrasion of the skin increases susceptibility. Eating meat from infected animals can result in gastrointestinal anthrax. Inhalation anthrax typically occurs when a person inhales spores aerosolized by industrial processing of contaminated materials, such as hides or wool, or by working with contaminated animal hides or wool in a way that can aerosolize dust and spores; it can also result from bioterrorism. Anthrax in humans is not generally considered to be contagious; person-to-person transmission of cutaneous anthrax has rarely been reported.

EPIDEMIOLOGY

Anthrax is a zoonotic disease that primarily affects herbivores such as cattle, sheep, goats, antelope, and deer, which become infected by ingesting contaminated vegetation, water, or soil; humans are generally incidental hosts.

Anthrax is most common in agricultural regions in Central and South America, sub-Saharan Africa, Central and Southwestern Asia, and southern and Eastern Europe. Anthrax is now rare in the United States and Canada; however, sporadic outbreaks occur every year in livestock and wild herbivores in these countries. Travelers to endemic areas have acquired anthrax through either direct or indirect contact with carcasses of animals that died from anthrax. Cases of cutaneous, gastrointestinal, and inhalation anthrax have

been reported among people who have handled or played drums made with contaminated goat hides from countries endemic for anthrax or who have been present at events where those drums have been played. Cases have also been reported among people making drums from contaminated goat hides imported from countries endemic for anthrax, as well as members of their households exposed to environments contaminated by the drum-making process.

Sepsis and severe soft tissue infection at injection sites have been reported in drug users in northern Europe and are suspected to be due to recreational use of heroin contaminated with *B. anthracis* spores. No associated cases have been identified in people who had not deliberately taken heroin. To date no heroin has been found to be contaminated with *B. anthracis* spores.

CLINICAL PRESENTATION

Cutaneous anthrax usually develops 1–7 days after exposure. The case-fatality ratio is as high as 20% if untreated, but typically is <1% with antimicrobial therapy. Cutaneous anthrax is characterized by localized itching, followed by the development of a painless papule, which turns vesicular and enlarges, ulcerates, and develops into a depressed black eschar within 7–10 days of the initial lesion. The head, neck, forearms, and hands are the most commonly affected sites. Edema usually surrounds the lesion, sometimes with secondary vesicles, hyperemia, and regional lymphadenopathy. Patients may have associated fever, malaise, and headache.

Gastrointestinal anthrax usually develops 1–7 days after consumption of contaminated meat and can present in either intestinal or oropharyngeal forms. Shock and death may occur within 2–5 days of onset; estimates of the case-fatality ratio for gastrointestinal anthrax are >50% if untreated, but <40% with treatment.

Inhalation anthrax usually develops within a week after exposure, but the incubation period may be prolonged (up to

2 months). Estimates for the case-fatality ratio are >85%; even with aggressive treatment, this ratio can be as high as 45%. Initial symptoms are nonspecific and may mimic those of influenza, including myalgia, fever, nonproductive cough, malaise, nausea, and vomiting; upper respiratory tract symptoms are rare. The patient's condition dramatically worsens 2–3 days after symptom onset, with the development of severe respiratory distress, diaphoresis, cyanosis, and shock.

Cases of anthrax in injection drug users reportedly developed within 1–4 days of exposure in most cases for which a suspected exposure could be identified; the case-fatality ratio was >25% in confirmed cases. Cases presented with severe soft tissue infection with or without localized swelling or with symptoms of sepsis, disseminated infection, and toxemia.

Hemorrhagic meningitis may develop with any of the clinical forms of anthrax from hematogenous spread. Anthrax meningitis is nearly always fatal.

DIAGNOSIS

Laboratory diagnosis depends on bacterial culture and isolation of B. anthracis; detection of bacterial DNA, antigens, or toxins; or detection of a host immune response to B. anthracis. Serologic testing of host antibody responses requires acute- and convalescent-phase sera for diagnosis. Anthrax lethal toxin can be detected from acute-phase serum. Confirmatory testing, including isolate identification, antigen detection in tissues, or quantitative serology, should be performed in the United States by the state health department or Laboratory Response Network laboratories, or internationally by the relevant national reference laboratory. Guidelines for collecting and submitting clinical specimens for testing and algorithms for laboratory diagnosis can be found at www.bt.cdc.gov/agent/anthrax/labtesting. Specimens for culture should be collected before initiating antimicrobial therapy. Diagnostic procedures for inhalation anthrax include thoracic imaging studies to detect a widened mediastinum or pleural effusion.

TREATMENT

Ciprofloxacin is the drug of choice. Because of intrinsic resistance, neither cephalosporins nor trimethoprim-sulfamethoxazole should be used. Localized or uncomplicated naturally occurring cutaneous anthrax can be treated with ciprofloxacin or oral doxycycline, except in children aged <2 years. If susceptibility testing is supportive, oral penicillin V or amoxicillin may be used to complete the regimen. Treatment recommendations for severe systemic or life-threatening disease (such as inhalation anthrax; gastrointestinal anthrax; anthrax meningitis; severe cutaneous anthrax with systemic involvement, extensive edema, or head and neck lesions; treatment of children aged <2 years; or cutaneous anthrax associated with aerosol exposure) are found at www.cdc.gov/mmwr/preview/mmwrhtml/mm5042a1.htm.

PREVENTION

Vaccination against anthrax is not recommended for travelers and is not available for civilian travelers. Travelers should not have direct or indirect contact with carcasses of animals found in anthrax-endemic regions or eat meat from animals that were not inspected by health officials and found to be healthy at the time of slaughter. The risk of acquiring anthrax from playing with or handling an animal hide drum is very low. Since 2006, 6 cases of anthrax (including all 3 forms: cutaneous, gastrointestinal, and inhalation) in the United States and United Kingdom have been associated with making animal-hide drums or participating in drumming workshops or events where animal-hide drums were played. Some of these cases were fatal. Travelers who wish to bring back animal hides from anthrax-endemic regions to make drums should strongly consider the health risks before importing the hides.

No tests are available to determine if animal products are free of contamination with B. anthracis spores. Animal-hide drum owners or players should report any unexplained fever or new skin lesions to their health care provider and describe their recent contact with animal-hide drums.

The importation of goat-hide souvenirs, such as goat-hide drums, from Haiti is prohibited by CDC (see Chapter 6, Taking Animals & Animal Products across International Borders). Importation of animal products, including processed or unprocessed cattle and goat hides, is regulated by the United States Department of Agriculture (USDA). Animal products, trophies, or souvenirs from anthrax-endemic regions must be accompanied by an international veterinary certificate stating that they were harvested from animals that were free of anthrax, or that they have been disinfected in accordance with international regulations, for them to be allowed to be imported into the United States. Cattle or goat hides that have been tanned, pickled in a solution of salt and mineral acid, or treated with lime are considered to pose less of a risk for infectious diseases and may be imported under certain conditions. For more information, consult the USDA website at www.aphis.usda.gov/import_export/animals/animal_import/animal_imports.shtml and the World Organisation for Animal Health (OIE) Terrestrial Animal Health Code at www.oie.int/en/international-standard-setting/terrestrial-code/access-online.

CDC website: http://emergency.cdc.gov/agent/anthrax

BIBLIOGRAPHY

1. Anaraki S, Addiman S, Nixon G, Krahe D, Ghosh R, Brooks T, et al. Investigations and control measures following a case of inhalation anthrax in east London in a drum maker and drummer, October 2008. Euro Surveill. 2008 Dec 18;13(51).
2. Bales ME, Dannenberg AL, Brachman PS, Kaufmann AF, Klatsky PC, Ashford DA. Epidemiologic response to anthrax outbreaks: field investigations, 1950–2001. Emerg Infect Dis. 2002 Oct;8(10):1163–74.
3. CDC. Cutaneous anthrax associated with drum making using goat hides from West Africa—Connecticut, 2007. MMWR Morb Mortal Wkly Rep. 2008 Jun 13;57(23):628–31.
4. CDC. Gastrointestinal anthrax after an animal-hide drumming event—New Hampshire and Massachusetts, 2009. MMWR Morb Mortal Wkly Rep. 2010 Jul 23;59(28):872–7.
5. CDC. Inhalation anthrax associated with dried animal hides—Pennsylvania and New York City, 2006. MMWR Morb Mortal Wkly Rep. 2006 Mar 17;55(10):280–2.
6. Eurosurveillance editorial team. Probable human anthrax death in Scotland. Euro Surveill. 2006;11(8):E060817.2.
7. Inglesby TV, O'Toole T, Henderson DA, Bartlett JG, Ascher MS, Eitzen E, et al. Anthrax as a biological weapon, 2002: updated recommendations for management. JAMA. 2002 May 1;287(17):2236–52.
8. National Anthrax Outbreak Control Team. An outbreak of anthrax among drug users in Scotland, December 2009 to December 2010. Glasgow: Health Protection Scotland; 2011 [cited 2012 Sep 18]. Available from: http://www.documents.hps.scot.nhs.uk/giz/anthrax-outbreak/anthrax-outbreak-report-2011-12.pdf.
9. Stern EJ, Uhde KB, Shadomy SV, Messonnier N. Conference report on public health and clinical guidelines for anthrax. Emerg Infect Dis [Internet]. 2008 Apr;14(4). Available from: http://wwwnc.cdc.gov/eid/article/14/4/07-0969.htm.
10. Van den Enden E, Van Gompel A, Van Esbroeck M. Cutaneous anthrax, Belgian traveler. Emerg Infect Dis. 2006 Mar;12(3):523–5.

BARTONELLA INFECTIONS
Christina A. Nelson

INFECTIOUS AGENT
Gram-negative bacteria in the genus *Bartonella*. Human illness is primarily caused by *Bartonella henselae* (cat-scratch disease [CSD]), *B. quintana* (trench fever), and *B. bacilliformis* (Carrión disease). A variety of *Bartonella* spp. can cause culture-negative endocarditis; other clinical syndromes due to *Bartonella* spp. have also been reported. For example, in 2007, a newly recognized species of *Bartonella* (*B. rochalimae*) was identified in an ill traveler returning from Peru.

TRANSMISSION
CSD is contracted through scratches from domestic or feral cats, particularly kittens. CSD may be transmitted directly to humans by the bite of infected cat fleas, although this has not yet been proven. Trench fever is transmitted by the human body louse. Carrión disease

is transmitted by sand flies (genus *Lutzomyia*) that are infected with *B. bacilliformis*.

EPIDEMIOLOGY

CSD and trench fever are distributed worldwide. In the United States, CSD is more common in children, and the incidence peaks from September through January. Trench fever typically occurs in populations that do not have access to proper hygiene, such as refugees and the homeless. Carrión disease has limited geographic distribution; transmission occurs in the Andes Mountains at 1–3 km (0.6–1.9 miles) elevation in western South America, including Peru, Colombia, and Ecuador. Most cases are reported in Peru.

CLINICAL PRESENTATION

CSD symptoms include fever; enlarged, tender lymph nodes that develop 1–3 weeks after exposure; and a papule or pustule at the inoculation site. Trench fever symptoms include fever, headache, transient rash, and bone pain (mainly in the shins, neck, and back).

Bacillary angiomatosis (caused by *B. henselae* or *B. quintana*) and peliosis hepatis (caused by *B. henselae*) occur primarily in people infected with HIV. Bacillary angiomatosis may present as skin, subcutaneous, or bone lesions. Many *Bartonella* spp. can cause signs and symptoms of subacute endocarditis, which is often culture-negative.

Carrión disease has 2 distinct phases: an acute phase (Oroya fever) characterized by fever, myalgia, headache, and anemia and an eruptive phase (verruga peruana) characterized by red-to-purple nodular skin lesions.

DIAGNOSIS

CSD can be diagnosed clinically in patients with typical presentation and a compatible exposure history. Serology can confirm the diagnosis, although cross-reactivity may limit interpretation. *B. henselae* DNA may also be detected by PCR or culture of pus or lymph node aspirates by using special techniques.

Trench fever can be diagnosed by isolating *B. quintana* from blood or by serology. PCR technology is improving the diagnosis of disseminated *Bartonella* infections. Endocarditis caused by *Bartonella* spp. can be diagnosed by elevated serology of the patient and by PCR or culture of excised heart valve tissue.

Oroya fever is typically diagnosed via blood culture or direct observation of the bacilli in peripheral blood smears.

TREATMENT

Most cases of CSD eventually resolve without treatment, but a small percentage of people will develop disseminated disease with severe complications. The use of antibiotics to shorten the course of disease is debated, although azithromycin speeds the decrease in lymph node volume.

Various antibiotics are effective against *Bartonella* infections, including penicillins, tetracyclines, cephalosporins, aminoglycosides, and fluoroquinolones. Recommended antibiotic regimens and duration of treatment vary by clinical disease.

PREVENTION

Avoid playing with cats, particularly strays. Protect against bites of sand flies and body lice (see Chapter 2, Protection against Mosquitoes, Ticks, & Other Insects & Arthropods).

CDC website: www.cdc.gov/healthypets/diseases/catscratch.htm

BIBLIOGRAPHY

1. Bass JW, Freitas BC, Freitas AD, Sisler CL, Chan DS, Vincent JM, et al. Prospective randomized double blind placebo-controlled evaluation of azithromycin for treatment of cat-scratch disease. Pediatr Infect Dis J. 1998 Jun;17(6):447–52.
2. Eremeeva ME, Gerns HL, Lydy SL, Goo JS, Ryan ET, Mathew SS, et al. Bacteremia, fever, and splenomegaly caused by a newly recognized bartonella species. N Engl J Med. 2007 Jun 7;356(23):2381–7.
3. Florin TA, Zaoutis TE, Zaoutis LB. Beyond cat scratch disease: widening spectrum of *Bartonella henselae* infection. Pediatrics. 2008 May;121(5):e1413–25.
4. Fournier PE, Thuny F, Richet H, Lepidi H, Casalta JP, Arzouni JP, et al. Comprehensive diagnostic strategy for blood culture-negative endocarditis: a prospective study of 819 new cases. Clin Infect Dis. 2010 Jul 15;51(2):131–40.
5. Guptill L, Wu CC, HogenEsch H, Slater LN, Glickman N, Dunham A, et al. Prevalence, risk factors, and genetic diversity of *Bartonella henselae* infections in pet cats in four regions of the United States. J Clin Microbiol. 2004 Feb;42(2):652–9.
6. Maguina C, Gotuzzo E. Bartonellosis. New and old. Infect Dis Clin North Am. 2000 Mar;14(1): 1–22, vii.

BRUCELLOSIS
Marta A. Guerra, Barun K. De

INFECTIOUS AGENT
Facultative, intracellular, gram-negative coccobacilli; known human pathogens include *Brucella abortus, B. melitensis, B. suis,* and *B. canis.*

TRANSMISSION
Most commonly through consumption of contaminated dairy products. *Brucella* can enter the body via skin wounds, mucous membranes, or inhalation. Person-to-person transmission is rare.

EPIDEMIOLOGY
High-risk regions include the Mediterranean Basin, South and Central America, Eastern Europe, Asia, Africa, and the Middle East.

CLINICAL PRESENTATION
Incubation period is 2–4 weeks (range, 5 days to 5 months). Initial presentation is nonspecific, including fever, muscle aches, fatigue, headache, and night sweats.

DIAGNOSIS
Blood culture is the diagnostic gold standard, but is not always positive. If blood or bone marrow culture is used, the laboratory must be informed that *Brucella* is suspected, so that they will process the sample for a longer period of time and protect laboratory personnel. A serum agglutination test is the most common serologic approach, but other serology, ELISA, and PCR have been used to make a diagnosis.

TREATMENT
Doxycycline, rifampin, and trimethoprim-sulfamethoxazole have been used in various combinations for treatment. Sometimes surgery is required.

PREVENTION
Avoid unpasteurized dairy products and undercooked meat.

CDC website: www.cdc.gov/nczved/divisions/dfbmd/diseases/brucellosis

BIBLIOGRAPHY
1. Ariza J, Bosilkovski M, Cascio A, Colmenero JD, Corbel MJ, Falagas ME, et al. Perspectives for the treatment of brucellosis in the 21st century: the Ioannina recommendations. PLoS Med. 2007 Dec;4(12):e317.
2. Arnow PM, Smaron M, Ormiste V. Brucellosis in a group of travelers to Spain. JAMA. 1984 Jan 27;251(4):505–7.
3. Memish ZA, Balkhy HH. Brucellosis and international travel. J Travel Med. 2004 Jan–Feb;11(1):49–55.
4. Pappas G, Papadimitriou P, Akritidis N, Christou L, Tsianos EV. The new global map of human brucellosis. Lancet Infect Dis. 2006 Feb;6(2):91–9.
5. World Health Organization. Brucellosis. Geneva: World Health Organization; 2012 [cited 2012 Sep 18]. Available from: http://www.who.int/zoonoses/diseases/brucellosis/en.

CAMPYLOBACTERIOSIS
Barbara E. Mahon

INFECTIOUS AGENT
Infection is caused by gram-negative, spiral-shaped microaerophilic bacteria of the family Campylobacteraceae. Most infections are caused by *Campylobacter jejuni*; other species, including *C. coli*, also cause infection. *C. jejuni* and *C. coli* are carried normally in the intestinal tracts of many domestic and wild animals.

TRANSMISSION

The major modes of transmission include eating contaminated foods (especially undercooked chicken and foods contaminated by raw chicken), drinking contaminated water or raw (unpasteurized) milk, and having contact with animals, particularly farm animals such as cows and chickens, as well as domestic cats and dogs. Campylobacter can also be transmitted from person to person by the fecal-oral route.

EPIDEMIOLOGY

Campylobacter is a leading cause of bacterial diarrheal disease worldwide; in the United States, it is estimated to cause 1.3 million human illnesses every year. Campylobacter is the most common laboratory-confirmed enteric pathogen reported in travelers returning to the United States from every region of the world. The risk of infection is highest in travelers to Africa and South America, especially in areas with poor restaurant hygiene and inadequate sanitation. The infectious dose is thought to be small, typically <500 organisms.

CLINICAL PRESENTATION

Incubation period is typically 2–4 days. Campylobacteriosis is characterized by diarrhea (frequently bloody), abdominal pain, fever, and occasionally nausea and vomiting. More severe illness can occur, including dehydration, bloodstream infection, and symptoms mimicking acute appendicitis or ulcerative colitis. Guillain-Barré syndrome is a well-established postinfectious complication of campylobacteriosis.

DIAGNOSIS

Diagnosis is traditionally based on isolation of the organism from stools by using selective media incubated under reduced oxygen tension at 42°C (107.6°F) for 72 hours. Visualization of motile and curved, spiral, or S-shaped rods by stool phase-contrast or darkfield microscopy can provide rapid presumptive evidence for *Campylobacter* enteritis. Rapid culture-independent tests are becoming more widely available and commonly used. Although these tests are convenient to use, their sensitivity and specificity are variable; in settings of low prevalence, the positive predictive value is likely to be low. When feasible, laboratories should confirm positive results by culture.

TREATMENT

The disease is generally self-limited, lasting a week or less. Antibiotic therapy decreases the duration of symptoms if administered early in the course of disease. Because campylobacteriosis generally cannot be distinguished from other causes of travelers' diarrhea without a diagnostic test, the use of empiric antibiotics in travelers should follow the guidelines for travelers' diarrhea.

Rates of antibiotic resistance, especially fluoroquinolone resistance, have risen sharply in the past 20 years, and high rates of resistance are now seen in many regions of the world. Travel abroad is a risk factor for infection with resistant *Campylobacter*. Clinicians should suspect resistant infection in returning travelers with campylobacteriosis in whom empiric fluoroquinolone treatment has failed. When fluoroquinolone resistance is proven or suspected, azithromycin is usually the next choice of treatment, although resistance to macrolides has also been reported.

PREVENTION

No vaccine is available; food and water precautions are recommended (see Chapter 2, Food & Water Precautions). CDC does not recommend antibiotic prophylaxis.

CDC website: www.cdc.gov/nczved/divisions/dfbmd/diseases/campylobacter

BIBLIOGRAPHY

1. Coker AO, Isokpehi RD, Thomas BN, Amisu KO, Obi CL. Human campylobacteriosis in developing countries. Emerg Infect Dis. 2002 Mar;8(3):237–44.
2. Friedman CR, Hoekstra RM, Samuel M, Marcus R, Bender J, Shiferaw B, et al. Risk factors for sporadic *Campylobacter* infection in the United States: a case-control study in FoodNet sites. Clin Infect Dis. 2004 Apr 15;38 Suppl 3:S285–96.
3. Humphrey T, O'Brien S, Madsen M. Campylobacters as zoonotic pathogens: a food production perspective. Int J Food Microbiol. 2007 Jul 15;117(3):237–57.
4. Kassenborg HD, Smith KE, Vugia DJ, Rabatsky-Ehr T, Bates MR, Carter MA, et al. Fluoroquinolone-resistant *Campylobacter* infections: eating poultry outside of the home and foreign travel are risk factors. Clin Infect Dis. 2004 Apr 15;38 Suppl 3:S279–84.
5. Moore JE, Barton MD, Blair IS, Corcoran D, Dooley JS, Fanning S, et al. The epidemiology of antibiotic resistance in *Campylobacter*. Microbes Infect. 2006 Jun;8(7):1955–66.

CHIKUNGUNYA

J. Erin Staples, Susan L. Hills, Ann M. Powers

INFECTIOUS AGENT

Chikungunya virus (CHIKV) is a single-stranded RNA virus that belongs to the family *Togaviridae*, genus *Alphavirus*.

TRANSMISSION

CHIKV is transmitted via the bite of an infected mosquito of the *Aedes* spp., predominantly *Aedes aegypti* and *Ae. albopictus*. Nonhuman and human primates are likely the main reservoirs of the virus, and anthroponotic (human-to-vector-to-human) transmission occurs during outbreaks of the disease. Bloodborne transmission is possible; cases have been documented among laboratory personnel handling infected blood and a health care worker drawing blood from an infected patient.

The risk of a person transmitting the virus to a biting mosquito or through blood is highest when the patient is viremic during the first 2–6 days of illness. Maternal-fetal transmission has been documented during pregnancy. The highest risk occurs when a woman is viremic at the time of delivery, with a vertical transmission rate of 49%. However, studies have not found CHIKV in breast milk.

EPIDEMIOLOGY

CHIKV has been identified in many countries in Africa and Asia and is responsible for numerous epidemics in these areas. Since the disease reemerged in 2004, millions of cases have occurred and continue to occur throughout countries in and around the Indian Ocean and in Southeast Asia. Transmission has also been documented periodically in temperate areas, such as in Italy in 2007 and France in 2010. Given the large CHIKV epidemics, high level of viremia in humans, and the worldwide distribution of *Ae. aegypti* and *Ae. albopictus*, there is a risk of importation of chikungunya virus into new areas by infected travelers.

Risk for travelers is highest with travel to areas experiencing ongoing epidemics of the disease. Most epidemics occur during the tropical rainy season and abate during the dry season. However, outbreaks in Africa have occurred after periods of drought, where open water containers served as vector-breeding sites. Risk of CHIKV infection exists throughout the day, as the primary vector, *Ae. aegypti*, aggressively bites during the daytime. *Ae. aegypti* mosquitoes bite indoors or outdoors near a dwelling. They typically breed in domestic containers that hold water, including buckets and flower pots.

Both adults and children can become infected and symptomatic with the disease. From 2006 through 2011, 117 cases of chikungunya fever were identified or reported among US travelers. Most cases occurred in travelers to areas with known ongoing outbreaks.

CLINICAL PRESENTATION

Approximately 3%–28% of people infected with CHIKV will remain asymptomatic. For people who develop symptomatic illness, the incubation period is typically 3–7 days (range, 2–12 days). Disease is most often characterized by sudden onset of high fever (temperature typically higher than 102°F [39°C]) and severe joint pain or stiffness. Other symptoms may include rash, headache, fatigue, nausea, vomiting, and myalgias. Fevers typically last from several days up to 1 week; the fever can be biphasic. Joint symptoms are severe and often debilitating. They are usually symmetric and occur most commonly in hands and feet, but they can affect more proximal joints. Rash usually occurs after onset of fever. It is typically maculopapular, involving the trunk and extremities, but can also include palms, soles, and face.

Abnormal laboratory findings can include thrombocytopenia, lymphopenia, and elevated creatinine and liver function tests. Rare but serious complications of the disease can occur, including myocarditis, ocular disease (uveitis, retinitis), hepatitis, acute renal disease, severe bulbous lesions, and neuroinvasive disease, such as meningoencephalitis, Guillain-Barré syndrome, paresis, or palsies. Fatalities related to CHIKV infection are rare. Older age and underlying medical conditions, such as hypertension, diabetes, or heart disease, are likely risk factors for poor outcomes.

After the acute illness, some patients have prolonged fatigue lasting several weeks. Additionally, some patients have reported incapacitating joint pain, stiffness, or tenosynovitis, which may last for weeks or months. Some studies have reported joint symptoms >1 year after the initial infection.

Pregnant women have symptoms and outcomes similar to those of other people, and most CHIKV infections that occur during pregnancy will not result in the virus being transmitted to the fetus. However, when intrapartum transmission occurs, it can result in complications for the baby, including neurologic disease, hemorrhagic symptoms, and myocardial disease. There are also rare reports of spontaneous abortions after maternal CHIKV infection.

DIAGNOSIS

The differential diagnosis of CHIKV infection is broad, as fever with or without arthralgia is a common manifestation of many diseases. In addition, patients with chikungunya fever may not have the typical manifestations, and CHIKV infection may coexist with other infectious diseases such as dengue or malaria. Diseases that should be considered in the differential diagnosis may vary on the basis of pertinent epidemiologic features, such as place of residence or travel locations and activities, and can include dengue, malaria, leptospirosis, erythema infectiosum, other alphavirus infections (including Mayaro, Ross River, Barmah Forest, O'nyong-nyong, and Sindbis viruses), and postinfectious arthritis.

Preliminary diagnosis is based on the patient's clinical features, places and dates of travel, and activities. Laboratory diagnosis is generally accomplished by testing serum to detect virus, viral nucleic acid, or virus-specific IgM and neutralizing antibodies. During the first week after onset of symptoms, CHIKV infection can often be diagnosed by using viral culture or nucleic acid amplification on serum. CHIKV-specific IgM and neutralizing antibodies normally develop toward the end of the first week of illness. Therefore, to definitively rule out the diagnosis, convalescent-phase samples should be obtained from patients whose acute-phase samples test negative.

Testing for CHIKV IgM and IgG is commercially available. However, confirmatory neutralizing antibody testing is only available through CDC (970-221-6400) and a few state health laboratories. Although reporting CHIKV infections is not mandatory in the United States, all clinicians are encouraged to notify their state or local health department of suspected CHIKV cases so that measures can be taken to mitigate the risk of local (anthroponotic) transmission.

TREATMENT

No specific antiviral treatment is available for chikungunya fever. Treatment is for symptoms and can include rest, fluids, and use of analgesics and antipyretics. Infected people should be protected from further mosquito exposure (staying indoors in areas with screens or under a mosquito net) during the first few days of the illness, so they do not contribute to the transmission cycle.

PREVENTIION

No vaccine or preventive drug is available. The best way to prevent CHIKV infection is to avoid mosquito bites (see Chapter 2, Protection against Mosquitoes, Ticks, & Other Insects & Arthropods). When counseling travelers going to areas with ongoing outbreaks of chikungunya fever, providers should use caution when advising travelers at increased risk for more severe disease, including travelers with underlying medical conditions and women who are late in their pregnancy (as their unborn infants are at increased risk).

CDC website: www.cdc.gov/chikungunya

BIBLIOGRAPHY

1. Burt FJ, Rolph MS, Rulli NE, Mahalingam S, Heise MT. Chikungunya: a re-emerging virus. Lancet. 2012 Feb 18;379(9816):662–71.
2. CDC. Chikungunya distribution and global map. Atlanta: CDC; 2012 [updated May 2012; cited 2012 Sep 10]. Available from: www.cdc.gov/chikungunya/map/index.html.
3. Gibney KB, Fischer M, Prince HE, Kramer LD, St George K, Kosoy OL, et al. Chikungunya fever in the United States: a fifteen year review of cases. Clin Infect Dis. 2011 Mar 1;52(5):e121–6.
4. Grandadam M, Caro V, Plumet S, Thiberge JM, Souares Y, Failloux AB, et al. Chikungunya virus, southeastern France. Emerg Infect Dis. 2011 May;17(5):910–3.

5. Kularatne SA, Gihan MC, Weerasinghe SC, Gunasena S. Concurrent outbreaks of chikungunya and dengue fever in Kandy, Sri Lanka, 2006–07: a comparative analysis of clinical and laboratory features. Postgrad Med J. 2009 Jul;85(1005):342–6.

6. Pan American Health Organization and CDC. Preparedness and response for chikungunya virus introduction in the Americas. Washington, DC: Pan American Health Organization; 2011 [cited 2012 Sep 18]. Available from: http://new.paho.org/hq/index.php?option=com_content&view=article&id=3545&Itemid=2545&lang=en.

7. Powers AM. Chikungunya. Clin Lab Med. 2010 Mar;30(1):209–19.

8. Rajapakse S, Rodrigo C, Rajapakse A. Atypical manifestations of chikungunya infection. Trans R Soc Trop Med Hyg. 2010 Feb;104(2):89–96.

9. Ramful D, Carbonnier M, Pasquet M, Bouhmani B, Ghazouani J, Noormahomed T, et al. Mother-to-child transmission of chikungunya virus infection. Pediatr Infect Dis J. 2007 Sep; 26(9):811–5.

10. Rezza G, Nicoletti L, Angelini R, Romi R, Finarelli AC, Panning M, et al. Infection with chikungunya virus in Italy: an outbreak in a temperate region. Lancet. 2007 Dec 1;370(9602):1840–6.

11. Tsetsarkin KA, Chen R, Sherman MB, Weaver SC. Chikungunya virus: evolution and genetic determinants of emergence. Curr Opin Virol. 2011 Oct;1(4):310–7.

CHOLERA

Joan M. Brunkard, Anna E. Newton, Eric Mintz

INFECTIOUS AGENT

Cholera is an acute bacterial, intestinal infection caused by toxigenic *Vibrio cholerae* O-group 1 or O-group 139. Many other serogroups of *V. cholerae*, with or without the cholera toxin gene (including the nontoxigenic strains of the O1 and O139 serogroups), can cause a choleralike illness. Only toxigenic strains of serogroups O1 and O139 have caused widespread epidemics and are reportable to the World Health Organization (WHO) as "cholera."

V. cholerae O1 has 2 biotypes, classical and El Tor, and each biotype has 2 distinct serotypes, Inaba and Ogawa. The symptoms of infection are indistinguishable, although more people infected with the El Tor biotype remain asymptomatic or have only a mild illness. Globally, most cases of cholera are caused by O1 El Tor organisms. In recent years, an El Tor variant that has characteristics of both classical and El Tor biotypes and may be more virulent than older El Tor strains has emerged in Asia and spread to Africa and the Caribbean.

TRANSMISSION

Toxigenic *V. cholerae* O1 and O139 are free-living bacterial organisms found in fresh and brackish water, often in association with copepods or other zooplankton, shellfish, and aquatic plants. Cholera infections are most commonly acquired from drinking water in which *V. cholerae* is found naturally or into which it has been introduced from the feces of an infected person. Other common vehicles include contaminated fish and shellfish. Other foods, including produce, are less commonly implicated. Direct transmission from person to person, even to health care workers during epidemics, has been reported but is not frequent.

EPIDEMIOLOGY

Since 1961, the seventh pandemic of cholera, caused by *V. cholerae* serogroup O1, biotype El Tor, has spread from Indonesia through most of Asia into Eastern Europe and Africa, and from North Africa to the Iberian Peninsula. In 1991, an extensive epidemic began in Peru and spread to neighboring countries in the Western Hemisphere. Although few cases of cholera occur in South or Central America, *V. cholerae* O1 remains endemic in much of Africa and South and Southeast Asia. *V. cholerae* O139 spread rapidly through Asia in the early 1990s but has since remained localized to a few areas in Asia. In October 2010, a cholera epidemic began in Haiti, just 10 months after a devastating earthquake destroyed the Haitian capital of Port-au-Prince and surrounding areas. During the first year of the outbreak, 480,577 cases and 6,673 deaths were reported. In the early weeks of the outbreak, the case-fatality ratio (CFR) was 3%–4%, but declined after improvements in access to care; the CFR for Haiti was 0.84% in 2011 compared with 2.22% in 2010. In November 2010, cholera was first reported in the neighboring Dominican Republic, with 21,432 cases and 363 deaths reported by December 2011. Cholera is likely to persist in Haiti at endemic levels because of the lack of safe water and sanitation infrastructure, with the potential for localized outbreaks and seasonal spikes in cases associated with heavy rainfall. Sporadic cases associated with travel to or from Hispaniola may continue to occur.

Most cholera cases go unreported. In 2011, 58 countries reported 589,854 cholera cases and 7,816 cholera deaths (CFR, 1.3%) to WHO. The 2011 global cholera case numbers represent an 85% increase from 2010. Since 2010, there has been a geographic shift in cholera incidence from Africa to the Americas as a result of the Haiti outbreak, which accounted for 55% and >57% of all cholera cases reported in 2010 and 2011, respectively. From 2001 through 2009, >90% of cholera cases were reported from Africa, including 98% of cases and 99% of deaths during 2009. Cholera has the potential to emerge in dramatic epidemics, as was seen with the massive outbreaks that affected Zimbabwe in 2008 and 2009, with close to 100,000 cases and >4,000 deaths reported, and with the current epidemic in Haiti, with >500,000 cases and 7,000 deaths reported during 2010 and 2011.

From 1999 through 2011, 86 confirmed cases of cholera in the United States were acquired abroad; of these, 40 were associated with the epidemic in Hispaniola in 2010 and 2011. Travelers who follow the usual tourist itineraries and who observe safe food and water recommendations and hygiene precautions while in countries reporting cholera have virtually no risk. The risk is increased for those who drink untreated water, do not follow proper hygiene recommendations, or eat raw or poorly cooked food, especially seafood, in endemic or outbreak settings.

Although rare, 2 cases of cholera have been reported among volunteer US health care workers caring for cholera patients during the peak period of the epidemic in Haiti; recent evidence shows that lack of hand-washing supplies at treatment centers may lead to diarrheal illness and other health care–associated infections.

Two reports of cholera have been associated with food served on international flights, most recently in 1992, during the Latin American epidemic, on a flight from Argentina to Los Angeles. CDC consequently advised the International Air Transport Association that prepackaged oral rehydration salts should be carried on international flights and that certain food items (such as shrimp) prepared in cities with cholera epidemics should not be served. Airline flights have not been implicated in any subsequent cases of cholera.

CLINICAL PRESENTATION

Cholera infection is most often asymptomatic or results in a mild gastroenteritis. Severe cholera is characterized by acute, profuse watery diarrhea, described as "rice-water stools," and often nausea and vomiting, leading to volume depletion. Signs and symptoms include tachycardia, loss of skin turgor, dry mucous membranes, hypotension, and thirst. Additional symptoms, including muscle cramps, are secondary to the resulting electrolyte imbalances. If untreated, rapid loss of body fluids can lead to severe dehydration, hypovolemic shock, and death within hours. With adequate and timely rehydration, CFRs are <1%. Most people infected with toxigenic V. cholerae will be asymptomatic or have mild diarrhea.

DIAGNOSIS

Cholera is confirmed through culture of a stool specimen or rectal swab. Cary-Blair medium can be used for transport, and selective media such as taurocholate-tellurite-gelatin agar and thiosulfate-citrate-bile salts (TCBS) agar may be used for isolation and identification. Reagents for serogrouping V. cholerae isolates are available in all state health department laboratories. Commercially available rapid test kits do not yield an isolate for antimicrobial susceptibility testing and subtyping and should not be used for routine diagnosis. All isolates obtained in the United States should be sent to CDC via state health department laboratories for cholera toxin testing and subtyping. Cholera is a nationally reportable disease.

TREATMENT

Rehydration is the cornerstone of cholera treatment. Oral rehydration solution and, when necessary, intravenous fluids and electrolytes, if administered in a timely manner and in adequate volumes, will reduce CFRs to well under 1%. Antibiotics reduce fluid requirements and duration of illness. Antimicrobial therapy is indicated for moderate and severe cases, which can be treated with doxycycline, tetracycline, erythromycin, azithromycin, or ciprofloxacin. Whenever possible, antimicrobial susceptibility testing should inform treatment choices. Zinc supplementation reduces the severity and duration of cholera and other diarrheal diseases in children in resource-limited areas.

PREVENTION

Safe food and water precautions and frequent handwashing are critical in preventing cholera (see Chapter 2, Food & Water Precautions). Chemoprophylaxis is not indicated.

No cholera vaccine is currently licensed in the United States. Two oral vaccines are prequalified by WHO and are available outside the United States: Dukoral (Crucell, the Netherlands) and Shanchol (Shantha Biotechnics, India). CDC does not recommend cholera vaccines for US travelers because of the low risk of cholera and the unavailability of vaccines in the United States. No country or territory requires vaccination against cholera as a condition for entry.

Further information on Dukoral can be obtained from Crucell (www.crucell.com). Information on Shanchol can be obtained from Shantha Biotechnics (www.shanthabiotech.com).

CDC website: www.cdc.gov/cholera

BIBLIOGRAPHY

1. CDC. Cholera associated with an international airline flight, 1992. MMWR Morb Mortal Wkly Rep. 1992 Feb 28;41(8):134–5.
2. CDC. Cholera outbreak—Haiti, October 2010. MMWR Morb Mortal Wkly Rep. 2010 Nov 5;59(43):1411.
3. CDC. Two cases of toxigenic Vibrio cholerae O1 infection after Hurricanes Katrina and Rita—Louisiana, October 2005. MMWR Morb Mortal Wkly Rep. 2006 Jan 20;55(2):31–2.
4. CDC. Update: cholera outbreak—Haiti, 2010. MMWR Morb Mortal Wkly Rep. 2010 Nov 19;59(45):1473–9.
5. Gaffga NH, Tauxe RV, Mintz ED. Cholera: a new homeland in Africa? Am J Trop Med Hyg. 2007 Oct;77(4):705–13.
6. Haitian Ministry of Public Health and Population (MSPP). Ministere de la Sante Publique et de la Population. Port-au-Prince, Haiti: Haitian Ministry of Public Health and Population; 2012 [cited 2012 Sep 18]. Available from: http://mspp.gouv.ht.
7. Harris JB, Larocque RC, Charles RC, Mazumder RN, Khan AI, Bardhan PK. Cholera's western front. Lancet. 2010 Dec 11;376(9757):1961–5.
8. Harris JB, LaRocque RC, Qadri F, Ryan ET, Calderwood SB. Cholera. Lancet. 2012 Jun 30;379(9835):2466–76.
9. Lucas ME, Deen JL, von Seidlein L, Wang XY, Ampuero J, Puri M, et al. Effectiveness of mass oral cholera vaccination in Beira, Mozambique. N Engl J Med. 2005 Feb 24;352(8):757–67.
10. Nelson EJ, Harris JB, Morris JG, Jr., Calderwood SB, Camilli A. Cholera transmission: the host, pathogen and bacteriophage dynamic. Nat Rev Microbiol. 2009 Oct;7(10):693–702.
11. Newton AE, Heiman KE, Schmitz A, Torok T, Apostolou A, Hanson H, et al. Cholera in United States associated with epidemic in Hispaniola. Emerg Infect Dis. 2011 Nov;17(11):2166–8.
12. Schilling K, Cartwright E, Stamper J er al. Diarrheal illness among US residents providing services in Haiti during the cholera epidemic, 2010–2011. Poster session presented at: International Conference on Emerging Infectious Diseases; 2012 Mar 11–14; Atlanta, GA. Abstract available: http://www.iceid.org/images/iceid_2012_finalprogram_final.pdf.
13. Sur D, Lopez AL, Kanungo S, Paisley A, Manna B, Ali M, et al. Efficacy and safety of a modified killed-whole-cell oral cholera vaccine in India: an interim analysis of a cluster-randomised, double-blind, placebo-controlled trial. Lancet. 2009 Nov 14;374(9702):1694–702.
14. Sutton RG. An outbreak of cholera in Australia due to food served in flight on an international aircraft. J Hyg (Lond). 1974 Jun;72(3):441–51.
15. World Health Organization. Cholera, 2011. Wkly Epidemiol Rec. 2012 Aug 3;87(31/32):289–304.

COCCIDIOIDOMYCOSIS
Tom M. Chiller

INFECTIOUS AGENT
The fungi *Coccidioides immitis* and *C. posadasii*.

TRANSMISSION
Inhalation of fungal conidia from dust found in ambient air or generated by soil-disrupting human activities or natural disasters. Not transmitted from person to person.

EPIDEMIOLOGY
Endemic in arid regions, including those in the southwestern United States. Outside the United States, coccidioidomycosis is endemic in parts of Central and South America. Travelers are at increased risk if they participate in activities that expose them to dust, such as construction, landscaping, mining, agriculture, archaeological excavation, military maneuvers, and recreational pursuits such as dirt biking.

CLINICAL PRESENTATION
The incubation period ranges from 7 to 21 days. Most infections (60%) are asymptomatic. Symptomatic infection will generally range from a self-limited influenzalike illness, characterized by fever, headache, rash, muscle aches, dry cough, weight loss, and malaise, to primary pulmonary coccidioidomycosis, characterized by pneumonia with changes on chest radiography.

In rare instances, severe lung disease (such as cavitary pneumonia) or dissemination to the central nervous system, joints, bones, or skin may develop. People at increased risk for severe pulmonary disease are the elderly, those with diabetes or recent smoking history, and people of low socioeconomic status. People at increased risk for disseminated disease include African Americans and Filipinos, those with immunocompromising conditions (such as HIV), and women in the third trimester of pregnancy.

DIAGNOSIS
Best diagnosed by using serologic, histopathologic, and culture methods. Serologic tests are useful to confirm diagnoses and provide prognostic information.

TREATMENT
Some experts feel that people without risk for severe or disseminated disease do not require treatment, because the illness is self-limited; others propose treatment to reduce the intensity or duration of symptoms. People at high risk for dissemination should receive antifungal therapy when diagnosed with acute coccidioidomycosis. Additionally, people with severe acute pulmonary disease, chronic pulmonary infection, or disseminated disease should receive antifungal therapy. Depending on the clinical situation, azole antifungal agents (such as fluconazole or itraconazole) or amphotericin B may be used.

PREVENTION
Limit exposure to outdoor dust in endemic areas.

CDC website: www.cdc.gov/fungal/coccidioido mycosis

BIBLIOGRAPHY
1. Ampel NM. Coccidioidomycosis: a review of recent advances. Clin Chest Med. 2009 Jun;30(2):241–51.
2. Chiller TM, Galgiani JN, Stevens DA. Coccidioidomycosis. Infect Dis Clin North Am. 2003 Mar;17(1):41–57, viii.
3. Crum NF, Lederman ER, Stafford CM, Parrish JS, Wallace MR. Coccidioidomycosis: a descriptive survey of a reemerging disease. Clinical characteristics and current controversies. Medicine (Baltimore). 2004 May;83(3):149–75.

CRYPTOSPORIDIOSIS

Michele C. Hlavsa

INFECTIOUS AGENT

Protozoan parasites in the genus *Crypto-sporidium*, most commonly *Cryptosporidium hominis* and *C. parvum*.

TRANSMISSION

Oral-fecal, primarily through contaminated food or water, including water swallowed while swimming, or through contact with an infected person or animal, most notably pre-weaned calves.

EPIDEMIOLOGY

Distributed worldwide. *Cryptosporidium* caused only a small proportion (6%) of cases of travelers' diarrhea in North American travelers to Mexico.

CLINICAL PRESENTATION

Symptoms usually begin 7–10 days (range, 2–26 days) after infection and are generally self-limited. The most common symptom is watery diarrhea. Other symptoms can include abdominal cramps, vomiting, weight loss, fever, decreased appetite, fatigue, joint pain, and headache. In immunocompetent people, symptoms most frequently resolve within 2–3 weeks; patients might experience a recurrence of symptoms after a brief period of recovery before complete symptom resolution. Clinical presentation of cryptosporidiosis in HIV-infected patients varies with level of immunosuppression, ranging from no symptoms or transient disease to relapsing or chronic diarrhea or cholera-like diarrhea, which can lead to life-threatening wasting and malabsorption. Extraintestinal cryptosporidiosis (in the biliary or respiratory tract or rarely the pancreas) has been documented in people who are immunocompromised.

DIAGNOSIS

Tests for *Cryptosporidium* are typically not included in routine ova and parasite testing. Therefore, clinicians should specifically request testing for this parasite, when suspected. Because *Cryptosporidium* can be excreted intermittently, multiple stool collections (3 stool specimens collected on separate days) increase test sensitivity. Diagnostic techniques include direct fluorescent antibody (considered the gold standard), EIA testing, rapid immunochromatographic cartridge assays, and microscopy with modified acid-fast staining. False-positive results might occur when using rapid immunochromatographic cartridge assays, and confirmation by microscopy should be considered.

TREATMENT

Most immunocompetent patients will recover without treatment. Diarrhea should be managed with fluid replacement. Nitazoxanide is approved to treat cryptosporidiosis in immunocompetent patients and is available for those aged ≥1 year. Nitazoxanide has not been shown to be an effective treatment of cryptosporidiosis in HIV-infected patients. However, dramatic clinical and parasitologic responses have been reported in these patients after the immune system has been reconstituted with active combination antiretroviral therapy. Protease inhibitors might have direct anti-*Cryptosporidium* activity.

PREVENTION

Food and water precautions (see Chapter 2, Food & Water Precautions) and handwashing. *Cryptosporidium* is extremely tolerant to halogens (such as chlorine or iodine), and alcohol-based hand sanitizers are not effective against the parasite. Water can be treated effectively by heating it to a rolling boil for 1 minute or filtering with an absolute 1-μm filter. More prevention recommendations can be found at www.cdc.gov/parasites/crypto/gen_info/prevent.html.

CDC website: www.cdc.gov/parasites/crypto

BIBLIOGRAPHY

1. Fayer R, Xiao L, editors. Cryptosporidium and Cryptosporidiosis. 2nd ed. Boca Raton, FL: CRC; 2008.
2. Lima AAM, Samie A, Guerrant RL. Cryptosporidiosis. In: Guerrant RL, Walker DH, Weller PF, editors. Tropical Infectious Diseases: Principles, Pathogens and Practice. 3rd ed. Philadelphia: Saunders Elsevier; 2011. p. 640–63.
3. Nair P, Mohamed JA, DuPont HL, Figueroa JF, Carlin LG, Jiang ZD, et al. Epidemiology of cryptosporidiosis in North American travelers to Mexico. Am J Trop Med Hyg. 2008 Aug;79(2):210–4.
4. Pantenburg B, Cabada MM, White AC, Jr. Treatment of cryptosporidiosis. Expert Rev Anti Infect Ther. 2009 May;7(4):385–91.

CUTANEOUS LARVA MIGRANS

Susan Montgomery

INFECTIOUS AGENT

Larval stages of dog and cat hookworms (*Ancylostoma* spp.).

TRANSMISSION

Skin contact with contaminated soil or sand.

EPIDEMIOLOGY

Most cases are reported in travelers to the Caribbean, Africa, Asia, and South America. Beaches are a common source of infection.

CLINICAL PRESENTATION

Creeping eruption usually appears 1–5 days after skin penetration, but the incubation period may be ≥1 month. Typically, a serpiginous, erythematous track appears in the skin and is associated with intense itchiness and mild swelling. Usual locations are the foot and buttocks, although any skin surface coming in contact with contaminated soil can be affected.

DIAGNOSIS

Diagnosed on the basis of characteristic skin lesions. Biopsy is not recommended.

TREATMENT

Albendazole is the treatment of choice. Ivermectin is effective but not approved for this indication.

PREVENTION

Reduce contact with contaminated soil by wearing shoes and protective clothing and using barriers such as towels when seated on the ground.

CDC website: www.cdc.gov/parasites/zoonotichookworm

BIBLIOGRAPHY

1. Caumes E. Treatment of cutaneous larva migrans. Clin Infect Dis. 2000 May;30(5):811–4.
2. Gillespie SH. Cutaneous larva migrans. Curr Infect Dis Rep. 2004 Feb;6(1):50–3.
3. Heukelbach J, Feldmeier H. Epidemiological and clinical characteristics of hookworm-related cutaneous larva migrans. Lancet Infect Dis. 2008 May;8(5):302–9.
4. Hochedez P, Caumes E. Hookworm-related cutaneous larva migrans. J Travel Med. 2007 Sep–Oct;14(5):326–33.
5. Lederman ER, Weld LH, Elyazar IR, von Sonnenburg F, Loutan L, Schwartz E, et al. Dermatologic conditions of the ill returned traveler: an analysis from the GeoSentinel Surveillance Network. Int J Infect Dis. 2008 Nov;12(6):593–602.

CYCLOSPORIASIS

Barbara L. Herwaldt

INFECTIOUS AGENT
Cyclospora cayetanensis, a coccidian protozoan parasite.

TRANSMISSION
Ingestion of infective *Cyclospora* oocysts, such as in contaminated food or water.

EPIDEMIOLOGY
Most common in tropical and subtropical regions where outbreaks are frequently seasonal (such as during summers and rainy season in Nepal). Outbreaks in the United States and Canada have been linked to imported fresh produce.

CLINICAL PRESENTATION
Incubation period averages 1 week (range, 2 days to >2 weeks). Onset of symptoms is often abrupt but can be gradual; some people have an influenzalike prodrome. The most common symptom is watery diarrhea, which can be profuse. Other symptoms can include anorexia, weight loss, abdominal cramps, bloating, nausea, body aches, vomiting, and low-grade fever.

DIAGNOSIS
Diagnosed by detecting *Cyclospora* oocysts in stool specimens. Stool examinations for ova and parasites usually do not include methods for detecting *Cyclospora*, so clinicians should specifically request *Cyclospora* testing. Diagnostic assistance is also available from CDC (www.dpd.cdc.gov/dpdx; 404-718-4745; parasites@cdc.gov).

TREATMENT
Trimethoprim-sulfamethoxazole; no highly effective alternatives have been identified.

PREVENTION
Food and water precautions (see Chapter 2, Food & Water Precautions); disinfection with chlorine or iodine is unlikely to be effective.

CDC website: www.cdc.gov/parasites/cyclosporiasis

BIBLIOGRAPHY
1. Herwaldt BL. *Cyclospora cayetanensis*: a review, focusing on the outbreaks of cyclosporiasis in the 1990s. Clin Infect Dis. 2000 Oct;31(4):1040–57.

2. Shlim DR. *Cyclospora cayetanensis*. Clin Lab Med. 2002 Dec;22(4):927–36.

CYSTICERCOSIS

Caryn Bern, Susan Montgomery, Paul T. Cantey

INFECTIOUS AGENT
Taenia solium, a cestode parasite.

TRANSMISSION
Ingestion of eggs, excreted by a human carrier of the pork tapeworm, on fecally contaminated food or through close contact with the carrier. Autoinfection is also possible. Eating undercooked pork with cysticerci results in tapeworm infection (taeniasis), not human cysticercosis.

EPIDEMIOLOGY
Common where sanitary conditions are poor and where pigs have access to human feces. Endemic areas include Mexico, Latin America,

sub-Saharan Africa, India, and East Asia. Uncommon in travelers. Seen in immigrants from endemic regions.

CLINICAL PRESENTATION

Median latent period of 5 years (range, 1–30 years). Symptoms depend on the number, location, and stage of cysts. The most common location is brain parenchyma, with late-onset seizures. Other presentations include increased intracranial pressure, encephalitis, symptoms of space-occupying lesion, and hydrocephalus. Cysticercosis should be ruled out in any adult with new-onset seizures who comes from an endemic area or has potential exposure to a tapeworm carrier.

DIAGNOSIS

Neuroimaging studies (CT or MRI) and confirmatory serologic testing. The most reliable serologic test is the enzyme-linked immuno-transfer blot, but this test may be negative in up to 30% of patients with a single parenchymal lesion.

TREATMENT

Control of symptoms is the cornerstone of therapy. Anticonvulsants, dexamethasone, or both may be indicated. For some lesions, surgical intervention may be the treatment of choice. Antiparasitic treatment (albendazole, praziquantel) should *not* be initiated in patients with heavy infections, cysticercotic encephalitis, or increased intracranial pressure, as dying cysts can cause or worsen some symptoms. In these cases, the priority is neurologic management (steroids, mannitol), neurosurgical management, or both. Physicians can consult with CDC to obtain more information about diagnosis and treatment (www.dpd.cdc.gov/dpdx; 404-718-4745; parasites@cdc.gov).

PREVENTION

Food and water precautions (see Chapter 2, Food & Water Precautions).

CDC website: www.cdc.gov/parasites/cysticercosis

BIBLIOGRAPHY

1. Garcia HH, Del Brutto OH. Neurocysticercosis: updated concepts about an old disease. Lancet Neurol. 2005 Oct;4(10):653–61.
2. Garcia HH, Del Brutto OH, Nash TE, White AC, Jr., Tsang VC, Gilman RH. New concepts in the diagnosis and management of neurocysticercosis (*Taenia solium*). Am J Trop Med Hyg. 2005 Jan;72(1):3–9.
3. Sorvillo FJ, DeGiorgio C, Waterman SH. Deaths from cysticercosis, United States. EID 2007 Feb;13(2):230–5.

DENGUE

Kay M. Tomashek, Harold S. Margolis

INFECTIOUS AGENT

Dengue is caused by infection with any 1 of 4 related positive-strand RNA viruses of the genus *Flavivirus*, dengue viruses (DENV) 1, 2, 3, or 4.

TRANSMISSION

Transmission occurs through the bite of an infected *Aedes* mosquito, primarily *Aedes aegypti* and *Ae. albopictus*. Humans are the main host and the primary source of virus for female mosquitoes, which become infective after an extrinsic incubation period of 8–12 days and can then transmit DENV for the rest of their approximately 1-month lifespan.

Because of the approximately 7-day viremia in humans, bloodborne transmission is possible through exposure to infected blood, organs, or other tissues (such as bone marrow). In addition, perinatal DENV transmission occurs, and the highest risk appears to be among infants whose mothers are acutely ill around the time of delivery. It is not known if DENV is transmitted through breast milk.

EPIDEMIOLOGY

Dengue is endemic throughout the tropics and subtropics and is a leading cause of febrile illness among travelers returning from the Caribbean, South America, and South and Southeast Asia, according to an analysis of data collected by the GeoSentinel Surveillance Network. Dengue occurs in >100 countries worldwide (Maps 3-1, 3-2, and 3-3), including Puerto Rico, the US Virgin Islands, and US-affiliated Pacific Islands. Sporadic outbreaks with local transmission have occurred in Florida, Hawaii, and along the Texas-Mexico border. Although the geographic distribution of dengue is similar to that of malaria, dengue is more of a risk in urban and residential areas than is malaria. The DengueMap (www.healthmap.org/dengue/index.php) shows areas of ongoing transmission.

CLINICAL PRESENTATION

About 75% of all DENV infections are asymptomatic. Symptomatic infection (dengue) most commonly presents as a mild to moderate, nonspecific, acute, febrile illness. However, as many as 5% of all dengue patients develop severe, life-threatening disease. Early clinical findings are nonspecific but require a high index of suspicion, because recognizing early signs of shock and promptly initiating intensive supportive therapy can reduce risk of death among patients with severe dengue from 10% to <1%. See Box 3-1 for information regarding the new World Health Organization (WHO) guidelines for classifying dengue.

Dengue begins abruptly after an incubation period of 4–7 days (range, 3–14 days), and the course follows 3 phases: febrile, critical, and convalescent. Fever typically lasts 2–7 days and can be biphasic. Other signs and symptoms may include severe headache; retroorbital pain; muscle, joint and bone pain; macular or maculopapular rash; and minor hemorrhagic manifestations, including petechiae, ecchymosis, purpura, epistaxis, bleeding gums, hematuria, or a positive tourniquet test result. Some patients have injected oropharynx and facial erythema in the first 24–48 hours after onset. Warning signs of progression to severe dengue occur in the late febrile phase around the time of defervescence and include persistent vomiting,

severe abdominal pain, mucosal bleeding, difficulty breathing, signs of hypovolemic shock, and rapid decline in platelet count with an increase in hematocrit (hemoconcentration).

The critical phase of dengue begins at defervescence and typically lasts 24–48 hours. Most patients clinically improve during this phase, but those with substantial plasma leakage develop severe disease as a result of a marked increase in vascular permeability. Initially, physiologic compensatory mechanisms maintain adequate circulation, which narrows pulse pressure as diastolic blood pressure increases. Patients with severe plasma leakage have pleural effusions or ascites, hypoproteinemia, and hemoconcentration. Patients may appear to be well despite early signs of shock. However, once hypotension develops, systolic blood pressure rapidly declines, and irreversible shock and death may ensue despite resuscitation. Patients can also develop hemorrhagic manifestations, including hematemesis, bloody stool, melena, or menorrhagia, especially if they have prolonged shock. Dengue patients can have atypical manifestations, including hepatitis, myocarditis, pancreatitis, and encephalitis.

As the plasma leakage subsides, the patient enters the convalescent phase and begins to reabsorb extravasated intravenous fluids and pleural and abdominal effusions. As a patient's well-being improves, hemodynamic status stabilizes (although he or she may manifest bradycardia), and diuresis ensues. The patient's hematocrit stabilizes or may fall because of the dilutional effect of the reabsorbed fluid, and the white cell count usually starts to rise, followed by a slow recovery of platelet count. The convalescent-phase rash may desquamate and be pruritic.

Laboratory findings commonly include leucopenia, thrombocytopenia, hyponatremia, elevated aspartate aminotransferase and alanine aminotransferase, and a normal erythrocyte sedimentation rate.

Data are limited on health outcomes of dengue in pregnancy and effects of maternal DENV infection on the developing fetus. Perinatal DENV transmission can occur, and peripartum maternal infection may increase the likelihood of symptomatic disease in the newborn. Of the 34 perinatal transmission cases described in the literature, all developed

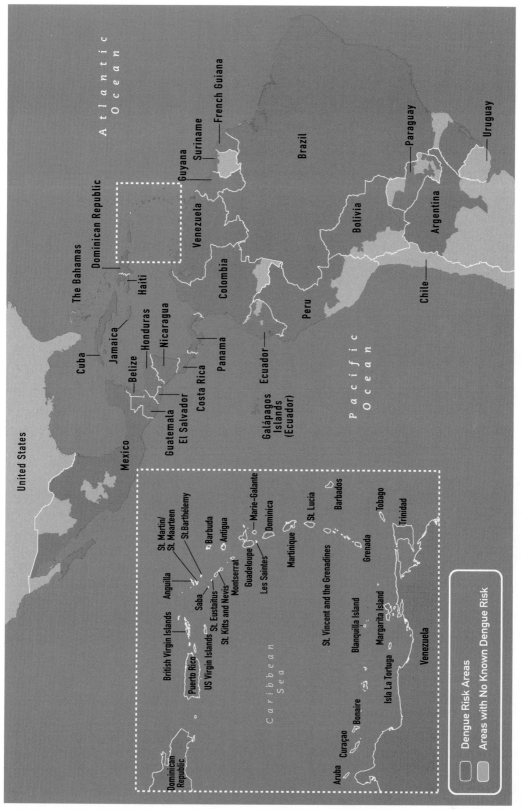

MAP 3-1. DISTRIBUTION OF DENGUE IN THE AMERICAS AND THE CARIBBEAN

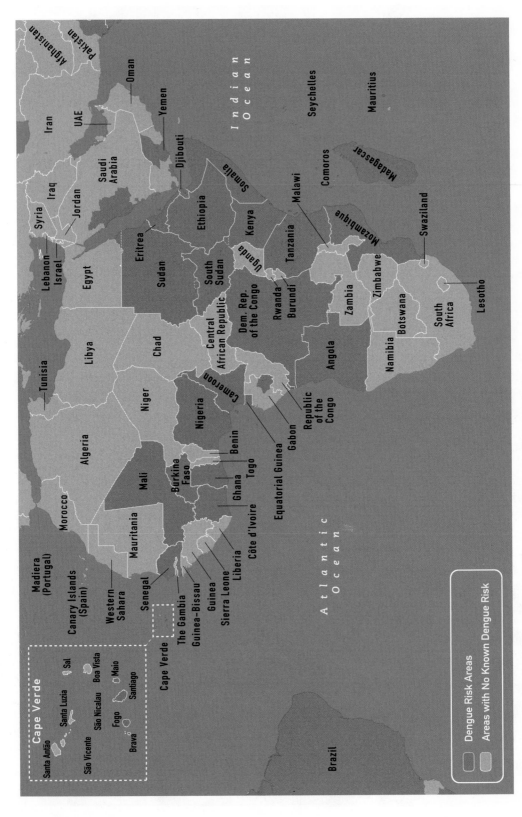

MAP 3-2. DISTRIBUTION OF DENGUE IN AFRICA AND THE MIDDLE EAST

Dengue Risk Areas

Areas with No Known Dengue Risk

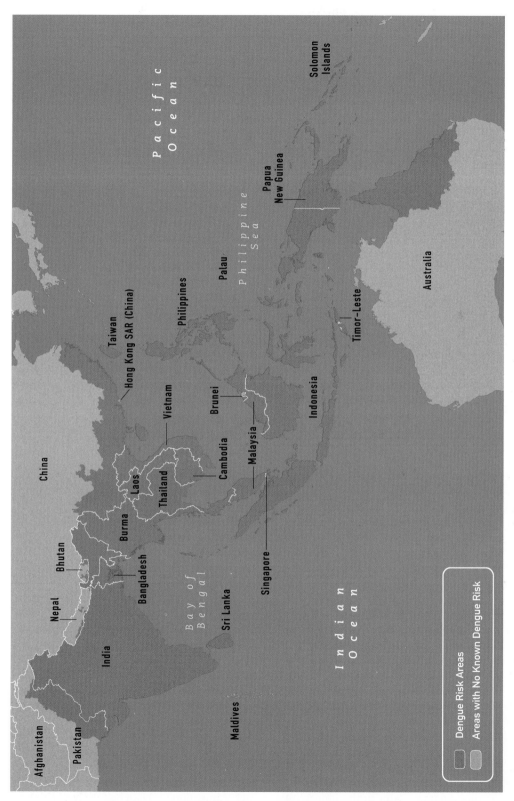

MAP 3-3. DISTRIBUTION OF DENGUE IN ASIA AND OCEANIA

Dengue Risk Areas

Areas with No Known Dengue Risk

BOX 3-1. NEW GUIDELINES FOR CLASSIFYING DENGUE

In November 2009, World Health Organization (WHO) issued a new guideline that classifies symptomatic cases as dengue or severe dengue.

Dengue is defined by a combination of ≥2 clinical findings in a febrile person who traveled to or lives in a dengue-endemic area. Clinical findings include nausea, vomiting, rash, aches and pains, a positive tourniquet test, leukopenia, and the following warning signs: abdominal pain or tenderness, persistent vomiting, clinical fluid accumulation, mucosal bleeding, lethargy, restlessness, and liver enlargement. The presence of a warning sign may predict severe dengue in a patient.

Severe dengue is classified as dengue with any of the following: severe plasma leakage leading to shock or fluid accumulation with respiratory distress; severe bleeding; or severe organ impairment such as elevated transaminases ≥1,000 IU/L, impaired consciousness, or heart impairment.

From 1975 through 2009, symptomatic dengue virus infections were classified according to the WHO guidelines as dengue fever, dengue hemorrhagic fever (DHF), and dengue shock syndrome (DSS, the most severe form of DHF). The case definition was changed to the 2009 clinical classification after reports that the case definition of DHF was both too difficult to apply in resource-limited settings and too specific, as it failed to identify a substantial proportion of severe dengue cases, including cases of hepatic failure and encephalitis. Many dengue experts felt that the original case definitions, which were developed based on data from pediatric cases in Southeast Asia, were not applicable to other regions and populations. The 2009 clinical classification has been criticized because it is felt to be overly inclusive, as it allows several different ways to qualify for severe dengue, and nonspecific warning signs are used as diagnostic criteria for dengue. Last, the new guidelines have been criticized because they do not define the clinical criteria for establishing severe dengue (with the exception of providing laboratory cutoff values for transaminase levels), thereby leaving severity determination up to individual clinical judgment.

thrombocytopenia and all but 1 had fever in the first 2 weeks after birth. Nearly 40% had a hemorrhagic manifestation, and one-fourth had hypotension. Transplacental transfer of maternal IgG anti-DENV (from a previous maternal infection) may increase risk for severe dengue among infants infected at 6–12 months of age.

DIAGNOSIS

Clinicians should consider dengue in a patient who was in an endemic area within 2 weeks before symptom onset. All suspected cases should be reported to the local health department, because dengue is a nationally reportable disease. Laboratory confirmation can be made from a single acute-phase serum specimen obtained early (≤5 days after fever onset) in the illness by detecting DENV genomic sequences with RT-PCR or DENV nonstructural protein 1 (NS1) antigen by immunoassay. Later in the illness (≥4 days after fever onset), IgM anti-DENV can be

detected with ELISA. For patients presenting during the first week after fever onset, diagnostic testing should include a test for DENV (PCR or NS1) and IgM anti-DENV. For patients presenting >1 week after fever onset, IgM anti-DENV is most useful, although NS1 has been reported positive up to 12 days after fever onset.

Presence of DENV by PCR or NS1 antigen in a single diagnostic specimen is considered laboratory confirmation in patients with a compatible clinical and travel history. IgM anti-DENV in a single serum sample suggests a probable, recent DENV infection. IgM anti-DENV seroconversion in acute- and convalescent-phase serum specimens is considered laboratory confirmation of dengue.

IgG anti-DENV by ELISA in a single serum sample is not useful for diagnostic testing, because it remains elevated for life after any DENV infection and can be falsely positive in people with antibodies to other flaviviruses (such as West Nile, yellow fever, Japanese encephalitis).

Dengue diagnostic testing (molecular and immunoassay) is available from several commercial reference diagnostic laboratories, state public health laboratories, and CDC (www.cdc.gov/Dengue/clinicalLab/index.html). Consultation on dengue diagnostic testing can be obtained from CDC at 787-706-2399.

TREATMENT

No specific antiviral agents exist for dengue. Patients should be advised to stay well hydrated and to avoid aspirin (acetylsalicylic acid), aspirin-containing drugs, and other nonsteroidal anti-inflammatory drugs (such as ibuprofen) because of their anticoagulant properties. Fever should be controlled with acetaminophen and tepid sponge baths. Febrile patients should avoid mosquito bites to reduce risk of further transmission. For those who develop severe dengue, close observation and frequent monitoring in an intensive care unit setting may be required. Prophylactic platelet transfusions in dengue patients are not beneficial and may contribute to fluid overload.

PREVENTION

No vaccine is available, although several are in clinical trials; no chemoprophylaxis is available to prevent dengue. Travelers to dengue-endemic areas are at risk of getting dengue; risk increases with longer duration of travel and disease incidence in the travel destination (such as during dengue season and during epidemics). Travelers should be advised to avoid mosquito bites by taking the following preventive measures:

- Select accommodations with well-screened windows and doors or air conditioning when possible. *Aedes* mosquitoes typically live indoors and are often found in dark, cool places, such as in closets, under beds, behind curtains, and in bathrooms. Travelers should be advised to use insecticides to get rid of mosquitoes in these areas.
- Wear clothing that adequately covers the arms and legs, especially during the early morning and late afternoon, when risk of being bitten is the highest.
- Use insect repellent (see Chapter 2, Protection against Mosquitoes, Ticks, & Other Insects & Arthropods).
- For long-term travelers, empty and clean or cover any standing water that can be mosquito-breeding sites in the local residence (such as water storage tanks or flowerpot trays).

CDC website: www.cdc.gov/dengue

BIBLIOGRAPHY

1. Baaten GG, Sonder GJ, Zaaijer HL, van Gool T, Kint JA, van den Hoek A. Travel-related dengue virus infection, The Netherlands, 2006–2007. Emerg Infect Dis. 2011 May;17(5):821–8.
2. Bandyopadhyay S, Lum LC, Kroeger A. Classifying dengue: a review of the difficulties in using the WHO case classification for dengue haemorrhagic fever. Trop Med Int Health. 2006 Aug;11(8):1238–55.
3. Carroll ID, Toovey S, Van Gompel A. Dengue fever and pregnancy—a review and comment. Travel Med Infect Dis. 2007 May;5(3):183–8.
4. Freedman DO, Weld LH, Kozarsky PE, Fisk T, Robins R, von Sonnenburg F, et al. Spectrum of disease and relation to place of exposure among ill returned travelers. N Engl J Med. 2006 Jan 12;354(2):119–30.
5. Guzman MG, Halstead SB, Artsob H, Buchy P, Farrar J, Gubler DJ, et al. Dengue: a continuing global threat. Nat Rev Microbiol. 2010 Dec;8(12 Suppl):S7–16.
6. Lindback H, Lindback J, Tegnell A, Janzon R, Vene S, Ekdahl K. Dengue fever in travelers to the tropics, 1998 and 1999. Emerg Infect Dis. 2003 Apr;9(4):438–42.
7. Mohammed HP, Ramos MM, Rivera A, Johansson M, Munoz-Jordan JL, Sun W, et al. Travel-associated dengue infections in the United States, 1996 to 2005. J Travel Med. 2010 Jan–Feb;17(1):8–14.
8. Pérez-Padilla J, Rosario-Casablanca R, Pérez-Cruz L, Rivera-Dipini C, Tomashek KM. Perinatal transmission of dengue virus in Puerto Rico: a case report. Open Journal of Obstetrics and Gynecology. 2011;1(3):90–3.
9. Radke EG, Gregory CJ, Kintziger KW, Sauber-Schatz EK, Hunsperger EA, Gallagher GR, et al. Dengue outbreak in Key West, Florida, USA, 2009. Emerg Infect Dis. 2012 Jan;18(1):135–7.
10. Schwartz E, Weld LH, Wilder-Smith A, von Sonnenburg F, Keystone JS, Kain KC, et al. Seasonality, annual trends, and characteristics of dengue among ill returned travelers, 1997–2006. Emerg Infect Dis. 2008 Jul;14(7):1081–8.

11. Simmons CP, Farrar JJ, van Vinh Chau N, Wills B. Dengue. N Engl J Med. 2012 Apr 12;366(15): 1423–32.

12. Srikiatkhachorn A, Rothman AL, Gibbons RV, Sittisombut N, Malasit P, Ennis FA, et al. Dengue—how best to classify it. Clin Infect Dis. 2011 Sep;53(6):563–7.

13. Streit JA, Yang M, Cavanaugh JE, Polgreen PM. Upward trend in dengue incidence among hospitalized patients, United States. Emerg Infect Dis. 2011 May;17(5):914–6.

14. Tomashek KM, Margolis HS. Dengue: a potential transfusion-transmitted disease. Transfusion. 2011 Aug;51(8):1654–60.

15. Wilder-Smith A, Schwartz E. Dengue in travelers. N Engl J Med. 2005 Sep 1;353(9):924–32.

16. World Health Organization. Dengue: guidelines for diagnosis, treatment, prevention and control. Geneva: World Health Organization; 2009.

DIPHTHERIA

Tejpratap S. P. Tiwari

INFECTIOUS AGENT

Toxigenic strains of *Corynebacterium diphtheriae* biotype *mitis, gravis, intermedius,* or *belfanti*.

TRANSMISSION

Person-to-person through oral or respiratory droplets, close physical contact, and rarely, by fomites. Cutaneous diphtheria is common in tropical countries, and contact with discharge from skin lesions may transmit infection in these environments.

EPIDEMIOLOGY

Endemic in many countries in Africa, South America, Asia, the South Pacific, the Middle East, and Eastern Europe and in Haiti and the Dominican Republic.

CLINICAL PRESENTATION

The incubation period is 2–5 days (range, 1–10 days). Affected anatomic sites include the mucous membrane of the upper respiratory tract (nose, pharynx, tonsils, larynx, and trachea [respiratory diphtheria]), skin (cutaneous diphtheria), or rarely, mucous membranes at other sites (eye, ear, vulva). Nasal diphtheria can be asymptomatic or mild, with a blood-tinged discharge.

Respiratory diphtheria has a gradual onset and is characterized by a mild fever (rarely >101°F [38.3°C]), sore throat, difficulty swallowing, malaise, loss of appetite, and if the larynx is involved, hoarseness. The hallmark of respiratory diphtheria is a pseudomembrane that appears within 2–3 days of illness over the mucous lining of the tonsils, pharynx, larynx, or nares and that can extend into the trachea. The pseudomembrane is firm, fleshy, grey, and adherent; it will bleed after attempts to remove or dislodge it. Fatal airway obstruction can result if the pseudomembrane extends into the larynx or trachea, or if a piece of it becomes dislodged.

DIAGNOSIS

A presumptive diagnosis is usually based on clinical features. Diagnosis is confirmed by isolating *C. diphtheriae* from culture of nasal or throat swabs or membrane tissue.

TREATMENT

Patients with respiratory diphtheria require hospitalization to monitor response to treatment and manage complications. Equine diphtheria antitoxin (DAT) is the mainstay of treatment and is administered after specimen testing, without waiting for laboratory confirmation. In the United States, DAT is available to physicians under an investigational new drug protocol by contacting CDC at 770-488-7100.

An antibiotic (erythromycin or penicillin) should be used to eliminate the causative organisms, stop exotoxin production, and reduce communicability. Supportive care (airway, cardiac monitoring) is required. Antimicrobial prophylaxis (erythromycin or penicillin) is recommended for close contacts of patients.

PREVENTION

All travelers should be up-to-date with diphtheria toxoid vaccine before departure. Routine booster doses with Td (tetanus-diphtheria) should be given to all adults every 10 years. This booster is particularly important for travelers who will live or work with local populations in countries where diphtheria is endemic.

BIBLIOGRAPHY

1. CDC. Fatal respiratory diphtheria in a US traveler to Haiti—Pennsylvania, 2003. MMWR Morb Mortal Wkly Rep. 2004 Jan 9;52(53):1285–6.
2. CDC. Updated recommendations for use of tetanus toxoid, reduced diphtheria toxoid and acellular pertussis (Tdap) vaccine from the Advisory Committee on Immunization Practices, 2010. MMWR Morb Mortal Wkly Rep. 2011 Jan 14;60(1):13–5.
3. Galazka A. The changing epidemiology of diphtheria in the vaccine era. J Infect Dis. 2000 Feb;181 Suppl 1:S2–9.

CDC website: www.cdc.gov/vaccines/vpd-vac/diphtheria

ECHINOCOCCOSIS
Pedro L. Moro

INFECTIOUS AGENT
Larval stages of taeniid cestodes of the genus *Echinococcus*.

TRANSMISSION
Oral contact with infected dog feces, particularly in the course of playful and close contact between children and dogs, or through contaminated food or water.

EPIDEMIOLOGY
Echinococcus granulosus is prevalent in broad regions of Eurasia, several South American countries, and Africa. *E. multilocularis* is endemic in the central part of Europe, parts of the Near East, Russia, the Central Asian Republics, China, northern Japan, and Alaska. *E. vogeli* is indigenous to the humid tropical forests in central and northern South America. A small number of polycystic echinococcosis cases in these areas are caused by *E. oligarthrus*.

CLINICAL PRESENTATION
Cystic Echinococcosis or Cystic Hydatid Disease
In humans, hydatid cysts of *E. granulosus* are slowly enlarging masses comparable to benign neoplasms; most human infections remain asymptomatic. Clinical manifestations are determined by the site, size, and condition of the cysts. Hydatid cysts in the liver and the lungs together account for 90% of affected localizations.

Alveolar Echinococcosis or Alveolar Hydatid Disease
The embryo of *E. multilocularis* seems to localize invariably in the liver of the intermediate host. Patients eventually die from hepatic failure, invasion of contiguous structures, or less frequently, metastases to the brain.

Polycystic Echinococcosis or Polycystic Hydatid Disease
Relatively large cysts develop over years and are primarily found in the liver and occasionally in the thorax or abdominal cavity. Those who are symptomatic may present with a painful right hypochondrial mass, progressive jaundice, or, as in the other forms of disease, liver abscess(es).

DIAGNOSIS
A presumptive diagnosis can be made on the basis of a combination of the individual's history and imaging studies, such as a CT scan. Lesions may be found incidentally in an asymptomatic person. Serologic assays may also be performed, and newer ones are under development. Additional information and diagnostic assistance are available through CDC (www.dpd.cdc.gov/dpdx; 404-718-4745; parasites@cdc.gov).

TREATMENT
Surgical removal is preferred when liver cysts are large (>10 cm), secondarily infected, or located in certain organs (brain, lung, or

kidney). PAIR (puncture, aspiration, injection, reaspiration) is a minimally invasive technique used to treat cysts in the liver and other abdominal locations. It is less risky and less expensive than surgery. Benzimidazoles (albendazole, mebendazole) should be given to prevent recurrence after surgery or PAIR. Albendazole should be given continuously, with no monthly treatment interruptions and in 2 divided doses, with a fat-rich meal to increase its bioavailability. Approximately 30% of patients treated with albendazole are cured after 3–6 months and even higher proportions (30%–50%) demonstrate regression of cyst size and alleviation of symptoms.

Alveolar hydatid disease may require both surgery and long-term albendazole, but has a high case-fatality rate. Praziquantel is used in some circumstances.

PREVENTION

Advise travelers to avoid contact with dogs or wild canids in endemic areas. Also advise them not to drink untreated water from streams, canals, lakes, or rivers and to observe food and water precautions (see Chapter 2, Food & Water Precautions).

CDC website: www.cdc.gov/parasites/echino coccosis

BIBLIOGRAPHY

1. Brunetti E, Kern P, Vuitton DA. Expert consensus for the diagnosis and treatment of cystic and alveolar echinococcosis in humans. Acta Trop. 2010 Apr;114(1):1–16.
2. Eckert J, Gottstein B, Heath D, Liu FJ. Prevention of echinococcosis in humans and safety precautions. In: Eckert J, Gemmell MA, Meslin FX, Pawlowski ZS, editors. WHO/OIE Manual on Echinococcosis in Humans and Animals: a Public Health Problem of Global Concern. Paris: World Organization for Animal Health; 2001. p. 238–45.
3. Moro PL, Schantz PM. Echinococcosis: historical landmarks and progress in research and control. Ann Trop Med Parasitol. 2006 Dec;100(8):703–14.

ESCHERICHIA COLI
Joanna Gaines, Rajal Mody, Ciara O'Reilly

INFECTIOUS AGENT

The species *Escherichia coli* consists of a diverse group of bacteria. Most *E. coli* strains do not cause illness; many are present as commensals in healthy human gut flora. However, some *E. coli* strains have acquired virulence genes and can cause disease in the intestinal tract or extraintestinally. Pathogenic *E. coli* strains are categorized into pathotypes on the basis of their virulence genes. Six pathotypes are associated with diarrhea (diarrheogenic): enterotoxigenic *E. coli* (ETEC), Shiga toxin–producing *E. coli* (STEC), enteropathogenic *E. coli* (EPEC), enteroaggregative *E. coli* (EAEC), enteroinvasive *E. coli* (EIEC), and possibly diffusely adherent *E. coli* (DAEC). Other pathotypes are common causes of urinary tract infections, bloodstream infections, and meningitis but will not be covered here. Many serotypes of *E. coli* are determined by surface antigens (H and O), and specific serotypes tend to cluster within a specific pathotype.

STEC are also called verotoxigenic *E. coli* (VTEC), and the term enterohemorrhagic *E. coli* (EHEC) is commonly used to specify STEC strains capable of causing human illness, especially bloody diarrhea and hemolytic uremic syndrome (HUS).

TRANSMISSION

Diarrheogenic pathotypes can be passed in the feces of humans and other animals. Transmission of *E. coli* occurs through the fecal-oral route, primarily via contaminated food or water. Transmission also occurs through person-to-person contact, as well as contact with animals or their environment. The intestinal tracts of animals, especially cattle and other ruminants, are the primary reservoirs of STEC.

EPIDEMIOLOGY

Travel to less-developed countries is associated with higher risk for travelers' diarrhea, including E. coli infection. ETEC is the most common cause of diarrhea among travelers returning from most regions, and other pathotypes can also cause travelers' diarrhea. ETEC was first recognized as a cause of human diarrheal illness in the 1960s. It has since emerged as a major bacterial cause of diarrhea among children in the developing world. Additionally, ETEC is a major bacterial cause of diarrhea in travelers to the developing world. ETEC produces 2 toxins, a heat-stable toxin (known as ST) and a heat-labile toxin (LT). Although different strains of ETEC can secrete either or both of these toxins, the illness caused by each toxin is similar. Both toxins stimulate the lining of the intestines to secrete excessive fluid, thus producing diarrhea. Due to limitations in detection, the relative contribution of pathotypes other than STEC to the prevalence of travelers' diarrhea is unclear and likely underrecognized. Additional information about travelers' diarrhea is available in Chapter 2, Travelers' Diarrhea.

STEC infections are mainly observed in industrialized countries, and most STEC infections do not occur as part of an outbreak. The serogroup most frequently isolated from patients in the United States is O157, but collectively, non-O157 serogroups are estimated to cause more infections. Compared with patients with STEC O157 infection, patients diagnosed with non-O157 STEC infections may be more likely to have recently traveled outside the United States. In 2011, a Shiga toxin–producing EAEC O104:H4 strain caused a large outbreak in Europe; several cases were identified among returning US travelers.

CLINICAL PRESENTATION

Where information is available, non-STEC diarrheogenic E. coli infections have an incubation period ranging from 9 hours to 3 days. The median incubation period of STEC infections is 3–4 days, with a range of 1–10 days. The clinical manifestations of diarrheogenic E. coli vary by pathotype (Table 3-1).

DIAGNOSIS

Many patients with travel-associated E. coli infections, especially those with nonbloody diarrhea, as commonly occurs with ETEC infection, are likely to be managed symptomatically and are unlikely to have the diagnosis confirmed by a laboratory. Most clinical laboratories in the United States do not use tests that can detect diarrheogenic E. coli other than STEC. Testing for non-STEC pathotypes is typically done at public health laboratories and only when an outbreak of diarrheal illness of unknown origin is being investigated. In this situation, isolates for testing may be submitted to CDC via state health departments. These tests typically involve PCR testing for the specific virulence genes of ETEC, EPEC, EAEC, EIEC, and DAEC.

When a decision is made to identify a cause of an acute diarrheal illness, in addition to routine culture for Salmonella, Shigella, and Campylobacter, the stool sample should be cultured for E. coli O157:H7 and simultaneously assayed for non-O157 STEC with a test that detects Shiga toxin. For more information, see www.cdc.gov/mmwr/preview/mmwrhtml/rr5812a1.htm.

All presumptive E. coli O157 isolates and Shiga toxin–positive specimens should be sent to a public health laboratory for further characterization. Rapid, accurate diagnosis of STEC infection is important, because treatment with parenteral volume expansion may decrease renal damage and improve patient outcome.

TREATMENT

Patients with profuse diarrhea or vomiting should be rehydrated. Evidence from pediatric studies indicates that early use of intravenous fluids (within the first 4 days of diarrhea onset) may decrease the risk of HUS in patients with STEC O157 infections. Some people choose to travel with an antibiotic (usually ciprofloxacin, rifaximin, or azithromycin) and take it if they develop loose stools. CDC does not recommend chemoprophylaxis with antibiotics to prevent travelers' diarrhea. (See Chapter 7, Traveling Safely with Infants & Children, for information about managing travelers' diarrhea in children.)

Non-STEC diarrheogenic E. coli are often resistant to traditional antimicrobial agents, including ampicillin and trimethoprim-sulfamethoxazole.

Clinicians treating a patient whose clinical syndrome suggests STEC infection (Table 3-1) should be aware that administering antimicrobial agents may increase the risk of HUS. Additionally, antimotility agents should

Table 3-1. Mechanism of pathogenesis and typical clinical syndrome of *Escherichia coli* pathotypes

PATHOTYPE	MECHANISM OF PATHOGENESIS	TYPICAL CLINICAL SYNDROME
ETEC	Heat stable/heat labile enterotoxin production	Acute watery diarrhea, afebrile, occasionally severe
EAEC	Small and large bowel adherence; enterotoxin and cytotoxin production	Watery diarrhea, bloody diarrhea; can cause prolonged or persistent diarrhea in children
EPEC	Small bowel adherence and epithelial cell effacement mediated by intimin	Severe acute watery diarrhea, bloody diarrhea; may be persistent; common cause of infant diarrhea in developing countries
EIEC	Adherence, mucosal invasion and inflammation of large bowel	Watery diarrhea, dysenterylike diarrhea, fever
DAEC	Diffuse adherence to epithelial cells	Pathogenicity not conclusively demonstrated but may be associated with watery diarrhea
STEC	Large bowel adherence (frequently mediated via intimin); Shiga toxin 1, Shiga toxin 2 production	Watery diarrhea that may progress to bloody diarrhea in 1–3 days; pain with defecation; abdominal tenderness; patients may report a history of fever but be afebrile on presentation, often >5 stools in 24 hours

Abbreviations: ETEC, enterotoxigenic *E. coli*; EAEC, enteroaggregative *E. coli*; EPEC, enteropathogenic *E. coli*; EIEC, enteroinvasive *E. coli*; DAEC, diffusely adherent *E. coli*; STEC, Shiga toxin–producing *E. coli*.

be avoided in patients with bloody diarrhea or patients with confirmed STEC infections, because some studies have found that these agents may increase the risk of HUS or neurologic complications.

PREVENTION

There is no vaccine for E. coli infection, nor is chemoprophylaxis recommended. Food and water are primary sources of E. coli infection, so travelers should be reminded of the importance of adhering to food and water precautions (see Chapter 2, Food & Water Precautions). People who may be exposed to livestock, especially ruminants, should be instructed on the importance of handwashing in preventing E. coli infection. During E. coli outbreaks, clinicians should alert people traveling to affected areas and be cognizant of possible infections among returning travelers.

CDC website: www.cdc.gov/ecoli

BIBLIOGRAPHY

1. Bennett WE, Jr., Tarr PI. Enteric infections and diagnostic testing. Curr Opin Gastroenterol. 2009 Jan;25(1):1–7.
2. DuPont HL. Systematic review: the epidemiology and clinical features of travellers' diarrhoea. Aliment Pharmacol Ther. 2009 Aug;30(3):187–96.
3. Frank C, Werber D, Cramer JP, Askar M, Faber M, an der Heiden M, et al. Epidemic profile of Shiga-toxin-producing *Escherichia coli* O104:H4 outbreak in Germany. N Engl J Med. 2011 Nov 10;365(19):1771–80.

4. Gomi H, Jiang ZD, Adachi JA, Ashley D, Lowe B, Verenkar MP, et al. In vitro antimicrobial susceptibility testing of bacterial enteropathogens causing traveler's diarrhea in four geographic regions. Antimicrob Agents Chemother. 2001 Jan;45(1):212–6.

5. Hedican EB, Medus C, Besser JM, Juni BA, Koziol B, Taylor C, et al. Characteristics of O157 versus non-O157 Shiga toxin-producing Escherichia coli infections in Minnesota, 2000–2006. Clin Infect Dis. 2009 Aug 1;49(3):358–64.

6. Hickey CA, Beattie TJ, Cowieson J, Miyashita Y, Strife CF, Frem JC, et al. Early volume expansion during diarrhea and relative nephroprotection during subsequent hemolytic uremic syndrome. Arch Pediatr Adolesc Med. 2011 Oct;165(10):884–9.

7. Holtz LR, Neill MA, Tarr PI. Acute bloody diarrhea: a medical emergency for patients of all ages. Gastroenterology. 2009 May;136(6):1887–98.

8. Kaper JB, Nataro JP, Mobley HL. Pathogenic Escherichia coli. Nat Rev Microbiol. 2004 Feb;2(2):123–40.

9. Mintz ED. Enterotoxigenic Escherichia coli: outbreak surveillance and molecular testing. Clin Infect Dis. 2006 Jun 1;42(11):1518–20.

10. Shah N, DuPont HL, Ramsey DJ. Global etiology of travelers' diarrhea: systematic review from 1973 to the present. Am J Trop Med Hyg. 2009 Apr;80(4):609–14.

11. Wong CS, Mooney JC, Brandt JR, Staples AO, Jelacic S, Boster DR, et al. Risk factors for the hemolytic uremic syndrome in children infected with Escherichia coli O157:H7: a multivariable analysis. Clin Infect Dis. 2012 Jul;55(1):33–41.

FASCIOLIASIS
Ronnie Henry, LeAnne M. Fox

INFECTIOUS AGENT
Trematode flatworms *Fasciola hepatica* and *F. gigantica*.

TRANSMISSION
Consumption of watercress or other aquatic plants contaminated with infective metacercariae or contaminated pond water.

EPIDEMIOLOGY
Broadly distributed. The highest rates of *F. hepatica* infection have been reported from Bolivia, Peru, Egypt, Iran, Portugal, and France. *F. gigantica* has a more limited distribution (parts of Africa, the Middle East, and South and East Asia).

CLINICAL PRESENTATION
The acute phase begins 6–12 weeks after infection and can last >4 months. Most patients are asymptomatic, but symptoms might include marked eosinophilia, abdominal pain, intermittent high fever, weight loss, or urticaria. Within weeks to months, symptoms of the acute phase subside as worms enter the bile ducts, beginning the chronic phase. Patients in this phase may also be asymptomatic or may present with biliary colic, epigastric pain, nausea, jaundice, or pruritus. The long-term prognosis depends on the extent of the liver and biliary damage.

DIAGNOSIS
Detection of eggs in stool or duodenal or biliary aspirates. Serologic tests may be useful during the acute phase, since egg production does not start until 3–4 months after exposure. Radiologic examinations, including ultrasonogram and CT of the liver, are helpful, especially during the hepatic or migratory acute phase.

TREATMENT
First-line treatment is with triclabendazole, which is not commercially available for human use in the United States. An alternative drug is nitazoxanide. Surgical resection or endoscopic retrograde cholangiopancreatographic removal of adult flukes can be done in cases with biliary tract obstruction.

PREVENTION
Avoid eating uncooked aquatic plants, including watercress, mint, and parsley; avoid drinking untreated freshwater.

CDC website: www.cdc.gov/parasites/fasciola

BIBLIOGRAPHY

1. Garcia HH, Moro PL, Schantz PM. Zoonotic helminth infections of humans: echinococcosis, cysticercosis and fascioliasis. Curr Opin Infect Dis. 2007 Oct;20(5):489–94.
2. Mas-Coma S, Bargues MD, Valero MA. Fascioliasis and other plant-borne trematode zoonoses. Int J Parasitol. 2005 Oct;35(11–12):1255–78.
3. Rowan SE, Levi ME, Youngwerth JM, Brauer B, Everson GT, Johnson SC. The variable presentations and broadening geographic distribution of hepatic fascioliasis. Clin Gastroenterol Hepatol. 2012 Jun;10(6):598–602.

FILARIASIS, LYMPHATIC

LeAnne M. Fox

INFECTIOUS AGENT

Filarial nematodes *Wuchereria bancrofti*, *Brugia malayi*, and *B. timori*.

TRANSMISSION

Through the bite of infected *Aedes*, *Culex*, *Anopheles*, and *Mansonia* mosquitoes.

EPIDEMIOLOGY

Found in sub-Saharan Africa, Egypt, southern Asia, the western Pacific Islands, the northeastern coast of Brazil, Guyana, Haiti, and the Dominican Republic. Travelers are at low risk.

CLINICAL PRESENTATION

Most infections are asymptomatic, but lymphatic dysfunction may lead to lymphedema of the leg, scrotum, penis, arm, or breast years after infection. Acute episodes are associated with painful swelling of an affected limb, fever, or chills due to bacterial superinfection. Tropical pulmonary eosinophilia is a potentially serious progressive lung disease that presents with nocturnal cough, wheezing, and fever, resulting from immune hyperresponsiveness to microfilariae in the pulmonary capillaries.

DIAGNOSIS

Microscopic detection of microfilariae on an appropriately timed thick blood film. Determination of serum antifilarial IgG is also a diagnostically useful test. This assay is available through the Parasitic Diseases Laboratory at the National Institutes of Health or through CDC (www.dpd.cdc.gov/dpdx; 404-718-4745; parasites@cdc.gov).

TREATMENT

The drug of choice, diethylcarbamazine, can be obtained from CDC under an investigational new drug protocol (404-718-4745; parasites@cdc.gov). Patients with lymphedema and hydrocele can benefit from lymphedema management and, in the case of hydrocele, surgical repair.

PREVENTION

Mosquito precautions (see Chapter 2, Protection against Mosquitoes, Ticks, & Other Insects & Arthropods).

CDC website: www.cdc.gov/parasites/lymphaticfilariasis

BIBLIOGRAPHY

1. Eberhard ML, Lammie PJ. Laboratory diagnosis of filariasis. Clin Lab Med. 1991 Dec;11(4):977–1010.
2. Lipner EM, Law MA, Barnett E, Keystone JS, von Sonnenburg F, Loutan L, et al. Filariasis in travelers presenting to the GeoSentinel Surveillance Network. PLoS Negl Trop Dis. 2007;1(3):e88.
3. Nutman TB, editor. Lymphatic Filariasis. London: Imperial College Press; 2000.

GIARDIASIS

Julia Warner Gargano, Jonathan S. Yoder

INFECTIOUS AGENT

The protozoan parasite *Giardia intestinalis* (formerly known as *G. lamblia* or *G. duodenalis*).

TRANSMISSION

By ingesting fecally contaminated food or water, including water swallowed while swimming; through contact with fecally contaminated environmental surfaces; or through person-to-person contact, such as caring for an infected person or sexual contact.

EPIDEMIOLOGY

Transmission occurs worldwide, most commonly diagnosed in travelers returning from south Asia, the Middle East, and South America. Risk of infection increases with duration of travel.

CLINICAL PRESENTATION

Symptoms typically develop 1–2 weeks after infection and generally resolve within 2–4 weeks. Signs and symptoms include diarrhea (often with foul-smelling, greasy stools), abdominal cramps, bloating, flatulence, fatigue, anorexia, and nausea. Typically, a patient presents with the gradual onset of 2–5 loose stools per day and gradually increasing fatigue. Sometimes upper gastrointestinal symptoms are more prominent. Weight loss may occur over time. Fever and vomiting are uncommon. Reactive arthritis, irritable bowel syndrome, and other chronic symptoms sometimes occur after infection with *Giardia* (see Chapter 5, Persistent Travelers' Diarrhea).

DIAGNOSIS

Giardia cysts or trophozoites are not consistently seen in the stools of infected patients. Diagnostic yield can be increased by examining up to 3 stool samples over several days. Direct fluorescent antibody (DFA) testing is extremely sensitive and specific. Other immunodiagnostic kits that do not require microscopy also detect *Giardia* antigens, but do not take the place of ova and parasite examinations.

TREATMENT

Tinidazole, metronidazole, nitazoxanide, paromomycin, furazolidone, and quinacrine are known to be effective in treating giardiasis. Because making a definitive diagnosis is difficult, empiric treatment can be used in patients with the appropriate history and typical symptoms.

PREVENTION

Food and water precautions (see Chapter 2, Food & Water Precautions) and hand hygiene.

CDC website: www.cdc.gov/parasites/giardia

BIBLIOGRAPHY

1. Greenwood Z, Black J, Weld L, O'Brien D, Leder K, Von Sonnenburg F, et al. Gastrointestinal infection among international travelers globally. J Travel Med. 2008 Jul–Aug;15(4):221–8.
2. Okhuysen PC. Traveler's diarrhea due to intestinal protozoa. Clin Infect Dis. 2001 Jul 1;33(1):110–4.
3. Swaminathan A, Torresi J, Schlagenhauf P, Thursky K, Wilder-Smith A, Connor BA, et al. A global study of pathogens and host risk factors associated with infectious gastrointestinal disease in returned international travellers. J Infect. 2009 Jul;59(1):19–27.

HAND, FOOT, & MOUTH DISEASE

Ronnie Henry, Eileen Schneider

INFECTIOUS AGENT

In the United States, coxsackievirus A16 is most commonly detected, but other enteroviruses (such as coxsackievirus A10) can cause hand, foot, and mouth disease. Recently, coxsackievirus A6 has been detected in outbreaks. Internationally, enterovirus 71 is a common etiologic agent.

TRANSMISSION

Person-to-person, through contact with saliva, sputum, fluid in blisters, or stool of an infected person.

EPIDEMIOLOGY

Distributed worldwide; recent large outbreaks have been reported in Cambodia, China, Japan, Korea, Malaysia, Singapore, Thailand, Taiwan, and Vietnam.

CLINICAL PRESENTATION

Incubation period is 4–6 days. Patients usually present with fever and malaise, followed by sore throat and the development of vesicles in the mouth and a rash, often vesicular, on the hands (palms) and feet (soles). In some cases, the rash may be more widespread. Lesions usually resolve in 1 week, but rare complications can include aseptic meningitis and encephalitis.

DIAGNOSIS

Diagnosis is most often made clinically. Laboratory testing (such as PCR) is available and is usually performed on atypical or severe cases.

TREATMENT

Supportive care.

PREVENTION

Avoiding close contact with infected people, maintaining good hand hygiene, and disinfecting potentially contaminated surfaces, including toys.

CDC website: www.cdc.gov/hand-foot-mouth

BIBLIOGRAPHY

1. Ooi MH, Wong SC, Lewthwaite P, Cardosa MJ, Solomon T. Clinical features, diagnosis, and management of enterovirus 71. Lancet Neurol. 2010 Nov;9(11):1097–105.
2. World Health Organization. A guide to clinical management and public health response for hand, foot and mouth disease (HFMD). Geneva: World Health Organization; 2011 [cited 2012 Sep 20]. Available from: http://www.wpro.who.int/publications/docs/GuidancefortheclinicalmanagementofHFMD.pdf.

HELICOBACTER PYLORI

Ezra J. Barzilay, Ryan P. Fagan

INFECTIOUS AGENT

Helicobacter pylori is a small, curved, microaerophilic, gram-negative, rod-shaped bacterium.

TRANSMISSION

Believed to be fecal-oral or possibly oral-oral.

EPIDEMIOLOGY

Common worldwide. Estimated prevalence is 70% in developing countries and 30%–40% in the United States and other industrialized countries.

CLINICAL PRESENTATION

Usually asymptomatic, but *H. pylori* is the major cause of peptic ulcer disease and gastritis, which presents as gnawing or burning epigastric pain. Less commonly, symptoms include nausea, vomiting, loss of appetite, or bleeding.

DIAGNOSIS

Fecal antigen assay, urea breath test, rapid urease test, or histology of biopsy specimen. A positive serology indicates present or past infection.

TREATMENT

Clarithromycin triple therapy (proton pump inhibitor [PPI] + clarithromycin + amoxicillin or metronidazole) or bismuth quadruple therapy (PPI or H_2-blocker + bismuth + metronidazole + tetracycline). See www.acg.gi.org/physicians/guidelines/ManagementofHpylori.pdf.

PREVENTION

No specific recommendations.

BIBLIOGRAPHY

1. Chey WD, Wong BC. American College of Gastroenterology guideline on the management of *Helicobacter pylori* infection. Am J Gastroenterol. 2007 Aug;102(8):1808–25.
2. Lindkvist P, Wadstrom T, Giesecke J. *Helicobacter pylori* infection and foreign travel. J Infect Dis. 1995 Oct;172(4):1135–6.
3. Peterson WL, Fendrick AM, Cave DR, Peura DA, Garabedian-Ruffalo SM, Laine L. *Helicobacter pylori*-related disease: guidelines for testing and treatment. Arch Intern Med. 2000 May 8;160(9):1285–91.

HELMINTHS, SOIL-TRANSMITTED
Els Mathieu

INFECTIOUS AGENTS

Ascaris lumbricoides (roundworm), *Ancylostoma duodenale* (hookworm), *Necator americanus* (hookworm), and *Trichuris trichiura* (whipworm) are helminths (parasitic worms) that infect the intestine and are transmitted via contaminated soil.

TRANSMISSION

Infection with roundworm and whipworm occurs when eggs in soil have become infective and are ingested. Hookworm infection usually occurs when larvae, hatched from eggs in the soil, penetrate the skin (for example, when people walk barefoot on contaminated soil) but can also occur when larvae are ingested.

EPIDEMIOLOGY

Widespread, but the prevalence is highest in tropical, developing countries. Travelers to these countries should be at low risk of infection if prevention measures are taken.

CLINICAL PRESENTATION

Most infections are asymptomatic, especially when few worms are present. Pulmonary symptoms occur in a small percentage of patients when roundworm larvae pass through the lungs. Roundworm can also cause intestinal discomfort, obstruction, and impaired nutritional status. Hookworm infection can lead to anemia and protein deficiency due to blood loss. Whipworm infection can cause blood loss, as well as dysentery and rectal prolapse. However, travelers are rarely at risk for these more severe manifestations because they are generally associated with high worm burdens seen in indigenous populations.

DIAGNOSIS

By identifying eggs in a stool specimen. Adult roundworms may occasionally be coughed up or found in stool or vomit.

TREATMENT

Albendazole or mebendazole.

PREVENTION

Food and water precautions (see Chapter 2, Food & Water Precautions) and by avoiding walking barefoot on soil that may be contaminated with sewage, where human feces may have been used as fertilizer, or where people may have defecated.

CDC website: www.cdc.gov/parasites/sth

BIBLIOGRAPHY

1. Bethony J, Brooker S, Albonico M, Geiger SM, Loukas A, Diemert D, et al. Soil-transmitted helminth infections: ascariasis, trichuriasis, and hookworm. Lancet. 2006 May 6;367(9521):1521–32.
2. Brooker S, Bundy DAP. Soil-transmitted helminths (geohelminths). In: Cook GC, Zumla A, editors. Manson's Tropical Diseases. 22nd ed. London: Saunders; 2009. p 1515–48.
3. Brooker S, Clements AC, Bundy DA. Global epidemiology, ecology and control of soil-transmitted helminth infections. Adv Parasitol. 2006;62:221–61.

HEPATITIS A

Umid M. Sharapov, Eyasu H. Teshale

INFECTIOUS AGENT

Hepatitis A virus (HAV) is an RNA virus classified as a picornavirus.

TRANSMISSION

Through direct person-to-person contact; contaminated water, ice, or shellfish harvested from sewage-contaminated water; or from contaminated raw fruits, vegetables, or other foods. HAV is shed in the feces of infected people. The virus reaches peak levels 1–2 weeks before onset of symptoms and diminishes rapidly after liver dysfunction or symptoms appear, which is concurrent with the appearance of circulating antibodies to HAV. Infants and children, however, may shed virus for up to 6 months after infection.

EPIDEMIOLOGY

Common throughout the developing world, where infections most frequently are acquired during early childhood and are usually asymptomatic or mild. In these countries, a high proportion of adults in the population are immune to HAV, and epidemics of hepatitis A are uncommon. In developed countries, infection is less common, but community-wide outbreaks may occur. Hepatitis A is one of the most common vaccine-preventable infections acquired during travel. In the United States the most frequently identified risk factor for hepatitis A is international travel. Risk is highest for those who live in or visit rural areas, trek in backcountry areas, or frequently eat or drink in settings of poor sanitation. However, cases of travel-related hepatitis A can also occur in travelers to developing countries with "standard" tourist itineraries, accommodations, and eating behaviors.

CLINICAL PRESENTATION

Incubation period averages 28 days (range, 15–50 days). Infection may be asymptomatic or may range in severity from a mild illness lasting 1–2 weeks to a severely disabling disease lasting several months. Clinical manifestations include the abrupt onset of fever, malaise, anorexia, nausea, and abdominal discomfort, followed within a few days by jaundice. The likelihood of having symptoms with HAV infection is related to the age of the infected person. In children aged <6 years, most (70%) infections are asymptomatic; if illness does occur, its duration is usually <2 months. Ten percent of infected people have prolonged or relapsing symptoms over a 6- to 9-month period. The overall case-fatality ratio is 0.3%; however, the ratio is 1.8% among adults aged >50 years.

DIAGNOSIS

Anti-HAV IgM in serum or ≥4-fold rise in specific antibodies in paired sera.

TREATMENT

Supportive care only.

PREVENTION

Vaccination or immune globulin (IG), and food and water precautions.

Vaccine

Two monovalent hepatitis A vaccines and a combined hepatitis A and hepatitis B (Twinrix) vaccine are licensed in the United States (Table 3-2). The immunogenicity of the combination vaccine is equivalent to that of the monovalent hepatitis vaccines when tested after completion of the licensed schedule.

Indications for Use

All susceptible people traveling for any purpose, frequency, or duration to countries with high or intermediate HAV endemicity should be vaccinated or receive IG before departure. Currently, international travel is considered the number one risk factor for HAV infection in the United States. Although the Advisory Committee for Immunization Practices recommends hepatitis A vaccination for people traveling to countries with high or intermediate HAV endemicity, published maps may not be the best guide in determining endemicity in developing countries. Prevalence patterns of HAV infection may vary among regions within a country, and missing or obsolete data present a challenge. Countries where the prevalence of HAV infection is decreasing have increasing numbers of susceptible people, and there is a risk of large outbreaks of hepatitis A. In addition, in recent years, large outbreaks of hepatitis A were reported in developed countries among people who had been exposed to either food handlers with hepatitis A or imported food contaminated with HAV. Taking into account the complexity involved with interpreting hepatitis A risk maps and potential foodborne hepatitis A risk in countries with low endemicity, some expert travel clinicians advise people traveling outside the United States to consider hepatitis A vaccination regardless of their destination.

Vaccination is recommended for unvaccinated household members and other people who will have close personal contact (such as regular babysitters) with an international adoptee from a country of high or intermediate endemicity (see Chapter 7, International Adoption).

Vaccine Administration

One dose of monovalent hepatitis A vaccine protects most healthy people aged ≤40 years. The vaccine series should be completed according to the licensed schedule for long-term protection.

Hepatitis A vaccine at the age-appropriate dose is preferred to IG; however, for optimal protection, adults aged >40 years, immunocompromised people, and people with chronic liver disease or other chronic medical conditions planning to depart to an area in <2 weeks should receive the initial dose of vaccine along with IG (0.02 mL/kg) at a separate injection site.

Travelers who are aged <12 months, are allergic to a vaccine component, or who otherwise elect not to receive vaccine should receive a single dose of IG (0.02 mL/kg), which provides effective protection against HAV infection for up to 3 months. Those who do not receive vaccination and plan to travel for >3 months should receive an IG dose of 0.06 mL/kg, which must be repeated if the duration of travel is >5 months.

Although vaccination of an immune traveler is not contraindicated and does not increase the risk for adverse effects, screening for total anti-HAV before travel can be useful in some circumstances to determine susceptibility and eliminate unnecessary vaccination. Postvaccination testing for serologic response is not indicated.

Other Vaccine Considerations

Using the vaccines according to the licensed schedules is preferable. However, an interrupted series does not need to be restarted. More than 95% of vaccinated people develop protective levels of anti-HAV 1 month after the first dose. Given their similar immunogenicity, a series that has been started with one brand of monovalent vaccine may be completed with the other brand. For children and adults who complete the primary series, booster doses of vaccine are not recommended.

Table 3-2. Vaccines to prevent hepatitis A

VACCINE	TRADE NAME (MANUFACTURER)	AGE (Y)	DOSE	ROUTE	SCHEDULE	BOOSTER
Hepatitis A vaccine, inactivated	Havrix (GlaxoSmithKline)	1–18	0.5 mL (720 ELU)	IM	0, 6–12 mo	None
		≥19	1.0 mL (1,440 ELU)	IM	0, 6–12 mo	None
Hepatitis A vaccine, inactivated	Vaqta (Merck & Co., Inc.)	1–18	0.5 mL (25 U)	IM	0, 6–18 mo	None
		≥19	1.0 mL (50 U)	IM	0, 6–18 mo	None
Combined hepatitis A and B vaccine	Twinrix (GlaxoSmithKline)	≥18 (primary)	1.0 mL (720 ELU HAV + 20 µg HBsAg)	IM	0, 1, 6 mo	None
		≥18 (accelerated)	same as above	IM	0, 7, 21–30 d	12 mo

Abbreviations: ELU, ELISA units of inactivated HAV; IM, intramuscular; U, units HAV antigen; HAV, hepatitis A virus; HBsAg, hepatitis B surface antigen.

Vaccine Safety and Adverse Reactions

Among adults, the most frequently reported side effects, occurring 3–5 days after a vaccine dose, are tenderness or pain at the injection site (53%–56%) or headache (14%–16%). Among children, the most common side effects reported are pain or tenderness at the injection site (15%–19%), feeding problems (8% in one study), or headache (4% in one study). No serious adverse events in children or adults have been found that could be attributed definitively to the vaccine, nor have increases in serious adverse events been identified among vaccinated people compared with baseline rates.

Precautions and Contraindications

These vaccines should not be administered to travelers with a history of hypersensitivity to any vaccine component. Twinrix should not be administered to people with a history of hypersensitivity to yeast. Because hepatitis A vaccine consists of inactivated virus and hepatitis B vaccine consists of a recombinant protein, no special precautions are needed for vaccination of immunocompromised travelers.

Pregnancy

The safety of hepatitis A vaccine for pregnant women has not been determined. However, because hepatitis A vaccine is produced from inactivated HAV, the theoretical risk to either the pregnant woman or the developing fetus is thought to be low. The risk of vaccination should be weighed against the risk of hepatitis A among female travelers who might be at high risk for exposure to HAV.

Postexposure Prophylaxis

Travelers who are exposed to HAV and who have not received hepatitis A vaccine or IG previously should be administered 1 dose of monovalent hepatitis A vaccine or IG (0.02 mL/kg) as soon as possible. The efficacy of IG or vaccine when administered >2 weeks after exposure has not been established. Information about the relative efficacy of vaccine compared with IG postexposure is limited.

For healthy people aged 12 months to 40 years, a dose of monovalent hepatitis A vaccine is recommended. For people aged >40 years, IG is preferred, but vaccine can be used if IG is unavailable. IG is recommended for people aged <12 months, people who are immunocompromised, people who have chronic liver disease, and people for whom vaccine is contraindicated. More detailed information can be found in the Advisory Committee on Immunization Practices recommendations at www.cdc.gov/mmwr/preview/mmwrhtml/mm5641a3.htm.

CDC website: www.cdc.gov/hepatitis/HAV

BIBLIOGRAPHY

1. Bacaner N, Stauffer B, Boulware DR, Walker PF, Keystone JS. Travel medicine considerations for North American immigrants visiting friends and relatives. JAMA. 2004 Jun 16;291(23):2856–64.
2. CDC. Update: Prevention of hepatitis A after exposure to hepatitis A virus and in international travelers. Updated recommendations of the Advisory Committee on Immunization Practices (ACIP). MMWR Morb Mortal Wkly Rep. 2007 Oct 19;56(41):1080–4.
3. CDC. Updated recommendations from the Advisory Committee on Immunization Practices (ACIP) for use of hepatitis A vaccine in close contacts of newly arriving international adoptees. MMWR Morb Mortal Wkly Rep. 2009 Sep 18;58(36):1006–7.
4. CDC, Division of Viral Hepatitis. Viral hepatitis surveillance: United States, 2009. Atlanta: CDC; 2009 [cited 2012 Sep 20]. Available from: http://www.cdc.gov/hepatitis/Statistics/2009Surveillance/PDFs/2009HepSurveillanceRpt.pdf.
5. Fiore AE. Hepatitis A transmitted by food. Clin Infect Dis. 2004 Mar 1;38(5):705–15.
6. Fiore AE, Wasley A, Bell BP. Prevention of hepatitis A through active or passive immunization: recommendations of the Advisory Committee on Immunization Practices (ACIP). MMWR Recomm Rep. 2006 May 19;55(RR-7):1–23.
7. Klevens RM, Miller JT, Iqbal K, Thomas A, Rizzo EM, Hanson H, et al. The evolving epidemiology of hepatitis A in the United States: incidence and molecular epidemiology from population-based surveillance, 2005–2007. Arch Intern Med. 2010 Nov 8;170(20):1811–8.
8. Mohd Hanafiah K, Jacobsen KH, Wiersma ST. Challenges to mapping the health risk of hepatitis A virus infection. Int J Health Geogr. 2011;10:57.
9. Murphy TV, Feinstone SM, Bell BP. Hepatitis A vaccines. In: Plotkin SA, Orenstein WA, Offit PA, editors. Vaccines. 6th ed. Philadelphia: Saunders Elsevier; 2012. p. 183–204.

10. Mutsch M, Spicher VM, Gut C, Steffen R. Hepatitis A virus infections in travelers, 1988–2004. Clin Infect Dis. 2006 Feb 15;42(4):490–7.
11. Van Damme P, Banatvala J, Fay O, Iwarson S, McMahon B, Van Herck K, et al. Hepatitis A booster vaccination: is there a need? Lancet. 2003 Sep 27;362(9389):1065–71.
12. Winokur PL, Stapleton JT. Immunoglobulin prophylaxis for hepatitis A. Clin Infect Dis. 1992 Feb;14(2):580–6.

HEPATITIS B
Francisco Averhoff

INFECTIOUS AGENT
Hepatitis B is a disease caused by hepatitis B virus (HBV), a small, circular, partially double-stranded DNA virus in the *Hepadnaviridae* family.

TRANSMISSION
HBV is transmitted by contact with contaminated blood, blood products, and other body fluids (such as semen). Activities associated with transmission include any that may increase the likelihood of contaminated blood or body fluid exposure. Travelers may be at increased risk due to engaging in casual and unprotected sex, having medical procedures in areas where blood may not be screened, or even through obtaining tattoos or having acupuncture.

EPIDEMIOLOGY
An estimated 240 million people have chronic HBV infection globally (Map 3-4). Nevertheless, no data show the specific risk of infection with HBV among US travelers. Published reports of travelers acquiring hepatitis are rare, and the risk for travelers who do not have high-risk behaviors or exposures is low. The risk for HBV infection in travelers may be higher in countries where the prevalence of chronic HBV infection is high or intermediate; expatriates, missionaries, and long-term development workers may be at increased risk for HBV infection in such countries. All travelers should be aware of how HBV is transmitted and take measures to minimize their exposures.

CLINICAL PRESENTATION
HBV infection primarily affects the liver. Typically, the incubation period for hepatitis B is 90 days (range, 60–150 days). The usual signs and symptoms include malaise, fatigue, anorexia, nausea, vomiting, abdominal pain, and jaundice. In some cases skin rashes, joint pain, and arthritis may occur. Among people aged ≥5 years, 30%–50% will develop signs and symptoms during acute infection. In children aged <5 years and immunocompromised adults, acute HBV infection is typically asymptomatic. The overall case-fatality ratio of acute hepatitis B is approximately 1%.

Acute hepatitis B progresses to chronic HBV infection in 30%–90% of people infected as infants or young children and in <5% of people infected during adolescence or adulthood. Chronic infection with HBV may result in chronic liver disease, including cirrhosis and liver cancer.

DIAGNOSIS
Serologic markers specific for hepatitis B are necessary to diagnose HBV infection and to identify the stage of infection (Table 3-3). These markers can be used to differentiate between acute, resolving, and chronic infection.

TREATMENT
No specific treatment is available for acute hepatitis B. Supportive treatment, including hospitalization, may be indicated for some people with severe clinical manifestations. Antiretroviral drugs are approved to treat chronic hepatitis B.

PREVENTION
Vaccine
Indications for Use
Hepatitis B vaccination should be administered to all unvaccinated people traveling to areas with

Table 3-3. Interpretation of serologic test results for hepatitis B virus infection[1]

SEROLOGIC MARKER				
HBsAg[2]	TOTAL ANTI-HBc	IgM ANTI-HBc	ANTI-HBs	INTERPRETATION
−	−	−	−	Never infected
+	−	−	−	Early acute infection; transient (up to 18 days) after vaccination
+	+	+	−	Acute infection
−	+	+	+ or −	Acute resolving infection
−	+	−	+	Recovered from past infection and immune
+	+	−	−	Chronic infection
−	+	−	−	False-positive (susceptible); past infection; occult infection;[3] or passive transfer of anti-HBc to infant born to HBsAg-positive mother
−	−	−	+	Immune if concentration is ≥10 mIU/mL after vaccine series completion; passive transfer after hepatitis B immune globulin administration

Abbreviations: HBsAg, hepatitis B surface antigen; anti-HBc, antibody to hepatitis B core antigen; anti-HBs, antibody to hepatitis B surface antigen.

[1] From: CDC. A comprehensive immunization strategy to eliminate transmission of hepatitis B virus infection in the United States: recommendations of the Advisory Committee on Immunization Practices (ACIP). Part II: immunization of adults. MMWR Recomm Rep. 2006 Dec 8;55(RR-16):1–33.

[2] To ensure that an HBsAg-positive test result is not a false positive, samples with reactive HBsAg results should be tested with a licensed neutralizing confirmatory test, if recommended in the manufacturer's package insert.

[3] People positive only for anti-HBc are unlikely to be infectious except under unusual circumstances in which they are the source for direct percutaneous exposure of susceptible recipients to large quantities of virus (such as blood transfusion or organ transplant).

intermediate to high prevalence of chronic hepatitis B (HBV surface antigen prevalence ≥2%). Complete vaccination recommendations are available at www.cdc.gov/vaccines/pubs/acip-list. htm#hepb. Vaccination may be considered for all international travelers, regardless of destination, depending on the traveler's behavioral risk as determined by the provider and traveler.

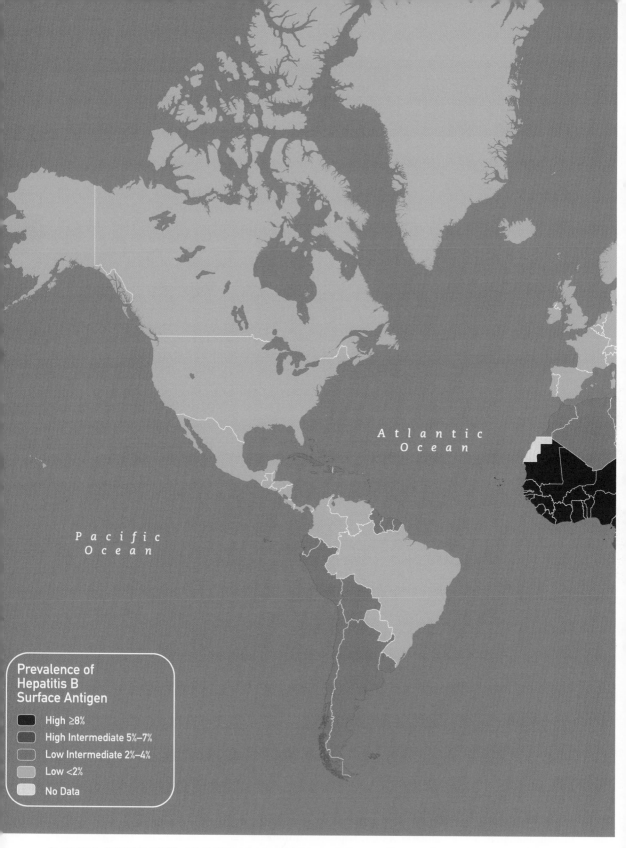

MAP 3-4. PREVALENCE OF CHRONIC HEPATITIS B VIRUS INFECTION AMONG ADULTS[1,2]

Prevalence of
Hepatitis B
Surface Antigen

- High ≥8%
- High Intermediate 5%–7%
- Low Intermediate 2%–4%
- Low <2%
- No Data

[1] Used with permission from: Ott JJ, Stevens GA, Groeger J, Wiersma ST. Global epidemiology of hepatitis B virus infection: new estimates of age-specific seroprevalence and endemicity. Vaccine. 2012.30(12):2212–9.

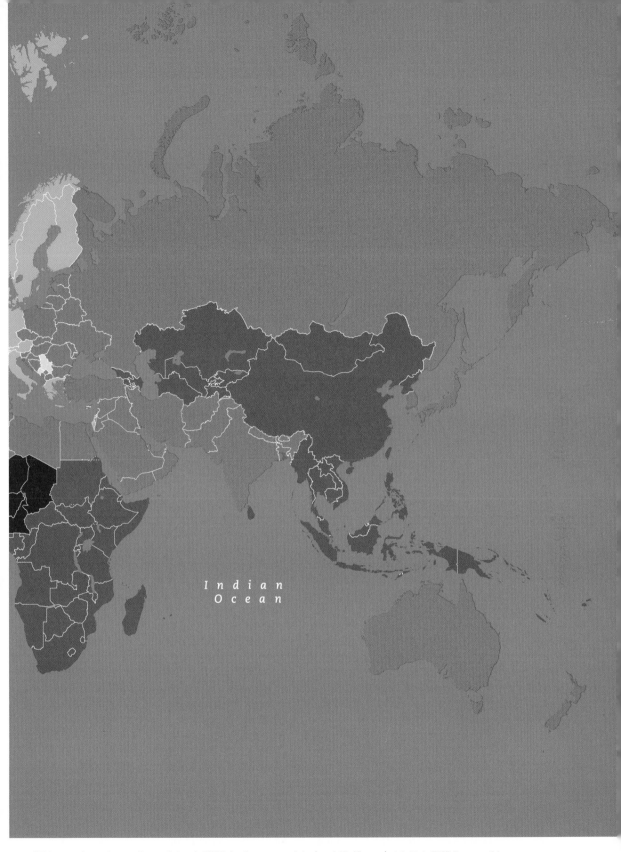

Indian Ocean

[2] This map shows the prevalence of chronic HBV infection among adults (aged 19–49 years) globally in 2005; because this analysis grouped countries together regionally, individual country prevalence may be higher or lower than reflected on the map.

Vaccine Administration

Hepatitis B vaccine (see Table 3-4) is usually administered as a 3-dose series on a 0-, 1-, 6-month schedule to achieve immunity. The second dose should be given ≥1 month after the first dose; the third dose should be given ≥2 months after the second dose and ≥4 months after the first dose. The third dose should not be given before age 24 weeks. Exceptions to this schedule are available with specific licensed products in the United States; Recombivax HB (Merck & Co.) is licensed for a 2-dose schedule for children aged 11–15 years, and Engerix-B (GlaxoSmithKline) is licensed for a 4-dose schedule (0, 1, and 2 months, plus a 12-month booster). Combination vaccines including hepatitis B are available for children, and a combination hepatitis A and hepatitis B vaccine, Twinrix (GlaxoSmithKline), is also licensed in the United States. Consult the prescribing information when administering alternate schedules and formulations. Vaccination series started with one brand may be completed with another brand. Protection from the primary vaccination series is robust, and >95% of healthy people achieve immunity with the 3-dose series. Serologic testing and booster vaccination are not recommended before travel for immunocompetent adults who have been previously vaccinated.

Special Situations

Ideally, hepatitis B vaccination should begin ≥6 months before travel so the full vaccine series can be completed before departure. Because some protection is provided by 1 or 2 doses, the vaccine series should be initiated, if indicated, even if it cannot be completed before departure. Optimal protection, however, is not conferred until after the final vaccine dose is received, and travelers should be advised to complete the vaccine series. An approved accelerated vaccination schedule can be used for people traveling on short notice who face imminent exposure or for emergency responders to disaster areas. The accelerated vaccination schedule calls for vaccine doses administered at days 0, 7, and 21–30; a booster should be administered at 12 months to promote long-term immunity. A combined hepatitis A and hepatitis B vaccine can also be used on the same 3-dose schedule (0, 7, 21–30 days).

Vaccine Safety and Adverse Reactions

Hepatitis B vaccines are safe for people of all ages. Pain at the injection site (3%–29%) and fever (temperature >99.9°F [37.7°C]; 1%–6%) are the most frequently reported side effects among vaccine recipients. Hepatitis B vaccines should not be administered to people with a history of hypersensitivity to any vaccine component, including yeast. The vaccine contains a recombinant protein (hepatitis B surface antigen) that is noninfectious.

Limited data indicate no apparent risk of adverse events to the mother or the developing fetus when hepatitis B vaccine is administered to pregnant women. HBV infection affecting a pregnant woman can result in serious disease for the mother and chronic infection for the newborn. Neither pregnancy nor lactation should be considered a contraindication for vaccination.

Personal Protection Measures

As part of the pre-travel education process, all travelers should be counseled and given information about the risks for hepatitis B and other bloodborne pathogens from contaminated equipment or items used during medical, dental, or cosmetic procedures; blood products; injection drug use; any activities or procedures that involve piercing the skin or mucosa; or unprotected sexual activity, and should be informed about prevention measures. When seeking medical or dental care or cosmetic procedures (such as tattooing or piercing), travelers should be alert to the use of equipment that has not been adequately sterilized or disinfected, reuse of contaminated equipment, and unsafe injecting practices (such as reuse of disposable needles and syringes). HBV and other bloodborne pathogens can be transmitted if tools are not sterile or if personnel do not follow proper infection control procedures. Travelers should consider the health risks when receiving medical or dental care. The health risks should be strongly considered when deciding to obtain a tattoo or body piercing in areas where adequate sterilization or disinfection procedures might not be available or practiced.

CDC website: www.cdc.gov/hepatitis/HBV

Table 3-4. Vaccines to prevent hepatitis B

VACCINE	TRADE NAME (MANUFACTURER)	AGE (Y)	DOSE	ROUTE	SCHEDULE	BOOSTER
Hepatitis B vaccine, recombinant[1]	Engerix-B (GlaxoSmithKline)	0–19 (primary)	0.5 mL (10 µg HBsAg)	IM	0, 1, 6 mo	None
		0–10 (accelerated)	0.5 mL (10 µg HBsAg)	IM	0, 1, 2 mo	12 mo
		11–19 (accelerated)	1.0 mL (20 µg HBsAg)	IM	0, 1, 2 mo	12 mo
		≥20 (primary)	1.0 mL (20 µg HBsAg)	IM	0, 1, 6 mo	None
		≥20 (accelerated)	1.0 mL (20 µg HBsAg)	IM	0, 1, 2 mo	12 mo
Hepatitis B vaccine, recombinant[1]	Recombivax HB (Merck & Co., Inc.)	0–19 (primary)	0.5 mL (5 µg HBsAg)	IM	0, 1, 6 mo	None
		11–15 (adolescent accelerated)	1.0 mL (10 µg HBsAg)	IM	0, 4–6 mo	None
		≥20 (primary)	1.0 mL (10 µg HBsAg)	IM	0, 1, 6 mo	None
Combined hepatitis A and B vaccine	Twinrix (GlaxoSmithKline)	≥18 (primary)	1.0 mL (720 ELU HAV + 20 µg HBsAg)	IM	0, 1, 6 mo	None
		≥18 (accelerated)	same as above	IM	0, 7, 21–30 d	12 mo

Abbreviations: HBsAg, hepatitis B surface antigen; IM, intramuscular; ELU, ELISA units of inactivated HAV; HAV, hepatitis A virus.
[1]Consult the package insert for differences in dosing for hemodialysis and other immunocompromised patients.

BIBLIOGRAPHY

1. CDC. Recommended adult immunization schedule—United States, 2012. MMWR. 2012;61(4):1–7.
2. CDC. Updated US Public Health Service guidelines for the management of occupational exposures to HBV, HCV, and HIV and recommendations for postexposure prophylaxis. MMWR Recomm Rep. 2001 Jun 29;50 (RR-11):1–42.
3. Connor BA, Patron DJ. Use of an accelerated immunization schedule for combined hepatitis A and B protection in the corporate traveler. J Occup Environ Med. 2008 Aug;50(8):945–50.
4. Croughs M, Van Gompel A, de Boer E, Van Den Ende J. Sexual risk behavior of travelers who consulted a pretravel clinic. J Travel Med. 2008 Jan–Feb;15(1):6–12.
5. Keystone J. Hepatitis B immunization for all travelers. J Travel Med. 2009 Jul–Aug;16(4):297.
6. Lok AS, McMahon BJ. Chronic hepatitis B: update of recommendations. Hepatology. 2004 Mar;39(3):857–61.
7. Mast EE, Margolis HS, Fiore AE, Brink EW, Goldstein ST, Wang SA, et al. A comprehensive immunization strategy to eliminate transmission of hepatitis B virus infection in the United States: recommendations of the Advisory Committee on Immunization Practices (ACIP) part 1: immunization of infants, children, and adolescents. MMWR Recomm Rep. 2005 Dec 23;54 (RR-16):1–31.
8. Mast EE, Weinbaum CM, Fiore AE, Alter MJ, Bell BP, Finelli L, et al. A comprehensive immunization strategy to eliminate transmission of hepatitis B virus infection in the United States: recommendations of the Advisory Committee on Immunization Practices (ACIP) Part II: immunization of adults. MMWR Recomm Rep. 2006 Dec 8;55 (RR-16):1–33.
9. Ott JJ, Stevens GA, Groeger J, Wiersma ST. Global epidemiology of hepatitis B virus infection: new estimates of age-specific HBsAg seroprevalence and endemicity. Vaccine. 2012 Mar 9;30(12):2212–9.
10. Simonsen L, Kane A, Lloyd J, Zaffran M, Kane M. Unsafe injections in the developing world and transmission of bloodborne pathogens: a review. Bull World Health Organ. 1999;77(10):789–800.
11. Sonder GJ, van Rijckevorsel GG, van den Hoek A. Risk of hepatitis B for travelers: is vaccination for all travelers really necessary? J Travel Med. 2009 Jan–Feb;16(1):18–22.
12. Van Damme P, Ward J, Shouval D, Wiersma S, Zanetti A. Hepatitis B vaccines. In: Plotkin SA, Orenstein WA, Offit PA, editors. Vaccines. 6th ed. Philadelphia: Saunders Elsevier; 2012. p. 205–34.

HEPATITIS C

Deborah Holtzman

INFECTIOUS AGENT

Hepatitis C is caused by the hepatitis C virus (HCV), a spherical, enveloped, positive-strand RNA virus, approximately 50 nm in diameter.

TRANSMISSION

Transmission of HCV is bloodborne and occurs mainly through sharing drug-injection equipment, from transfusion of unscreened blood, or from untreated clotting factors. In developing countries, unsterile medicinal and other injection practices account for many HCV infections. Although infrequent, HCV can be transmitted through other procedures that involve blood exposure (such as tattooing) and during sexual contact.

EPIDEMIOLOGY

Approximately 2%–3% (130–170 million) of the world's population has been infected with HCV. In many developed countries, including the United States, the prevalence of HCV infection is <2%. The prevalence is higher (>2%) in several countries in Latin America, Eastern Europe, and the former Soviet Union, and certain countries in Africa, the Middle East, and South Asia; the prevalence is reported to be highest (>10%) in Egypt (Map 3-5). The most frequent mode of transmission in the United States is through sharing drug-injection equipment. Travelers' risk for contracting HCV infection is generally low, but travelers should exercise caution when traveling to countries where the prevalence of HCV infection is ≥2%, as the following activities can result in blood exposure:

- Receiving blood transfusions that have not been screened for HCV
- Having medical or dental procedures
- Activities such as acupuncture, tattooing, public shaving, or injection drug use in which equipment has not been adequately sterilized or disinfected, or in which contaminated equipment is reused
- Working in health care fields (medical, dental, or laboratory) that entail direct exposure to human blood

CLINICAL PRESENTATION

Most people (80%) with acute HCV infection have no symptoms. If symptoms do occur, they may include loss of appetite, abdominal pain, fatigue, nausea, dark urine, and jaundice. Of those who develop chronic HCV infection, the most common symptom is fatigue; severe liver disease develops in about 10%–20% of infected people. HCV is a major cause of cirrhosis and hepatocellular cancer and is the leading reason for liver transplantation in the United States.

DIAGNOSIS

Two major types of tests are available: IgG assays for anti-HCV antibodies and nucleic acid amplification testing to detect HCV RNA in blood (viremia). Assays for IgM, to detect early or acute infection, are not available. Approximately 75%–85% of people who seroconvert to anti-HCV, indicative of acute infection, will progress to chronic infection and persistently detectable viremia. False-negative antibody test results, while rare, may occur early in acute infection, usually in the first 15 weeks after exposure and infection.

TREATMENT

Treatment for hepatitis C is rapidly evolving. Currently, sustained virologic response (SVR), which is considered a cure, is achieved in 50% of patients taking the previous standard treatment of pegylated interferon and ribavirin for 24–48 weeks. In May 2011, 2 new protease inhibitors, telaprevir and boceprevir, were approved to treat hepatitis C in the United States. When these drugs were added to a regimen of pegylated interferon and ribavirin in clinical trials, SVR rates increased to 75% for those also receiving telaprevir and to 63% for those also receiving boceprevir among people with HCV genotype 1 (the most common genotype in the United States). Treatment is most effective for people diagnosed within the first year of infection. However, this is difficult as serologic markers of acute infection are lacking and most acute cases are only mildly symptomatic or asymptomatic.

PREVENTION

No vaccine is available to prevent HCV infection, nor does immune globulin provide protection. Before traveling, people should check with their health care providers to understand the potential risk of infection and any precautions they should take. When seeking medical or dental care, travelers should be alert to the use of medical, surgical, and dental equipment that has not been adequately sterilized or disinfected, reuse of contaminated equipment, and unsafe injection practices (such as reuse of disposable needles and syringes). HCV and other bloodborne pathogens can be transmitted if instruments are not sterile or the clinician does not follow other proper infection-control procedures (washing hands, using latex gloves, and cleaning and disinfecting surfaces and instruments). There are still a few areas of the world, such as parts of sub-Saharan Africa, where blood donors may not be screened for HCV. Travelers should be advised to consider the health risks if they are thinking about getting a tattoo or body piercing or having a medical procedure in areas where adequate sterilization or disinfection procedures might not be practiced. Travelers should be advised to seek testing for HCV upon return if they received blood transfusions or sustained other blood exposures for which they could not assess the risks.

CDC website: www.cdc.gov/hepatitis/HCV

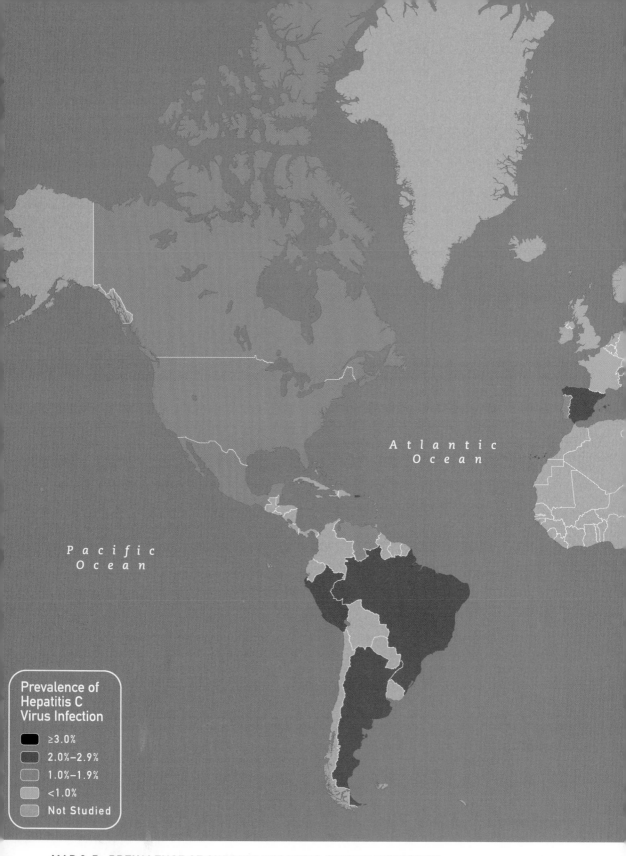

Prevalence of Hepatitis C Virus Infection

- ≥3.0%
- 2.0%–2.9%
- 1.0%–1.9%
- <1.0%
- Not Studied

Atlantic Ocean

Pacific Ocean

MAP 3-5. PREVALENCE OF CHRONIC HEPATITIS C VIRUS INFECTION[1]

[1] Negro F, Alberti A. The global health burden of hepatitis C virus infection. Liver Int. 2011 Jul;31(2 Suppl):1–3. Data used with permission from John Wiley and Sons.

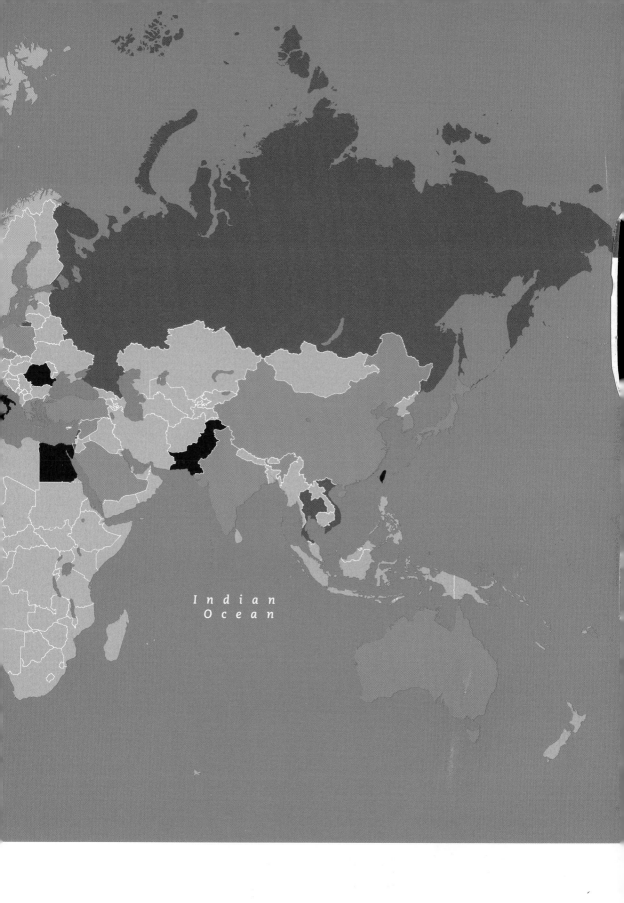

*Indian
Ocean*

BIBLIOGRAPHY

1. Alter MJ. Epidemiology of hepatitis C virus infection. World J Gastroenterol. 2007 May 7;13(17):2436–41.

2. Averhoff FM, Glass N, Holtzman D. Global burden of hepatitis C: considerations for healthcare providers in the United States. Clin Infect Dis. 2012 Jul;55 Suppl 1:S10–5.

3. Cornberg M, Razavi HA, Alberti A, Bernasconi E, Buti M, Cooper C, et al. A systematic review of hepatitis C virus epidemiology in Europe, Canada and Israel. Liver Int. 2011 Jul;31 Suppl 2:30–60.

4. Global Burden Of Hepatitis C Working Group. Global burden of disease (GBD) for hepatitis C. J Clin Pharmacol. 2004 Jan;44(1):20–9.

5. Jacobson IM, McHutchison JG, Dusheiko G, Di Bisceglie AM, Reddy KR, Bzowej NH, et al. Telaprevir for previously untreated chronic hepatitis C virus infection. N Engl J Med. 2011 Jun 23;364(25):2405–16.

6. Kershenobich D, Razavi HA, Sanchez-Avila JF, Bessone F, Coelho HS, Dagher L, et al. Trends and projections of hepatitis C virus epidemiology in Latin America. Liver Int. 2011 Jul;31 Suppl 2:18–29.

7. Madhava V, Burgess C, Drucker E. Epidemiology of chronic hepatitis C virus infection in sub-Saharan Africa. Lancet Infect Dis. 2002 May;2(5):293–302.

8. Poordad F, McCone J, Jr., Bacon BR, Bruno S, Manns MP, Sulkowski MS, et al. Boceprevir for untreated chronic HCV genotype 1 infection. N Engl J Med. 2011 Mar 31;364(13):1195–206.

9. Prati D. Transmission of hepatitis C virus by blood transfusions and other medical procedures: a global review. J Hepatol. 2006 Oct;45(4):607–16.

10. Shepard CW, Finelli L, Alter MJ. Global epidemiology of hepatitis C virus infection. Lancet Infect Dis. 2005 Sep;5(9):558–67.

11. Shimakami T, Lanford RE, Lemon SM. Hepatitis C: recent successes and continuing challenges in the development of improved treatment modalities. Curr Opin Pharmacol. 2009 Oct;9(5):537–44.

12. Sievert W, Altraif I, Razavi HA, Abdo A, Ahmed EA, Alomair A, et al. A systematic review of hepatitis C virus epidemiology in Asia, Australia and Egypt. Liver Int. 2011 Jul;31 Suppl 2:61–80.

13. Simonsen L, Kane A, Lloyd J, Zaffran M, Kane M. Unsafe injections in the developing world and transmission of bloodborne pathogens: a review. Bull World Health Organ. 1999;77(10):789–800.

HEPATITIS E
Chong-Gee Teo

INFECTIOUS AGENT
Infection is caused by hepatitis E virus (HEV), a single-stranded, RNA virus belonging to the *Hepeviridae* family.

TRANSMISSION
HEV is transmitted primarily by the fecal-oral route. In regions with poor sanitation and limited access to safe drinking water, epidemics and interepidemic occurrences of hepatitis E are largely waterborne. Transmission to fetuses and neonates by women infected during pregnancy is common. In Japan, sporadic disease can be zoonotic and foodborne, associated with eating meat and offal (including liver) of deer, boars, and pigs. In France, disease can be acquired from eating *figatellu*, a sausage delicacy prepared from raw pig liver. Sporadic disease is also observed in other temperate countries, including the United States, but its cause is generally unknown. Shellfish can transmit HEV. Disease from blood transfusion has been reported, although rare.

EPIDEMIOLOGY
Waterborne outbreaks (often large, involving hundreds to thousands of people) have occurred in South and Central Asia, tropical East Asia, Africa, and Central America (Map 3-6). Clinical attack rates are highest in young adults aged 15–49 years. In outbreak-prone areas, interepidemic disease is sporadically encountered. In these areas, pregnant women—whether infected sporadically or during an epidemic—are at risk of progressing to liver failure and death after infection. Miscarriages and neonatal deaths also commonly occur as a result of HEV infection.

Sporadic disease also occurs in regions that are not prone to outbreaks, such as the Middle East, temperate East Asia (including China), North and South America, and Europe. Symptomatic disease is observed most frequently in adults aged >50 years. Primary infection acquired by people who are immunosuppressed, particularly solid-organ transplant recipients, may progress to chronic infection.

People living in the United States are at risk of HEV infection when they travel to areas where epidemics have occurred. When traveling in Japan and Europe, eating raw or inadequately cooked venison, boar meat, pig liver, or food products derived from these, is a risk factor for infection.

CLINICAL PRESENTATION
The incubation period is 2–9 weeks (mean 6 weeks). Signs and symptoms of disease during primary infection include jaundice, fever, loss of appetite, abdominal pain, and lethargy. Acute hepatitis E is frequently self-limited. Pregnant women (particularly those infected during the second or third trimester) may present with or progress to liver failure, and the fetus is at risk for spontaneous abortion and premature delivery. People with preexisting chronic liver disease may undergo further hepatic decompensation when infected with HEV. Recipients of organ transplants may have no symptoms when infected by HEV but can occasionally develop neurologic deficits.

DIAGNOSIS
The diagnosis of acute hepatitis E is established by detecting anti-HEV IgM and IgG in serum. Detecting HEV RNA in serum or stools further confirms the serologic diagnosis but is seldom required. Longer-term, serial detection of HEV RNA in serum or stools, regardless of the HEV antibody serostatus, suggests chronic HEV infection. No diagnostic test has been approved by the Food and Drug Administration for use in the United States.

TREATMENT
Treatment is supportive.

PREVENTION
No vaccine is available, nor are drugs for preventing infection. Travelers should avoid

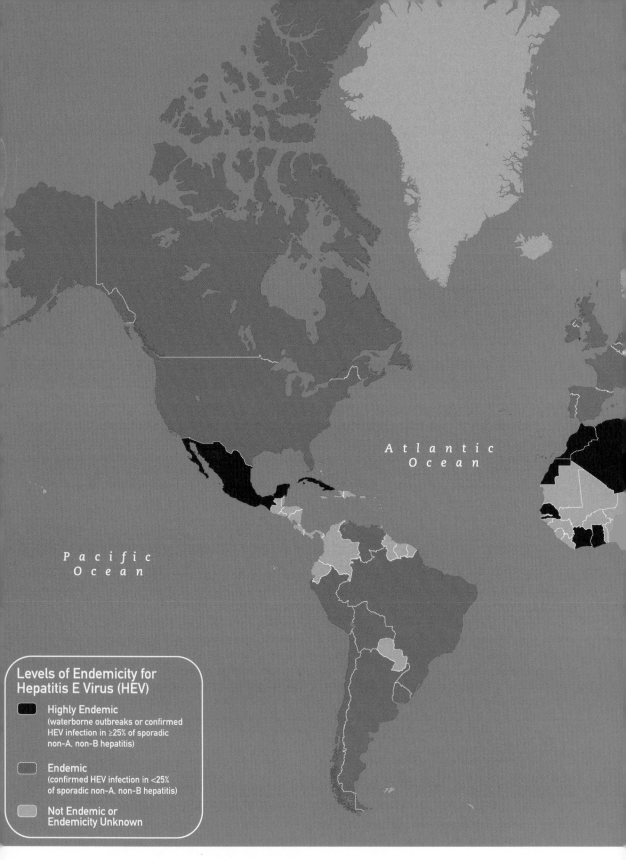

Levels of Endemicity for
Hepatitis E Virus (HEV)

Highly Endemic
(waterborne outbreaks or confirmed
HEV infection in ≥25% of sporadic
non-A, non-B hepatitis)

Endemic
(confirmed HEV infection in <25%
of sporadic non-A, non-B hepatitis)

**Not Endemic or
Endemicity Unknown**

MAP 3-6. DISTRIBUTION OF HEPATITIS E VIRUS INFECTION, 2012

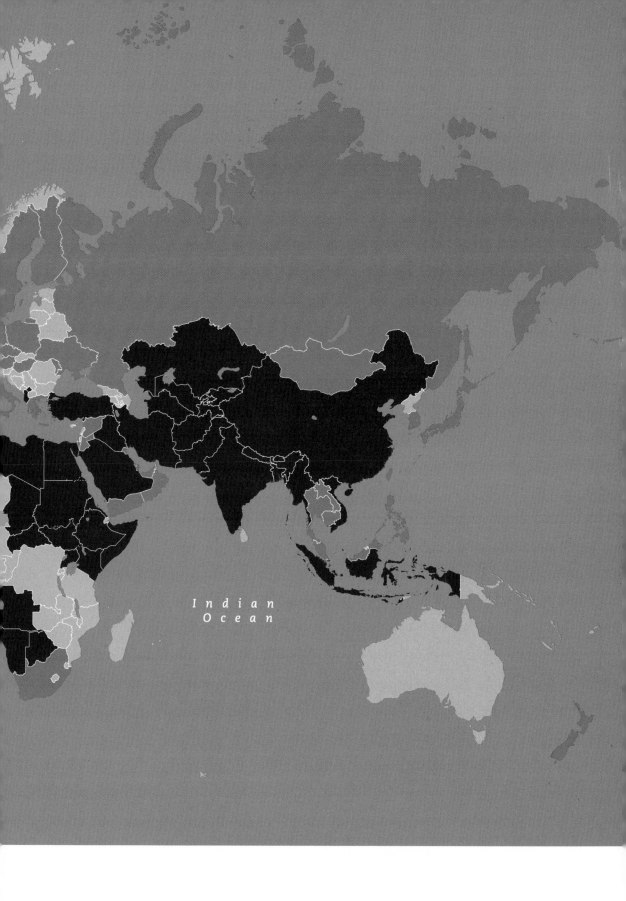

Indian Ocean

drinking unboiled or unchlorinated water and beverages that contain unboiled water or ice. Travelers should eat only thoroughly cooked food, including seafood, meat, offal,

and products derived from these (see Chapter 2, Food & Water Precautions).

CDC website: www.cdc.gov/hepatitis/HEV

BIBLIOGRAPHY

1. Aggarwal R, Jameel S. Hepatitis E. Hepatology. 2011 Dec;54(6):2218–26.
2. Nelson KE, Kmush B, Labrique AB. The epidemiology of hepatitis E virus infections in developed countries and among immunocompromised patients. Expert Rev Anti Infect Ther. 2011 Dec;9(12):1133–48.

HISTOPLASMOSIS
Tom M. Chiller

INFECTIOUS AGENT
Histoplasma capsulatum, a dimorphic fungus that grows as a mold in soil and as a yeast in animal and human hosts.

TRANSMISSION
Through inhalation of spores (conidia) from soil that may be contaminated with bat guano or bird droppings; not transmitted directly from person to person.

EPIDEMIOLOGY
Distributed worldwide, except in Antarctica, but most often associated with river valleys. Activities such as spelunking, mining, construction, excavation, demolition, roofing, chimney cleaning, farming, gardening, and installing heating and air-conditioning systems are associated with histoplasmosis. Activities that expose people to areas where bats live and birds roost also increase risk. Outbreaks have been reported associated with travel to many countries in Central and South America, most often associated with visiting caves.

CLINICAL PRESENTATION
Incubation period is typically 3–17 days for acute disease. Ninety percent of infections are asymptomatic or result in a mild influenzalike illness. Some infections may cause acute pulmonary histoplasmosis, manifested by high fever, headache, nonproductive cough, chills, weakness, pleuritic chest pain, and fatigue. Most people spontaneously recover 2–3 weeks after onset of symptoms, although fatigue may persist longer. Dissemination, especially to the gastrointestinal tract and central nervous system, can occur in people who are immunocompromised.

DIAGNOSIS
Culture of *H. capsulatum* from bone marrow, blood, sputum, and tissue specimens is the definitive method. Demonstration of the typical intracellular yeast forms by microscopic examination strongly supports the diagnosis of histoplasmosis when clinical, epidemiologic, and other laboratory studies are compatible. EIA on urine, serum, plasma, bronchoalveolar lavage, or cerebrospinal fluid is a rapid diagnostic test commercially available in the United States.

TREATMENT
Treatment is not usually indicated for healthy, immunocompetent people with acute, localized pulmonary infection. People with more extensive disease or persistent symptoms beyond 1 month are generally treated with an azole drug, such as itraconazole, for mild to moderate illness or amphotericin B for severe infection.

PREVENTION
People at increased risk for severe disease should avoid high-risk areas, such as bat-inhabited caves.

CDC website: www.cdc.gov/fungal/histoplasmosis

BIBLIOGRAPHY

1. CDC. Outbreak of histoplasmosis among travelers returning from El Salvador—Pennsylvania and Virginia, 2008. MMWR Morb Mortal Wkly Rep. 2008 Dec 19;57(50):1349–53.
2. Kauffman CA. Histoplasmosis. Clin Chest Med. 2009 Jun;30(2):217–25.
3. Kauffman CA. Histoplasmosis: a clinical and laboratory update. Clin Microbiol Rev. 2007 Jan;20(1):115–32.
4. Morgan J, Cano MV, Feikin DR, et al. A large outbreak of histoplasmosis among American travelers associated with a hotel in Acapulco, Mexico, spring 2001. Am J Trop Med Hyg. 2003;69:663–9.
5. Weinberg M, Weeks J, Lance-Parker S, Traeger M, Wiersma S, Phan QN, et al. Severe histoplasmosis in travelers to Nicaragua. Emerg Infect Dis. 2003 Oct;9(10):1322–5.
6. Wheat LJ. Histoplasmosis: a review for clinicians from non-endemic areas. Mycoses. 2006 Jul;49(4):274–82.

HIV INFECTION

John T. Brooks

INFECTIOUS AGENT

HIV, a single-stranded, positive-sense, enveloped RNA virus in the genus *Lentivirus*.

TRANSMISSION

HIV can be transmitted through sexual contact, needle- or syringe-sharing, medical use of blood or blood components, organ or tissue transplantation, and artificial insemination. It can also be transmitted from mother to child during pregnancy, at birth, and postpartum through breastfeeding. HIV may be transmitted occupationally to health care workers who are exposed to blood and other potentially infectious bodily fluids via percutaneous injury or splash exposures to mucous membranes or nonintact skin (see Chapter 2, Occupational Exposure to HIV). HIV is not transmitted through casual person-to-person contact; air, food, or water; contact with inanimate objects; or by mosquitoes or other arthropod vectors. The use of any public conveyance (such as airplanes, automobiles, boats, buses, or trains) by people with HIV infection does not pose a risk of HIV infection for the crew members or other travelers.

EPIDEMIOLOGY

HIV infection occurs worldwide. As of the end of 2010, an estimated 34 million people were living with HIV infection. Although sub-Saharan Africa remains the most affected part of the world (24.8 million cases or 68% of all people living with HIV infection), notable increases in HIV infection have occurred in Eastern Europe and Central Asia, where the number of people living with HIV infection from 2001 to 2010 rose 250% (Map 3-7). Most new infections come from low- and middle-income countries. Many countries lack comprehensive surveillance systems and, despite improvements, the true number of cases may be higher than officially reported, particularly in developing countries.

The risk of HIV infection for international travelers is generally low, although the risk is determined less by geographic destination and more by behaviors such as drug use and unprotected sex. Travelers who might undergo medical procedures, whether scheduled or in an emergency, should be aware that in developing countries the blood supply (and organs and tissues used for transplantation) might not be adequately screened, increasing the risk of HIV transmission.

DIAGNOSIS

Any person who suspects that she or he may have been exposed to HIV should be tested. Most people develop detectable antibodies within 2–8 weeks (mean, 25 days). Ninety-seven percent of people develop antibodies in the first 3 months after infection. In rare cases, it can take up to 6 months to develop antibodies to HIV. After infection, a person remains antibody positive for life, except when people lose the capacity to mount detectable antibodies in the latest stages of the disease. The earliest time after exposure that HIV infection can

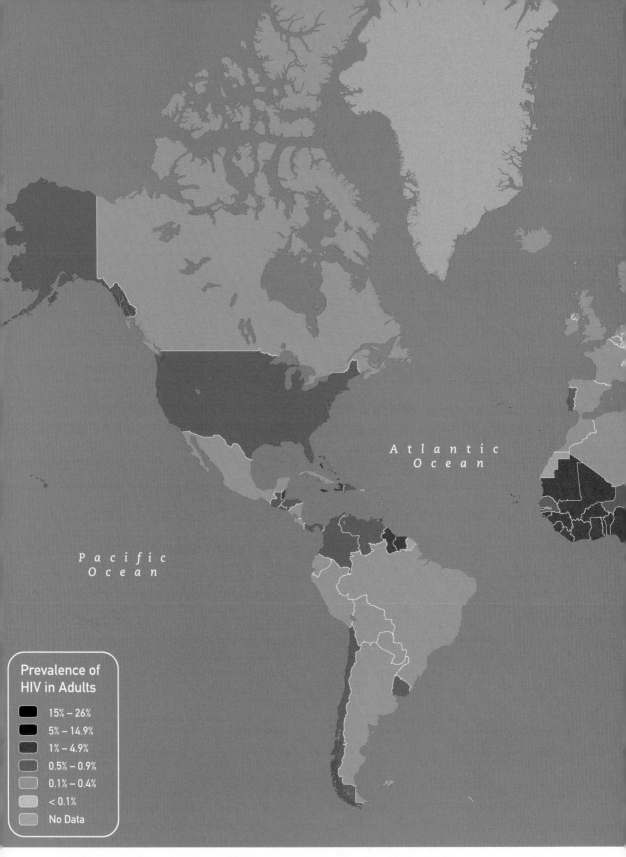

Prevalence of HIV in Adults

- 15% – 26%
- 5% – 14.9%
- 1% – 4.9%
- 0.5% – 0.9%
- 0.1% – 0.4%
- < 0.1%
- No Data

Atlantic Ocean

Pacific Ocean

MAP 3-7. HIV PREVALENCE IN ADULTS, 2011[1]

[1] From: UNAIDS/ONUSIDA 2012. AIDSinfo database. Available from: www.unaids.org/en/dataanalysis/datatools/aidsinfo. Data used by kind permission of Joint United Nations Programme on HIV/AIDS (UNAIDS).

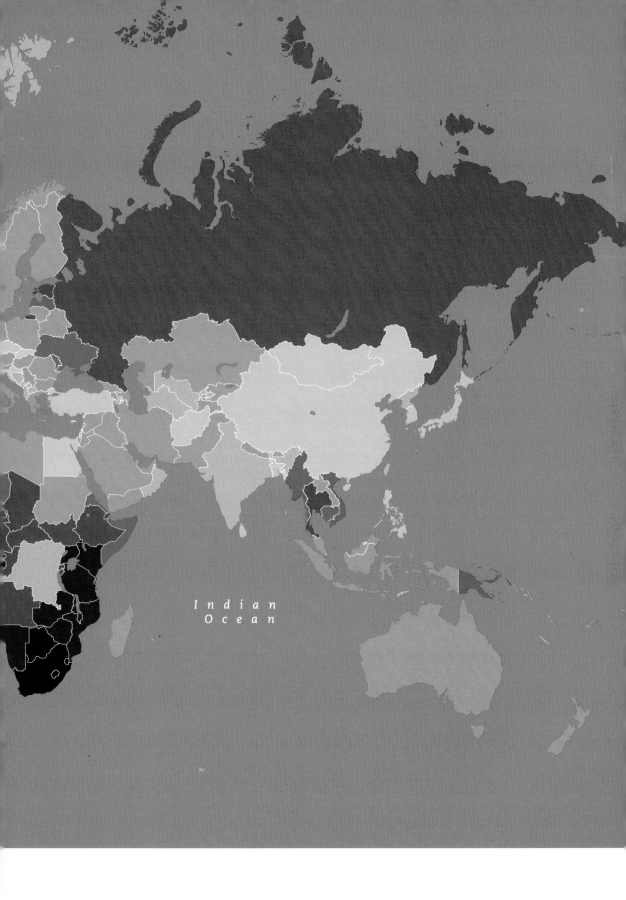

*Indian
Ocean*

be diagnosed is about 9 days, when HIV RNA becomes detectable in blood; however, the tests needed to measure HIV RNA are costly and may not be available. Any person not known to be HIV-infected who is diagnosed with an AIDS-compatible illness, such as *Pneumocystis* pneumonia, should be tested for HIV. For further information on HIV testing, travelers should talk to their health care provider or identify an HIV testing site near them by visiting the National HIV Testing Resources website at www.hivtest.org or call CDC-INFO toll-free at 800-CDC-INFO (800-232-4636) or 888-232-6348 (TTY). Both these resources are confidential.

TREATMENT

Prompt medical care and effective treatment with antiretrovirals can inhibit HIV from damaging the immune system and delay progression of disease. US guidelines recommend all people with HIV infection be treated for their own health and to prevent transmission to others. Detailed information on specific treatments is available from the Department of Health and Human Services AIDSinfo (www.aidsinfo.nih.gov). Information on enrolling in clinical trials is also available at AIDSinfo. Travelers may contact AIDSinfo toll-free at 800-448-0440 (English or Spanish) or 888-480-3739 (TTY).

PREVENTION

No vaccine is available to prevent infection with HIV. Travelers should be advised that they are at risk if they:

- Have sexual contact (heterosexual or homosexual) with an infected person.
- Use or allow the use of contaminated, unsterilized syringes or needles for any injections or other procedures that pierce the skin, including acupuncture, use of illicit drugs, steroid or vitamin injections, medical or dental procedures, ear or body piercing, or tattooing.
- Receive infected blood, blood components, or clotting factor concentrates. HIV infection by this route is rare in countries or cities where donated blood and plasma are screened for antibodies to HIV.
- Work in a health care setting. Typically, exposures occur as a result of percutaneous exposure to contaminated sharps, including needles, lancets, scalpels, and broken glass (from capillary or test tubes). See Chapter 2, Occupational Exposure to HIV.

To reduce their risk of acquiring HIV, travelers should:

- Avoid sexual encounters with people who are infected with HIV, whose HIV infection status is unknown, or who are at high risk for HIV infection, such as intravenous drug users, commercial sex workers (both male and female), and other people with multiple sexual partners.
- Use condoms consistently and correctly, especially if engaging in vaginal, anal, or oral-genital sexual contact with a person who is HIV-infected or whose HIV status is unknown.
- Avoid injecting drugs.
- Avoid sharing needles or other devices that can puncture skin.
- Avoid, if at all possible, blood transfusions or use of clotting factor concentrates.
- Ensure that if traveling for purposes of medical treatment ("medical tourism"), the blood and blood products used in the facility where the traveler will be treated are screened for HIV and that such facilities exercise proper infection control practices.
- Consider, particularly if at high risk for acquiring HIV infection (such as men who have sex with men) discussing preexposure prophylaxis with a health care provider (see www.cdc.gov/hiv/prep).

Condoms

People who are sensitive to latex should use condoms made of polyurethane or other synthetic materials and should carry their own supply of male or female condoms. If no condom is available, travelers should abstain from sex with people who are HIV-infected or whose HIV status is unknown. Barrier methods other than condoms do not prevent HIV transmission. Spermicides alone are also not effective. The widely used spermicide nonoxynol-9 can increase the risk of HIV transmission and should not be used.

Needles

Needles used to draw blood or administer injections should be sterile, single use, disposable, and prepackaged in a sealed container. If at all possible, travelers should avoid receiving medications from multidose vials, which may have become contaminated by used needles. Travelers with type 1 diabetes, hemophilia, or other conditions that necessitate routine or frequent injections should be advised to carry a supply of medication, syringes, needles, and disinfectant swabs sufficient to last their entire stay abroad. These travelers should request documentation of the medical necessity for traveling with these items (a doctor's letter) to avoid having them confiscated, such as by inspection personnel at ports of entry (see Chapter 2, Travel Health Kits, for more information about traveling with medications).

Transfusions

In many developed countries, the risk of HIV infection through transfusion of blood or blood products has been virtually eliminated through required testing of all donated blood. Developing countries may have no formal program or may have inadequate technology for testing blood or biological products for contamination with HIV. If transfusion is necessary, the blood should be tested for HIV antibodies by trained laboratory technicians using a reliable test.

Postexposure Prophylaxis

Travelers who will be working in a medical setting (such as a nurse volunteer drawing blood or medical missionary performing surgeries) may have contact with HIV-infected or potentially infected biological materials. These travelers should ensure that they will have access to all personal protective equipment necessary (latex gloves, goggles, face shield, gowns) and that this equipment meets established international quality standards. Such travelers should also become familiar with the principles of postexposure prophylaxis (note: this

treatment must be initiated within 72 hours after exposure), establish a plan for seeking medical consultation, and bring a supply of antiretroviral medication sufficient to provide postexposure prophylaxis until medical care can be obtained. For more information, see Chapter 2, Occupational Exposure to HIV.

People who have been exposed to HIV in a nonoccupational setting should seek immediate medical consultation to consider postexposure prophylaxis. Postexposure prophylaxis for potential exposure to HIV as a result of mass-casualty events is generally not warranted, except in special circumstances (for example, a blast injury in a facility that contained a large archive of HIV-infected blood specimens). Clinicians seeking advice on postexposure prophylaxis can call the US National HIV/AIDS Clinicians' Consultation Center PEPline toll-free at 888-448-4911 (www. nccc.ucsf.edu).

HIV TESTING REQUIREMENTS FOR US TRAVELERS ENTERING FOREIGN COUNTRIES

International travelers should be advised that some countries screen incoming travelers for HIV infection and may deny entry to people with AIDS or evidence of HIV infection. These countries usually screen only people planning extended visits, such as for work or study. People intending to visit a country for an extended stay should review that country's policies and requirements. This information is usually available from the consular officials of the individual nations. Information about entry and exit requirements compiled by the Department of State can be found at http://travel.state.gov/travel/tips/tips_1232. html#requirement.

CDC website: www.cdc.gov/hiv

BIBLIOGRAPHY

1. Chapman LE, Sullivent EE, Grohskopf LA, Beltrami EM, Perz JF, Kretsinger K, et al. Recommendations for postexposure interventions to prevent infection with hepatitis B virus, hepatitis C virus, or human immunodeficiency virus, and tetanus in persons wounded during bombings and other mass-casualty events—United States, 2008: recommendations of the Centers for Disease Control and Prevention (CDC). MMWR Recomm Rep. 2008 Aug 1;57(RR-6):1–21.

2. Joint United Nations Programme on HIV/AIDS (UNAIDS). UNAIDS World AIDS Day report, 2012. Geneva: Joint United Nations Programme on HIV/AIDS (UNAIDS); 2012 [cited 2012 Dec 20]. Available from: http://www.unaids.org/en/resources/campaigns/20121120_globalreport2012/.

3. Panlilio AL, Cardo DM, Grohskopf LA, Heneine W, Ross CS. Updated US Public Health Service guidelines for the management of occupational exposures

to HIV and recommendations for postexposure prophylaxis. MMWR Recomm Rep. 2005 Sep 30;54(RR-9):1–17.

4. Rice B, Gilbart VL, Lawrence J, Smith R, Kall M, Delpech V. Safe travels? HIV transmission among Britons travelling abroad. HIV Med. 2012 May;13(5):315–7.

5. Smith DK, Grohskopf LA, Black RJ, Auerbach JD, Veronese F, Struble KA, et al. Antiretroviral postexposure prophylaxis after sexual, injection-drug use, or other nonoccupational exposure to HIV in the United States: recommendations from the US Department of Health and Human Services. MMWR Recomm Rep. 2005 Jan 21;54(RR-2):1–20.

HUMAN PAPILLOMAVIRUS

Eileen F. Dunne, Lauri Markowitz

INFECTIOUS AGENT

Human papillomavirus (HPV) is a small DNA virus.

TRANSMISSION

Primarily by sexual contact, most commonly intercourse.

EPIDEMIOLOGY

Common worldwide; no unique or inherent risks for travelers.

CLINICAL PRESENTATION

Usually subclinical and asymptomatic; persistent infection can lead to cervical cancer.

DIAGNOSIS

Usually diagnosed when genital warts are seen or by results of a Papanicolaou test, HPV test, or colposcopy. Definitive diagnosis is made by biopsy.

TREATMENT

There is no treatment for HPV; the goal of therapy is to reduce or eliminate clinical manifestations.

PREVENTION

Two vaccines, a quadrivalent HPV vaccine (HPV4) and a bivalent HPV vaccine (HPV2), are licensed and recommended for use in adolescents and young adults.

CDC website: www.cdc.gov/hpv

BIBLIOGRAPHY

1. CDC. FDA licensure of bivalent human papillomavirus vaccine (HPV2, Cervarix) for use in females and updated HPV vaccination recommendations from the Advisory Committee on Immunization Practices (ACIP). MMWR Morb Mortal Wkly Rep. 2010 May 28;59(20):626–9.

2. CDC. Recommendations on the use of quadrivalent human papillomavirus vaccine in males—Advisory Committee on Immunization Practices (ACIP), 2011. MMWR Morb Mortal Wkly Rep. 2011 Dec 23;60(50):1705–8.

3. Markowitz LE, Dunne EF, Saraiya M, Lawson HW, Chesson H, Unger ER. Quadrivalent human papillomavirus vaccine: recommendations of the Advisory Committee on Immunization Practices (ACIP). MMWR Recomm Rep. 2007 Mar 23;56(RR-2):1–24.

INFLUENZA

Adena Greenbaum, Joseph Bresee

INFECTIOUS AGENT

Influenza is caused by infection of the respiratory tract with influenza viruses, which are classified into 3 types: A, B, and C. Only virus types A and B, however, commonly cause illness in humans. Influenza A(H1N1), A(H3N2), and influenza B viruses currently circulate globally among humans. In the spring of 2009, a new influenza A(H1N1) virus with a combination of genes not previously detected was identified. This virus, now called influenza A(H1N1)pdm09, resulted in an influenza pandemic in 2009–2010. Travelers aided the rapid global spread of this virus, which continues to circulate worldwide and behave as a seasonal human influenza A virus. The predominant types and subtypes in circulation can vary from year to year and can differ between geographic areas and time of year. Information on current circulating virus strains in various regions can be found via CDC (www.cdc.gov/flu/weekly/fluactivitysurv. htm) or the World Health Organization (www. who.int/influenza).

TRANSMISSION

Influenza viruses spread from person to person, primarily through large-particle respiratory droplet transmission (such as when an infected person coughs or sneezes near a susceptible person). Transmission via large-particle droplets requires close contact between the source and the recipient, because droplets generally travel only short distances (approximately 6 feet or less) through the air, before settling onto surfaces. Airborne transmission via small-particle aerosols in the vicinity of the infectious person may also occur. Indirect transmission through hand transfer of influenza virus from virus-contaminated surfaces to mucosal surfaces of the face (such as the nose or mouth) may also occur. However, the relative contribution of the different modes of transmission to the spread of influenza viruses is unclear.

Most healthy adults who are ill with influenza shed the virus in the upper respiratory tract and are infectious from the day before symptom onset to approximately 5–7 days after symptom onset. Generally, people are most contagious in the 3 days after illness onset. Children and those who are immunocompromised or severely ill, including those who are hospitalized, may shed influenza virus for 10 days or more after the onset of symptoms. Seasonal influenza viruses have rarely been detected from nonrespiratory sources such as diarrheal stool or blood.

EPIDEMIOLOGY

Seasonal Influenza

Influenza season varies geographically and by climate. In temperate climates, influenza activity generally occurs during the winter months. The influenza season in the Northern Hemisphere may begin as early as October and can extend until May. The influenza season in the Southern Hemisphere may begin in April and last through September. In tropical and subtropical areas, influenza may occur throughout the year, but most countries will have defined seasonal peaks.

Influenza virus infections can cause disease in all age groups. Infection rates are highest in children, and rates of severe illness and death are highest among people aged ≥65, children <2 years, and people of any age who have underlying medical conditions that place them at increased risk for complications of influenza. Children aged <2 years have rates of influenza-related hospitalizations that are as high as those in the elderly, although with much lower death rates. CDC estimates that from 1976 through 2006, annual influenza-associated deaths in the United States ranged from a low of approximately 3,000 people to a high of approximately 49,000 people; about 90% of these deaths occurred among people aged ≥65 years.

Zoonotic Influenza

While influenza B viruses circulate among humans, influenza A viruses circulate among many animal populations. The primary reservoir for influenza A viruses is wild birds, especially waterfowl. Influenza A viruses found in birds are typically referred to as avian influenza viruses. Swine influenza A viruses circulate widely among pigs worldwide. Influenza A viruses can also be found in other animal species such as domestic poultry, cats, dogs, horses, and bats.

Human infections with animal-origin influenza A viruses are uncommon, but they do occur. From 2005 through early 2012, 36 human influenza illnesses caused by swine-origin influenza A virus were reported in the United States (called "variant" influenza virus infections). A large increase in cases of an influenza A(H3N2) variant virus that contains the M gene from the influenza A(H1N1)pdm09 virus was identified starting in July 2012. As of September 2012, over 300 confirmed cases have been identified in the United States. Most occurred after direct or indirect contact with an infected animal, and though limited person-to-person transmission has occurred, no sustained community spread of H3N2v has been detected as of September 2012. The severity of illness has been similar to that seen with seasonal influenza.

Although avian influenza A viruses do not commonly infect humans, sporadic cases of human infection with these viruses have been reported. From 2003 through mid-2012, >600 human cases of illness from infection with highly pathogenic avian influenza (HPAI) virus (H5N1) have been reported globally, with approximately 60% mortality. Most human infections with HPAI H5N1 virus have occurred after direct or close contact with sick or dead infected poultry. HPAI H5N1 virus is widespread among poultry in some countries in Asia and the Middle East and is considered to be endemic among poultry in 6 countries: Bangladesh, China, Egypt, India (West Bengal), Indonesia, and Vietnam. From 2003 through mid-2012, 87% of all recognized human cases have occurred in these countries. Rare instances of limited, nonsustained human-to-human transmission of HPAI H5N1 virus have been reported. Human infections with other avian influenza A viruses, although rare, have been reported, including H7N2, H7N3, H7N7, and H9N2 viruses.

CLINICAL PRESENTATION

Uncomplicated influenza illness is characterized by the abrupt onset of signs and symptoms that include fever, muscle aches, headache, malaise, nonproductive cough, sore throat, vomiting, and rhinitis. Illness without fever can occur, especially in elderly people. Children are more likely than adults to also experience nausea, vomiting, or diarrhea when ill with influenza. Physical findings are predominantly localized to the respiratory tract and include nasal discharge, pharyngeal inflammation without exudates, and occasionally rales on chest auscultation. The incubation period is usually 1–4 days after exposure. Influenza illness typically resolves within 1 week for most previously healthy children and adults who do not receive antiviral medication, although cough and malaise can persist for >2 weeks, especially in the elderly. Complications of influenza virus infection include primary influenza viral pneumonia, secondary bacterial pneumonia, exacerbation of underlying medical conditions (such as pulmonary and cardiac disease), encephalopathy, myocarditis, myositis, or coinfections with other viral or bacterial pathogens.

DIAGNOSIS

Influenza can be difficult to distinguish from respiratory illnesses caused by other pathogens on the basis of signs and symptoms alone. The positive predictive value of clinical signs and symptoms for influenzalike illness for laboratory-confirmed influenza virus infection is 30%–88%, depending on the level of influenza activity.

Diagnostic tests available for influenza include viral culture, rapid diagnostic tests, immunofluorescence assays, and RT-PCR. Most patients with clinical illness consistent with uncomplicated influenza in an area where influenza viruses are circulating do not require diagnostic influenza testing for clinical management. For individual patients, tests are most useful when they are likely to help with diagnosis and treatment decisions. Patients who should be considered for influenza diagnostic testing include:

- Hospitalized patients with suspected influenza
- Patients for whom a diagnosis of influenza will inform decisions regarding

clinical care, especially those with high-risk conditions

- Patients for whom results of influenza testing would affect infection control or management of close contacts, including other patients, such as in institutional outbreaks or other settings (cruise ships or tour groups, for example)

The sensitivity of rapid influenza diagnostic tests is substantially lower than for RT-PCR or viral culture. Therefore, a negative rapid test result does not rule out influenza virus infection, and clinicians should not rely on a negative rapid test to make decisions about treatment.

TREATMENT

Early antiviral treatment can shorten the duration of fever and other symptoms and reduce the risk of complications from influenza. Antiviral treatment is recommended as early as possible for any patient with confirmed or suspected influenza who is hospitalized; has severe, complicated, or progressive illness; or is at a higher risk for influenza complications (see www.cdc.gov/flu/professionals/antivirals/summary-clinicians.htm). Antiviral treatment can also be considered for any previously healthy patient not at high risk of complications, with confirmed or suspected influenza, if treatment can be initiated within 48 hours of illness onset.

Although antiviral therapy is ideally initiated within the first 48 hours of illness, for hospitalized patients, those with severe illness, or those at higher risk of complications, antiviral therapy may still be beneficial if started >48 hours after illness onset. Two neuraminidase inhibitors are available for antiviral treatment and chemoprophylaxis of influenza: oral oseltamivir (Tamiflu) and inhaled zanamivir (Relenza). Both are active against influenza A and B viruses. Oseltamivir is approved for treatment and chemoprophylaxis of patients aged ≥1 year. Zanamivir is approved for treatment in those aged ≥7 years and for chemoprophylaxis in those aged ≥5 years (Table 3-5). Two other medications, amantadine and rimantadine, which belong to the adamantane class of antivirals, are active only against influenza A but not influenza B viruses and are not recommended for treatment or chemoprophylaxis because of widespread viral resistance among circulating influenza A viruses. People at increased risk for complications of influenza should discuss antiviral treatment and chemoprophylaxis with their health care provider before travel, if traveling to areas where influenza activity is occurring.

The effectiveness of antivirals for treating HPAI H5N1 virus infections has not been fully studied, although limited observational evidence suggests that early treatment has been associated with lower risk of death. CDC recommends treatment with oseltamivir for human infection with avian or swine influenza A viruses.

PREVENTION
Vaccine
Indications for Use
Annual influenza vaccination for those aged ≥6 months is the most effective way to prevent influenza and its complications.

Two types of influenza vaccines are available for use in the United States: trivalent inactivated vaccine (TIV) and trivalent live attenuated influenza vaccine (LAIV). TIV can be administered by intramuscular or intradermal injection and is available for people ≥6 months of age. Specific age indications vary by manufacturer and product; label instructions should be followed. For adults aged ≥65 years, a high-dose TIV is also available, containing higher levels of antigen. LAIV, administered by nasal spray, is approved for use only in healthy people aged 2–49 years who are not pregnant. Within indicated groups for each vaccine, there is no preference for TIV, high-dose TIV, or LAIV. In February 2012, the Food and Drug Administration approved the first quadrivalent LAIV (approved for ages 2–49 years), which is administered by nasal spray.

In the United States, annual influenza vaccination is recommended by the Advisory Committee on Immunization Practices for all US residents aged ≥6 months who do not have contraindications. Vaccination of pregnant women and household contacts of children aged <6 months can reduce the risk of influenza in children who are too young to receive influenza vaccine. Travelers, especially those who are part of large tourist groups, may be exposed to influenza at any time of year through exposure to others from areas of the world where influenza viruses are circulating.

Table 3-5. Recommended dosage and schedule of influenza antiviral medications[1] for treatment[2] and chemoprophylaxis[3]

Antiviral Agent		AGE GROUP (Y)			
		1–6	7–9	10–12	≥13
Zanamivir	Treatment, influenza A and B	NA	10 mg[4] bid	10 mg[4] bid	10 mg[4] bid
	Chemoprophylaxis, influenza A and B	NA for ages 1–4; ages 5–6, 10 mg[4] qd	10 mg[4] qd	10 mg[4] qd	10 mg[4] qd
Oseltamivir[5]	Treatment,[6] influenza A and B	Dose varies by child's weight[6]	Dose varies by child's weight[6]	Dose varies by child's weight;[6] >40 kg, give adult dose	75 mg bid
	Chemoprophylaxis,[7] influenza A and B	Dose varies by child's weight[7]	Dose varies by child's weight[7]	Dose varies by child's weight;[7] >40 kg, give adult dose	75 mg qd

Abbreviations: NA, not approved.

[1] Zanamivir is approved to treat people aged ≥7 years and approved for chemoprophylaxis of people aged ≥5 years. Zanamivir is not recommended for people with underlying airway disease. Oseltamivir is approved for treatment or chemoprophylaxis of people aged ≥1 year. No antiviral medications are approved for treatment or chemoprophylaxis of influenza among children aged <1 year. This information is based on data published by the Food and Drug Administration, available at www.fda.gov/Drugs/DrugSafety/InformationbyDrugClass/ucm100228.htm.

[2] Recommended duration for antiviral treatment is 5 days. Longer treatment courses can be considered for patients who remain severely ill after 5 days of treatment.

[3] Recommended duration for prophylaxis is 10 days when administered after a household exposure and 7 days after the most recent known exposure in other situations. For control of outbreaks in long-term care facilities and hospitals, CDC recommends antiviral chemoprophylaxis for a minimum of 2 weeks and up to 1 week after the most recent known case was identified.

[4] 10 mg Zanamivir is 2 inhalations.

[5] See Antiviral Agents for the Treatment and Chemoprophylaxis of Influenza, Recommendations of the Advisory Committee on Immunization Practices (ACIP) for information about use of oseltamivir for infants aged <1 year. A reduction in the dose of oseltamivir is recommended for people with creatinine clearance <30 mL/min.

[6] The treatment dosing recommendation for oseltamivir for children aged ≥1 year who weigh ≤15 kg is 30 mg bid. For children who weigh >15 kg but ≤23 kg, the dose is 45 mg bid. For children who weigh >23 kg but ≤40 kg, the dose is 60 mg bid. For children who weigh >40 kg, the dose is 75 mg bid.

[7] The chemoprophylaxis dosing recommendation for oseltamivir for children aged ≥1 year who weigh ≤15 kg is 30 mg qd. For children who weigh >15 kg but ≤23 kg, the dose is 45 mg qd. For children who weigh >23 kg but ≤40 kg, the dose is 60 mg qd. For children who weigh >40 kg, the dose is 75 mg qd.

To maximize the protective benefit, travelers being vaccinated against influenza should receive their vaccine ≥2 weeks before departure if vaccine is available. In order to optimize the immune response, children aged 6 months through 8 years being vaccinated for the first time are recommended to receive 2 doses of influenza vaccine administered a minimum of 4 weeks apart.

Vaccine Safety and Adverse Reactions
TIV

The most frequent side effects of vaccination with intramuscular and intradermal TIV in adults are soreness and redness at the vaccination site. These local reactions are slightly more common with intradermal vaccine and high-dose TIV. They generally are mild and rarely interfere with the ability to conduct usual activities. Fever, malaise, myalgia, and other systemic symptoms sometimes occur after vaccination; these may be more frequent in those with no previous exposure to the influenza virus antigens in the vaccine (such as young children) and are generally short-lived.

Guillain-Barré syndrome (GBS) was associated with the 1976 swine influenza vaccine, with an increased risk of 1 additional case of GBS per 100,000 people vaccinated. None of the studies of influenza vaccines other than the 1976 influenza vaccine has demonstrated a similar increase in GBS. Currently, the estimated risk for vaccine-related GBS is low, approximately 1 additional case per 1 million vaccinated.

LAIV

The most frequent side effects of trivalent and quadrivalent LAIV reported in healthy adults include minor upper respiratory symptoms, runny nose, and sore throat, which are generally well tolerated. Some children and adolescents have reported fever, vomiting, myalgia, and wheezing. These symptoms, particularly fever, are more often associated with the first administered LAIV dose and are self-limited.

LAIV should not be administered to any child aged <2 years or to children aged 2–4 years who have a history of wheezing in the past year or who have a diagnosis of asthma. People aged 5–49 years who have conditions that increase the risk of severe influenza, including pregnancy, should receive TIV and not LAIV.

Precautions and Contraindications
Egg allergy

Immediate hypersensitivity reactions (such as hives, angioedema, allergic asthma, and systemic anaphylaxis) rarely occur after influenza vaccination. These reactions likely result from hypersensitivity to vaccine components, one of which is residual egg protein. People who have developed only hives from egg exposure may receive the influenza vaccine. CDC recommends they receive TIV, administered by a provider familiar with egg allergies, and are observed after vaccine administration. Those who have had a severe reaction to eggs, including angioedema, acute respiratory distress, or required epinephrine after egg exposure, should consult a physician experienced in allergic reactions for evaluation to determine if vaccine should be administered. Influenza vaccine is contraindicated in those who have had a previous severe allergic reaction to influenza vaccine, regardless of which vaccine component was responsible for the reaction.

Personal Protection Measures

Measures that may help prevent influenza virus infection and other infections during travel include avoiding contact with others while sick; avoiding close contact with sick people; washing hands often with soap and water (where soap and water are not available, using an alcohol-based hand sanitizer containing ≥60% alcohol); avoiding touching one's eyes, nose, and mouth; and covering coughs and sneezes with a tissue, then disposing of the tissue. In countries where HPAI H5N1 virus outbreaks are occurring among poultry, travelers should avoid markets and farms where live poultry are sold or raised, avoid contact with dead poultry, and not drink chicken blood or eat undercooked chicken.

CDC website: www.cdc.gov/flu

BIBLIOGRAPHY

1. Block SL, Yi T, Sheldon E, Dubovsky F, Falloon J. A randomized, double-blind noninferiority study of quadrivalent live attenuated influenza vaccine in adults. Vaccine. 2011 Nov 21;29(50):9391–7.
2. CDC. Estimates of deaths associated with seasonal influenza—United States, 1976–2007. MMWR Morb Mortal Wkly Rep. 2010 Aug 27;59(33):1057–62.
3. CDC. Influenza antiviral medications: summary for clinicians. Atlanta: CDC; 2011 [cited 2012 Sep 20].

Available from: http://www.cdc.gov/flu/professionals/antivirals/summary-clinicians.htm.
4. CDC. Influenza symptoms and the role of laboratory diagnostics. Atlanta: CDC; 2011 [cited 2012 Sep 20]. Available from: http://www.cdc.gov/flu/professionals/diagnosis/labrolesprocedures.htm.
5. CDC. Prevention and control of influenza with vaccines: recommendations of the Advisory Committee on Immunization Practices (ACIP),

2011. MMWR Morb Mortal Wkly Rep. 2011 Aug 26;60(33):1128–32.

6. Dawood FS, Jain S, Finelli L, Shaw MW, Lindstrom S, Garten RJ, et al. Emergence of a novel swine-origin influenza A (H1N1) virus in humans. N Engl J Med. 2009 Jun 18;360(25):2605–15.

7. Fiore AE, Uyeki TM, Broder K, Finelli L, Euler GL, Singleton JA, et al. Prevention and control of influenza with vaccines: recommendations of the Advisory Committee on Immunization Practices (ACIP), 2010. MMWR Recomm Rep. 2010 Aug 6;59(RR-8):1–62.

8. Jain S, Kamimoto L, Bramley AM, Schmitz AM, Benoit SR, Louie J, et al. Hospitalized patients with 2009 H1N1 influenza in the United States, April–June 2009. N Engl J Med. 2009 Nov 12;361(20):1935–44.

9. McGeer A, Green KA, Plevneshi A, Shigayeva A, Siddiqi N, Raboud J, et al. Antiviral therapy and outcomes of influenza requiring hospitalization in Ontario, Canada. Clin Infect Dis. 2007 Dec 15;45(12):1568–75.

10. World Health Organization. New influenza A (H1N1) virus: global epidemiological situation, June 2009. Wkly Epidemiol Rec. 2009 Jun 19;84(25):249–57.

JAPANESE ENCEPHALITIS

Susan L. Hills, Ingrid B. Weber, Marc Fischer

INFECTIOUS AGENT

Japanese encephalitis (JE) virus is a single-stranded RNA virus that belongs to the genus *Flavivirus* and is closely related to West Nile and Saint Louis encephalitis viruses.

TRANSMISSION

JE virus is transmitted to humans through the bite of an infected mosquito, primarily *Culex* species. The virus is maintained in an enzootic cycle between mosquitoes and amplifying vertebrate hosts, primarily pigs and wading birds. Humans are incidental or dead-end hosts, because they usually do not develop a level or duration of viremia sufficient to infect mosquitoes.

EPIDEMIOLOGY

JE virus is the most common vaccine-preventable cause of encephalitis in Asia, occurring throughout most of Asia and parts of the western Pacific (Map 3-8). Local transmission of JE virus has not been detected in Africa, Europe, or the Americas. Transmission principally occurs in rural agricultural areas, often associated with rice cultivation and flood irrigation. In some areas of Asia, these ecologic conditions may occur near, or occasionally within, urban centers. In temperate areas of Asia, transmission is seasonal, and human disease usually peaks in summer and fall. In the subtropics and tropics, seasonal transmission varies with monsoon rains and irrigation practices and may be prolonged or even occur year-round.

In endemic countries, where adults have acquired immunity through natural infection, JE is primarily a disease of children. However, travel-associated JE can occur among people of any age. For most travelers to Asia, the risk for JE is extremely low but varies based on destination, duration, season, and activities.

From 1973 through 2011, there were 58 published reports of travel-associated JE among travelers from nonendemic countries. From the time of licensure of a JE vaccine in the United States in 1992 through 2011, only 7 JE cases among US travelers have been reported to CDC.

The overall incidence of JE among people from nonendemic countries traveling to Asia is estimated to be <1 case per 1 million travelers. However, expatriates and travelers who stay for prolonged periods in rural areas with active JE virus transmission are likely at similar risk as the susceptible resident population (5–50 cases per 100,000 children per year). Travelers on even brief trips might be at increased risk if they have extensive outdoor or nighttime exposure in rural areas during periods of active transmission. Short-term (<1 month) travelers whose visits are restricted to major urban areas are at minimal risk for JE. In some endemic areas there are few human cases among residents because of natural immunity among older people or vaccination; however, JE virus is usually still maintained in these areas in an

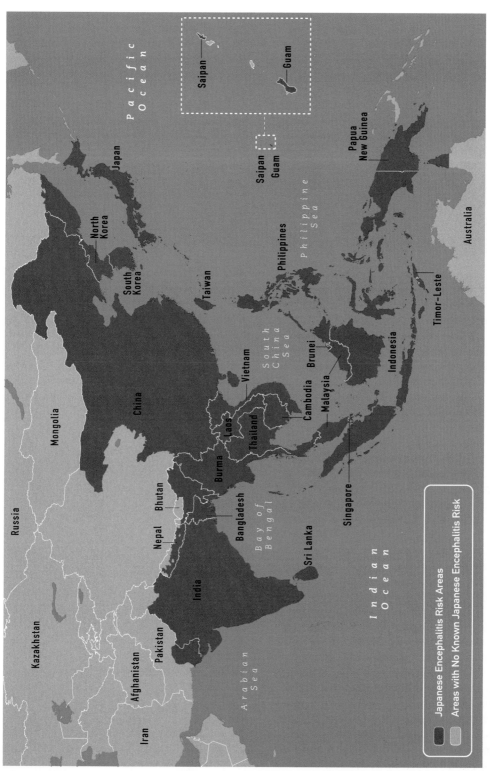

MAP 3-8. GEOGRAPHIC DISTRIBUTION OF JAPANESE ENCEPHALITIS

Japanese Encephalitis Risk Areas

Areas with No Known Japanese Encephalitis Risk

enzootic cycle between animals and mosquitoes. Therefore, susceptible visitors may be at risk for infection.

CLINICAL PRESENTATION

Most human infections with JE virus are asymptomatic; <1% of people infected with JE virus develop clinical disease. Acute encephalitis is the most commonly recognized clinical manifestation of JE virus infection. Milder forms of disease, such as aseptic meningitis or undifferentiated febrile illness, can also occur. The incubation period is 5–15 days. Illness usually begins with sudden onset of fever, headache, and vomiting. Mental status changes, focal neurologic deficits, generalized weakness, and movement disorders may develop over the next few days.

- The classical description of JE includes a parkinsonian syndrome with mask-like facies, tremor, cogwheel rigidity, and choreoathetoid movements.
- Acute flaccid paralysis, with clinical and pathological features similar to those of poliomyelitis, has also been associated with JE virus infection.
- Seizures are common, especially among children.
- Common clinical laboratory findings include moderate leukocytosis, mild anemia, and hyponatremia. Cerebrospinal fluid (CSF) typically has a mild to moderate pleocytosis with a lymphocytic predominance, slightly elevated protein, and normal ratio of CSF to plasma glucose.

The case-fatality ratio is approximately 20%–30%. Among survivors, 30%–50% have serious neurologic, cognitive, or psychiatric sequelae.

DIAGNOSIS

JE should be suspected in a patient with evidence of a neurologic infection (such as encephalitis, meningitis, or acute flaccid paralysis) who has recently traveled to or resided in an endemic country in Asia or the western Pacific. Laboratory diagnosis of JE virus infection should be performed by using a JE virus–specific IgM-capture ELISA on CSF or serum. JE virus–specific IgM can be measured in the CSF of most patients by 4 days after onset of symptoms and in serum by 7 days after onset. A ≥4-fold rise in JE virus–specific neutralizing antibodies between acute- and convalescent-phase serum specimens may be used to confirm the diagnosis. Vaccination history, date of onset of symptoms, and information regarding other flaviviruses known to circulate in the geographic area that may cross-react in serologic assays need to be considered when interpreting results.

Humans have low levels of transient viremia and usually have neutralizing antibodies by the time distinctive clinical symptoms are recognized. Virus isolation and nucleic-acid amplification tests are insensitive in detecting JE virus or viral RNA in blood or CSF and should not be used for ruling out a diagnosis of JE. Clinicians should contact their state or local health department or CDC at 970-221-6400 for assistance with diagnostic testing.

TREATMENT

There is no specific antiviral treatment for JE; therapy consists of supportive care and management of complications.

PREVENTION

Personal Protection Measures

The best way to prevent mosquitoborne diseases, including JE, is to avoid mosquito bites (see Chapter 2, Protection against Mosquitoes, Ticks, & Other Insects & Arthropods).

Vaccine

One JE vaccine is licensed and available in the United States—an inactivated Vero cell culture–derived vaccine, Ixiaro (Table 3-6). Ixiaro, manufactured by Intercell and distributed by Novartis Vaccines, was approved in March 2009 for use in people aged ≥17 years. Pediatric clinical trials are being conducted to enable licensure of Ixiaro for use in children. Information on current options for use of JE vaccine in children is available on the CDC website. Other inactivated and live attenuated JE vaccines are manufactured and used in other countries but are not licensed for use in the United States.

Indications for Use of JE Vaccine for Travelers

When making recommendations regarding the use of JE vaccine for travelers, clinicians must weigh the overall low risk of travel-associated JE, the high rate of death and disability when JE occurs, the low probability of serious

Table 3-6. Vaccine to prevent Japanese encephalitis (JE)

VACCINE	TRADE NAME (MANUFACTURER)	AGE	DOSE	ROUTE	SCHEDULE	BOOSTER[1]
JE vaccine, inactivated	Ixiaro (Intercell)	≥17 years	0.5 mL	IM	0, 28 days	≥1 year after primary series

Abbreviation: IM, intramuscular.
[1] If potential for JE virus exposure continues.

adverse events after immunization, and the cost of the vaccine. Evaluation of a traveler's risk should take into account the planned itinerary, including travel location, duration, activities, and seasonal patterns of disease in the areas to be visited (Table 3-7). The data in the table should be interpreted cautiously, because JE virus transmission activity varies within countries and from year to year.

The Advisory Committee on Immunization Practices recommends JE vaccine for travelers who plan to spend ≥1 month in endemic areas during the JE virus transmission season. This includes long-term travelers, recurrent travelers, or expatriates who will be based in urban areas but are likely to visit endemic rural or agricultural areas during a high-risk period of JE virus transmission. Vaccine should also be considered for the following:

- Short-term (<1 month) travelers to endemic areas during the JE virus transmission season, if they plan to travel outside an urban area and their activities will increase the risk of JE virus exposure. Examples of higher-risk activities or itineraries include 1) spending substantial time outdoors in rural or agricultural areas, especially during the evening or night; 2) participating in extensive outdoor activities (such as camping, hiking, trekking, biking, fishing, hunting, or farming); and 3) staying in accommodations without air conditioning, screens, or bed nets.
- Travelers to an area with an ongoing JE outbreak.
- Travelers to endemic areas who are uncertain of specific destinations, activities, or duration of travel.

JE vaccine is not recommended for short-term travelers whose visits will be restricted to urban areas or times outside a well-defined JE virus transmission season.

Vaccine Efficacy and Immunogenicity

There are no efficacy data for Ixiaro. The vaccine was licensed in the United States on the basis of its ability to induce JE virus neutralizing antibodies as a surrogate for protection, as well as safety evaluations in almost 5,000 adults. In the pivotal noninferiority immunogenicity study, 96% of adults developed protective neutralizing antibodies after receiving a primary immunization series of 2 doses administered 28 days apart.

Vaccine Administration

The primary immunization schedule for Ixiaro is 2 doses administered intramuscularly on days 0 and 28. The 2-dose series should be completed ≥1 week before travel.

The full duration of protection after primary immunization with Ixiaro is unknown. In one clinical trial assessing duration of protection, 83% of people who received 2 doses of Ixiaro maintained protective levels of antibodies at 12 months after the first vaccine dose. In a second study, 58% and 48% of people had protective antibodies at 12 and 24 months, respectively, and in a third, 69% of subjects had protective antibodies at 15 months.

If the primary series of Ixiaro was administered ≥1 year previously, a booster dose should be given before potential reexposure or if there is a continued risk for JE virus infection. Data on the response to a booster dose administered ≥2 years after the primary

Table 3-7. Risk for Japanese encephalitis (JE), by country[1]

COUNTRY	AFFECTED AREAS	TRANSMISSION SEASON	COMMENTS
Australia	Outer Torres Strait islands	December–May; all human cases reported February–April	1 human case reported from north Queensland mainland
Bangladesh	Presumed widespread	Most human cases reported May–October	Sentinel surveillance has identified human cases in Chittagong, Dhaka, Khulna, Rajshahi, and Sylhet Divisions; highest incidence reported from Rajshahi Division; outbreak reported from Tangail District, Dhaka Division, in 1977
Bhutan	Very rare reports; probably endemic in nonmountainous areas	No data	Proximity to other endemic areas and presence of vectors suggests virus transmission is likely
Brunei	No data; presumed to be endemic countrywide	Unknown; presumed year-round transmission	Proximity to other endemic areas suggests virus transmission is likely
Burma (Myanmar)	Limited data; presumed to be endemic countrywide	Unknown; most human cases reported from May–October	Outbreaks of human disease documented in Shan State; antibodies documented in animals and humans in other areas
Cambodia	Presumed to be endemic countrywide	Year-round with peaks reported May–October	Sentinel surveillance has identified human cases in at least 15 of 23 provinces, including Phnom Penh, Takeo, Kampong Cham, Battambang, Svay Rieng, and Siem Reap; case reported recently in a traveler who visited Phnom Penh and Angkor Wat/Siem Reap only
China	Human cases reported from all provinces except Xizang (Tibet), Xinjiang, and Qinghai; not considered endemic in Hong Kong and Macau, but rare cases reported from the New Territories	Most human cases reported June–October	Highest rates reported from Guizhou, Shaanxi, Sichuan, and Yunnan provinces, and Chongqing City; vaccine not routinely recommended for travel limited to Beijing or other major cities

continued

TABLE 3-7. RISK FOR JAPANESE ENCEPHALITIS, BY COUNTRY[1] (continued)

COUNTRY	AFFECTED AREAS	TRANSMISSION SEASON	COMMENTS
India	Human cases reported from all states except Dadra, Daman, Diu, Gujarat, Himachal Pradesh, Jammu and Kashmir, Lakshadweep, Meghalaya, Nagar Haveli, Punjab, Rajasthan, and Sikkim	Most human cases reported May–October, especially in northern India; the season may be extended or year-round in some areas, especially in southern India	Highest rates of human disease reported from the states of Andhra Pradesh, Assam, Bihar, Goa, Haryana, Karnataka, Kerala, Tamil Nadu, Uttar Pradesh, and West Bengal
Indonesia	Presumed to be endemic countrywide	Human cases reported year-round; peak season varies by island	Sentinel surveillance has identified human cases in Bali, Kalimantan, Java, Nusa Tenggara, Papua, and Sumatra
Japan[2]	Rare sporadic human cases on all islands except Hokkaido; enzootic activity ongoing	Most human cases reported July–October	Large number of human cases reported until JE vaccination program introduced in late 1960s; most recent small outbreak reported from Chugoku district in 2002; enzootic transmission without human cases observed on Hokkaido; vaccine not routinely recommended for travel limited to Tokyo or other major cities
Korea, North	Limited data; presumed to be endemic countrywide	No data; proximity to South Korea suggests peak transmission is likely to occur May–October	
Korea, South[2]	Rare sporadic human cases countrywide; enzootic activity ongoing	Most human cases reported May–October	Large number of human cases reported until routine JE vaccination program introduced in mid-1980s; highest rates of disease were reported from the southern provinces; last major outbreak reported in 1982; vaccine not routinely recommended for travel limited to Seoul or other major cities
Laos	Limited data; presumed to be endemic countrywide	Year-round, with peak June–September	Sentinel surveillance has identified human cases in north, central, and southern Laos

continued

TABLE 3-7. RISK FOR JAPANESE ENCEPHALITIS, BY COUNTRY[1] (continued)

COUNTRY	AFFECTED AREAS	TRANSMISSION SEASON	COMMENTS
Malaysia	Endemic in Sarawak; sporadic cases reported from all other states; occasional outbreaks reported	Year-round transmission; peak October–December in Sarawak	Most human cases reported from Sarawak; vaccine not routinely recommended for travel limited to Kuala Lumpur or other major cities
Mongolia	Not considered endemic		Vaccine not recommended
Nepal	Endemic in southern lowlands (Terai); cases also reported from hill and mountain districts, including the Kathmandu valley	Most human cases reported June–October	Highest rates of human disease reported from western Terai districts, including Banke, Bardiya, Dang, and Kailali; vaccine not routinely recommended for those trekking in high-altitude areas or spending short periods in Kathmandu or Pokhara en route to such trekking routes
Pakistan	Limited data; human cases reported from around Karachi	Unknown	
Papua New Guinea	Limited data; probably widespread	Unknown; probably year-round	Sporadic human cases reported from Western Province; serologic evidence of disease from Gulf and Southern Highland Provinces; a case of JE was reported from near Port Moresby in 2004
Philippines	Limited data; presumed to be endemic on all islands	Unknown; probably year-round	Outbreaks reported in Nueva Ecija and Manila; sentinel surveillance has identified human cases in other areas of Luzon and the Visayas
Russia	Rare human cases reported from the Far Eastern maritime areas south of Khabarovsk	Most human cases reported July–September	
Singapore	Rare sporadic human cases reported	Year-round	Vaccine not routinely recommended
Sri Lanka	Endemic countrywide except in mountainous areas	Year-round with variable peaks based on monsoon rains	Highest rates of human disease reported from Anuradhapura, Gampaha, Kurunegala, Polonnaruwa, and Puttalam districts

continued

TABLE 3-7. RISK FOR JAPANESE ENCEPHALITIS, BY COUNTRY[1] (continued)

COUNTRY	AFFECTED AREAS	TRANSMISSION SEASON	COMMENTS
Taiwan[2]	Rare sporadic human cases islandwide	Most human cases reported May–October	Large number of human cases reported until routine JE vaccination introduced in 1968; vaccine not routinely recommended for travel limited to Taipei or other major cities
Thailand	Endemic countrywide; seasonal epidemics in the northern provinces	Year-round with seasonal peaks May–October, especially in the north	Highest rates of human disease reported from the Chiang Mai Valley; sporadic human cases reported from Bangkok suburbs; several cases reported recently in travelers who visited resort or coastal areas of southern Thailand.
Timor-Leste	Sporadic human cases reported; presumed to be endemic countrywide	No data; cases reported year-round in neighboring West Timor	
Vietnam	Endemic countrywide; seasonal epidemics in the northern provinces	Year-round with seasonal peaks May–October, especially in the north	Highest rates of disease in the northern provinces around Hanoi and northwestern and northeastern provinces bordering China
Western Pacific Islands	Outbreaks of human disease reported in Guam in 1947–1948 and Saipan in 1990	Unknown; most human cases reported October–March	Enzootic cycle might not be sustainable; outbreaks may follow introductions of virus; vaccine not recommended

[1] Data are based on published reports and personal correspondence. Risk assessments should be performed cautiously, because risk can vary within areas and from year to year, and surveillance data regarding human cases and JEV transmission are incomplete.

[2] In some endemic areas, human cases among residents are limited because of natural immunity among older people or vaccination. However, because JEV is maintained in an enzootic cycle between animals and mosquitoes, susceptible visitors to these areas still may be at risk for infection.

series are not available. Data on the need for and timing of additional booster doses are also not available.

There are limited data on the use of Ixiaro as a booster dose after a primary series with the mouse brain–derived inactivated JE vaccine. Two studies have been conducted, one in US military personnel and the other at 2 travel clinics in Europe. Both studies demonstrated that in people who had previously received at least a primary series of mouse brain–derived inactivated JE vaccine, a single dose of Ixiaro adequately boosted neutralizing antibody levels and provided at least short-term protection. Both studies measured antibody responses at 4–8 weeks after the booster dose; therefore, additional studies are needed to determine the duration of protection after a single dose of Ixiaro in prior recipients of a mouse brain–derived vaccine. Until those data are available, people who have received JE-Vax, the mouse brain–derived vaccine formerly used in the United States, and require further vaccination against JE virus, should receive a 2-dose primary series of Ixiaro.

Vaccine Safety and Adverse Reactions

Local symptoms of pain and tenderness were the most commonly reported symptoms in a safety study with 1,993 participants who received 2 doses of Ixiaro. Headache, myalgia, fatigue, and an influenzalike illness were each reported at a rate of >10%. Because Ixiaro was licensed after study in <5,000 recipients, the possibility of rare serious adverse events cannot be excluded. Postlicensure studies and surveillance are ongoing to further evaluate the safety of Ixiaro in a larger population.

Precautions and Contraindications

A severe allergic reaction after a previous dose of Ixiaro is a contraindication to administration of further doses. Ixiaro contains protamine sulfate, a compound known to cause hypersensitivity reactions in some people. No studies of Ixiaro in pregnant women have been conducted. Therefore, administration of Ixiaro to pregnant women usually should be deferred. However, pregnant women who must travel to an area where risk for JE virus infection is high should be vaccinated when the theoretical risk of immunization is outweighed by the risk of infection.

CDC website: www.cdc.gov/ncidod/dvbid/jencephalitis

BIBLIOGRAPHY

1. Campbell GL, Hills SL, Fischer M, Jacobson JA, Hoke CH, Hombach JM, et al. Estimated global incidence of Japanese encephalitis: a systematic review. Bull World Health Organ. 2011 Oct 1;89(10):766–74, 74A–74E.
2. CDC. Japanese encephalitis among three US travelers returning from Asia, 2003–2008. MMWR Morb Mortal Wkly Rep. 2009 Jul 17;58(27):737–40.
3. CDC. Japanese encephalitis in two children—United States, 2010. MMWR Morb Mortal Wkly Rep. 2011 Mar 11;60(9):276–8.
4. CDC. Recommendations for use of a booster dose of inactivated Vero cell culture–derived Japanese encephalitis vaccine: advisory committee on immunization practices, 2011. MMWR Morb Mortal Wkly Rep. 2011 May 27;60(20):661–3.
5. Fischer M, Lindsey N, Staples JE, Hills S. Japanese encephalitis vaccines: recommendations of the Advisory Committee on Immunization Practices (ACIP). MMWR Recomm Rep. 2010 Mar 12;59(RR-1):1–27.
6. Hills SL, Griggs AC, Fischer M. Japanese encephalitis in travelers from non-endemic countries, 1973–2008. Am J Trop Med Hyg. 2010 May;82(5):930–6.
7. Jeurissen A, Strauven T. A case of aseptic meningitis due to Japanese encephalitis virus in a traveller returning from the Philippines. Acta Neurol Belg. 2011 Jun;111(2):143–5.
8. Schuller E, Klingler A, Dubischar-Kastner K, Dewasthaly S, Muller Z. Safety profile of the Vero cell–derived Japanese encephalitis virus (JEV) vaccine IXIARO(®). Vaccine. 2011 Nov 3;29(47):8669–76.
9. Shlim DR, Solomon T. Japanese encephalitis vaccine for travelers: exploring the limits of risk. Clin Infect Dis. 2002 Jul 15;35(2):183–8.
10. Tauber E, Kollaritsch H, Korinek M, Rendi-Wagner P, Jilma B, Firbas C, et al. Safety and immunogenicity of a Vero-cell-derived, inactivated Japanese encephalitis vaccine: a non-inferiority, phase III, randomised controlled trial. Lancet. 2007 Dec 1;370(9602):1847–53.
11. Tauber E, Kollaritsch H, von Sonnenburg F, Lademann M, Jilma B, Firbas C, et al. Randomized, double-blind, placebo-controlled phase 3 trial of the safety and tolerability of IC51, an inactivated Japanese encephalitis vaccine. J Infect Dis. 2008 Aug 15;198(4):493–9.
12. Werlinrud AM, Christiansen CB, Koch A. Japanese encephalitis in a Danish short-term traveler to Cambodia. J Travel Med. 2011 Nov–Dec;18(6):411–3.
13. Woolpert T, Staples JE, Faix DJ, Nett RJ, Kosoy OI, Biggerstaff BJ, et al. Immunogenicity of one dose of Vero cell culture–derived Japanese encephalitis (JE) vaccine in adults previously vaccinated with mouse brain–derived JE vaccine. Vaccine. 2012 Apr 26;30(20):3090–6.
14. World Health Organization. Japanese encephalitis vaccines. Wkly Epidemiol Rec. 2006 Aug 25;81(34/35):331–40.

LEGIONELLOSIS (LEGIONNAIRES' DISEASE & PONTIAC FEVER)

Laurel E. Garrison, Lauri A. Hicks

INFECTIOUS AGENT

Gram-negative bacteria of the genus *Legionella*.

TRANSMISSION

Inhalation of a water aerosol containing the bacteria. The bacterium grows in warm freshwater environments. Person-to-person transmission does not occur with either Legionnaires' disease or Pontiac fever.

EPIDEMIOLOGY

Legionellae are ubiquitous worldwide. Most cases of legionellosis are caused by *Legionella pneumophila*. Disease occurs after exposure to aquatic settings that promote bacterial growth—the aquatic environment is somewhat stagnant, the water is warm (77°F–108°F [25°C–42°C]), and the water must be aerosolized so that the bacteria can be inhaled into the lungs. These 3 conditions are met almost exclusively in developed or industrialized settings. Disease does not occur in association with natural freshwater settings such as waterfalls, lakes, or streams.

Outbreaks of legionellosis have been described in numerous countries throughout the world. The largest outbreak (449 cases) ever reported was traced to a cooling tower on the roof of a city hospital in Murcia, Spain, in 2001. Travel-associated outbreaks are commonly recognized.

Despite the presence of *Legionella* bacteria in many aquatic environments, the risk of developing legionellosis for most people is low. Travelers who are exposed to aerosolized, warm water containing *Legionella* are at risk for infection. Travelers who are aged >50 years, are current or former smokers, have chronic lung conditions, or are immunocompromised are at higher risk of developing illness after exposure. Many outbreaks have been associated with exposure to cruise ships, hotels, and resorts. Exposures can occur during recreation in or near a whirlpool spa, while showering in a hotel, or touring in cities with buildings that have cooling towers. Patients often do not recall specific water exposures, as they frequently occur during normal activities.

CLINICAL PRESENTATION

Legionnaires' disease typically presents with pneumonia, which usually requires hospitalization and can be fatal in 10%–15% of cases. Symptom onset occurs 2–14 days after exposure. In outbreak settings, <5% of people exposed to the source of the outbreak develop Legionnaires' disease.

Pontiac fever is milder than Legionnaires' disease and presents as an influenzalike illness, with fever, headache, and muscle aches, but no signs of pneumonia. Pontiac fever can affect healthy people, as well as those with underlying illnesses, and symptoms occur within 72 hours of exposure. Most patients fully recover. Up to 95% of people exposed in outbreak settings can develop symptoms of Pontiac fever.

DIAGNOSIS

Isolation of *Legionella* from respiratory secretions, lung tissue, pleural fluid, or a normally sterile site is an important method for diagnosis of Legionnaires' disease. Clinical isolates are often necessary to interpret the findings of an investigation through comparison with isolates obtained from environmental sources. Because of differences in mechanism of disease, *Legionella* cannot be isolated in people who have Pontiac fever.

The most used diagnostic method is the *Legionella* urinary antigen assay. However, the assay can only detect *L. pneumophila* serogroup 1, the most common cause of legionellosis. Paired serology showing a 4-fold rise in antibody titer between acute- and convalescent-phase specimens also confirms the diagnosis. A single antibody titer of any level is not diagnostic of legionellosis.

TREATMENT

For travelers with suspected Legionnaires' disease, specific antibiotic treatment is necessary and should be administered promptly while diagnostic tests are being processed. Appropriate antibiotics include fluoroquinolones and macrolides. Treatment may be necessary for up to 3 weeks. In severe cases, patients may have prolonged stays in intensive care units. Consultation with an infectious diseases specialist is advised. Pontiac fever is a self-limited illness that requires supportive care only; antibiotics have no benefit.

PREVENTION

There is no vaccine for legionellosis, and antibiotic prophylaxis is not effective. Travelers at increased risk for infection, such as the elderly or those with immunocompromising conditions such as cancer or diabetes, may choose to avoid high-risk areas, such as whirlpool spas. If exposure cannot be avoided, travelers should be advised to seek medical attention promptly if they develop symptoms of Legionnaires' disease or Pontiac fever.

CDC website: www.cdc.gov/legionella

BIBLIOGRAPHY

1. Burnsed LJ, Hicks LA, Smithee LM, Fields BS, Bradley KK, Pascoe N, et al. A large, travel-associated outbreak of legionellosis among hotel guests: utility of the urine antigen assay in confirming Pontiac fever. Clin Infect Dis. 2007 Jan 15;44(2):222–8.
2. CDC. Cruise ship-associated Legionnaires' disease, November 2003–May 2004. MMWR Morb Mortal Wkly Rep. 2005 Nov 18;54(45):1153–5.
3. CDC. Legionellosis—United States, 2000–2009. MMWR Morb Mortal Wkly Rep. 2011 Aug 19;60(32):1083–6.
4. CDC. Surveillance for travel-associated Legionnaires' disease—United States, 2005–2006. MMWR Morb Mortal Wkly Rep. 2007 Dec 7;56(48):1261–3.
5. Fields BS, Benson RF, Besser RE. *Legionella* and Legionnaires' disease: 25 years of investigation. Clin Microbiol Rev. 2002 Jul;15(3):506–26.
6. Garcia-Fulgueiras A, Navarro C, Fenoll D, Garcia J, Gonzalez-Diego P, Jimenez-Bunuales T, et al. Legionnaires' disease outbreak in Murcia, Spain. Emerg Infect Dis. 2003 Aug;9(8):915–21.
7. Jernigan DB, Hofmann J, Cetron MS, Genese CA, Nuorti JP, Fields BS, et al. Outbreak of Legionnaires' disease among cruise ship passengers exposed to a contaminated whirlpool spa. Lancet. 1996 Feb 24;347(9000):494–9.
8. Joseph CA, Ricketts KD, Yadav R, Patel S, European Working Group for *Legionella* Infections. Travel-associated Legionnaires' disease in Europe in 2009. Euro Surveill. 2010 Oct 14;15(41):19683.

LEISHMANIASIS, CUTANEOUS

Barbara L. Herwaldt, Alan J. Magill

Leishmaniasis is a parasitic disease found in parts of the tropics, subtropics, and southern Europe. Leishmaniasis has several different forms. This section focuses on cutaneous leishmaniasis (CL), the most common form, both in general and in travelers.

INFECTIOUS AGENT

Leishmaniasis is caused by obligate intracellular protozoan parasites; approximately 20 *Leishmania* species cause CL.

TRANSMISSION

CL is transmitted through the bite of an infected female phlebotomine sand fly. CL also can occur after accidental occupational (laboratory) exposures to *Leishmania* parasites.

EPIDEMIOLOGY

In the Old World (Eastern Hemisphere), CL is found in parts of the Middle East, Asia (particularly southwest and central Asia), Africa (particularly the tropical region and North Africa), and southern Europe. In the New World (Western Hemisphere), CL is found in parts of Mexico, Central America, and South America. Occasional cases have been reported in Texas and Oklahoma. CL is not found in Chile, Uruguay, or Canada. Overall, CL is found in focal areas of >90 countries. Most (up to 90%)

of the world's cases of CL occur in only a few of those countries: Afghanistan, Algeria, Iran, Iraq, Saudi Arabia, and Syria in the Old World; and Bolivia, Brazil, Colombia, Nicaragua, and Peru in the New World.

The geographic distribution of cases of CL evaluated in countries such as the United States reflects travel and immigration patterns. More than 75% of the cases diagnosed in US civilians have been acquired in Latin America, including popular tourist destinations such as Costa Rica. Cases in US service personnel have reflected military activities (such as in Afghanistan and Iraq). CL is usually more common in rural than urban areas, but it is found in some periurban and urban areas (such as in Kabul, Afghanistan). The ecologic settings range from rainforests to arid regions.

The risk is highest from dusk to dawn because sand flies typically feed (bite) at night and during twilight hours. Although sand flies are less active during the hottest time of the day, they may bite if they are disturbed (for example, if hikers brush against tree trunks or other sites where sand flies are resting). Vector activity can easily be overlooked: sand flies do not make noise, they are small (approximately one-third the size of mosquitoes), and their bites might not be noticed.

Examples of types of travelers who might have an increased risk for CL include ecotourists, adventure travelers, bird watchers, Peace Corps volunteers, missionaries, military personnel, construction workers, and people who do research outdoors at night or twilight. However, even short-term travelers in endemic areas have developed CL.

CLINICAL PRESENTATION

CL is characterized by skin lesions (open or closed sores), which typically develop within several weeks or months after exposure. In some people, the sores first appear months or years later, in the context of trauma (such as skin wounds or surgery). The sores can change in size and appearance over time. They typically progress from small papules to nodular plaques, and eventually lead to open sores with a raised border and central crater (ulcer), which can be covered with scales or crust. The lesions usually are painless but can be painful, particularly if open sores become infected with bacteria. Satellite lesions, regional lymphadenopathy (swollen glands),

and nodular lymphangitis can be noted. The sores usually heal eventually, even without treatment. However, they can last for months or years and typically result in scarring.

A potential concern applies to some of the *Leishmania* species in South and Central America: some parasites can spread from the skin to the mucosal surfaces of the nose or mouth and cause sores there. This form of leishmaniasis, mucosal leishmaniasis (ML), might not be noticed until years after the original skin sores appear to have healed. Although ML is uncommon, it has occurred in travelers and expatriates whose cases of CL were not treated or were inadequately treated. The initial clinical manifestations typically involve the nose (chronic stuffiness, bleeding, and inflamed mucosa or sores) and less often the mouth; in advanced cases, ulcerative destruction of the nose, mouth, and pharynx can be noted (such as perforation of the nasal septum).

DIAGNOSIS

Clinicians should consider CL in people with chronic (nonhealing) skin lesions who have been in areas where leishmaniasis is found. Laboratory confirmation of the diagnosis is achieved by detecting *Leishmania* parasites (or DNA) in infected tissue, through light-microscopic examination of stained specimens, culture techniques, or molecular methods.

CDC can assist in all aspects of the diagnostic evaluation. Identification of the *Leishmania* species can be important, particularly if more than one species is found where the patient traveled and if the species can have different clinical and prognostic implications. Serologic testing generally is not useful for CL but can provide supportive evidence for the diagnosis of ML.

For consultative services, contact CDC Parasitic Diseases Inquiries (404-718-4745; parasites@cdc.gov).

TREATMENT

Decisions about whether and how to treat CL should be individualized. All cases of ML should be treated; there are several therapeutic options. Clinicians may consult with CDC staff about the relative merits of various approaches (see the Diagnosis section above for contact information).

The pentavalent antimonial compound sodium stibogluconate (Pentostam) is available to US-licensed physicians through the CDC Drug Service (404-639-3670) for intravenous or intramuscular administration under an investigational new drug protocol (see www.cdc.gov/laboratory/drugservice/index.html).

PREVENTION

No vaccines or drugs to prevent infection are available. Preventive measures are aimed at reducing contact with sand flies by using personal protective measures (see Chapter 2, Protection against Mosquitoes, Ticks, & Other Insects & Arthropods). Travelers should be advised to:

- Avoid outdoor activities, especially from dusk to dawn, when sand flies generally are the most active.
- Wear protective clothing and apply insect repellent to exposed skin and under the edges of clothing, such as sleeves and

pant legs, according to the manufacturer's instructions.

- Sleep in air-conditioned or well-screened areas. Spraying the quarters with insecticide might provide some protection. Fans or ventilators might inhibit the movement of sand flies, which are weak fliers.

Sand flies are so small (approximately 2–3 mm, less than one-eighth of an inch) that they can pass through the holes in ordinary bed nets. Although closely woven nets are available, they may be uncomfortable in hot climates. The effectiveness of bed nets can be enhanced by treatment with a pyrethroid-containing insecticide. The same treatment can be applied to window screens, curtains, bed sheets, and clothing.

CDC website: www.cdc.gov/parasites/leishmaniasis

BIBLIOGRAPHY

1. Ahluwalia S, Lawn SD, Kanagalingam J, Grant H, Lockwood DN. Mucocutaneous leishmaniasis: an imported infection among travellers to central and South America. BMJ. 2004 Oct 9;329(7470):842–4.
2. Blum J, Desjeux P, Schwartz E, Beck B, Hatz C. Treatment of cutaneous leishmaniasis among travellers. J Antimicrob Chemother. 2004 Feb;53(2):158–66.
3. Herwaldt BL. Leishmaniasis. Lancet. 1999 Oct 2;354(9185):1191–9.
4. Herwaldt BL, Stokes SL, Juranek DD. American cutaneous leishmaniasis in US travelers. Ann Intern Med. 1993 May 15;118(10):779–84.
5. Magill AJ. Cutaneous leishmaniasis in the returning traveler. Infect Dis Clin North Am. 2005 Mar;19(1):241–66, x–xi.
6. Murray HW. Leishmaniasis in the United States: treatment in 2012. Am J Trop Med Hyg. 2012 Mar;86(3):434–40.
7. Murray HW, Berman JD, Davies CR, Saravia NG. Advances in leishmaniasis. Lancet. 2005 Oct 29–Nov 4;366(9496):1561–77.
8. Schwartz E, Hatz C, Blum J. New World cutaneous leishmaniasis in travellers. Lancet Infect Dis. 2006 Jun;6(6):342–9.
9. World Health Organization. Control of the leishmaniases. Geneva: World Health Organization; 2010 [cited 2012 Sep 21]. Available from: http://whqlibdoc.who.int/trs/WHO_TRS_949_eng.pdf.

LEISHMANIASIS, VISCERAL

Barbara L. Herwaldt, Alan J. Magill

Leishmaniasis is a parasitic disease found in parts of the tropics, subtropics, and southern Europe. Leishmaniasis has several different forms. This section focuses on visceral leishmaniasis (VL), which affects some of the internal organs of the body (such as the spleen, liver, and bone marrow).

INFECTIOUS AGENT

VL is caused by obligate intracellular protozoan parasites, particularly by the species *Leishmania donovani* and *L. infantum/L. chagasi*.

TRANSMISSION

VL is predominantly transmitted through the bite of an infected female phlebotomine sand fly, although congenital and parenteral transmission (through blood transfusions and needle sharing) have been reported.

EPIDEMIOLOGY

VL is usually more common in rural than urban areas, but it is found in some periurban areas (such as in northeastern Brazil). In the Old World (Eastern Hemisphere), VL is found in parts of Asia (particularly the Indian subcontinent and southwest and central Asia), the Middle East, Africa (particularly East Africa), and southern Europe. In the New World (Western Hemisphere), most cases occur in Brazil; some cases occur in scattered foci elsewhere in Latin America. Overall, VL is found in focal areas of >60 countries. Most (>90%) of the world's cases of VL occur in the Indian subcontinent (India, Bangladesh, and Nepal), East Africa (Sudan, South Sudan, and Ethiopia), and Brazil; none of the affected areas in these 7 countries are common tourist destinations.

The geographic distribution of cases of VL evaluated in countries such as the United States reflects travel and immigration patterns. VL is uncommon in US travelers and expatriates. Occasional cases have been diagnosed in short-term travelers (tourists) to southern Europe and also in longer-term travelers (such as expatriates and deployed soldiers) to the Mediterranean region and other areas where VL is found.

CLINICAL PRESENTATION

Among symptomatic people, the incubation period typically ranges from weeks to months. The onset of illness can be abrupt or gradual. Stereotypical manifestations of VL include fever, weight loss, hepatosplenomegaly (especially splenomegaly), and pancytopenia (anemia, leukopenia, and thrombocytopenia). If untreated, severe (advanced) cases of VL typically are fatal. Latent infection can become clinically manifest years to decades after exposure in people who become immunocompromised for other medical reasons.

DIAGNOSIS

Clinicians should consider VL in people with a relevant travel history (even in the distant past) and a persistent, unexplained febrile illness, especially if accompanied by other suggestive manifestations (such as splenomegaly and pancytopenia). Laboratory confirmation of the diagnosis is achieved by detecting *Leishmania* parasites (or DNA) in infected tissue (such as in bone marrow, liver, lymph node, or blood), through light-microscopic examination of stained specimens, culture techniques, or molecular methods. Serologic testing can provide supportive evidence for the diagnosis.

CDC can assist in all aspects of the diagnostic evaluation, including species identification. For consultative services, contact CDC Parasitic Diseases Inquiries (404-718-4745; parasites@cdc.gov) or see www.dpd.cdc.gov/dpdx.

TREATMENT

Infected travelers should be advised to consult an infectious disease or tropical medicine specialist. Therapy for VL should be individualized with expert consultation. The relative merits of various approaches can be discussed with CDC staff (see the Diagnosis section above for contact information).

Liposomal amphotericin B (AmBisome) is approved by the Food and Drug Administration to treat VL. The pentavalent antimonial compound sodium stibogluconate (Pentostam) is available to US-licensed physicians through the CDC Drug Service (404-639-3670) under an investigational new drug protocol (see www.cdc.gov/laboratory/drugservice/index.html).

PREVENTION

No vaccines or drugs to prevent infection are available. Preventive measures are aimed at reducing contact with sand flies (see the Protection against Mosquitoes, Ticks, & Other Insects & Arthropods section in Chapter 2 and Prevention in the previous section, Cutaneous Leishmaniasis). In particular, travelers should be advised to avoid outdoor activities, especially from dusk to dawn, when sand flies generally are the most active, and to sleep in air-conditioned or well-screened quarters. Preventive measures also include wearing protective clothing, applying insect repellent to exposed skin, using bed nets treated with a pyrethroid-containing insecticide, and spraying dwellings with residual-action insecticides.

CDC website: www.cdc.gov/parasites/leishmaniasis

BIBLIOGRAPHY

1. Herwaldt BL. Leishmaniasis. Lancet. 1999 Oct 2;354(9185):1191–9.

2. Malik AN, John L, Bryceson AD, Lockwood DN. Changing pattern of visceral leishmaniasis, United Kingdom, 1985–2004. Emerg Infect Dis. 2006 Aug;12(8):1257–9.

3. Murray HW. Leishmaniasis in the United States: treatment in 2012. Am J Trop Med Hyg. 2012 Mar;86(3):434–40.

4. Murray HW, Berman JD, Davies CR, Saravia NG. Advances in leishmaniasis. Lancet. 2005 Oct 29–Nov 4;366(9496):1561–77.

5. Myles O, Wortmann GW, Cummings JF, Barthel RV, Patel S, Crum-Cianflone NF, et al. Visceral leishmaniasis: clinical observations in 4 US army soldiers deployed to Afghanistan or Iraq, 2002–2004. Arch Intern Med. 2007 Sep 24;167(17):1899–901.

6. Weisser M, Khanlari B, Terracciano L, Arber C, Gratwohl A, Bassetti S, et al. Visceral leishmaniasis: a threat to immunocompromised patients in non-endemic areas? Clin Microbiol Infect. 2007 Aug;13(8):751–3.

7. World Health Organization. Control of the leishmaniases. Geneva: World Health Organization; 2010 [cited 2012 Sep 21]. Available from: http://whqlibdoc.who.int/trs/WHO_TRS_949_eng.pdf.

LEPTOSPIROSIS

Robyn A. Stoddard, Marta A. Guerra

INFECTIOUS AGENT

Obligate aerobic spirochete bacteria in the genus *Leptospira*.

TRANSMISSION

Infection occurs through abrasions or cuts in the skin, or through the conjunctiva and mucous membranes. Humans may be infected by direct contact with urine or reproductive fluids from infected animals, or with water or soil contaminated with those fluids. Prolonged immersion in contaminated water increases the risk for infection. Infection rarely occurs through animal bites or human-to-human contact.

EPIDEMIOLOGY

Leptospirosis has worldwide distribution, with a higher incidence in tropical climates, especially after heavy rainfall or flooding due to hurricanes. Outbreaks of leptospirosis have occurred in the United States after flooding in Hawaii and Puerto Rico. Travelers participating in recreational water activities are at increased risk, particularly after heavy rainfall or flooding.

CLINICAL PRESENTATION

The incubation period is 2 days to 3 weeks. The acute phase (approximately 7 days) presents as an acute febrile illness with symptoms including headache (can be severe and include retroorbital pain and photophobia), fever, chills, myalgia, nausea, diarrhea, abdominal pain, uveitis, conjunctival suffusion, and occasionally, a skin rash. The second or immune phase is characterized by antibody production and the presence of leptospires in the urine. The icteric or severe form of the disease (Weil disease) occurs in 5%–10% of patients with leptospirosis. Symptoms include jaundice, renal failure, hemorrhage (especially pulmonary), cardiac arrhythmias, pneumonitis, and hemodynamic collapse.

DIAGNOSIS

Diagnosis of leptospirosis is usually based on clinical recognition and serology; microscopic agglutination test is the gold standard. Culture is relatively insensitive, but detection of the organism using real-time PCR can provide a more timely diagnosis.

TREATMENT

Doxycycline is effective in decreasing the severity and duration of leptospirosis and should be initiated early in the course of the disease if leptospirosis is suspected. Intravenous penicillin is a drug of choice for patients with severe leptospirosis. Patients with severe leptospirosis may require hospitalization, supportive therapy, and close monitoring.

PREVENTION

No vaccine is available in the United States. Travelers who might be at an increased risk for infection should be advised to consider preventive measures such as chemoprophylaxis, wearing protective clothing, especially footwear, and covering cuts and abrasions with occlusive dressings. Until further data become available, CDC recommends chemoprophylaxis with doxycycline (200 mg orally, weekly), begun 1–2 days before and continuing through the period of exposure for people at high risk of leptospirosis. Doxycycline is not recommended for pregnant women or children aged <8 years.

CDC website: www.cdc.gov/leptospirosis

BIBLIOGRAPHY

1. Bajani MD, Ashford DA, Bragg SL, Woods CW, Aye T, Spiegel RA, et al. Evaluation of four commercially available rapid serologic tests for diagnosis of leptospirosis. J Clin Microbiol. 2003 Feb;41(2):803–9.
2. Haake DA, Dundoo M, Cader R, Kubak BM, Hartskeerl RA, Sejvar JJ, et al. Leptospirosis, water sports, and chemoprophylaxis. Clin Infect Dis. 2002 May 1;34(9):e40–3.
3. Levett PN. Leptospirosis. Clin Microbiol Rev. 2001 Apr;14(2):296–326.
4. Pappas G, Cascio A. Optimal treatment of leptospirosis: queries and projections. Int J Antimicrob Agents. 2006 Dec;28(6):491–6.
5. Stoddard RA, Gee JE, Wilkins PP, McCaustland K, Hoffmaster AR. Detection of pathogenic *Leptospira* spp. through TaqMan polymerase chain reaction targeting the LipL32 gene. Diagn Microbiol Infect Dis. 2009 Jul;64(3):247–55.

LYME DISEASE
Paul S. Mead

INFECTIOUS AGENT
Spirochetes belonging to the *Borrelia burgdorferi* sensu lato complex, including *B. afzelii*, *B. burgdorferi* sensu stricto, and *B. garinii*.

TRANSMISSION
Through the bite of *Ixodes* ticks; infected people are often unaware that they have been bitten.

EPIDEMIOLOGY
In Europe, endemic from southern Scandinavia into the northern Mediterranean countries of Italy, Spain, and Greece. Incidence is highest in central and Eastern European countries. In North America, highly endemic areas are the northeastern and north-central United States. Transmission has not been documented in the tropics. Lyme disease is rarely reported in returning travelers.

CLINICAL PRESENTATION
Incubation period is typically 3–30 days. Approximately 80% of people infected with *B. burgdorferi* develop a characteristic rash, erythema migrans (EM), within 30 days of exposure. EM is a red, expanding rash, with or without central clearing, that is often accompanied by symptoms of fatigue, fever, headache, mild stiff neck, arthralgia, or myalgia. Within days or weeks, infection can spread to other parts of the body, causing more serious neurologic conditions (meningitis, radiculopathy, and facial palsy) or cardiac abnormalities (myocarditis with atrioventricular heart block). Untreated, infection can progress over a period of months to cause monoarticular or oligoarticular arthritis, peripheral neuropathy, or encephalopathy. These long-term sequelae can be typically observed over a number of months, ranging from 1 week to a few years.

DIAGNOSIS
Observation of an EM rash with a history of recent travel to an endemic area (with or without history of tick bite) is sufficient. For patients with evidence of disseminated infection (musculoskeletal, neurologic, or cardiac manifestations), 2-tiered serologic testing, consisting of an ELISA/IFA and confirmatory

Western blot, is recommended. Patients suspected of acquiring Lyme disease overseas should be tested by using a C6-based ELISA, as other serologic tests may not detect infection with European species of *Borrelia*.

TREATMENT

Most patients can be treated with either oral doxycycline or intravenous ceftriaxone. See http://cid.oxfordjournals.org/content/43/9/1089.full.

BIBLIOGRAPHY

1. O'Connell S. Lyme borreliosis: current issues in diagnosis and management. Curr Opin Infect Dis. 2010 Jun;23(3):231–5.
2. Stanek G, Strle F. Lyme disease: European perspective. Infect Dis Clin North Am. 2008 Jun;22(2):327–39.
3. Steere AC. Lyme disease. N Engl J Med. 2001 Jul 12;345(2):115–25.

PREVENTION

Avoid tick habitats, use insect repellent on exposed skin and clothing, and carefully check every day for attached ticks. Minimize areas of exposed skin by wearing long-sleeved shirts, long pants, and closed shoes; tucking shirts in and tucking pants into socks may also reduce risk (see Chapter 2, Protection against Mosquitoes, Ticks, & Other Insects & Arthropods).

CDC website: www.cdc.gov/lyme

MALARIA
Paul M. Arguin, Kathrine R. Tan

INFECTIOUS AGENT

Malaria in humans is caused by 1 of 4 protozoan species of the genus *Plasmodium*: *Plasmodium falciparum*, *P. vivax*, *P. ovale*, or *P. malariae*. In addition, *P. knowlesi*, a parasite of Old World (Eastern Hemisphere) monkeys, has been documented as a cause of human infections and some deaths in Southeast Asia.

TRANSMISSION

All species are transmitted by the bite of an infective female *Anopheles* mosquito. Occasionally, transmission occurs by blood transfusion, organ transplantation, needle sharing, or congenitally from mother to fetus.

EPIDEMIOLOGY

Malaria is a major international public health problem, causing an estimated 215 million infections worldwide and 655,000 deaths annually. Although these numbers are decreasing, the numbers of cases of malaria in travelers has been increasing steadily for the past 3 years. Despite the apparent progress in reducing the global prevalence of malaria, many areas remain malaria endemic, and the use of prevention measures by travelers is still inadequate. Information about malaria transmission in specific countries (see Travel Vaccines & Malaria Information, by Country later in this chapter) is derived from various sources, including the World Health Organization. The information presented herein was accurate at the time of publication; however, factors that can change rapidly and from year to year (such as local weather conditions, mosquito vector density, and prevalence of infection) can markedly affect local malaria transmission patterns. Updated information may be found on the CDC website at www.cdc.gov/malaria. Tools such as the Malaria Map Application can assist in locating more unusual destinations and determining if malaria transmission occurs there (www.cdc.gov/malaria/map).

Malaria transmission occurs in large areas of Africa, Central and South America, parts of the Caribbean, Asia (including South Asia, Southeast Asia, and the Middle East), Eastern Europe, and the South Pacific (Maps 3-9 and 3-10).

The risk for acquiring malaria differs substantially from traveler to traveler and from

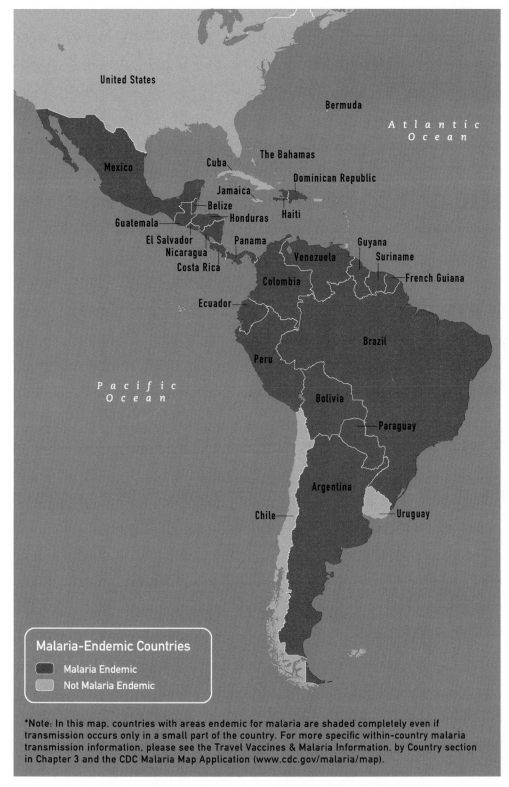

Malaria-Endemic Countries

■ Malaria Endemic
□ Not Malaria Endemic

*Note: In this map, countries with areas endemic for malaria are shaded completely even if transmission occurs only in a small part of the country. For more specific within-country malaria transmission information, please see the Travel Vaccines & Malaria Information, by Country section in Chapter 3 and the CDC Malaria Map Application (www.cdc.gov/malaria/map).

MAP 3-9. MALARIA-ENDEMIC COUNTRIES IN THE WESTERN HEMISPHERE

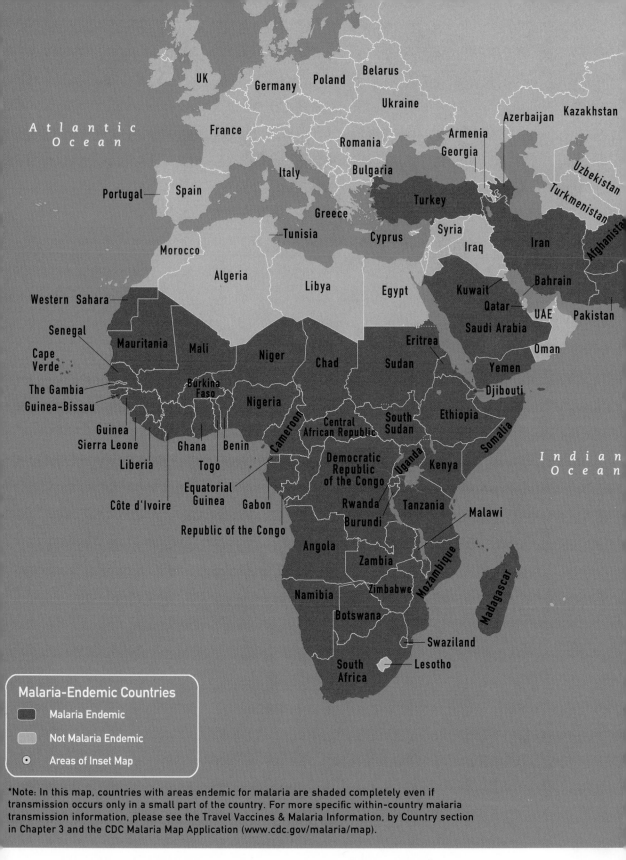

Malaria-Endemic Countries

■ Malaria Endemic

■ Not Malaria Endemic

◉ Areas of Inset Map

*Note: In this map, countries with areas endemic for malaria are shaded completely even if transmission occurs only in a small part of the country. For more specific within-country malaria transmission information, please see the Travel Vaccines & Malaria Information, by Country section in Chapter 3 and the CDC Malaria Map Application (www.cdc.gov/malaria/map).

MAP 3-10. MALARIA-ENDEMIC COUNTRIES IN THE EASTERN HEMISPHERE

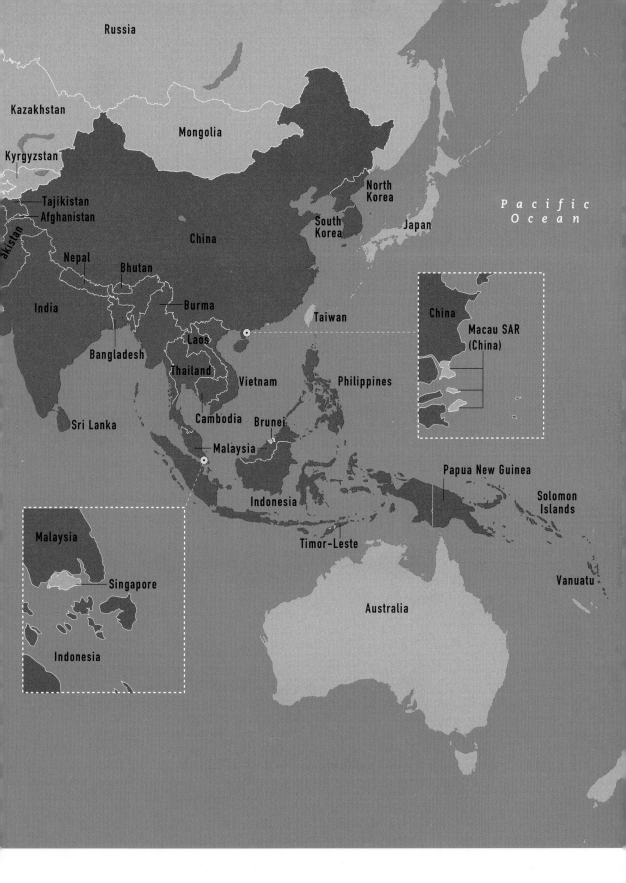

region to region, even within a single country. This variability is a function of the intensity of transmission within the various regions and the itinerary, duration, season, and type of travel. In 2010, almost 1,700 cases of malaria (including 9 deaths) were reported to CDC, the largest number since 1980. Of these, 65% were acquired in Africa, 19% in Asia, 15% in the Caribbean and the Americas, and <1% in Oceania. These absolute numbers of cases should be considered in the context of the volume of travel to these locations. Travelers with the highest estimated relative risk for infection are those going to West Africa and Oceania. Travelers going to other parts of Africa, South Asia, and South America have a moderate estimated relative risk for infection. Travelers with lower estimated relative risk are those going to Central America and other parts of Asia.

CLINICAL PRESENTATION

Malaria is characterized by fever and influenzalike symptoms, including chills, headache, myalgias, and malaise; these symptoms can occur at intervals. Uncomplicated disease may be associated with anemia and jaundice. In severe disease, seizures, mental confusion, kidney failure, acute respiratory distress syndrome, coma, and death may occur. Malaria symptoms can develop as early as 7 days (usually ≥14 days) after initial exposure in a malaria-endemic area and as late as several months or more after departure. Suspected or confirmed malaria, especially P. falciparum, is a medical emergency, requiring urgent intervention as clinical deterioration can occur rapidly and unpredictably. See Box 3-2 detailing some clinical highlights for malaria.

DIAGNOSIS

Travelers who have symptoms of malaria should seek medical evaluation **as soon as possible**. Physicians should consider malaria in any patient with a febrile illness who has recently returned from a malaria-endemic country.

Smear microscopy remains the gold standard for malaria diagnosis. Microscopy can also be used to determine the species of malaria parasite and quantify the parasitemia—both of which are necessary pieces of information for providing the most appropriate treatment. Microscopy results should

be available within a few hours. It is an unacceptable practice to send these tests to an offsite laboratory or batch them with results provided days later.

Various test kits are available to detect antigens derived from malaria parasites. Such immunologic (immunochromatographic) tests most often use a dipstick or cassette format and provide results in 2–15 minutes. These rapid diagnostic tests (RDTs) offer a useful alternative to microscopy in situations where reliable microscopic diagnosis is not immediately available. Although RDTs can detect malaria antigens within minutes, they cannot determine the species or quantify parasitemia. In addition, positive and negative results must always be confirmed by microscopy. While confirmation does not have to occur simultaneously with the RDT, the information from microscopy, including the actual presence of malaria parasites, the species, and parasitemia, will be most useful if it is available as soon as possible. The Food and Drug Administration (FDA) has approved one RDT for use in the United States by hospital and commercial laboratories, not by individual clinicians or by patients themselves. This RDT, called BinaxNOW Malaria test, is produced by Inverness Medical Professional Diagnostics, located in Scarborough, Maine.

PCR tests are also available for detecting malaria parasites. Although these tests are slightly more sensitive than routine microscopy, results are not usually available as quickly as microscopy results should be, thus limiting the utility of this test for acute diagnosis. PCR testing is most useful for definitively identifying the species of malaria parasite and detecting mixed infections. Species confirmation by PCR is available at the CDC malaria laboratory.

In sub-Saharan Africa, clinical overdiagnosis and the rate of false-positive microscopy for malaria may be high. Travelers to this region should be warned they may be diagnosed with malaria incorrectly, even though they are taking a reliable antimalarial regimen. In such cases, acutely ill travelers should be advised to seek the best available medical services and follow the treatment offered locally (except the use of halofantrine, which is not recommended; see below) but *not* to stop their chemoprophylaxis regimen.

BOX 3-2. CLINICAL HIGHLIGHTS FOR MALARIA

- Overdose of antimalarial drugs, particularly chloroquine, can be fatal. Medication should be stored in childproof containers out of the reach of infants and children.
- Chemoprophylaxis can be started earlier if there are particular concerns about tolerating one of the medications. For example, mefloquine can be started 3–4 weeks in advance to allow potential adverse events to occur before travel. If unacceptable side effects develop, there would be time to change the medication before the traveler's departure.
- The drugs used for antimalarial chemoprophylaxis are generally well tolerated. However, side effects can occur. Minor side effects usually do not require stopping the drug. Travelers who have serious side effects should see a clinician who can determine if their symptoms are related to the medicine and make a medication change.
- In comparison with drugs with short half-lives, which are taken daily, drugs with longer half-lives, which are taken weekly, offer the advantage of a wider margin of error if the traveler is late with a dose. For example, if a traveler is 1–2 days late with a weekly drug, prophylactic blood levels can remain adequate; if the traveler is 1–2 days late with a daily drug, protective blood levels are less likely to be maintained.
- In those who are G6PD deficient, primaquine can cause hemolysis, which can be fatal. Be sure to document a normal G6PD level before prescribing primaquine.
- Travelers should be informed that malaria could be fatal if treatment is delayed. Medical help should be sought promptly if malaria is suspected, and a blood sample should be taken and examined for malaria parasites on one or more occasions.
- Travelers should also be informed that malaria could be fatal even when treated, which is why it is always preferable to prevent malaria cases rather than rely on treating infections after they occur.
- Malaria smear results or a rapid diagnostic test must be available immediately (within a few hours). Sending specimens to offsite laboratories where results are not available for extended periods of time (days) is not acceptable. If a patient has an illness suggestive of severe malaria and a compatible travel history in an area where malaria transmission occurs, it is advisable to start treatment as soon as possible, even before the diagnosis is established. CDC recommendations for malaria treatment can be found at www.cdc.gov/malaria/diagnosis_treatment/index.html.

TREATMENT

Malaria can be treated effectively early in the course of the disease, but delay of therapy can have serious or even fatal consequences. Travelers who have symptoms of malaria should be advised to seek medical evaluation **as soon as possible**. Specific treatment options depend on the species of malaria, the likelihood of drug resistance (based on where the infection was acquired), the age of the patient, pregnancy status, and the severity of infection.

Detailed CDC recommendations for malaria treatment can be found at www.cdc.gov/malaria/diagnosis_treatment/treatment.html. Clinicians who require assistance with the diagnosis or treatment of malaria should call the CDC Malaria Hotline (770-488-7788 or toll-free at 855-856-4713) from 9 AM to 5 PM Eastern Time. After hours or on weekends and holidays, clinicians requiring assistance should call the CDC Emergency Operations Center at 770-488-7100 and ask the operator to page the person on call for the Malaria Branch. In addition, it is advisable to consult with a clinician who has specialized travel or tropical medicine expertise or with an infectious disease physician.

Medications that are not used in the United States for the treatment of malaria, such as halofantrine, are widely available overseas. CDC does not recommend halofantrine for treatment because of cardiac adverse events, including deaths, which have been documented after treatment. These adverse events have occurred in people with and without preexisting cardiac problems and both in the presence and absence of other antimalarial drugs (such as mefloquine).

Travelers who reject the advice to take prophylaxis, who choose a suboptimal drug regimen (such as chloroquine in an area with chloroquine-resistant *P. falciparum*), or who require a less-than-optimal drug regimen for medical reasons are at increased risk for acquiring malaria and needing prompt treatment while overseas. In addition, some travelers who are taking effective prophylaxis but who will be in remote areas may decide, in consultation with their travel health provider, to take along a reliable supply of a full course of an approved malaria treatment regimen (see Box 3-3 for a definition of *reliable supply*). In the event that they are diagnosed with malaria, they will have immediate access to this treatment regimen, which if acquired in the United States is unlikely to be counterfeit and will not deplete local resources. In rare instances when access to medical care is not available and the traveler develops a febrile illness consistent with malaria, the reliable supply medication can be self-administered presumptively. **Travelers should be advised that this self-treatment of a possible malarial infection is only a temporary measure and that prompt medical evaluation is imperative.**

Two malaria treatment regimens can be prescribed as a reliable supply: atovaquone-proguanil and artemether-lumefantrine. The use of the same or related drugs that have been taken for prophylaxis is not recommended to treat malaria. For example, atovaquone-proguanil may be used as a reliable supply medication by travelers not taking atovaquone-proguanil for prophylaxis. See Table 3-8 for the dosing recommendation.

PREVENTION

The goal of these malaria prevention guidelines is to prevent malaria caused by all species, not only *P. falciparum*. These guidelines apply to both short-term and long-term travelers. Malaria prevention consists of a combination of mosquito avoidance measures and chemoprophylaxis. Although efficacious, the recommended interventions are not 100% effective. For details about how CDC determines malaria prevention recommendations for travelers, see Box 3-4.

Preventing malaria involves striking a balance between ensuring that all people at risk for infection use the recommended prevention measures, while preventing rare occurrences of adverse effects of these interventions among people using them unnecessarily. An individual risk assessment should be conducted for every traveler, taking into account not only the destination country but also the detailed itinerary, including specific cities, types of accommodation, season, and style of travel. In addition, conditions such as pregnancy or antimalarial drug resistance at the destination may modify the risk assessment.

Depending on the level of risk, it may be appropriate to recommend no specific interventions, mosquito avoidance measures only, or mosquito avoidance measures plus chemoprophylaxis. For areas of intense transmission, such as West Africa, exposure for even short periods of time can result in transmission, so travelers to this area should be considered at high risk for infection. Malaria transmission is not distributed homogeneously throughout all countries. Some destinations have malaria transmission occurring only in certain areas. If travelers are going to the high-transmission areas

---

BOX 3-3. WHAT IS A RELIABLE SUPPLY?

A reliable supply is a complete course of an approved malaria treatment regimen obtained in the United States before travel. A reliable supply—

- Is not counterfeit
- Will not interact adversely with the patient's other medicines, including chemoprophylaxis
- Will not deplete local resources in the destination country

INFECTIOUS DISEASES RELATED TO TRAVEL

Table 3-8. Reliable supply regimens for the treatment of malaria

DRUG[1]	ADULT DOSE	PEDIATRIC DOSE	COMMENTS
Atovaquone-proguanil The adult tablet contains 250 mg atovaquone and 100 mg proguanil. The pediatric tablet contains 62.5 mg atovaquone and 25 mg proguanil.	4 adult tablets, orally as a single daily dose for 3 consecutive days	Daily dose to be taken for 3 consecutive days: 5–8 kg: 2 pediatric tablets 9–10 kg: 3 pediatric tablets 11–20 kg: 1 adult tablet 21–30 kg: 2 adult tablets 31–40 kg: 3 adult tablets >41 kg: 4 adult tablets	Contraindicated in people with severe renal impairment (creatinine clearance <30 mL/min) Not recommended for people on atovaquone-proguanil prophylaxis Not recommended for children weighing <5 kg, pregnant women, and women breastfeeding infants weighing <5 kg
Artemether-lumefantrine One tablet contains 20 mg artemether and 120 mg lumefantrine.	A 3-day treatment schedule with a total of 6 oral doses is recommended for both adult and pediatric patients based on weight. The patient should receive the initial dose, followed by the second dose 8 hours later, then 1 dose twice per day for the following 2 days. 5–<15 kg: 1 tablet per dose 15–<25 kg: 2 tablets per dose 25–<35 kg: 3 tablets per dose ≥35 kg: 4 tablets per dose		Not for people on mefloquine prophylaxis Not recommended for children weighing <5 kg, pregnant women, and women breastfeeding infants weighing <5 kg

[1] If used for presumptive self-treatment, medical care should be sought as soon as possible.

BOX 3-4. HOW CDC ARRIVES AT RECOMMENDATIONS FOR PREVENTING MALARIA AMONG TRAVELERS

Countries are not required to submit malaria surveillance data to CDC. On an ongoing basis, we actively solicit data from multiple sources, including World Health Organization (main and regional offices); national malaria control programs; international organizations, such as the International Society of Travel Medicine; CDC overseas staff; US Military; academic, research, and aid organizations; and published records from the medical literature. We also make judgments about the reliability and accuracy of those data. When possible, we assess trends and consider the data in the context of what we know about the malaria control activities within that country or other mitigating factors, such as natural disasters, wars, and other events that may be affecting the ability to control malaria or accurately count and report it. We consider factors such as the volume of travel to that country and the number of acquired cases reported in the US surveillance system. Based on all those considerations, we then try to accurately describe areas of that country where transmission occurs, substantial occurrences of antimalarial drug resistance, the proportions of species present, and the recommended chemoprophylaxis options.

during peak transmission times, even though the country as a whole may have lower amounts of malaria transmission, they may be at high risk for infection while there.

Geography is just one part of determining a traveler's risk for infection. Risk can differ substantially for different travelers if their behaviors and circumstances differ. For example, travelers staying in air-conditioned hotels may be at lower risk than backpackers or adventure travelers. Similarly, long-term residents living in screened and air-conditioned housing are less likely to be exposed than are people living without such amenities. The highest risk is associated with first- and second-generation immigrants living in non-endemic countries who return to their countries of origin to visit friends and relatives (VFRs). VFR travelers often consider themselves to be at no risk, because they grew up in a malarious country and consider themselves immune. However, acquired immunity is lost quickly, and VFRs should be considered to have the same risk as otherwise non-immune travelers (see Chapter 8, Immigrants Returning Home to Visit Friends & Relatives [VFRs]). Travelers should also be reminded that even if one has had malaria before, one can get it again, and preventive measures are still necessary.

Mosquito Avoidance Measures

Because of the nocturnal feeding habits of *Anopheles* mosquitoes, malaria transmission occurs primarily between dusk and dawn. Contact with mosquitoes can be reduced by remaining in well-screened areas, using mosquito bed nets (preferably insecticide-treated nets), using an effective insecticide spray in living and sleeping areas during evening and nighttime hours, and wearing clothes that cover most of the body.

All travelers should use an effective mosquito repellent (see Chapter 2, Protection against Mosquitoes, Ticks, & Other Insects & Arthropods). Repellents should be applied to exposed parts of the skin when mosquitoes are likely to be present. If travelers are also wearing sunscreen, sunscreen should be applied first and insect repellent second. In addition to using a topical insect repellent, a permethrin-containing product may be applied to bed nets and clothing for additional protection against mosquitoes.

Chemoprophylaxis

All recommended primary chemoprophylaxis regimens involve taking a medicine before, during, and after travel to an area with malaria. Beginning the drug before travel allows the antimalarial agent to be in the blood before the traveler is exposed to malaria parasites. In choosing a chemoprophylaxis regimen before travel, the traveler and the travel health provider should consider several factors. The travel itinerary should be reviewed in detail and compared with the information on where malaria transmission occurs within a given country, to determine whether the traveler will be traveling in a part of the country where malaria occurs and if antimalarial drug resistance has been reported in that location (see the Travel Vaccines & Malaria Information, by Country section later in this chapter). Additional factors to consider are the patient's other medical conditions, medications being taken (to assess potential drug interactions), the cost of the medicines, and the potential side effects. Table 3-9 lists some of the benefits and limitations of medicines used for malaria chemoprophylaxis; additional information about choosing a malaria chemoprophylaxis regimen can be found at www.cdc.gov/malaria/travelers/drugs.html.

The resistance of P. *falciparum* to chloroquine has been confirmed in all areas with P. *falciparum* malaria except the Caribbean, Central America west of the Panama Canal, and some countries in the Middle East. In addition, resistance to sulfadoxine-pyrimethamine is widespread in the Amazon River Basin area of South America, much of Southeast Asia, other parts of Asia, and in large parts of Africa. Resistance to mefloquine has been confirmed on the borders of Thailand with Burma (Myanmar) and Cambodia, in the western provinces of Cambodia, in the eastern states of Burma on the border between Burma and China, along the borders of Laos and Burma, the adjacent parts of the Thailand-Cambodia border, and in southern Vietnam. The resistance of P. *vivax* to chloroquine has been confirmed in Papua New Guinea and Indonesia.

In addition to primary prophylaxis, presumptive antirelapse therapy (also known as terminal prophylaxis) uses a medication toward the end of the exposure period (or immediately thereafter) to prevent relapses or

Table 3-9. Considerations when choosing a drug for malaria prophylaxis

DRUG	REASONS TO CONSIDER USE OF THIS DRUG	REASONS TO CONSIDER AVOIDING USE OF THIS DRUG
Atovaquone-proguanil	• Good for last-minute travelers because the drug is started 1–2 days before travel • Some people prefer to take a daily medicine • Good choice for shorter trips because the traveler takes the medicine for only 7 days after traveling rather than 4 weeks • Well tolerated—side effects uncommon • Pediatric tablets are available and may be more convenient	• Cannot be used by women who are pregnant or breastfeeding a child that weighs <5 kg • Cannot be taken by people with severe renal impairment • Tends to be more expensive than some of the other options (especially for long trips) • Some people (including children) would rather not take a medicine every day
Chloroquine	• Some people would rather take medicine weekly • Good choice for long trips because it is taken only weekly • Some people are already taking hydroxychloroquine chronically for rheumatologic conditions; in those instances, they may not have to take an additional medicine • Can be used in all trimesters of pregnancy	• Cannot be used in areas with chloroquine or mefloquine resistance • May exacerbate psoriasis • Some people would rather not take a weekly medication • For short trips, some people would rather not take medication for 4 weeks after travel • Not a good choice for last-minute travelers, because drug needs to be started 1–2 weeks before travel
Doxycycline	• Some people prefer to take a daily medicine • Good for last-minute travelers because the drug is started 1–2 days before travel • Tends to be the least expensive antimalarial • People who are already taking doxycycline chronically to prevent acne do not have to take an additional medicine • Doxycycline also can prevent some additional infections (such as rickettsial infections and leptospirosis), so it may be preferred by people planning to hike, camp, and swim in fresh water	• Cannot be used by pregnant women and children aged <8 years • Some people would rather not take a medicine every day • For short trips, some people would rather not take medication for 4 weeks after travel • Women prone to getting vaginal yeast infections when taking antibiotics may prefer taking a different medicine • People may want to avoid the increased risk of sun sensitivity • Some people are concerned about the potential of getting an upset stomach from doxycycline
Mefloquine	• Some people would rather take medicine weekly • Good choice for long trips because it is taken only weekly • Can be used in all trimesters of pregnancy	• Cannot be used in areas with mefloquine resistance • Cannot be used in patients with certain psychiatric conditions • Cannot be used in patients with a seizure disorder • Not recommended for people with cardiac conduction abnormalities • Not a good choice for last-minute travelers because drug needs to be started ≥2 weeks before travel • Some people would rather not take a weekly medication • For short trips, some people would rather not take medication for 4 weeks after travel

continued

TABLE 3-9. CONSIDERATIONS WHEN CHOOSING A DRUG FOR MALARIA PROPHYLAXIS (continued)

DRUG	REASONS TO CONSIDER USE OF THIS DRUG	REASONS TO CONSIDER AVOIDING USE OF THIS DRUG
Primaquine	• It is the most effective medicine for preventing *P. vivax*, so it is a good choice for travel to places with more than 90% *P. vivax* • Good choice for shorter trips because the traveler takes the medicine for 7 days after traveling rather than 4 weeks • Good for last-minute travelers because the drug is started 1–2 days before travel • Some people prefer to take a daily medicine	• Cannot be used in patients with glucose-6-phosphate dehydrogenase (G6PD) deficiency • Cannot be used in patients who have not been tested for G6PD deficiency • There are costs and delays associated with getting a G6PD test; however, it only has to be done once. Once a normal G6PD level is verified and documented, the test does not have to be repeated the next time primaquine is considered • Cannot be used by pregnant women • Cannot be used by women who are breastfeeding, unless the infant has also been tested for G6PD deficiency • Some people (including children) would rather not take a medicine every day • Some people are concerned about the potential of getting an upset stomach from primaquine

delayed-onset clinical presentations of malaria caused by hypnozoites (dormant liver stages) of *P. vivax* or *P. ovale*. Because most malarious areas of the world (except the Caribbean) have at least 1 species of relapsing malaria, travelers to these areas have some risk for acquiring either *P. vivax* or *P. ovale*, although the actual risk for an individual traveler is difficult to define. Presumptive antirelapse therapy is generally indicated only for people who have had prolonged exposure in malaria-endemic areas (such as missionaries, military personnel, or Peace Corps volunteers).

The medications recommended for chemoprophylaxis of malaria may also be available at overseas destinations. However, combinations of these medications and additional drugs that are not recommended may be commonly prescribed and used in other countries. Travelers should be strongly discouraged from obtaining chemoprophylaxis medications while abroad. The quality of these products is not known; they may not be protective and could be dangerous. These medications may have been produced by substandard manufacturing practices, may be counterfeit, or may contain contaminants.

Additional information on this topic can be found in Chapter 2, *Perspectives*: Pharmaceutical Quality & Counterfeit Drugs, and on the FDA website (www.fda.gov/Drugs/ResourcesForYou/Consumers/BuyingUsingMedicineSafely/BuyingMedicinefromOutsidetheUnitedStates/default.htm).

Medications Used for Chemoprophylaxis
Atovaquone-Proguanil

Atovaquone-proguanil is a fixed combination of the drugs atovaquone and proguanil. Prophylaxis should begin 1–2 days before travel to malarious areas and should be taken daily, at the same time each day, while in the malarious areas, and daily for 7 days after leaving the areas (see Table 3-10 for recommended dosages). Atovaquone-proguanil is well tolerated, and side effects are rare. The most common adverse effects reported in people using atovaquone-proguanil for prophylaxis or treatment are abdominal pain, nausea, vomiting, and headache. Atovaquone-proguanil is not recommended for prophylaxis in children weighing <5 kg (11 lb), pregnant women, or patients with severe renal impairment (creatinine clearance <30 mL/min). Proguanil may increase the effect of warfarin, so international normalized ratio monitoring or dosage adjustment may be needed.

Chloroquine and Hydroxychloroquine

Chloroquine phosphate or hydroxychloroquine sulfate can be used for prevention of malaria only in destinations where chloroquine resistance is not present (see Maps 3-9 and 3-10 and the Travel Vaccines & Malaria Information, by Country section later in this chapter). Prophylaxis should begin 1–2 weeks before travel to malarious areas. It should be continued by taking the drug once a week, on the same day of the week, during travel in malarious areas and for 4 weeks after a traveler leaves these areas (see Table 3-10 for recommended dosages). Reported side effects include gastrointestinal disturbance, headache, dizziness, blurred vision, insomnia, and pruritus, but generally these effects do not require that the drug be discontinued. High doses of chloroquine, such as those used to treat rheumatoid arthritis, have been associated with retinopathy; this serious side effect appears to be extremely unlikely when chloroquine is used for routine weekly malaria prophylaxis. Chloroquine and related compounds have been reported to exacerbate psoriasis. People who experience uncomfortable side effects after taking chloroquine may tolerate the drug better by taking it with meals. As an alternative, the related compound hydroxychloroquine sulfate may be better tolerated.

Doxycycline

Doxycycline prophylaxis should begin 1–2 days before travel to malarious areas. It should be continued once a day, at the same time each day, during travel in malarious areas and daily for 4 weeks after the traveler leaves such areas. Insufficient data exist on the antimalarial prophylactic efficacy of related compounds such as minocycline (commonly prescribed for the treatment of acne). People on a long-term regimen of minocycline who need malaria prophylaxis should stop taking minocycline 1–2 days before travel and start doxycycline instead. Minocycline can be restarted after the full course of doxycycline is completed (see Table 3-10 for recommended dosages).

Doxycycline can cause photosensitivity, usually manifested as an exaggerated sunburn reaction. The risk for such a reaction can be minimized by avoiding prolonged, direct exposure to the sun and by using sunscreen. In addition, doxycycline use is associated with an increased frequency of vaginal yeast infections. Gastrointestinal side effects (nausea or vomiting) may be minimized by taking the drug with a meal or by specifically prescribing doxycycline monohydrate or the enteric-coated doxycycline hyclate, rather than the generic doxycycline hyclate, which is often less expensive. To reduce the risk for esophagitis, travelers should be advised to swallow the medicine with sufficient fluids and not to take doxycycline before going to bed. Doxycycline is contraindicated in people with an allergy to tetracyclines, during pregnancy, and in infants and children aged <8 years. Vaccination with the oral typhoid vaccine Ty21a should be delayed for ≥24 hours after taking a dose of doxycycline.

Mefloquine

Mefloquine prophylaxis should begin ≥2 weeks before travel to malarious areas. It should be continued once a week, on the same day of the week, during travel in malarious areas and for 4 weeks after a traveler leaves such areas (see Table 3-10 for recommended dosages). Mefloquine has been associated with rare but serious adverse reactions (such as psychoses or seizures) at prophylactic doses; these reactions are more frequent with the higher doses used for treatment. Other side effects that have occurred in chemoprophylaxis studies include gastrointestinal disturbance, headache, insomnia, abnormal dreams, visual disturbances, depression, anxiety disorder, and dizziness. Other more severe neuropsychiatric disorders occasionally reported during postmarketing surveillance include sensory and motor neuropathies (including paresthesia, tremor, and ataxia), agitation or restlessness, mood changes, panic attacks, forgetfulness, confusion, hallucinations, aggression, paranoia, and encephalopathy. On occasion, psychiatric symptoms have been reported to continue long after mefloquine has been stopped. Mefloquine is contraindicated for use by travelers with a known hypersensitivity to mefloquine or related compounds (such as quinine or quinidine) and in people with active depression, a recent history of depression, generalized anxiety disorder, psychosis,

Table 3-10. Drugs used in the prophylaxis of malaria

DRUG	USAGE	ADULT DOSE	PEDIATRIC DOSE	COMMENTS
Atovaquone-proguanil	Prophylaxis in all areas	Adult tablets contain 250 mg atovaquone and 100 mg proguanil hydrochloride. 1 adult tablet orally, daily	Pediatric tablets contain 62.5 mg atovaquone and 25 mg proguanil hydrochloride. 5–8 kg: 1/2 pediatric tablet daily >8–10 kg: 3/4 pediatric tablet daily >10–20 kg: 1 pediatric tablet daily >20–30 kg: 2 pediatric tablets daily >30–40 kg: 3 pediatric tablets daily >40 kg: 1 adult tablet daily	Begin 1–2 days before travel to malarious areas. Take daily at the same time each day while in the malarious area and for 7 days after leaving such areas. Contraindicated in people with severe renal impairment (creatinine clearance <30 mL/min). Atovaquone-proguanil should be taken with food or a milky drink. Not recommended for prophylaxis for children weighing <5 kg, pregnant women, and women breastfeeding infants weighing <5 kg. Partial tablet doses may need to be prepared by a pharmacist and dispensed in individual capsules, as described in the text.
Chloroquine phosphate	Prophylaxis only in areas with chloroquine-sensitive malaria	300 mg base (500 mg salt) orally, once/week	5 mg/kg base (8.3 mg/kg salt) orally, once/week, up to a maximum adult dose of 300 mg base	Begin 1–2 weeks before travel to malarious areas. Take weekly on the same day of the week while in the malarious area and for 4 weeks after leaving such areas. May exacerbate psoriasis.
Doxycycline	Prophylaxis in all areas	100 mg orally, daily	≥8 years of age: 2.2 mg/kg up to adult dose of 100 mg/day	Begin 1–2 days before travel to malarious areas. Take daily at the same time each day while in the malarious area and for 4 weeks after leaving such areas. Contraindicated in children aged <8 years and pregnant women.
Hydroxychloroquine sulfate	An alternative to chloroquine for prophylaxis only in areas with chloroquine-sensitive malaria	310 mg base (400 mg salt) orally, once/week	5 mg/kg base (6.5 mg/kg salt) orally, once/week, up to a maximum adult dose of 310 mg base	Begin 1–2 weeks before travel to malarious areas. Take weekly on the same day of the week while in the malarious area and for 4 weeks after leaving such areas.

Mefloquine	Prophylaxis in areas with mefloquine-sensitive malaria	228 mg base (250 mg salt) orally, once/week	≤9 kg: 4.6 mg/kg base (5 mg/kg salt) orally, once/week >9–19 kg: 1/4 tablet once/week >19–30 kg: 1/2 tablet once/week >30–45 kg: 3/4 tablet once/week >45 kg: 1 tablet once/week	Begin ≥2 weeks before travel to malarious areas. Take weekly on the same day of the week while in the malarious area and for 4 weeks after leaving such areas. Contraindicated in people allergic to mefloquine or related compounds (quinine, quinidine) and in people with active depression, a recent history of depression, generalized anxiety disorder, psychosis, schizophrenia, other major psychiatric disorders, or seizures. Use with caution in people with psychiatric disturbances or a previous history of depression. Not recommended for people with cardiac conduction abnormalities.
Primaquine[1]	Prophylaxis for short-duration travel to areas with principally *P. vivax*	30 mg base (52.6 mg salt) orally, daily	0.5 mg/kg base (0.8 mg/kg salt) up to adult dose orally, daily	Begin 1–2 days before travel to malarious areas. Take daily at the same time each day while in the malarious area and for 7 days after leaving such areas. Contraindicated in people with G6PD deficiency. Also contraindicated during pregnancy and lactation, unless the infant being breastfed has a documented normal G6PD level.
	Used for presumptive antirelapse therapy (terminal prophylaxis) to decrease the risk for relapses of *P. vivax* and *P. ovale*	30 mg base (52.6 mg salt) orally, daily for 14 days after departure from the malarious area	0.5 mg/kg base (0.8 mg/kg salt) up to adult dose orally, daily for 14 days after departure from the malarious area	Indicated for people who have had prolonged exposure to *P. vivax*, *P. ovale*, or both. Contraindicated in people with G6PD deficiency. Also contraindicated during pregnancy and lactation, unless the infant being breastfed has a documented normal G6PD level.

Abbreviation: G6PD, glucose-6-phosphate dehydrogenase.
[1]All people who take primaquine should have a documented normal G6PD level before starting the medication.

schizophrenia, other major psychiatric disorders, or seizures. It should be used with caution in people with psychiatric disturbances or a history of depression. A review of available data suggests that mefloquine may be used in people concurrently on β-blockers, if they have no underlying arrhythmia. However, mefloquine is not recommended for people with cardiac conduction abnormalities. Any traveler receiving a prescription for mefloquine must also receive a copy of the FDA medication guide, which can be found at www.accessdata.fda.gov/drugsatfda_docs/label/2008/019591s023lbl.pdf.

Primaquine

Primaquine phosphate has 2 distinct uses for malaria prevention: primary prophylaxis in areas with primarily P. *vivax* and presumptive antirelapse therapy (terminal prophylaxis).

When taken for primary prophylaxis, primaquine should be taken 1–2 days before travel to malarious areas, daily, at the same time each day, while in the malarious areas, and daily for 7 days after leaving the areas (see Table 3-10 for recommended dosages). Primary prophylaxis with primaquine obviates the need for presumptive antirelapse therapy.

When used for presumptive antirelapse therapy, primaquine is administered for 14 days after the traveler has left a malarious area. When chloroquine, doxycycline, or mefloquine is used for primary prophylaxis, primaquine is usually taken during the last 2 weeks of postexposure prophylaxis. When atovaquone-proguanil is used for prophylaxis, primaquine may be taken during the final 7 days of atovaquone-proguanil, and then for an additional 7 days. Primaquine should be given concurrently with the primary prophylaxis medication. However, if that is not feasible, the primaquine course should still be administered after the primary prophylaxis medication has been completed.

The most common adverse event in people with normal glucose-6-phosphate dehydrogenase (G6PD) levels is gastrointestinal upset if primaquine is taken on an empty stomach. This problem is minimized or eliminated if primaquine is taken with food. In G6PD-deficient people, primaquine can cause hemolysis that can be fatal. **Before primaquine is used, G6PD deficiency MUST be ruled out by laboratory testing.**

Travel to Areas with Limited Malaria Transmission

For destinations where malaria cases occur sporadically and risk for infection to travelers is assessed as being low, CDC recommends that travelers use mosquito avoidance measures only, and no chemoprophylaxis should be prescribed (see the Travel Vaccines & Malaria Information, by Country section later in this chapter).

Travel to Areas with Mainly P. vivax Malaria

For destinations where the main species of malaria present is P. *vivax*, in addition to mosquito avoidance measures, primaquine is a good choice for primary prophylaxis for travelers who are not G6PD deficient. Its use for this indication is considered off-label in the United States. The predominant species of malaria and the recommended chemoprophylaxis medicines are listed in the Travel Vaccines & Malaria Information, by Country section later in this chapter. For people unable to take primaquine, other drugs can be used as described below, depending on the presence of antimalarial drug resistance.

Travel to Areas with Chloroquine-Sensitive Malaria

For destinations where chloroquine-sensitive malaria is present, in addition to mosquito avoidance measures, the many effective chemoprophylaxis options include chloroquine, atovaquone-proguanil, doxycycline, mefloquine, and in some instances, primaquine for travelers who are not G6PD-deficient. Longer-term travelers may prefer the convenience of weekly chloroquine, while shorter-term travelers may prefer the shorter course of atovaquone-proguanil or primaquine.

Travel to Areas with Chloroquine-Resistant Malaria

For destinations where chloroquine-resistant malaria is present, in addition to mosquito avoidance measures, chemoprophylaxis options are atovaquone-proguanil, doxycycline, and mefloquine.

Travel to Areas with Mefloquine-Resistant Malaria

For destinations where mefloquine-resistant malaria is present, in addition to mosquito avoidance measures, chemoprophylaxis options are either atovaquone-proguanil or doxycycline.

Chemoprophylaxis for Infants, Children, and Adolescents

Infants of any age or weight or children and adolescents of any age can contract malaria. Therefore, all children traveling to malaria-endemic areas should use the recommended prevention measures, which often include taking an antimalarial drug. In the United States, antimalarial drugs are available only in oral formulations and may taste bitter. Pediatric doses should be carefully calculated according to body weight but should never exceed adult dose. Pharmacists can pulverize tablets and prepare gelatin capsules for each measured dose. If the child is unable to swallow the capsules or tablets, parents should prepare the child's dose of medication by breaking open the gelatin capsule and mixing the drug with a small amount of something sweet, such as applesauce, chocolate syrup, or jelly, to ensure the entire dose is delivered to the child. Giving the dose on a full stomach may minimize stomach upset and vomiting.

Chloroquine and mefloquine are options for use in infants and children of all ages and weights, depending on drug resistance at their destination. Primaquine can be used for children who are not G6PD-deficient traveling to areas with principally P. vivax. Doxycycline may be used for children who are aged ≥8 years. Atovaquone-proguanil may be used for prophylaxis for infants and children weighing ≥5 kg (11 lb). Prophylactic dosing for children weighing <11 kg (24 lb) constitutes off-label use in the United States. Pediatric dosing regimens are contained in Table 3-10.

Chemoprophylaxis during Pregnancy and Breastfeeding

Malaria infection in pregnant women can be more severe than in non-pregnant women. Malaria can increase the risk for adverse pregnancy outcomes, including prematurity, spontaneous abortion, and stillbirth. For these reasons, and because no chemoprophylaxis regimen is completely effective, women who are pregnant or likely to become pregnant should be advised to avoid travel to areas with malaria transmission if possible (see Chapter 8, Pregnant Travelers). If travel to a malarious area cannot be deferred, use of an effective chemoprophylaxis regimen is essential.

Pregnant women traveling to areas where chloroquine-resistant P. falciparum has not been reported may take chloroquine prophylaxis. Chloroquine has not been found to have any harmful effects on the fetus when used in the recommended doses for malaria prophylaxis; therefore, pregnancy is not a contraindication for malaria prophylaxis with chloroquine phosphate or hydroxychloroquine sulfate. For travel to areas where chloroquine resistance is present, mefloquine is the only medication recommended for malaria chemoprophylaxis during pregnancy. In 2011, the FDA reviewed available data for mefloquine use during pregnancy and reclassified it from category C (animal reproduction studies have shown an adverse effect on the fetus and there are no adequate and well-controlled studies in humans, but potential benefits may warrant use of the drug in pregnant women despite potential risks) to category B (animal reproduction studies have failed to demonstrate a risk to the fetus and there are no adequate and well-controlled studies in pregnant women).

Because of insufficient data regarding its use during pregnancy, atovaquone-proguanil is not recommended to prevent malaria in pregnant women. Doxycycline is contraindicated for malaria prophylaxis during pregnancy because of the risk for adverse effects seen with tetracycline, a related drug, on the fetus, which include discoloration and dysplasia of the teeth and inhibition of bone growth. Primaquine should not be used during pregnancy because the drug may be passed transplacentally to a G6PD-deficient fetus and cause hemolytic anemia in utero.

Very small amounts of antimalarial drugs are excreted in the breast milk of lactating women. Because the quantity of antimalarial drugs transferred in breast milk is insufficient to provide adequate protection against malaria, infants who require chemoprophylaxis must receive the recommended dosages of antimalarial drugs listed in Table 3-10. Because chloroquine and mefloquine may be safely prescribed to infants, it is also safe for infants to be exposed to the small amounts excreted in breast milk. Although data are very limited about the use of doxycycline in lactating women, most experts consider the theoretical possibility of adverse events to the infant to be remote.

Although no information is available on the amount of primaquine that enters human breast milk, the mother and infant should be tested for G6PD deficiency before primaquine is given to a woman who is breastfeeding. Because data are not yet available on the safety of atovaquone-proguanil prophylaxis in infants weighing <5 kg (11 lb), CDC does not recommend it to prevent malaria in women breastfeeding infants weighing <5 kg. However, it can be used to treat women who are breastfeeding infants of any weight when the potential benefit outweighs the potential risk to the infant (such as treating a breastfeeding woman who has acquired P. falciparum malaria in an area of multidrug-resistant strains and who cannot tolerate other treatment options).

Choosing a Drug to Prevent Malaria

Recommendations for drugs to prevent malaria differ by country of travel and can be found in the Travel Vaccines & Malaria Information, by Country section later in this chapter. Recommended drugs for each country are listed in alphabetical order and have comparable efficacy in that country. No antimalarial drug is 100% protective; therefore, prophylaxis must be combined with the use of personal protective measures (such as insect repellent, long sleeves, long pants, sleeping in a mosquito-free setting or using an insecticide-treated bed net). When several different drugs are recommended for an area, Table 3-9 may help in the decision-making process.

Changing Medications as a Result of Side Effects during Chemoprophylaxis

Medications recommended for prophylaxis against malaria have different modes of action that affect the parasites at different stages of the life cycle. Thus, if the medication needs to be changed because of side effects before a full course has been completed, there are some special considerations (see Table 3-11).

BLOOD DONATION AFTER TRAVEL TO MALARIOUS AREAS

People who have been in an area where malaria transmission occurs are not permitted to donate blood in the United States for a period of time after returning from the malarious area to prevent transmission of malaria through blood transfusion (Table 3-12).

Risk assessments may differ between travel health providers and blood banks. A travel health provider advising a traveler going to a country with a relatively low amount of malaria transmission for a short period of time and engaging in low-risk behaviors may appropriately choose insect avoidance only and no chemoprophylaxis for the traveler. However, upon the traveler's return, a blood bank may still choose to defer that traveler for 1 year because of the travel to an area where transmission occurs.

CDC website: www.cdc.gov/malaria

Table 3-11. Changing medications as a result of side effects during chemoprophylaxis

DRUG BEING STOPPED	DRUG BEING STARTED	COMMENTS
Mefloquine	Doxycycline	Begin doxycycline, continue daily while in malaria-endemic area, and continue for 4 weeks after leaving malaria-endemic area.
	Atovaquone-proguanil	• If the switch occurs ≥3 weeks before departure from the endemic area, atovaquone-proguanil should be taken daily for the rest of the stay in the endemic area and for 1 week thereafter. • If the switch occurs <3 weeks before departure from the endemic area, atovaquone-proguanil should be taken daily for 4 weeks after the switch. • If the switch occurs after departure from the endemic area, atovaquone-proguanil should be taken daily until 4 weeks after the date of departure.
	Chloroquine	Not recommended
	Primaquine	Not recommended

continued

TABLE 3-11. CHANGING MEDICATIONS AS A RESULT OF SIDE EFFECTS DURING CHEMOPROPHYLAXIS (continued)

DRUG BEING STOPPED	DRUG BEING STARTED	COMMENTS
Doxycycline	Mefloquine Atovaquone-proguanil	Not recommended • If the switch occurs ≥3 weeks before departure from the endemic area, atovaquone-proguanil should be taken daily for the rest of the stay in the endemic area and for 1 week thereafter. • If the switch occurs <3 weeks before departure from the endemic area, atovaquone-proguanil should be taken daily for 4 weeks after the switch. • If the switch occurs after departure from the endemic area, atovaquone-proguanil should be taken daily until 4 weeks after the date of departure.
	Chloroquine	Not recommended
	Primaquine	Not recommended
Atovaquone-proguanil	Doxycycline	Begin doxycycline, continue daily while in malaria-endemic area, and continue for 4 weeks after leaving malaria-endemic area.
	Mefloquine	Not recommended
	Chloroquine	Not recommended
	Primaquine	This switch would be unlikely as primaquine is only recommended for primary prophylaxis in areas with mainly *P. vivax* for people with normal G6PD activity. Should that be the case, begin primaquine, continue daily while in malaria-endemic area, and continue for 7 days after leaving malaria-endemic area.
Chloroquine	Doxycycline	Begin doxycycline, continue daily while in malaria-endemic area, and continue for 4 weeks after leaving malaria-endemic area.
	Atovaquone-proguanil	• If the switch occurs ≥3 weeks before departure from the endemic area, atovaquone-proguanil should be taken daily for the rest of the stay in the endemic area and for 1 week thereafter. • If the switch occurs <3 weeks before departure from the endemic area, atovaquone-proguanil should be taken daily for 4 weeks after the switch. • If the switch occurs following departure from the endemic area, atovaquone-proguanil should be taken daily until 4 weeks after the date of departure.
	Mefloquine	Not recommended
	Primaquine	Not recommended
Primaquine	Doxycycline	Begin doxycycline, continue daily while in malaria-endemic area, and continue for 4 weeks after leaving malaria-endemic area.
	Atovaquone-proguanil	Begin atovaquone-proguanil, continue daily while in malaria-endemic area, and continue for 7 days after leaving malaria-endemic area.
	Chloroquine	Not recommended
	Mefloquine	Not recommended

Table 3-12. Food and Drug Administration recommendations for deferring blood donation in people returning from malarious areas

GROUP	BLOOD DONATION DEFERRAL
Travelers to malaria-endemic areas	May not donate blood for 1 year after travel
Former residents of malaria-endemic areas	May not donate blood for 3 years after departing
People diagnosed with malaria	May not donate for 3 years after treatment

BIBLIOGRAPHY

1. Baird JK, Fryauff DJ, Hoffman SL. Primaquine for prevention of malaria in travelers. Clin Infect Dis. 2003 Dec 15;37(12):1659–67.

2. Boggild AK, Parise ME, Lewis LS, Kain KC. Atovaquone-proguanil: report from the CDC expert meeting on malaria chemoprophylaxis (II). Am J Trop Med Hyg. 2007 Feb;76(2):208–23.

3. CDC. CDC malaria map application. Atlanta: CDC; 2010 [updated 2012 Mar 6; cited 2012 Sep 21]. Available from: http://www.cdc.gov/malaria/map/index.html.

4. CDC. Malaria. Atlanta: CDC; 2010 [updated 2012 Aug 9; cited 2012 Sep 21]. Available from: http://www.cdc.gov/malaria.

5. Fradin MS, Day JF. Comparative efficacy of insect repellents against mosquito bites. N Engl J Med. 2002 Jul 4;347(1):13–8.

6. Hill DR, Baird JK, Parise ME, Lewis LS, Ryan ET, Magill AJ. Primaquine: report from CDC expert meeting on malaria chemoprophylaxis I. Am J Trop Med Hyg. 2006 Sep;75(3):402–15.

7. Kitchen AD, Chiodini PL. Malaria and blood transfusion. Vox Sang. 2006 Feb;90(2):77–84.

8. Kochar DK, Saxena V, Singh N, Kochar SK, Kumar SV, Das A. Plasmodium vivax malaria. Emerg Infect Dis. 2005 Jan;11(1):132–4.

9. Leder K, Black J, O'Brien D, Greenwood Z, Kain KC, Schwartz E, et al. Malaria in travelers: a review of the GeoSentinel surveillance network. Clin Infect Dis. 2004 Oct 15;39(8):1104–12.

10. Leder K, Tong S, Weld L, Kain KC, Wilder-Smith A, von Sonnenburg F, et al. Illness in travelers visiting friends and relatives: a review of the GeoSentinel Surveillance Network. Clin Infect Dis. 2006 Nov 1;43(9):1185–93.

11. Mali S, Kachur SP, Arguin PM. Malaria surveillance—United States, 2010. MMWR Surveill Summ. 2012 Mar 2;61(2):1–17.

12. Newman RD, Parise ME, Barber AM, Steketee RW. Malaria-related deaths among US travelers, 1963–2001. Ann Intern Med. 2004 Oct 5;141(7):547–55.

13. Reyburn H, Mbatia R, Drakeley C, Carneiro I, Mwakasungula E, Mwerinde O, et al. Overdiagnosis of malaria in patients with severe febrile illness in Tanzania: a prospective study. BMJ. 2004 Nov 20;329(7476):1212.

14. Schwartz E, Parise M, Kozarsky P, Cetron M. Delayed onset of malaria—implications for chemoprophylaxis in travelers. N Engl J Med. 2003 Oct 16;349(16):1510–6.

15. Steinhardt LC, Magill AJ, Arguin PM. Review: Malaria chemoprophylaxis for travelers to Latin America. Am J Trop Med Hyg. 2011 Dec;85(6):1015–24.

16. Tan KR, Magill AJ, Parise ME, Arguin PM. Doxycycline for malaria chemoprophylaxis and treatment: report from the CDC expert meeting on malaria chemoprophylaxis. Am J Trop Med Hyg. 2011 Apr;84(4):517–31.

17. Whitty CJ, Edmonds S, Mutabingwa TK. Malaria in pregnancy. BJOG. 2005 Sep;112(9):1189–95.

18. World Health Organization. World malaria report 2011. Geneva: World Health Organization; 2011 [cited 2012 Sep 21]. Available from: http://www.who.int/malaria/world_malaria_report_2011/en/.

For the Record

A HISTORY OF MALARIA CHEMOPROPHYLAXIS

Alan J. Magill

Among the many dreaded fevers that plague man, "marsh fever" was distinguished by its periodicity, enlarged spleen, and pattern of attacking those exposed to wet, warm, boggy areas. In the mid-1700s, it became known by its Italian name, *mal'aria* ("bad air"), referring to bad or foul air emanating from swampy lands. The discovery and development of drugs to treat and prevent malaria have been driven for centuries by the desire and need to protect travelers, military personnel, explorers, and the commercial interest of imperial powers when they went into the malaria-endemic tropics.

HISTORICAL MILESTONES IN ANTIMALARIAL CHEMOPROPHYLAXIS

- 1620s: Jesuit missionaries living in Peru learned the healing power of powdered bark, often known as "Jesuits bark," from the cinchona trees growing in the high forests of Peru and Bolivia.
- 1768: James Lind, a British naval surgeon, recommended that "every man receive a daily ration of cinchona powder" as long as a ship lay at anchor in any tropical port. His advice, however, was not widely accepted, and it would be almost 100 years before the concept of chemoprophylaxis would be accepted.
- Early 1800s: Crews of the British Royal Navy manning the blockade of the West African coast to suppress the Atlantic slave trade were decimated by malaria.
- 1820: French chemists isolated quinine, the most active compound in cinchona bark, which allowed for quinine's expanded availability and use.
- 1854: The Scottish surgeon William Balfour Baikie gave 6–8 grains (1 grain = 65 mg) of quinine, half in the morning and half in the evening, dissolved in sherry, to all the ship's crew during a 118-day expedition up the river Benue in modern-day Nigeria. No men died. This unprecedented accomplishment gradually led to acceptance that malaria could be prevented by chemoprophylaxis.
- 1861: Quinine first saw widespread use as a prophylactic agent in the American Civil War when both the Union and Confederate Armies, plagued with malaria, used massive quantities to prevent the disease.
- 1880: A French military physician working in Algeria, Alphonse Laveran, discovered parasites in the blood of a French soldier. The identification of the infectious agent and its life cycle was an essential step in opening the way to the development of effective prophylactic agents.
- 1914–1918: During World War I, both Allied and Axis militaries suffered terribly from malaria. German armies were denied access to quinine, as most was held by a monopoly of Dutch growers on the island of Java.
- 1920s: German chemists pursued a synthetic route to new antimalarial drugs to circumvent the Dutch monopoly, achieving spectacular success with the introduction of pamaquine and mepacrine during the 1930s.
- 1941: With America's entry into World War II, trade between the United States and Germany ceased, and mepacrine was no longer available to the Allies.
- 1942: Japanese armies overran the Dutch cinchona plantations on Java, cutting off the supply of quinine and leaving the Allies with no antimalarial drugs.
- 1943: American scientists quickly devised a manufacturing process for mepacrine, and the drug was given as a treatment and as a prophylactic under the name Atabrine. Meanwhile, the Allies, especially the Americans, launched the largest antimalarial drug discovery and development program the world had seen. By 1945, several new antimalarial drugs had been introduced, including chloroquine and proguanil. Chloroquine went on to assume a role both in prophylaxis for travelers and as a treatment drug for endemic areas.
- 1959: Chloroquine-resistant *Plasmodium falciparum* malaria was first reported.
- 1965: Large-scale American military involvement began in South Vietnam, reaching almost 200,000 soldiers by the end of 1965. Chloroquine-resistant malaria caused illness and death in US forces.

- 1967: A second massive US government–sponsored antimalarial drug discovery effort centered at the Walter Reed Army Institute of Research began and led to the discovery of mefloquine.
- 1971: During studies of volunteers with experimentally induced malaria infections, it was observed that tetracycline, administered to treat intercurrent bacterial infections, appeared to exert blood schizontocidal activity against chloroquine-resistant *P. falciparum*. A few additional studies were performed with tetracycline, doxycycline, and minocycline, but no formal development of the drug as an antimalarial was pursued.
- Early 1980s: The Wellcome Research Laboratories developed atovaquone as an antimalarial drug. Clinical trials in uncomplicated *P. falciparum* malaria as monotherapy were disappointing, with early treatment failures due to the emergence of atovaquone-resistant parasites. However, combining atovaquone with proguanil led to an efficacious combination therapy.
- 1982: The fixed combination of pyrimethamine and sulfadoxine (Fansidar) became available in the United States and was recommended by CDC for prophylactic use in travelers at risk of acquiring chloroquine-resistant *P. falciparum*.
- 1985: Pyrimethamine-sulfadoxine as weekly malaria chemoprophylaxis was abruptly withdrawn because of fatal cases of Stevens-Johnson syndrome. Since no alternative drugs were licensed to prevent chloroquine-resistant *P. falciparum* malaria, CDC recommended daily doxycycline for antimalarial prophylaxis.
- Late 1980s: The US Army conducted several field and human challenge clinical trials demonstrating the efficacy of doxycycline as malaria prophylaxis.
- 1989: The US Food and Drug Administration (FDA) approved mefloquine (Lariam).
- 1992: Pfizer, at the request of FDA, submitted a supplemental new drug application for doxycycline for malaria chemoprophylaxis.
- 2000: Combination of fixed dose atovaquone-proguanil (Malarone) approved by FDA.

The 3 largest antimalarial drug development efforts of modern times occurred during and after major conflicts of the 20th Century—World War I, World War II, and the Vietnam War. The modern history of developing drugs to prevent malaria grew almost entirely from the need to protect military personnel and keep them healthy to conduct combat operations in malaria-endemic areas. Those massive government-funded efforts produced the drugs now used to keep modern civilian travelers safe from the sickness and death that mark malaria's march through time.

BIBLIOGRAPHY

1. Greenwood D. Conflicts of interest: the genesis of synthetic antimalarial agents in peace and war. J Antimicrob Chemother. 1995 Nov;36(5):857–72.
2. Kitchen LW, Vaughn DW, Skillman DR. Role of US military research programs in the development of US Food and Drug Administration—approved antimalarial drugs. Clin Infect Dis. 2006 Jul 1;43(1):67–71.
3. Smith DC. Quinine and fever: The development of the effective dosage. J Hist Med Allied Sci. 1976 Jul;31(3):343–67.
4. Smith DC, Sanford LB. Laveran's germ: the reception and use of a medical discovery. Am J Trop Med Hyg. 1985 Jan;34(1):2–20.
5. Sweeney AW. Wartime research on malaria chemotherapy. Parassitologia. 2000 Jun;42(1–2):33–45.

MEASLES (RUBEOLA)

Amy Parker Fiebelkorn, James L. Goodson

INFECTIOUS AGENT

Measles virus is a member of the genus *Morbillivirus* of the family Paramyxoviridae.

TRANSMISSION

Measles is transmitted primarily from person to person by large respiratory droplets but can also spread by the airborne route as aerosolized droplet nuclei. Infected people are usually contagious from 4 days before until 4 days after rash onset. Measles is one of the most contagious viral diseases known; secondary attack rates are >90% in susceptible household and institutional contacts. Humans are the only natural host for sustaining measles virus transmission, which makes global eradication of measles feasible.

EPIDEMIOLOGY

The number of reported measles cases in the United States has declined from nearly 900,000 annually in the early 1940s to an average of 83 cases annually from 2001 through 2011. As a result of high vaccination coverage and better measles control in the Americas, in 2000, measles was declared eliminated (no disease transmission for at least 12 months) in the United States. Indigenous measles virus circulation was interrupted in 2002 in the rest of the Western Hemisphere. However, measles virus continues to be imported into the United States from other parts of the world. Globally, an estimated 20 million measles cases occur each year. Given the large global incidence and high communicability of the disease, travelers may be exposed to the virus in almost any country they visit, particularly those outside the Western Hemisphere, where measles is endemic or where large outbreaks are occurring. Of the 222 reported measles cases in the United States in 2011, 200 (90%) were associated with importations from other countries, including 72 direct importations (52 among US residents traveling abroad and 20 among foreign visitors). The largest percentage of importations (46%) was among people who acquired the disease in Europe. However, importations consistently occur from other countries and regions, including India and the Philippines. Additional information on global measles control efforts is available on the Measles Initiative website at www.measlesinitiative.org.

CLINICAL PRESENTATION

The incubation period ranges from 7 to 21 days from exposure to onset of fever; rash usually appears about 14 days after exposure. Symptoms include prodromal fever that can rise as high as 105°F (40.6°C), conjunctivitis, coryza (runny nose), cough, and small spots with white or bluish-white centers on an erythematous base on the buccal mucosa (Koplik spots). A characteristic red, blotchy (maculopapular) rash appears on the third to seventh day after the prodromal symptoms appear. The rash begins on the face, becomes generalized, and lasts 4–7 days. Common complications include diarrhea (8%), middle ear infection (7%–9%), and pneumonia (1%–6%). Encephalitis, which can result in permanent brain damage, occurs in approximately 1 per 1,000–2,000 cases of measles.

Subacute sclerosing panencephalitis (SSPE), a rare but serious degenerative central nervous system disease caused by a persistent infection with a defective measles virus, is estimated to occur in 1 per 100,000 cases. However, among people who became infected with measles during the 1989–1991 measles resurgence in the United States, the estimated risk of SSPE was 22 per 100,000 reported measles cases. SSPE is manifested by mental and motor deterioration that starts an average of 7–10 years after measles virus infection (most frequently in children who were infected at age <2 years), progressing to coma and death. The risk of serious complications and death is highest for children aged ≤5 years and adults aged ≥20 years. It is also higher in populations with poor nutritional status.

DIAGNOSIS

Laboratory criteria for diagnosis include any of the following: a positive serologic test for measles IgM, IgG seroconversion, a significant rise in measles IgG level by any standard serologic assay, isolation of measles virus, or identification by PCR of measles virus RNA from a clinical specimen.

A clinical case of measles illness is characterized by all of the following:

- Generalized maculopapular rash lasting ≥3 days
- Temperature of ≥101°F (38.3°C)
- Cough, coryza, or conjunctivitis

A confirmed case is one that is either laboratory-confirmed or that meets the clinical case definition and is epidemiologically linked to a confirmed case. A laboratory-confirmed case does not need to meet the clinical case definition.

TREATMENT

Treatment is supportive. The World Health Organization recommends vitamin A for all children with acute measles, regardless of their country of residence, to reduce the risk of complications. Vitamin A is administered once a day for 2 days at the following doses:

- 50,000 IU for infants aged <6 months
- 100,000 IU for infants aged 6–11 months
- 200,000 IU for children aged ≥12 months

An additional (third) age-specific dose of vitamin A should be given 2–4 weeks later to children with clinical signs and symptoms of vitamin A deficiency. Parenteral and oral formulations of vitamin A are available in the United States.

PREVENTION

Measles has been preventable since 1963 through vaccination. People who do not have evidence of measles immunity should be considered at risk for measles during international travel. Acceptable presumptive evidence of immunity to measles for international travelers includes meeting any of the following criteria:

- For infants aged 6–11 months, documented administration of 1 dose of live measles-containing vaccine (MCV) and for people

aged ≥12 months, 2 doses of MCV ≥28 days apart, on or after the first birthday
- Laboratory evidence of immunity
- Birth before 1957
- Documented physician-diagnosed measles

Vaccine

Measles vaccine contains live, attenuated measles virus. In the United States, it is available only in combination formulations, such as measles-mumps-rubella (MMR) and measles-mumps-rubella-varicella (MMRV) vaccine. MMRV vaccine is licensed for children aged 12 months to 12 years and may be used in place of MMR vaccine if vaccination for measles, mumps, rubella, and varicella is needed.

International travelers, including people traveling to industrialized countries, who do not have presumptive evidence of measles immunity and who have no contraindications to MCV, should receive MCV before travel according to the following guidelines:

- Infants aged 6–11 months should receive 1 MCV dose. Infants vaccinated before age 12 months must be revaccinated on or after the first birthday with 2 doses of MCV separated by ≥28 days. MMRV is not licensed for children aged <12 months.
- Preschool and school-age children (aged ≥12 months) should be given 2 MCV doses separated by ≥28 days.
- Adults born in or after 1957 should be given 2 MCV doses separated by ≥28 days.

One dose of MCV is approximately 85% effective if administered at age 9 months and up to 95% effective if administered at age ≥1 year. More than 99% of people who receive 2 doses of MCV develop serologic evidence of measles immunity.

MCV and immune globulin (IG) may be effective as postexposure prophylaxis. MCV, if administered within 72 hours after initial exposure to measles virus, may provide some protection. If the exposure does not result in infection, the vaccine should induce protection against subsequent measles virus infection. IG can be used to prevent or mitigate measles in a susceptible person when administered within 6 days of exposure. However, any immunity conferred is temporary unless modified or typical measles occurs, and the person should receive MCV 5–6 months after IG administration.

Vaccine Safety and Adverse Reactions

In rare circumstances, MMR vaccination has been associated with the following adverse events:

- Anaphylaxis (approximately 1–3.5 occurrences per million doses administered)
- Thrombocytopenia (a rate of 1 case in every 25,000 doses during the 6 weeks after immunization)
- Febrile seizures (The risk of febrile seizures increases approximately 3-fold 8–14 days after receipt of MMR vaccine, but overall, the rate of febrile seizure after MCV is much lower than the rate after measles disease.)
- Joint symptoms (Arthralgia develops among approximately 25% of susceptible postpubertal women from the rubella component of the MMR vaccination. Approximately 10% have acute arthritislike signs and symptoms that generally persist for 1 day to 3 weeks and rarely recur. Chronic joint symptoms are rare, if they occur at all.)

Evidence does not support a causal link between MMR vaccination and any of the following: hearing loss, retinopathy, optic neuritis, ocular palsies, Guillain-Barré syndrome, cerebellar ataxia, Crohn disease, or autism. A published report on MMR vaccination and inflammatory bowel disease and pervasive developmental disorders (such as autism) has never been replicated by other studies, and has subsequently been widely discredited and retracted by the journal.

Compared with use of MMR and varicella vaccines at the same visit, use of MMRV vaccine is associated with a higher risk for fever and febrile seizures 5–12 days after the first dose among children aged 12–23 months, and approximately 1 additional febrile seizure for every 2,300–2,600 MMRV vaccine doses administered. Use of separate MMR and varicella vaccines avoids this increased risk for fever and febrile seizures.

Precautions and Contraindications
Allergy

People with severe allergy (hives, swelling of the mouth or throat, difficulty breathing, hypotension, and shock) to gelatin or neomycin, or who have had a severe allergic reaction to a prior dose of MMR or MMRV vaccine, should not be revaccinated. MMR or MMRV vaccines may be administered to people who are allergic to eggs without prior routine skin testing or the use of special protocols.

Immunosuppression

Enhanced replication of vaccine viruses can occur in people who have immune deficiency disorders. Death related to vaccine-associated measles virus infection has been reported among severely immunocompromised people. Therefore, severely immunosuppressed people should not be vaccinated with MMR or MMRV vaccines (for a thorough discussion of recommendations for immunocompromised travelers, see Chapter 8, Immunocompromised Travelers):

- People with leukemia in remission, and off chemotherapy, who were not immune to measles when diagnosed with leukemia may receive MMR vaccine. At least 3 months should elapse after termination of chemotherapy before administration of the first dose.
- MMR vaccination is recommended for all asymptomatic HIV-infected people who do not have evidence of severe immunosuppression (age-specific CD4 T-lymphocyte percentages of ≥15% of total) and for whom measles vaccination would otherwise be indicated. MMR vaccination should also be considered for all symptomatic HIV-infected people who do not have evidence of severe immunosuppression.
- People who have received high-dose corticosteroid therapy (in general, considered to be >20 mg prednisone or equivalent daily or on alternate days for an interval of ≥14 days) should avoid vaccination with MMR or MMRV for ≥1 month after cessation of steroid therapy.
- People who have received high-dose corticosteroid therapy daily or on alternate days for an interval of <14 days generally can be vaccinated with MMR or MMRV immediately after cessation of treatment, although some experts prefer waiting until 2 weeks after completion of therapy.
- Other immunosuppressive therapy: in general, MMR or MMRV vaccines should be withheld for ≥3 months after cessation of the immunosuppressive therapy and remission of the underlying disease. This interval is based on the assumptions that the immune response will have been

restored in 3 months and the underlying disease for which the therapy was given remains in remission.

Thrombocytopenia

The benefits of primary immunization are usually greater than the potential risks of thrombocytopenia. However, avoiding a subsequent dose of MMR or MMRV vaccine may be prudent if an episode of thrombocytopenia occurred within approximately 6 weeks after a previous dose of vaccine.

CDC website: www.cdc.gov/measles

BIBLIOGRAPHY

1. American Academy of Pediatrics. Measles. In: Pickering LK, editor. Red Book: 2012 Report of the Committee on Infectious Diseases. 29th ed. Elk Grove Village, IL: American Academy of Pediatrics; 2012. p. 489–99.
2. Bellini WJ, Rota JS, Lowe LE, Katz RS, Dyken PR, Zaki SR, et al. Subacute sclerosing panencephalitis: more cases of this fatal disease are prevented by measles immunization than was previously recognized. J Infect Dis. 2005 Nov 15;192(10):1686–93.
3. CDC. General recommendations on immunization—recommendations of the Advisory Committee on Immunization Practices (ACIP). MMWR Recomm Rep. 2011 Jan 28;60(2):1–64.
4. CDC. Measles—United States, 2011. MMWR Morb Mortal Wkly Rep. 2012 Apr 20;61:253–7.
5. CDC. Public health reporting and national notification for measles. Atlanta: CDC; 2009 [updated 2010 Jun 10; cited 2012 Sep 21]. Available from: http://www.cste.org/ps2009/09-ID-48.pdf.
6. CDC. Recommended adult immunization schedule—United States, 2012. MMWR Morb Mortal Wkly Rep. 2012;61(04):1–7.
7. CDC. Recommended immunization schedules for persons aged 0 through 18 Years—United States, 2012. MMWR Morb Mortal Wkly Rep. 2012 Feb 10;61(5):1–4.
8. European Centre for Disease Prevention and Control. European monthly measles monitoring (EMMO). Surveillance Report [Internet]. 2012 Feb 21 [cited 2012 Sep 21](8). Available from: http://ecdc.europa.eu/en/publications/Publications/SUR_EMMO_European-monthly-measles-monitoring-February-2012.pdf.
9. King GE, Markowitz LE, Patriarca PA, Dales LG. Clinical efficacy of measles vaccine during the 1990 measles epidemic. Pediatr Infect Dis J. 1991 Dec;10(12):883–8.
10. Marin M, Broder KR, Temte JL, Snider DE, Seward JF. Use of combination measles, mumps, rubella, and varicella vaccine: recommendations of the Advisory Committee on Immunization Practices (ACIP). MMWR Recomm Rep. 2010 May 7;59(RR-3):1–12.
11. MeaslesRubellaInitiative.org [Internet]. Washington, DC: American National Red Cross; 2012 [cited 2012 Sep 21]. Available from: http://www.measlesrubellainitiative.org/mi/.
12. Perry RT, Halsey NA. The clinical significance of measles: a review. J Infect Dis. 2004 May 1;189 Suppl 1:S4–16.
13. Strebel PM, Papania MJ, Fiebelkorn AP, Halsey NA. Measles vaccines. In: Plotkin SA, Orenstein WA, Offit PA, editors. Vaccines. 6th ed. Philadelphia: Saunders Elsevier; 2012. p. 352–87.
14. Sudfeld CR, Navar AM, Halsey NA. Effectiveness of measles vaccination and vitamin A treatment. Int J Epidemiol. 2010 Apr;39 Suppl 1:i48–55.
15. Watson JC, Hadler SC, Dykewicz CA, Reef S, Phillips L. Measles, mumps, and rubella—vaccine use and strategies for elimination of measles, rubella, and congenital rubella syndrome and control of mumps: recommendations of the Advisory Committee on Immunization Practices (ACIP). MMWR Recomm Rep. 1998 May 22;47 (RR-8):1–57.
16. Watson JC, Pearson JA, Markowitz LE, Baughman AL, Erdman DD, Bellini WJ, et al. An evaluation of measles revaccination among school-entry-aged children. Pediatrics. 1996 May;97(5):613–8.
17. World Health Organization. Measles [fact sheet no. 286]. Geneva: World Health Organization; 2012 [cited 2012 Sep 21]. Available from: http://www.who.int/mediacentre/factsheets/fs286/en/index.html.

MELIOIDOSIS

David D. Blaney, Jay E. Gee, Theresa L. Smith

INFECTIOUS AGENT

Burkholderia pseudomallei is a saprophytic, gram-negative bacillus widely distributed in tropical soil and water.

TRANSMISSION

Through inhalation or subcutaneous inoculation, occasionally by ingestion; person-to-person transmission is rare via contact with the blood or body fluids of an infected person.

EPIDEMIOLOGY

Endemic in Southeast Asia, northern Australia, Papua New Guinea, much of the Indian subcontinent, southern China, Hong Kong, and Taiwan. It is considered highly endemic in northeast Thailand, Malaysia, Singapore, and northern Australia. Melioidosis has been reported in Puerto Rico, suspected in El Salvador, and may be underdiagnosed in India, Africa, the Caribbean, and Central and South America. In northern Brazil, clusters of melioidosis have recently been recognized and are associated with periods of heavy rainfall. The risk is highest for military personnel, adventure travelers, ecotourists, construction and resource extraction workers, and other people whose contact with contaminated soil or water may expose them to the bacteria. Risk factors for systemic melioidosis include diabetes, excessive alcohol use, chronic renal disease, chronic lung disease (such as associated with cystic fibrosis or chronic obstructive pulmonary disease), thalassemia, and malignancy or other non-HIV-related immune suppression.

CLINICAL PRESENTATION

Incubation period is generally 1–21 days, although it may extend for months or years; with a high inoculum, symptoms can develop in a few hours. Melioidosis may occur as a subclinical infection, localized infection (such as cutaneous), pneumonia, meningoencephalitis, sepsis, or chronic suppurative infection. The latter may mimic tuberculosis, with fever, weight loss, productive cough, and upper lobe infiltrate, with or without cavitation. More than 50% of cases present with pneumonia.

DIAGNOSIS

Culture from blood, sputum, pus, urine, synovial fluid, peritoneal fluid, or pericardial fluid. Indirect hemagglutination assay is a widely used serologic test. Diagnostic assistance is available through CDC (www.cdc.gov/ncezid/dhcpp/bacterial_special/zoonoses_lab.html).

TREATMENT

Ceftazidime, imipenem, meropenem, trimethoprim-sulfamethoxazole, and doxycycline are commonly used. Relapse may be seen, especially in patients who choose a shorter than recommended course of therapy.

PREVENTION

Thoroughly clean skin lacerations, abrasions, or burns that have been contaminated with soil or surface water.

CDC website: www.cdc.gov/melioidosis

BIBLIOGRAPHY

1. Cheng AC, Currie BJ. Melioidosis: epidemiology, pathophysiology, and management. Clin Microbiol Rev. 2005 Apr;18(2):383–416.
2. Currie BJ, Dance DA, Cheng AC. The global distribution of *Burkholderia pseudomallei* and melioidosis: an update. Trans R Soc Trop Med Hyg. 2008 Dec;102 Suppl 1:S1–4.
3. Peacock SJ. Melioidosis. Curr Opin Infect Dis. 2006 Oct;19(5):421–8.

MENINGOCOCCAL DISEASE

Amanda Cohn, Jessica R. MacNeil

INFECTIOUS AGENT

Neisseria meningitidis is a gram-negative diplococcus. Meningococci are classified into serogroups on the basis of the composition of the capsular polysaccharide. The 5 major meningococcal serogroups associated with disease are A, B, C, Y, and W-135.

TRANSMISSION

Person-to-person transmission occurs by close contact with respiratory secretions or saliva.

EPIDEMIOLOGY

N. meningitidis is found worldwide. At any time, 5%–10% of the population may be carriers of *N. meningitidis*. Invasive disease is rare in nonepidemic areas, occurring at a rate of 0.5–10 cases per 100,000 population per year, but can occur at a rate of up to 1,000 cases per 100,000 population per year in epidemic regions.

The incidence of meningococcal disease is highest in the "meningitis belt" of sub-Saharan Africa (Map 3-11). The incidence of meningococcal disease is several times higher in the meningitis belt than in the United States, with periodic epidemics during the dry season (December–June). During nonepidemic periods, the rate of meningococcal disease in this region is roughly 5–10 cases per 100,000 population per year. During epidemics, the rate can be as high as 1,000 cases per 100,000 population. Although most common in the African meningitis belt, meningococcal outbreaks can occur anywhere in the world. Serogroup A predominates in the meningitis belt, although serogroups C, X, and W-135 are also found.

Young children have the highest risk for meningococcal disease, but 60% of cases occur in adolescents and adults. Risk is highest in travelers to the meningitis belt who have prolonged contact with local populations during an epidemic. The Hajj pilgrimage to Saudi Arabia has been associated with outbreaks of meningococcal disease in returning pilgrims and their contacts.

CLINICAL PRESENTATION

Meningococcal disease generally occurs 1–14 days after exposure and presents as meningitis in ≥50% of cases. Meningococcal meningitis is characterized by sudden onset of headache, fever, and stiffness of the neck, sometimes accompanied by nausea, vomiting, photophobia, or altered mental status. Up to 20% of people with meningococcal disease present with meningococcal sepsis, known as meningococcemia. Meningococcemia is characterized by an abrupt onset of fever and a petechial or purpuric rash. The rash may progress to purpura fulminans. Meningococcemia often involves hypotension, acute adrenal hemorrhage, and multiorgan failure. Among infants and children aged <2 years, meningococcal disease may have nonspecific symptoms. Neck stiffness, usually seen in people with meningitis, may be absent in this age group.

DIAGNOSIS

Early diagnosis and treatment are critical. A lumbar puncture should be done to examine the cerebrospinal fluid (CSF) and perform a Gram stain. If possible, the lumbar puncture should be done before starting antibiotic therapy to ensure that bacteria, if any, can be cultured from CSF. Diagnosis is generally made by isolating *N. meningitidis* from blood or CSF, by detecting meningococcal antigen in CSF by latex agglutination, or by evidence of *N. meningitidis* DNA by PCR.

The signs and symptoms of meningococcal meningitis are similar to those of other causes of bacterial meningitis, such as *Haemophilus influenzae* and *Streptococcus pneumoniae*. The causative organism should be identified so that the correct antibiotics can be used for treatment and prophylaxis.

TREATMENT

Meningococcal disease is potentially fatal and should always be viewed as a medical emergency. Antibiotic treatment must be started early in the course of the disease, and empirically prior to the diagnostic test results.

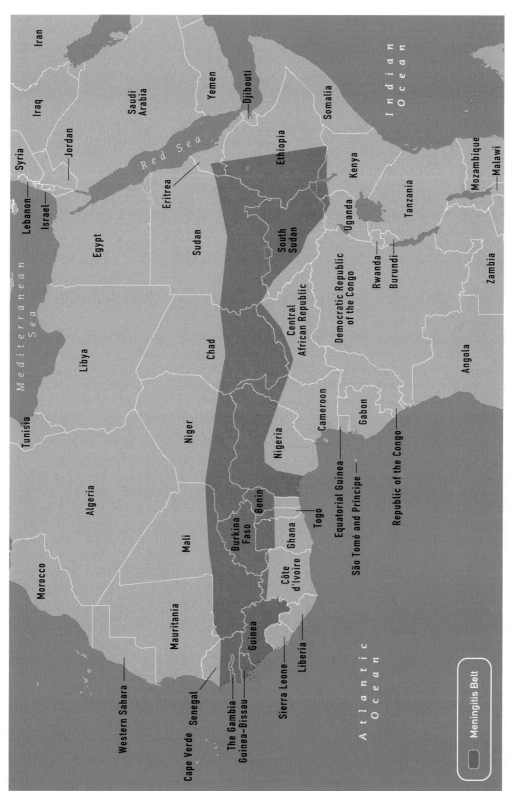

MAP 3-11. AREAS WITH FREQUENT EPIDEMICS OF MENINGOCOCCAL MENINGITIS

Several antibiotic choices are available, including third-generation cephalosporins.

PREVENTION
Vaccine
Indications for Use

The Advisory Committee on Immunization Practices (ACIP) recommends vaccination against meningococcal disease for people who travel to or reside in countries where *N. meningitidis* is hyperendemic or epidemic, particularly if contact with the local population will be prolonged. Hyperendemic regions include the meningitis belt of Africa during the dry season (December–June). Advisories for travelers to other countries are issued when epidemics of meningococcal disease caused by vaccine-preventable serogroups are recognized (see the CDC Travelers' Health website at www.cdc.gov/travel). Note that proof of receipt of quadrivalent vaccination against meningococcal disease is required for people traveling to Mecca during the annual Hajj and Umrah pilgrimages.

Vaccine Administration

Two quadrivalent meningococcal polysaccharide–protein conjugate vaccines are licensed for use in the United States: Menactra (Sanofi Pasteur) and Menveo (Novartis). A 1-dose primary series of Menactra is licensed for people aged 2–55 years; a 2-dose primary series of Menactra is licensed for children aged 9–23 months. Menveo is licensed for people aged 2–55 years. Quadrivalent meningococcal polysaccharide vaccine (Menomune, Sanofi-Pasteur) is licensed for use among people aged ≥2 years. These vaccines protect against meningococcal disease caused by serogroups A, C, Y, and W-135. No vaccine is available in the United States to prevent serogroup B meningococcal disease. Approximately 7–10 days are required after vaccination for development of protective antibody levels. Refer to Table 3-13 for more information about available meningococcal vaccines.

Menactra is the only meningococcal vaccine licensed for children aged 9–23 months. Either of the conjugate vaccines is preferred

Table 3-13. Vaccines to prevent meningococcal disease

VACCINE	TRADE NAME (MANUFACTURER)	AGE	DOSE	ROUTE	SCHEDULE	BOOSTER
Meningococcal polysaccharide diphtheria toxoid conjugate vaccine	Menactra (Sanofi Pasteur)	9–23 mo	0.5 mL	IM	0, 3 mo	If at continued risk[1]
		2–55 y	0.5 mL	IM	1 dose	
Meningococcal oligosaccharide diphtheria CRM$_{197}$ conjugate vaccine	Menveo (Novartis)	2–55 y	0.5 mL	IM	1 dose	If at continued risk[1]
Meningococcal polysaccharide vaccine	Menomune (Sanofi Pasteur)	≥2 y	0.5 mL	SC	1 dose	If at continued risk[2]

Abbreviations: IM, intramuscular; SC, subcutaneous.

[1] Revaccination with meningococcal conjugate vaccine is recommended after 3 years for children who were previously vaccinated at ages 9 months to 6 years. Revaccination with meningococcal conjugate vaccine is recommended after 5 years for people who were previously vaccinated at ages 7–55 years, and every 5 years thereafter for people who are at continued risk.

[2] Revaccination with meningococcal polysaccharide vaccine is recommended for adults >55 years who remain at increased risk 3–5 years after the last dose.

for people aged 2–55 years; polysaccharide vaccine should be used for people >55 years. In the United States, there is no licensed vaccine for children <9 months.

CDC recommends routine vaccination of people with conjugate vaccine at age 11 or 12 years, with a booster dose at age 16 years. For adolescents who receive the first dose at age 13–15 years, a one-time booster dose should be administered, preferably at age 16–18 years. People who receive their first dose at or after age 16 years do not need a booster dose, unless they remain at continued risk for meningococcal disease.

Travelers who were vaccinated previously and are living in or returning to Africa's meningitis belt may need to be revaccinated. ACIP recommends that children previously vaccinated at ages 9 months through 6 years who remain at an increased risk for meningococcal disease receive an additional dose of conjugate vaccine 3 years after their previous meningococcal vaccine and every 5 years thereafter, if at continued risk. Likewise, people who were previously vaccinated at ages 7–55 years and who remain at an increased risk for meningococcal disease should receive an additional dose of conjugate vaccine 5 years after their previous dose and every 5 years thereafter, if at continued risk. Travelers aged >55 years should be vaccinated or revaccinated with polysaccharide vaccine if it has been >5 years since their last meningococcal vaccine. Previously unvaccinated travelers <56 years of age who have a history of complement component deficiency (C3, properdin, factor D, or late component), functional or anatomic asplenia, or HIV should receive a 2-dose primary series of conjugate vaccine, 8–12 weeks apart. For those aged ≥56 years with these conditions, a single dose of polysaccharide vaccine should be given before travel if possible.

Travelers to the Hajj must show proof of vaccination in the previous 3 years.

Vaccine Safety and Adverse Reactions

For polysaccharide vaccine, the incidence of local reactions (such as pain and redness at the injection site) has ranged from 4% to 56% across studies. Severe reactions are rare, with an incidence of <0.1 per 100,000 vaccinees. In comparison trials, the incidence of severe reactions after conjugate vaccination was similar to the incidence after polysaccharide vaccination; however, local reactions (including pain that limited movement of the arm of injection) were more common after conjugate vaccination.

Precautions and Contraindications

People with moderate or severe acute illness should defer vaccination until their condition improves. Vaccination is contraindicated for people who have severe allergic reaction to any component of the vaccines. People with dry natural rubber latex allergy should not receive Menactra. Polysaccharide vaccine is an acceptable alternative for protection against meningococcal disease in these people. All meningococcal vaccines are inactivated and may be given to immunosuppressed people.

Antibiotic Chemoprophylaxis

In the United States and most industrialized countries, antibiotic chemoprophylaxis among close contacts of a patient with invasive meningococcal disease is recommended to prevent secondary cases. Chemoprophylaxis ideally should be initiated within 24 hours after the index patient is identified; prophylaxis given >2 weeks after exposure has little value. Antibiotic regimens for prophylaxis include rifampin, ciprofloxacin, and ceftriaxone. Ceftriaxone is recommended for pregnant women.

CDC website: www.cdc.gov/meningitis/bacterial.html

BIBLIOGRAPHY

1. American Academy of Pediatrics. Meningococcal infections. In: Pickering LK, editor. Red Book: 2012 Report of the Committee on Infectious Diseases. 29th ed. Elk Grove Village, IL: American Academy of Pediatrics; 2012. p. 500–9.
2. Bilukha OO, Rosenstein N. Prevention and control of meningococcal disease. Recommendations of the Advisory Committee on Immunization Practices (ACIP). MMWR Recomm Rep. 2005 May 27;54(RR-7):1–21.
3. CDC. Recommendation of the Advisory Committee on Immunization Practices (ACIP) for use of quadrivalent meningococcal conjugate vaccine (MenACWY-D) among children aged 9 through 23

months at increased risk for invasive meningococcal disease. MMWR Morb Mortal Wkly Rep. 2011 Oct 14;60(40):1391–2.

4. CDC. Updated recommendation from the Advisory Committee on Immunization Practices (ACIP) for revaccination of persons at prolonged increased risk for meningococcal disease. MMWR Morb Mortal Wkly Rep. 2009 Sep 25;58(37):1042–3.

5. CDC. Updated recommendations for use of meningococcal conjugate vaccines—Advisory Committee on Immunization Practices (ACIP), 2010. MMWR Morb Mortal Wkly Rep. 2011 Jan 28;60(3):72–6.

6. Greenwood B. Manson Lecture. Meningococcal meningitis in Africa. Trans R Soc Trop Med Hyg. 1999 Jul–Aug;93(4):341–53.

7. Rosenstein NE, Perkins BA, Stephens DS, Popovic T, Hughes JM. Meningococcal disease. N Engl J Med. 2001 May 3;344(18):1378–88.

8. Stephens DS, Greenwood B, Brandtzaeg P. Epidemic meningitis, meningococcaemia, and *Neisseria meningitidis*. Lancet. 2007 Jun 30;369(9580):2196–210.

9. Wilder-Smith A. Meningococcal disease: risk for international travellers and vaccine strategies. Travel Med Infect Dis. 2008 Jul;6(4):182–6.

MUMPS

Preeta K. Kutty, Albert E. Barskey IV

INFECTIOUS AGENT

An enveloped, negative-strand RNA virus (a paramyxovirus) of the genus *Rubulavirus*.

TRANSMISSION

By respiratory droplets, saliva, or contact with contaminated fomites.

EPIDEMIOLOGY

Endemic in many countries throughout the world. The risk of exposure among travelers is high in many countries, including industrialized countries.

CLINICAL PRESENTATION

Incubation period is 16–18 days (range, 12–25 days). Mumps is characterized by parotitis (swelling of the parotid salivary glands), either unilateral or bilateral. Onset of illness is usually nonspecific, with symptoms of fever, headache, malaise, myalgia, and anorexia. Complications may occur such as orchitis, aseptic meningitis, encephalitis, and pancreatitis. Approximately 30% of cases are asymptomatic.

DIAGNOSIS

Usually clinical, defined as illness with acute onset of unilateral or bilateral tender, self-limited swelling of the parotid glands, other salivary glands, or both, lasting ≥2 days, and without other apparent cause. A positive mumps laboratory confirmation for mumps virus is with RT-PCR or culture. For further information on laboratory testing, see www.cdc.gov/mumps/lab/index.html.

TREATMENT

Supportive care.

PREVENTION

All travelers aged ≥12 months should have evidence of mumps immunity, as documented by 2 doses of live mumps virus vaccine ≥28 days apart on or after the first birthday, laboratory evidence of immunity, birth before 1957, or history of physician-diagnosed mumps.

CDC website: www.cdc.gov/mumps

BIBLIOGRAPHY

1. CDC. Notice to readers: updated recommendations of the Advisory Committee on Immunization Practices (ACIP) for the control and elimination of mumps. MMWR Morb Mortal Wkly Rep. 2006 Jun 9;55(22):629–30.

2. CDC. Update: mumps outbreak—New York and New Jersey, June 2009–January 2010. MMWR Morb Mortal Wkly Rep. 2010 Feb 12; 59(5):125–9.

3. Dayan GH, Quinlisk MP, Parker AA, Barskey AE, Harris ML, Schwartz JM, et al. Recent resurgence of mumps in the United States. N Engl J Med. 2008 Apr 10;358(15):1580–9.

NOROVIRUS

Aron J. Hall, Ben Lopman

INFECTIOUS AGENT

Norovirus infection is caused by nonenveloped, single-stranded RNA viruses of the genus *Norovirus*, which have also been referred to as "Norwalk-like viruses," Norwalk viruses, and small round-structured viruses. Norovirus gastroenteritis is sometimes incorrectly referred to as "stomach flu"; however, there is no biologic association with influenza or influenza viruses.

TRANSMISSION

Transmission occurs primarily through the fecal-oral route, either through direct person-to-person contact or indirectly via contaminated food or water. Norovirus is also indirectly spread through aerosols of vomitus and contaminated environmental surfaces and objects.

EPIDEMIOLOGY

Seroprevalence studies in the Amazon, southern Africa, Mexico, Chile, and Canada have shown that norovirus infections are common throughout the world, and most children will have experienced ≥1 infection by the age of 5 years. Norovirus infections can occur year round, but in temperate climates, norovirus activity peaks during the winter. In the United States, norovirus is the leading cause of sporadic cases and outbreaks of gastroenteritis, estimated to cause 21 million illnesses a year and approximately 50% of all foodborne outbreaks. Noroviruses are common in both developing and developed countries.

Norovirus is a cause of travelers' diarrhea; prevalence ranges from 3% to 17% of travelers returning with diarrhea. However, coinfection and asymptomatic infection with norovirus are common, so focused studies are needed to determine exactly how frequently norovirus is the cause of disease. Risk for infection is present anywhere food is prepared in an unsanitary manner and may become contaminated, or where drinking water is inadequately treated. Of particular risk are "ready-to-eat" cold foods, such as sandwiches and salads.

Raw shellfish, especially oysters, are also a frequent source of infection, because virus from contaminated water concentrates in the gut of these filter feeders. Contaminated ice has also been implicated in outbreaks.

Large norovirus outbreaks are associated with settings where people live in close quarters and can easily infect each other, such as hotels, cruise ships, camps, and hospitals. Viral contamination of inanimate objects (fomites) may persist during outbreaks and be a source of infection. On cruise ships, for instance, such environmental contamination has caused recurrent norovirus outbreaks on successive cruises with newly boarded passengers. Transmission of norovirus on airplanes has been reported during both domestic and international flights and likely results from contamination of lavatories or from symptomatic passengers in the cabin.

CLINICAL PRESENTATION

Infected people usually have an acute onset of vomiting with nonbloody diarrhea. The incubation period is 12–48 hours. Other symptoms include abdominal cramps, nausea, and occasionally a low-grade fever. Illness is generally self-limited, and full recovery can be expected in 1–3 days. In some cases, dehydration, especially in patients who are very young or elderly, may require medical attention.

DIAGNOSIS

Norovirus infection is generally diagnosed based on symptoms. No laboratory tests have been approved by the Food and Drug Administration to guide clinical management of individual patients, but laboratory testing is used during outbreak investigations by public health agencies. Norovirus diagnostic testing is usually not available in developing countries.

The most common diagnostic test used at state public health laboratories and CDC is RT-PCR, which rapidly and reliably detects the virus in stool specimens. Several commercial EIAs are available to detect the virus in stool specimens. The specificity and sensitivity of these assays are poor compared with RT-PCR.

These tests have been used occasionally by cruise lines during outbreaks on ships.

TREATMENT

Supportive care, especially oral or intravenous rehydration. Antimotility agents should be avoided in children aged <3 years, but may be a useful adjunct to rehydration in older children and adults. Antiemetic agents should generally be reserved for adults. Antibiotics are not useful in treating patients with norovirus disease.

PREVENTION

No vaccine is currently available, although vaccine development efforts are advancing. Noroviruses are common and highly contagious, but the risk for infection can be minimized by frequent and proper handwashing and avoiding possibly contaminated food and water. Washing hands with soap and water for at least 20 seconds is considered the most effective way to reduce norovirus contamination; alcohol-based hand sanitizers (containing ≥60% alcohol) might be useful between handwashings but should not be considered a substitute for soap and water.

In addition to handwashing, measures to prevent transmission of noroviruses between people traveling together include carefully cleaning up fecal material or vomit and disinfecting contaminated surfaces and toilet areas. Products should be approved by the Environmental Protection Agency for norovirus disinfection; alternatively, a high concentration of domestic bleach (5–25 tablespoons bleach per gallon of water) may be used. Soiled articles of clothing should be washed at the maximum available cycle length and machine-dried at high heat.

To help prevent the spread of noroviruses, ill people have been isolated on cruise ships and in institutional settings.

CDC website: www.cdc.gov/norovirus

BIBLIOGRAPHY

1. Apelt N, Hartberger C, Campe H, Loscher T. The prevalence of norovirus in returning international travelers with diarrhea. BMC Infect Dis. 2010;10:131.
2. Atmar RL, Bernstein DI, Harro CD, Al-Ibrahim MS, Chen WH, Ferreira J, et al. Norovirus vaccine against experimental human Norwalk virus illness. N Engl J Med. 2011 Dec 8;365(23):2178–87.
3. Glass RI, Parashar UD, Estes MK. Norovirus gastroenteritis. N Engl J Med. 2009 Oct 29;361(18):1776–85.
4. Hall AJ, Vinjé J, Lopman B, Park GW, Yen C, Gregoricus N, et al. Updated norovirus outbreak management and disease prevention guidelines. MMWR Recomm Rep. 2011 Mar 4;60(RR-3):1–18.
5. Kirking HL, Cortes J, Burrer S, Hall AJ, Cohen NJ, Lipman H, et al. Likely transmission of norovirus on an airplane, October 2008. Clin Infect Dis. 2010 May 1;50(9):1216–21.
6. Koo HL, Ajami NJ, Jiang ZD, Neill FH, Atmar RL, Ericsson CD, et al. Noroviruses as a cause of diarrhea in travelers to Guatemala, India, and Mexico. J Clin Microbiol. 2010 May;48(5):1673–6.
7. Patel MM, Widdowson MA, Glass RI, Akazawa K, Vinje J, Parashar UD. Systematic literature review of role of noroviruses in sporadic gastroenteritis. Emerg Infect Dis. 2008 Aug;14(8):1224–31.
8. Scallan E, Hoekstra RM, Angulo FJ, Tauxe RV, Widdowson MA, Roy SL, et al. Foodborne illness acquired in the United States—major pathogens. Emerg Infect Dis. 2011 Jan;17(1):7–15.
9. Thornley CN, Emslie NA, Sprott TW, Greening GE, Rapana JP. Recurring norovirus transmission on an airplane. Clin Infect Dis. 2011 Sep;53(6):515–20.
10. Widdowson MA, Cramer EH, Hadley L, Bresee JS, Beard RS, Bulens SN, et al. Outbreaks of acute gastroenteritis on cruise ships and on land: identification of a predominant circulating strain of norovirus—United States, 2002. J Infect Dis. 2004 Jul 1;190(1):27–36.

ONCHOCERCIASIS (RIVER BLINDNESS)

LeAnne M. Fox

INFECTIOUS AGENT

Onchocerca volvulus, a filarial nematode.

TRANSMISSION

Through female blackflies (genus *Simulium*), which typically bite during the day and near rapidly flowing rivers and streams.

EPIDEMIOLOGY

Endemic in central Africa. Small endemic foci are also present in the Arabian Peninsula (Yemen) and in the Americas (Brazil, Colombia, Ecuador, Guatemala, southern Mexico, and Venezuela). Most infections, outside those in endemic populations, occur in expatriate groups, such as missionaries, field scientists, and Peace Corps volunteers.

CLINICAL PRESENTATION

Highly pruritic, papular dermatitis; subcutaneous nodules; lymphadenitis; and ocular lesions, which can progress to visual loss and blindness. Symptoms in travelers are primarily dermatologic and may occur months to years after departure from endemic areas.

DIAGNOSIS

Presence of microfilariae in superficial skin shavings or punch biopsy, adult worms in histologic sections of excised nodules, or characteristic eye lesions. Serologic testing is most useful for detecting infection when microfilariae are not identifiable. Determination of serum antifilarial IgG is available through the National Institutes of Health (301-496-5398) or CDC (www.dpd.cdc.gov/dpdx; 404-718-4745; parasites@cdc.gov).

TREATMENT

Ivermectin is the drug of choice. Repeated annual or semiannual doses may be required, as the drug kills the microfilariae but not the adult worms. Some experts recommend treating patients with 1 dose of ivermectin followed by 6 weeks of doxycycline. Diethylcarbamazine is contraindicated in onchocerciasis, because it has been associated with severe and fatal post-treatment reactions. An expert in tropical medicine should be consulted to help manage these patients.

PREVENTION

Avoid blackfly habitats (free-flowing rivers and streams) and use protection measures against biting insects (see Chapter 2, Protection against Mosquitoes, Ticks, & Other Insects & Arthropods).

CDC website: www.cdc.gov/parasites/onchocerciasis

BIBLIOGRAPHY

1. Hoeraif A. Filariasis: new drugs and new opportunities for lymphatic filariasis and onchocerciasis. Curr Opin Infect Dis. 2008 Dec;21(6):673–81.
2. Tielsch JM, Beeche A. Impact of ivermectin on illness and disability associated with onchocerciasis. Trop Med Int Health. 2004 Apr;9(4):A45–56.
3. WHO Expert Committee. Onchocerciasis and its control. Report of a WHO Expert Committee on Onchocerciasis Control. World Health Organ Tech Rep Ser. 1995;852:1–104.

PERTUSSIS

Tami H. Skoff, Jennifer L. Liang

INFECTIOUS AGENT

Fastidious gram-negative coccobacillus, *Bordetella pertussis*.

TRANSMISSION

Person-to-person transmission via aerosolized respiratory droplets or by direct contact with respiratory secretions.

EPIDEMIOLOGY

Pertussis is endemic worldwide, even in areas with high vaccination rates. From 2004 through 2010, the annual number of reported pertussis cases in the United States ranged from approximately 8,000 to >27,000. Disease rates are highest among young children in countries where vaccination coverage is low, which is primarily in the developing world. In developed countries, the incidence of pertussis is highest among infants too young to be vaccinated.

Immunity from childhood vaccination and natural disease wanes with time; therefore, adolescents and adults who have not received a tetanus-diphtheria-pertussis (Tdap) booster vaccination can become infected or reinfected. US travelers are not at increased risk for disease specifically because of international travel, but they are at risk if they come in close contact with infected people. Infants too young to be protected by a complete vaccination series are at highest risk for severe pertussis that requires hospitalization.

CLINICAL PRESENTATION

In classic disease, mild upper respiratory tract symptoms begin 7–10 days (range, 6–21 days) after exposure, followed by a cough that becomes paroxysmal. Coughing paroxysms can vary in frequency and are often followed by vomiting. Fever is absent or minimal. The clinical case definition for pertussis includes cough for ≥2 weeks with paroxysms, whoop, or posttussive vomiting.

Disease in infants aged <6 months can be atypical, with a short catarrhal stage, gagging, gasping, or apnea as early manifestations. Among infants aged <2 months, the case-fatality ratio is approximately 1%. Recently immunized children who develop disease may have mild cough illness; older children and adults may have prolonged cough with or without paroxysms. The cough gradually wanes over several weeks to months.

DIAGNOSIS

Factors such as prior vaccination status, stage of disease, antibiotic use, specimen collection and transport conditions, and use of nonstandardized tests may affect the sensitivity, specificity, and interpretation of available diagnostic tests for *B. pertussis*. CDC guidelines for the laboratory confirmation of pertussis cases include culture and PCR (when the above clinical case definition is met); serology and direct fluorescent antibody (DFA) tests are not confirmatory tests included in the case definition.

TREATMENT

Macrolide antibiotics (azithromycin, clarithromycin, and erythromycin) are recommended for the treatment of pertussis in people aged ≥1 month; for infants aged <1 month, azithromycin is the preferred antibiotic. Antimicrobial therapy with a macrolide antibiotic administered <3 weeks after cough onset can limit transmission to others. Postexposure prophylaxis is recommended for close contacts of cases and for people at high risk of developing severe disease (such as infants and those who will have contact with young infants). The recommended agents and dosing regimens for prophylaxis are the same as for the treatment of pertussis.

PREVENTION

Vaccine

Travelers should be up-to-date with pertussis vaccinations before departure. Multiple pertussis vaccines are available in the United States for infants and children, and 2 vaccines are available for adolescents and adults. A complete listing of licensed vaccines can be found at www.fda.gov/BiologicsBloodVaccines/Vaccines/ApprovedProducts/ucm093833.htm.

Complete vaccination of children aged <7 years with 5 doses of acellular pertussis vaccine in combination with diphtheria and tetanus toxoids (DTaP) is recommended; an accelerated schedule of doses may be used to complete the DTaP series. Children aged 7–10 years who are not fully vaccinated against pertussis and for whom no contraindication to pertussis vaccine exists should receive a single dose of Tdap to provide protection against pertussis. If additional doses of tetanus and diphtheria toxoid-containing vaccines are needed, then children aged 7–10 years should be vaccinated according to catch-up guidance, with Tdap preferred as the first dose. Adolescents aged 11–18 years who have completed the recommended childhood DTwP/DTaP vaccination series and who have not previously received Tdap and adults aged ≥19 years who have not previously received Tdap should receive a single dose of Tdap instead of tetanus and diphtheria toxoids (Td) vaccine for booster immunization against tetanus, diphtheria, and pertussis. Tdap vaccine, when indicated, should be administered to adolescents and adults regardless of interval since the last dose of Td vaccine.

To provide pertussis protection before travel, Tdap can be given regardless of the interval from the last Td, except to people for whom pertussis vaccination is contraindicated or for people who have previously received Tdap. Adolescents and adults who have never been immunized against pertussis, tetanus, or diphtheria, who have incomplete immunization, or whose immunity is uncertain should follow the catch-up schedule established for Td/Tdap. Tdap can be substituted for any one of the Td doses in the series.

CDC website: www.cdc.gov/pertussis

BIBLIOGRAPHY

1. American Academy of Pediatrics. Pertussis (whooping cough). In: Pickering LK, editor. Red Book: 2012 Report of the Committee on Infectious Diseases. 29th ed. Elk Grove Village, IL: American Academy of Pediatrics; 2012. p. 553–66.
2. Broder KR, Cortese MM, Iskander JK, Kretsinger K, Slade BA, Brown KH, et al. Preventing tetanus, diphtheria, and pertussis among adolescents: use of tetanus toxoid, reduced diphtheria toxoid and acellular pertussis vaccines. Recommendations of the Advisory Committee on Immunization Practices (ACIP). MMWR Recomm Rep. 2006 Dec 15;55(RR-17):1–33.
3. CDC. Updated recommendations for use of tetanus toxoid, reduced diphtheria toxoid and acellular pertussis (Tdap) vaccine from the Advisory Committee on Immunization Practices, 2010. MMWR Morb Mortal Wkly Rep. 2011 Jan 14;60(1):13–5.
4. Edwards KM, Decker MD. Pertussis vaccines. In: Plotkin SA, Orenstein WA, Offit PA, editors. Vaccines. 6th ed. Philadelphia: Saunders Elsevier; 2012. p. 447–92.
5. Tiwari T, Murphy TV, Moran J. Recommended antimicrobial agents for the treatment and postexposure prophylaxis of pertussis: 2005 CDC Guidelines. MMWR Recomm Rep. 2005 Dec 9;54 (RR-14):1–16.

PINWORM (ENTEROBIASIS, OXYURIASIS, THREADWORM)

Els Mathieu

INFECTIOUS AGENT

The intestinal nematode (roundworm) *Enterobius vermicularis*.

TRANSMISSION

Direct transfer of eggs by hand from anus to mouth, which can reinfect the same person or infect a different person, or indirect transmission via objects such as clothes and bedding that are contaminated with eggs.

EPIDEMIOLOGY

Endemic worldwide. Travelers are at risk if staying in crowded conditions with infected people. Frequently transmitted within families.

CLINICAL PRESENTATION

Incubation period is usually 1–2 months, but successive reinfections may be needed before symptoms appear. The most common symptom is perianal itching, which can disturb sleep. Adult worms can migrate from the anal area to other sites, including the vulva, vagina, and urethra. Secondary bacterial infection of scratched skin can also occur.

DIAGNOSIS

Direct visualization of adult worms near the anus, best done 2–3 hours after the infected person has fallen asleep, or microscopic identification of worm eggs collected by touching transparent tape to the anal area when the person first awakens in the morning.

TREATMENT

Drugs of choice are mebendazole, albendazole, and pyrantel pamoate (can be purchased without prescription). Treatment is repeated 2 weeks after the initial dose. In households where >1 member is infected or where repeated, symptomatic infections occur, all household members should be treated at the same time.

PREVENTION

Handwashing; maintaining clean, short fingernails; avoiding nail biting; avoiding scratching the perianal or perineal region; daily morning bathing (showers or stand-up baths best): and frequent changing and laundering of underclothes, nightclothes, and bedding with hot water help prevent the spread of the infection and reinfection of the same person.

CDC website: www.cdc.gov/parasites/pinworm

BIBLIOGRAPHY

1. American Academy of Pediatrics. Pinworm infection (*Enterobius vermicularis*). In: Pickering LK, editor. Red Book: 2012 Report of the Committee on Infectious Diseases. 29th ed. Elk Grove Village, IL: American Academy of Pediatrics; 2012. p. 566–7.

2. American Public Health Association. Enterobiasis. In: Heyman DL, editor. Control of Communicable Diseases Manual. 19th ed. Washington, DC: American Public Health Association; 2008. p. 223–5.

3. Kucik CJ, Martin GL, Sortor BV. Common intestinal parasites. Am Fam Physician. 2004 Mar 1;69(5):1161–8.

PLAGUE (BUBONIC, PNEUMONIC, SEPTICEMIC)

Paul S. Mead

INFECTIOUS AGENT

The gram-negative bacterium *Yersinia pestis*.

TRANSMISSION

Usually through the bite of infected rodent fleas. Less common exposures include handling infected animal tissues (hunters, wildlife personnel), inhalation of infectious droplets from cats or dogs with plague, and rarely, contact with a pneumonic plague patient.

EPIDEMIOLOGY

Endemic in rural areas in central and southern Africa, central Asia and the Indian subcontinent, the northeastern part of South America, and parts of the southwestern United States.

CLINICAL PRESENTATION

Incubation period is typically 1–6 days. Symptoms and signs of the 3 clinical presentations of plague illness are as follows:

- Bubonic (most common)—rapid onset of fever; painful, swollen, and tender lymph nodes, usually inguinal, axillary, or cervical
- Pneumonic—high fever, overwhelming pneumonia, cough, bloody sputum, chills

- Septicemic—fever, prostration, hemorrhagic or thrombotic phenomena, progressing to acral gangrene

DIAGNOSIS

Y. pestis can be isolated from bubo aspirates, blood cultures, or sputum culture if pneumonic. Diagnosis can be confirmed in public health laboratories by culture or serologic tests for the Y. pestis F1 antigen.

BIBLIOGRAPHY

1. Neerinckx S, Bertherat E, Leirs H. Human plague occurrences in Africa: an overview from 1877 to 2008. Trans R Soc Trop Med Hyg. 2010 Feb;104(2):97–103.
2. Perry RD, Fetherston JD. Yersinia pestis—etiologic agent of plague. Clin Microbiol Rev. 1997 Jan;10(1):35–66.
3. World Health Organization. Human plague: review of regional morbidity and mortality, 2004–2009. Wkly Epidemiol Rec. 2009 Feb 5;85(6):40–5.

TREATMENT

Parenteral antibiotic therapy with streptomycin is the recommended first-line therapy; alternatively, gentamicin or, where treatment is limited to oral therapy, doxycycline can be used.

PREVENTION

Reduce contact with fleas and potentially infected rodents and other wildlife.

CDC website: www.cdc.gov/plague

PNEUMOCOCCAL DISEASE
Ronnie Henry

INFECTIOUS AGENT

The gram-positive coccus *Streptococcus pneumoniae*.

TRANSMISSION

Person to person through close contact via respiratory droplets.

EPIDEMIOLOGY

Occurs worldwide, but prevalence is higher in developing than in industrialized countries. Risk is highest in young children, the elderly, and those with chronic illnesses or immune suppression.

CLINICAL PRESENTATION

Sudden onset of fever and malaise, cough, pleuritic chest pain, purulent or blood-tinged sputum. In the elderly, fever, shortness of breath, or altered mental status may be initial symptoms. Pneumococcal meningitis may present as a stiff neck, headache, lethargy, or seizures.

DIAGNOSIS

Isolation from blood or cerebrospinal fluid, but most patients do not have detectable bacteremia. Pneumococcal urine antigen test can be used in adults. Infection can be suspected if a sputum specimen contains gram-positive diplococci, polymorphonuclear leukocytes, and few epithelial cells. High white blood cell counts should raise suspicion for bacterial infection.

TREATMENT

Empiric therapy depends on the syndrome. Many strains are resistant to penicillin, cephalosporins, and macrolides, so definitive treatment should be targeted on the basis of antimicrobial susceptibility results. In the United States and other countries where β-lactam resistance is common, the initial regimen for pneumococcal meningitis might include vancomycin or a fluoroquinolone, plus a third-generation cephalosporin.

PREVENTION

The 13-valent pneumococcal conjugate vaccine (PCV13) is recommended for all children aged <5 years and children aged <72 months with chronic medical conditions; the vaccine may also be given to children aged <18 years with immunocompromising conditions.

A 23-valent pneumococcal polysaccharide vaccine (PPSV23) is recommended for adults aged ≥65 years and people aged 2–64 years with underlying medical conditions. Adults with immunocompromising conditions, functional or anatomic asplenia, cerebrospinal fluid leaks, or cochlear implants should receive PCV13 followed by PPSV23. See www.cdc.gov/vaccines/pubs/ACIP-list.htm#pcv.

CDC website: www.cdc.gov/vaccines/vpd-vac/pneumo

BIBLIOGRAPHY

1. CDC. Licensure of a 13-valent pneumococcal conjugate vaccine (PCV13) and recommendations for use among children—Advisory Committee on Immunization Practices (ACIP), 2010. MMWR Morb Mortal Wkly Rep. 2010 Mar 12;59(9):258–61.
2. CDC. Prevention of pneumococcal disease: recommendations of the Advisory Committee on Immunization Practices (ACIP). MMWR Recomm Rep. 1997 Apr 4;46(RR-8):1–24.
3. Fedson DS, Scott JA. The burden of pneumococcal disease among adults in developed and developing countries: what is and is not known. Vaccine. 1999 Jul 30;17 Suppl 1:S11–8.

POLIOMYELITIS

Gregory S. Wallace, James P. Alexander, Steven G. F. Wassilak

INFECTIOUS AGENT

Poliovirus (genus *Enterovirus*) types 1, 2, and 3. Polioviruses are small (27–30 nm), nonenveloped viruses with capsids enclosing a single-stranded, positive-sense RNA genome about 7,500 nucleotides long. Most of the properties of polioviruses are shared with the other enteroviruses.

TRANSMISSION

Fecal-oral or oral transmission. Acute infection involves the oropharynx, gastrointestinal tract, and occasionally the central nervous system.

EPIDEMIOLOGY

In the prevaccine era, infection with poliovirus was common worldwide, with seasonal peaks and epidemics in the summer and fall in temperate areas. The incidence of poliomyelitis in the United States declined rapidly after the licensure of inactivated polio vaccine (IPV) in 1955 and live oral polio vaccine (OPV) in the 1960s. The last cases of indigenously acquired polio in the United States occurred in 1979. The Global Polio Eradication Initiative (GPEI) subsequently eliminated polio in the Americas, where the last wild poliovirus (WPV)–associated polio case was detected in 1991. In January 2000, a change in vaccination policy in the United States from use of live OPV to exclusive use of IPV eliminated the 8–10 vaccine-associated paralytic poliomyelitis (VAPP) cases that had occurred annually since the introduction of OPV in the 1960s.

GPEI has built upon the success in the Americas and made great progress in eradicating WPVs, reducing the number of reported polio cases worldwide by more than 99% since the mid-1980s. As of March 2012, WPV circulation has never been interrupted in only 3 countries: Afghanistan, Nigeria, and Pakistan. In 3 African countries (Angola, Chad, and Democratic Republic of the Congo), WPV transmission has been reestablished after importations and outbreaks in 2008 and 2009. In spite of progress made in eradicating WPVs globally, countries are still at risk for imported cases. In 2010 and 2011, WPV outbreaks from importations occurred in 18 countries in Africa, Eastern Europe, and Asia.

Because of polio eradication efforts, the number of countries where travelers are at risk for polio has decreased dramatically. The last documented case of WPV-associated paralysis in a US resident traveling abroad occurred in 1986 in a 29-year-old vaccinated adult who had been traveling in South and

Southeast Asia. In 2005, an unvaccinated US adult traveling abroad acquired VAPP after contact with an infant recently vaccinated with OPV.

For additional information on the status of polio eradication efforts and vaccine recommendations, consult the travel notices on the CDC Travelers' Health website (www.cdc.gov/travel) or the GPEI website (www.polioeradication.org).

CLINICAL PRESENTATION

Clinical manifestations of poliovirus infection range from asymptomatic (most infections) to symptomatic, including acute flaccid paralysis of a single limb to quadriplegia, respiratory failure, and rarely, death.

DIAGNOSIS

The diagnosis is made by identifying poliovirus in clinical specimens (usually stool) obtained from an acutely ill patient. Poliovirus may be detected by culture of cell lines followed by identification using neutralization tests or PCR. Poliovirus may also be identified by direct amplification from stool specimens followed by genomic sequencing to identify the possible source of the virus. Shedding in fecal specimens can be intermittent, but usually poliovirus can be detected for up to 4 weeks after onset of illness. During the first 3–10 days of the illness, poliovirus can also be detected from oropharyngeal specimens. Poliovirus is rarely detected in the blood or cerebrospinal fluid.

TREATMENT

Only treatment for symptoms is available, ranging from pain and fever relief to intubation and mechanical ventilation for patients with respiratory insufficiency.

PREVENTION

Vaccine

In the United States, infants and children should be vaccinated against polio as part of a routine immunization series (see Infants and Children below). Polio vaccination is recommended for all travelers to polio-endemic or epidemic areas, including countries with recent proven WPV circulation in the previous 12 months and neighboring countries. For countries with WPV cases in the previous 12 months, consult the weekly update of

reported WPV cases at the GPEI website (http://www.polioeradication.org/Dataandmonitoring/Poliothisweek.aspx). Before traveling to areas where poliomyelitis cases are still occurring, travelers should ensure that they have completed the recommended age-appropriate polio vaccine series and have received a booster dose, if necessary (see Infants and Children and Adults below). To eliminate the risk for VAPP, IPV has been the only polio vaccine available in the United States since 2000; however, OPV continues to be used in many countries and for global polio eradication activities. For complete information on recommendations for poliomyelitis vaccination, consult the Advisory Committee on Immunization Practices recommendations website (http://www.cdc.gov/vaccines/pubs/acip-list.htm#polio).

Infants and Children

In the United States, all infants and children should receive 4 doses of IPV at ages 2, 4, and 6–18 months and 4–6 years. The final dose should be administered at age ≥4 years, regardless of the number of previous doses, and should be given ≥6 months after the previous dose. A fourth dose in the routine IPV series is not necessary if the third dose was administered at age ≥4 years and ≥6 months after the previous dose. If the routine series cannot be administered within the recommended intervals before protection is needed, the following alternatives are recommended:

- The first dose should be given to infants ≥6 weeks old.
- The second and third doses should be administered ≥4 weeks after the previous doses.
- The minimum interval between the third and fourth doses is 6 months.

If the age-appropriate series is not completed before departure, the remaining IPV doses to complete a full series should be administered when feasible, at the intervals recommended above, if the child remains at increased risk for poliovirus exposure.

Adults

Adults who are traveling to areas where poliomyelitis cases are still occurring and who are unvaccinated, incompletely vaccinated, or whose vaccination status is unknown should receive a series of 3 doses: 2 doses of IPV administered at an interval of 4–8 weeks; a third dose should be administered 6–12 months after the second. If 3 doses of IPV cannot be administered within the recommended intervals before protection is needed, the following alternatives are recommended:

- If >8 weeks is available before protection is needed, 3 doses of IPV should be administered ≥4 weeks apart.
- If <8 weeks but >4 weeks is available before protection is needed, 2 doses of IPV should be administered ≥4 weeks apart.
- If <4 weeks is available before protection is needed, a single dose of IPV is recommended.

If <3 doses are administered, the remaining IPV doses to complete a 3-dose series should be administered when feasible, at the intervals recommended above, if the person remains at increased risk for poliovirus exposure.

Adults who have completed a routine series of polio vaccine are considered to have lifelong immunity to poliomyelitis, but data are lacking. As a precaution, adults (≥18 years of age) who are traveling to areas where poliomyelitis cases are occurring and who have received a routine series with either IPV or OPV in childhood should receive another dose of IPV before departure. For adults, available data do not indicate the need for more than a single lifetime booster dose with IPV.

Vaccine Safety and Adverse Reactions

Minor local reactions (pain and redness) can occur after IPV administration. No serious adverse reactions to IPV have been documented. IPV should not be administered to people who have experienced a severe allergic reaction (such as anaphylaxis) after a previous dose of IPV or after receiving streptomycin, polymyxin B, or neomycin, which IPV contains in trace amounts; hypersensitivity reactions can occur after IPV administration among people sensitive to these 3 antibiotics.

Pregnancy and Breastfeeding

If a pregnant woman is unvaccinated or incompletely vaccinated and requires immediate protection against polio because of planned travel to a country or area where polio cases are occurring, IPV can be administered as recommended for adults. Breastfeeding is not a contraindication to administration of polio vaccine to an infant or mother.

Precautions and Contraindications

IPV may be administered to people with diarrhea. Minor upper respiratory illnesses with or without fever, mild to moderate local reactions to a previous dose of IPV, current antimicrobial therapy, and the convalescent phase of acute illness are not contraindications for vaccination.

Immunosuppression

IPV may be administered safely to immunocompromised travelers and their household contacts. Although a protective immune response cannot be ensured, IPV might confer some protection to the immunocompromised person. People with certain primary immunodeficiency diseases should not be given OPV and should avoid contact with excreted OPV virus (such as exposure to a child vaccinated with OPV in the previous 6 weeks); however, this situation no longer occurs in the United States unless a child receives OPV overseas.

CDC website: www.cdc.gov/vaccines/vpd-vac/polio

BIBLIOGRAPHY

1. Alexander JP, Ehresmann K, Seward J, Wax G, Harriman K, Fuller S, et al. Transmission of imported vaccine-derived poliovirus in an undervaccinated community in Minnesota. J Infect Dis. 2009 Feb 1;199(3):391–7.
2. Alexander LN, Seward JF, Santibanez TA, Pallansch MA, Kew OM, Prevots DR, et al. Vaccine policy changes and epidemiology of poliomyelitis in the United States. JAMA. 2004 Oct 13;292(14):1696–701.
3. CDC. Certification of poliomyelitis eradication—the Americas, 1994. MMWR Morb Mortal Wkly Rep. 1994 Oct 7;43(39):720–2.
4. CDC. Immunization schedules. Atlanta: CDC; 2012 [cited 201 Sep 21]. Available from: http://www.cdc.gov/vaccines/schedules/index.html.
5. CDC. Imported vaccine-associated paralytic poliomyelitis—United States, 2005. MMWR Morb Mortal Wkly Rep. 2006 Feb 3;55(4):97–9.

6. CDC. Outbreaks following wild poliovirus importations—Europe, Africa, and Asia, January 2009–September 2010. MMWR Morb Mortal Wkly Rep. 2010 Nov 5;59(43):1393–9.

7. CDC. Poliomyelitis. In: Atkinson W, Wolfe S, Hamborsky J, editors. Epidemiology and Prevention of Vaccine-Preventable Diseases. 12th ed. Washington, DC: Public Health Foundation; 2012. p. 249–62.

8. CDC. Poliomyelitis—United States, 1975–1984. MMWR Morb Mortal Wkly Rep. 1986 Mar 21;35(11):180–2.

9. CDC. Progress toward interrupting wild poliovirus circulation in countries with reestablished transmission—Africa, 2009–2010. MMWR Morb Mortal Wkly Rep. 2011 Mar 18;60(10):306–11.

10. CDC. Progress toward interruption of wild poliovirus transmission—worldwide, January 2010–March 2011. MMWR Morb Mortal Wkly Rep. 2011 May 13;60(18):582–6.

11. CDC. Tracking progress toward global polio eradication—worldwide, 2009–2010. MMWR Morb Mortal Wkly Rep. 2011 Apr 15;60(14):441–5.

12. CDC. Update on vaccine-derived polioviruses—worldwide, July 2009–March 2011. MMWR Morb Mortal Wkly Rep. 2011 Jul 1;60(25):846–50.

13. CDC. Updated recommendations of the Advisory Committee on Immunization Practices (ACIP) regarding routine poliovirus vaccination. MMWR Morb Mortal Wkly Rep. 2009 Aug 7;58(30):829–30.

14. Prevots DR, Burr RK, Sutter RW, Murphy TV. Poliomyelitis prevention in the United States. Updated recommendations of the Advisory Committee on Immunization Practices (ACIP). MMWR Recomm Rep. 2000 May 9;49(RR-5):1–22.

15. Sutter RW, Kew OM, Cochi SL, Aylward RB. Poliovirus vaccine—live. In: Plotkin SA, Orenstein WA, Offit PA, editors. Vaccines. 6th ed. Philadelphia: Saunders Elsevier; 2012. p. 598–645.

16. Vidor E, Plotkin SA. Poliovirus vaccine—inactivated. In: Plotkin SA, Orenstein WA, Offit PA, editors. Vaccines. 6th ed. Philadelphia: Saunders Elsevier; 2012. p. 573–97.

17. World Health Organization. Wild poliovirus weekly update. World Health Organization; 2010 [updated 2010 Mar 6; cited 2010 Apr 6]. Available from: http://www.polioeradication.org/Dataandmonitoring/Poliothisweek.aspx.

18. World Health Organization. Meeting of the Strategic Advisory Group of Experts on Immunization, November 2011—conclusions and recommendations. Wkly Epidemiol Rec. 2012 Jan 6:1–16.

19. World Health Organization. Wild poliovirus weekly update. World Health Organization; 2012 [cited 2012 Sep 21]. Available from: http://www.polioeradication.org/Dataandmonitoring/Poliothisweek.aspx.

Q FEVER

Alicia Anderson, Jennifer McQuiston

INFECTIOUS AGENT

The gram-negative intracellular bacterium *Coxiella burnetii*.

TRANSMISSION

Most commonly, through inhalation of aerosols or dust contaminated with dried birth fluids or excreta from infected animals (usually cattle, sheep, or goats). Infections via ingestion of contaminated, unpasteurized dairy products and human-to-human transmission via sexual contact have been rarely reported.

EPIDEMIOLOGY

Distributed worldwide; the prevalence is highest in African and Middle Eastern countries. Travelers who visit rural areas or farms with cattle, sheep, goats, or other livestock may be exposed to Q fever. Occupational exposure to infected animals (such as in farmers, veterinarians, butchers, meat packers, and seasonal or migrant farm workers), particularly during parturition, poses a high risk for disease transmission.

CLINICAL PRESENTATION

Approximately half of acute infections are mild or asymptomatic. Incubation period is typically 2–3 weeks but may be shorter after exposure to large numbers of organisms. The most common presentation of acute infection is a mild, self-limiting influenzalike illness, with pneumonia or hepatitis in more severe acute infections. Chronic infections occur primarily in patients with preexisting cardiac valvulopathies, vascular abnormalities, or immunosuppression. Women infected during pregnancy are at high risk for adverse pregnancy outcomes unless treated. The most common manifestations of chronic disease are endocarditis and endovascular infections.

DIAGNOSIS
Serologic evidence of a 4-fold rise in phase II IgG by indirect immunofluorescent assay (IFA) between paired sera taken 3–4 weeks apart is the gold standard for diagnosis of acute infection. A single high serum phase II IgG titer (>1:128) by IFA in conjunction with clinical evidence of infection may be considered evidence of probable infection. C. burnetii may be detected in infected tissues by using immunohistochemical staining or DNA detection methods or by direct isolation of the agent via culture. PCR assays may be used on whole blood samples in the early stages of illness and before initiation of antibiotic therapy.

TREATMENT
Doxycycline is the treatment of choice for acute Q fever. Pregnant women, children aged <8 years with mild illness, and patients allergic to doxycycline may be treated with alternative antibiotics such as trimethoprim-sulfamethoxazole. Treatment for acute Q fever is not recommended for asymptomatic people or for those whose symptoms have resolved. Chronic Q fever endocarditis is more difficult to treat effectively and typically requires long-term combination therapy.

PREVENTION
Avoid areas where potentially infected animals are kept, and avoid consumption of unpasteurized dairy products. A human vaccine for Q fever has been developed and used in Australia, but it is not available in the United States.

CDC website: www.cdc.gov/qfever

BIBLIOGRAPHY
1. Cohen NJ, Papernik M, Singleton J, Segreti J, Eremeeva ME. Q fever in an American tourist returned from Australia. Travel Med Infect Dis. 2007 May;5(3):194–5.
2. Kobbe R, Kramme S, Gocht A, Werner M, Lippert U, May J, et al. Travel-associated Coxiella burnetii infections: three cases of Q fever with different clinical manifestation. Travel Med Infect Dis. 2007 Nov;5(6):374–9.
3. Maurin M, Raoult D. Q fever. Clin Microbiol Rev. 1999 Oct;12(4):518–53.
4. McQuiston JH, Childs JE, Thompson HA. Q fever. J Am Vet Med Assoc. 2002 Sep 15;221(6):796–9.
5. Schimmer B, Morroy G, Dijkstra F, Schneeberger PM, Weers-Pothoff G, Timen A, et al. Large ongoing Q fever outbreak in the south of The Netherlands, 2008. Euro Surveill. 2008 Jul 31;13(31).
6. Ta TH, Jimenez B, Navarro M, Meije Y, Gonzalez FJ, Lopez-Velez R. Q Fever in returned febrile travelers. J Travel Med. 2008 Mar–Apr;15(2):126–9.

RABIES
Charles E. Rupprecht, David R. Shlim

INFECTIOUS AGENTS
Rabies is an acute, progressive encephalomyelitis caused by neurotropic viruses in the family Rhabdoviridae, genus Lyssavirus. Regardless of the viral variants found throughout the world, all lyssaviruses cause rabies, resulting in tens of millions of human exposures and tens of thousands of human deaths each year.

TRANSMISSION
Virus is present in the saliva of the biting rabid mammal. Transmission almost always occurs by an animal bite that inoculates virus into wounds. Virus inoculated into a wound does not enter the bloodstream but is taken up at a nerve synapse to travel to the central nervous system, where it causes encephalitis. Virus may enter the nervous system fairly rapidly

or may remain at the bite site for an extended period. The approximate density of nerve endings in the region of the bite may increase the risk of developing encephalitis more rapidly. The hands and face, because of the relative density of nerve endings, are considered higher-risk exposures. Rarely, virus has been transmitted by exposures other than bites that introduce the agent into open wounds or mucous membranes.

All mammals are believed to be susceptible to infection, but major reservoirs are carnivores and bats. Although dogs are the main reservoir in developing countries, the epidemiology of the disease from one region or country to another differs enough to warrant the medical evaluation of all mammal bites. *Bat bites anywhere in the world are a cause of concern and an indication for prophylaxis.*

EPIDEMIOLOGY

Rabies is found on all continents, except Antarctica. Regionally, different viral variants are adapted to various mammalian hosts and perpetuate in dogs and wildlife, such as bats and some carnivores, including foxes, jackals, mongooses, raccoons, and skunks. In certain areas of the world, canine rabies remains enzootic, including, but not limited to, parts of Africa, Asia, and Central and South America. Table 3-14 lists countries that have reported no cases of rabies during the most recent period for which information is available (formerly referred to as "rabies-free" countries).

Additional information about the global occurrence of rabies can be obtained from the following sources:

- World Health Organization (www.who.int/topics/rabies/en)

Table 3-14. Countries and political units that reported no indigenous cases of rabies during 2012[1]

REGION	COUNTRIES/LOCALITIES
Africa	Cape Verde, Mauritius, Réunion, São Tomé and Príncipe, and Seychelles
Americas	North: Bermuda, Saint Pierre and Miquelon Caribbean: Antigua and Barbuda, Aruba, The Bahamas, Barbados, Cayman Islands, Dominica, Guadeloupe, Jamaica, Martinique, Montserrat, Netherlands Antilles, Saint Kitts (Saint Christopher) and Nevis, Saint Lucia, Saint Martin, Saint Vincent and Grenadines, Turks and Caicos, and Virgin Islands (UK and US)
Asia and the Middle East	Hong Kong, Japan, Kuwait, Malaysia (Sabah), Qatar, Singapore, Taiwan, United Arab Emirates
Europe[2]	Albania, Austria, Belgium, Corsica, Cyprus, Czech Republic, Denmark, Finland, France, Germany, Gibraltar, Greece, Hungary, Iceland, Ireland, Isle of Man, Liechtenstein, Luxembourg, Monaco, Netherlands, Norway (except Svalbard), Portugal, Slovakia, Slovenia, Spain (except Ceuta and Melilla), Sweden, Switzerland, and United Kingdom
Oceania[3]	Australia,[3] Cook Islands, Fiji, French Polynesia, Guam, Hawaii, Kiribati, Micronesia, New Caledonia, New Zealand, Northern Mariana Islands, Palau, Papua New Guinea, Samoa, and Vanuatu

[1] Global surveillance efforts and reporting standards differ dramatically, conditions may change rapidly because of animal translocation, and bat rabies may exist in some areas that are reportedly "free" of rabies in other mammals.
[2] Bat lyssaviruses have been reported throughout Europe, including areas that are reportedly free of rabies in other wild mammals.
[3] Most of Pacific Oceania is reportedly "rabies-free," with the exception of Australia, where lyssaviruses in bats have been reported, as well as fatal human rabies cases.

- Rabies Bulletin—Europe (www.who-rabies-bulletin.org)
- World Organisation for Animal Health (www.oie.int/en/animal-health-in-the-world/rabies-portal)
- Local health authorities of the country, the embassy, or the local consulate's office in the United States

These lists are provided only as a guide, because up-to-date information may not be available, surveillance standards vary, and reporting status can change suddenly as a result of disease reintroduction or emergence. The actual rate of possible rabies exposure in travelers has not been calculated with accuracy. However, studies have found a range of roughly 16–200 per 100,000 travelers based on differing criteria.

CLINICAL PRESENTATION

Most patients will present after a documented, highly suspected, or likely exposure from a rabid animal. Clinical illness is compatible with acute, progressive encephalitis. After infection, the incubation period is highly variable, but it lasts approximately 1–3 months. The disease progresses acutely from a nonspecific, prodromal phase with fever and vague symptoms, to a neurologic phase, characterized by anxiety, paresis, paralysis, and other signs of encephalitis; spasms of swallowing muscles can be stimulated by the sight, sound, or perception of water (hydrophobia); and delirium and convulsions can develop, followed rapidly by coma and death. Once clinical signs manifest, most patients die in 7–14 days.

DIAGNOSIS

Diagnosis is straightforward in an encephalitic patient recently exposed to a rabid animal. However, in lieu of a history of a documented exposure and the potential for long incubation periods of weeks to months after initial viral transmission, clinical diagnosis may be complicated by the variety of symptoms and the differential exclusion of other etiologic agents associated with encephalitis.

Definitive diagnosis can be made by demonstrating virus in neuronal tissue, corneal impressions, or nuchal biopsy, either by detecting viral antigens or amplicons. Additional detailed information on diagnostic testing may be obtained from CDC (www.cdc.gov/rabies). A specific serologic response to virus can also support the diagnosis in an unvaccinated encephalitic patient.

TREATMENT

There is no known cure after the onset of clinical signs. One experimental approach, known as the Milwaukee protocol, involves coma induction and antiviral drug treatment and has been used in approximately 40 rabies patients around the world, with at least 4 reported survivors (www.chw.org/display/PPF/DocID/33223/router.asp). Despite these observations, rabies must still be considered 100% fatal for practical purposes, and preventive measures remain the only way to guarantee survival after a bite by a rabid animal.

PREVENTION

Prevention of rabies in travelers is best accomplished by having a comprehensive strategy. Such a strategy consists of 1) avoiding animal bites; 2) knowing how to prevent rabies after a bite; and 3) being able to travel (even to another country) to wherever postexposure prophylaxis (PEP) is available. To our knowledge, no traveler has died while trying to obtain PEP. The few travelers who have died of rabies received either no or inadequate PEP.

Avoiding Animal Bites

Travelers to rabies-enzootic countries should be warned about the risk of acquiring rabies and educated in animal bite-prevention strategies. Travelers should avoid feral animals, be aware of their surroundings so that they do not accidentally surprise a dog, and avoid contact with bats and other wildlife. A particular risk for a bite exposure is from monkeys who live near temples and other urban areas of Asia. Tourists to these sites should not carry any food on their person or in their backpack, purse, or other bag and should be careful not to approach or otherwise interact with monkeys. Casual exposure to cave air is not a concern, but visitors should be educated not to handle bats or other wildlife. Many bats have tiny teeth, and not all wounds may be apparent, compared with the lesions caused by carnivores. Any suspected or documented bite or scratch from a bat should be grounds for seeking PEP.

Children are at higher risk for rabies exposures because of their smaller stature, which makes extensive bites more likely; their curiosity and attraction to animals; and the possibility that they may not report a possible exposure. Although licks to fresh wounds or mucus membranes are a theoretical risk of acquiring rabies and PEP should be considered, there are no documented examples of rabies in travelers who were exposed in this manner.

Preexposure Vaccination

For certain international travelers, preexposure rabies vaccine may be recommended, based on the prevalence of rabies in the country to be visited, the availability of appropriate antirabies biologics, intended activities, and duration of stay. A decision to receive preexposure rabies immunization may also be based on the likelihood of repeat travel to at-risk destinations or taking up residence in a high-risk destination. Preexposure vaccination may be recommended for veterinarians, animal handlers, field biologists, cavers, missionaries, and certain laboratory workers. Table 3-15 provides criteria for preexposure vaccination. Serology for rabies virus neutralizing antibodies is used as one gauge

Table 3-15. Criteria for preexposure immunization for rabies

RISK CATEGORY	NATURE OF RISK	TYPICAL POPULATIONS	PREEXPOSURE REGIMEN
Continuous	Virus present continuously, often in high concentrations Specific exposures likely to go unrecognized Bite, nonbite, or aerosol exposure	Rabies research laboratory workers,[1] rabies biologics production workers	Primary course; serologic testing every 6 months; booster vaccination if antibody titer is below acceptable level[2]
Frequent	Exposure usually episodic with source recognized, but exposure might also be unrecognized Bite, nonbite, or aerosol exposure possible	Rabies diagnostic laboratory workers,[1] cavers, veterinarians and staff, and animal control and wildlife workers in rabies-epizootic areas	Primary course; serologic testing every 2 years; booster vaccination if antibody titer is below acceptable level[2]
Infrequent (more than general population)	Exposure nearly always episodic with source recognized Bite or nonbite exposure	Veterinarians, animal control, and wildlife workers in areas with low rabies rates; veterinary students; and travelers visiting areas where rabies is enzootic and immediate access to medical care, including biologics, is limited	Primary course; no serologic testing or booster vaccination
Rare (general population)	Exposure always episodic, with source recognized	US population at large, including people in rabies-epizootic areas	No preexposure immunization necessary

[1] Judgment of relative risk and extra monitoring of vaccination status of laboratory workers are the responsibility of the laboratory supervisor (see www.cdc.gov/biosafety/publications/bmbl5 for more information).

[2] Preexposure booster immunization consists of 1 dose of human diploid cell (rabies) vaccine or purified chick embryo cell vaccine, 1.0-mL dose, intramuscular (deltoid area). Per Advisory Committee on Immunization Practices recommendations, minimum acceptable antibody level is complete virus neutralization at a 1:5 serum dilution by the rapid fluorescent focus inhibition test, which is equivalent to approximately 0.1 IU/mL. A booster dose should be administered if titer falls below this level in populations that remain at risk.

for revaccination considerations. Lists of US laboratories performing rabies serology may be found on the CDC website (www.cdc.gov/rabies). Regardless of whether preexposure vaccine is administered, travelers going to areas with a high risk for rabies should be encouraged to purchase medical evacuation insurance (see Chapter 2, Travel Insurance, Travel Health Insurance, & Medical Evacuation Insurance).

In the United States, preexposure vaccination consists of a series of 3 injections with human diploid cell rabies vaccine (HDCV) or purified chick embryo cell (PCEC) vaccine. The schedule for this series is given in Table 3-16. Travelers should receive all 3 preexposure immunizations before travel. If 3 doses of rabies vaccine cannot be completed before travel, the traveler should not start the series, as it would be problematic to plan PEP after a partial immunization series.

Preexposure vaccination does not eliminate the need for additional medical attention after a rabies exposure, but it simplifies PEP. Preexposure vaccination may also provide some degree of protection when there is an unrecognized exposure to rabies virus and when PEP might be delayed. Travelers who have completed a 3-dose preexposure rabies immunization series or have received full PEP are considered preimmunized and do not require routine boosters, except after a suspected rabies exposure. Periodic serum testing for rabies virus neutralizing antibody is not necessary in routine international travelers.

Wound Management

Any animal bite or scratch should be thoroughly cleaned with copious amounts of soap and water. This local care will substantially reduce the risk for rabies. Wounds that might require suturing should have the suturing delayed for a few days. If suturing is necessary to control bleeding or for functional or cosmetic reasons, rabies immune globulin (RIG), if indicated, should be administered into the wound before closing. The use of local anesthetic is not contraindicated in wound management.

Postexposure Prophylaxis
In Travelers Who Received Preexposure Vaccination

In the event of a possible rabies exposure in someone who received preexposure rabies vaccination, 2 boosters of an acceptable rabies vaccine are given on days 0 and 3 after the exposure. The booster doses should be modern cell culture vaccines, but they do not have to be the same brand as the vaccine given in the original preexposure immunization series.

In Travelers Who Did Not Receive Preexposure Vaccination

If preexposure rabies vaccination has not been given, PEP consists of injections of RIG (20 IU/kg) and a series of 4 injections of rabies vaccine over 14 days (or 5 doses over a 1-month period in immunosuppressed patients, Table 3-17). After wound cleansing, as much of the calculated amount of RIG (Table 3-17) as is anatomically feasible should be infiltrated around the wound, striving to put the RIG in the areas where the animal's teeth and saliva have come in contact with the wound. The dose injected around the wound may be as small as 0.5 mL if the wound is small or

Table 3-16. Preexposure immunization for rabies[1]

VACCINE	DOSE (ML)	NUMBER OF DOSES	SCHEDULE (DAYS)	ROUTE
HDCV, Imovax (Sanofi)	1.0	3	0, 7, and 21 or 28	IM
PCEC, RabAvert (Novartis)	1.0	3	0, 7, and 21 or 28	IM

Abbreviations: HDCV, human diploid cell vaccine; IM, intramuscular; PCEC, purified chick embryo cell.
[1] Patients who are immunosuppressed by disease or medications should postpone preexposure vaccinations and consider avoiding activities for which rabies preexposure prophylaxis is indicated. When this course is not possible, immunosuppressed people who are at risk for rabies should have their antibody titers checked after vaccination.

Table 3-17. Postexposure immunization for rabies[1]

IMMUNIZATION STATUS	VACCINE/ PRODUCT	DOSE	NUMBER OF DOSES	SCHEDULE (DAYS)	ROUTE
Not previously immunized	RIG plus	20 IU/kg body weight	1	0	Infiltrated at bite site (if possible); remainder IM
	HDCV or PCEC	1.0 mL	4[2]	0, 3, 7, 14	IM
Previously immunized[3,4]	HDCV or PCEC	1.0 mL	2	0, 3	IM

Abbreviations: RIG, rabies immune globulin; IM, intramuscular; HDCV, human diploid cell vaccine; PCEC, purified chick embryo cell.

[1] All postexposure prophylaxis should begin with immediate, thorough cleansing of all wounds with soap and water.

[2] Five vaccine doses for the immunosuppressed patient. The first 4 vaccine doses are given on the same schedule as for an immunocompetent patient, and the fifth dose is given on day 28.

[3] Preexposure immunization with HDCV or PCEC, prior postexposure prophylaxis with HDCV or PCEC, or people previously immunized with any other type of rabies vaccine and a documented history of positive rabies virus neutralizing antibody response to the prior vaccination.

[4] RIG should not be administered.

on a finger. If the wounds are extensive, the calculated dose of RIG must not be exceeded. If the calculated dose is inadequate to inject all the wounds, the RIG should be diluted with normal saline to extend the number of wounds that can be injected. This is a particular issue in children, whose body weight may be small in relation to the size and number of wounds.

The remainder of the RIG dose, if any, should be injected intramuscularly. Care should be taken to guarantee that this remaining amount of RIG is deposited in a muscle and not injected subcutaneously, which may decrease its effectiveness. The remaining RIG can be given in the deltoid muscle, on the opposite side of the initial vaccine dose. The anterior thigh is an alternative site.

RIG should not be given >7 days after the start of the PEP series. This 7-day period does not relate to the time of the bite exposure itself. Initiation of PEP, including RIG infiltration, should begin after a bite exposure, even if there has been a considerable delay between the exposure and the traveler presenting for evaluation.

Human RIG is manufactured by plasmapheresis of blood from hyperimmunized volunteers. The manufactured quantity of human RIG falls short of worldwide requirements, and it is not available in many developing countries. Equine RIG or purified fractions of equine RIG have been used effectively in some developing countries where human RIG might not be available. If necessary, such heterologous products are preferable to no RIG.

The incidence of adverse events after the use of modern equine-derived RIG is low (0.8%–6.0%), and most reactions are minor. However, such products are not evaluated by US standards or regulated by the Food and Drug Administration, and their use cannot be recommended unequivocally. In addition, unpurified antirabies serum of equine origin might still be used in some countries where neither human nor equine RIG is available. The use of this antirabies serum is associated with higher rates of serious adverse reactions, including anaphylaxis.

Different PEP schedules, alternative routes of administration, and other rabies vaccines besides HDCV and PCEC may be used abroad. Although not approved for sale in the United States, purified Vero cell rabies vaccine and purified chick embryo cell vaccine (manufactured abroad) are acceptable alternatives if available in a destination country. Assistance in managing complicated PEP scenarios may be obtained from experienced travel medicine professionals, health departments, and CDC.

Rabies vaccine was once manufactured from viruses grown in animal brains, and some of these vaccines are still in use in developing countries. Typically, the brain-derived vaccines can be identified if the traveler is offered a large injection (5 mL) daily for approximately 14–21 days. The traveler should not accept these vaccines, but rather travel to where acceptable vaccines and RIG are available.

Rabies Vaccine
Vaccine Safety and Adverse Reactions
Travelers should be advised that they may experience local reactions after vaccination, such as pain, erythema, swelling, or itching at the injection site, or mild systemic reactions,

such as headache, nausea, abdominal pain, muscle aches, and dizziness. Approximately 6% of people receiving booster vaccinations with HDCV may experience an immune complex–like reaction characterized by urticaria, pruritus, and malaise. The likelihood of these reactions may be less with PCEC. Once initiated, rabies PEP should not be interrupted or discontinued because of local or mild systemic reactions to rabies vaccine.

Precautions and Contraindications
Pregnancy is not a contraindication to PEP. In infants and children, the dose of HDCV or PCEC for preexposure or PEP is the same as that recommended for adults. The dose of RIG for PEP is based on body weight (Table 3-17).

CDC website: www.cdc.gov/rabies

BIBLIOGRAPHY

1. Gautret P, Adehossi E, Soula G, Soavi MJ, Delmont J, Rotivel Y, et al. Rabies exposure in international travelers: do we miss the target? Int J Infect Dis. 2010 Mar;14(3):e243–6.
2. Gautret P, Parola P. Rabies vaccination for international travelers. Vaccine. 2012 Jan 5;30(2):126–33.
3. Gautret P, Tantawichien T, Vu Hai V, Piyaphanee W. Determinants of pre-exposure rabies vaccination among foreign backpackers in Bangkok, Thailand. Vaccine. 2011 May 23;29(23):3931–4.
4. Malerczyk C, Detora L, Gniel D. Imported human rabies cases in Europe, the United States, and Japan, 1990 to 2010. J Travel Med. 2011 Nov–Dec;18(6):402–7.
5. Mills DJ, Lau CL, Weinstein P. Animal bites and rabies exposure in Australian travellers. Med J Aust. 2011 Dec 19;195(11–12):673–5.
6. Pavli A, Saroglou G, Hadjianastasiou S, Patrinos S, Vakali A, Ouzounidou Z, et al. Knowledge and practices about rabies among travel medicine consultants in Greece. Travel Med Infect Dis. 2011 Jan;9(1):32–6.
7. Rupprecht CE, Briggs D, Brown CM, Franka R, Katz SL, Kerr HD, et al. Use of a reduced (4-dose) vaccine schedule for postexposure prophylaxis to prevent human rabies: recommendations of the advisory committee on immunization practices. MMWR Recomm Rep. 2010 Mar 19;59(RR-2):1–9.
8. Rupprecht CE, Gibbons RV. Clinical practice. Prophylaxis against rabies. N Engl J Med. 2004 Dec 16;351(25):2626–35.
9. Shaw MT, O'Brien B, Leggat PA. Rabies postexposure management of travelers presenting to travel health clinics in Auckland and Hamilton, New Zealand. J Travel Med. 2009 Jan–Feb;16(1):13–7.
10. Smith A, Petrovic M, Solomon T, Fooks A. Death from rabies in a UK traveller returning from India. Euro Surveill. 2005 Jul;10(30):pii=2761.
11. Strauss R, Granz A, Wassermann-Neuhold M, Krause R, Bago Z, Revilla-Fernandez S, et al. A human case of travel-related rabies in Austria, September 2004. Euro Surveill. 2005 Nov;10(11):225–6.
12. van Thiel PP, de Bie RM, Eftimov F, Tepaske R, Zaaijer HL, van Doornum GJ, et al. Fatal human rabies due to Duvenhage virus from a bat in Kenya: failure of treatment with coma-induction, ketamine, and antiviral drugs. PLoS Negl Trop Dis. 2009;3(7):e428.
13. Warrell MJ, Warrell DA. Rabies and other lyssavirus diseases. Lancet. 2004 Mar 20;363(9413):959–69.
14. Wijaya L, Ford L, Lalloo D. Rabies postexposure prophylaxis in a UK travel clinic: ten years' experience. J Travel Med. 2011 Jul–Aug;18(4):257–61.
15. World Health Organization. WHO expert consultation on rabies. World Health Organ Tech Rep Ser. 2005;931:1–88.
16. Yamamoto S, Iwasaki C, Oono H, Ninomiya K, Matsumura T. The first imported case of rabies into Japan in 36 years: a forgotten life-threatening disease. J Travel Med. 2008 Sep–Oct;15(5):372–4.

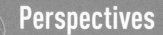
INTRADERMAL RABIES PREEXPOSURE IMMUNIZATION
David R. Shlim

Few topics in travel medicine prompt more concern and persistent questions than the prevention of rabies in travelers. Although we understand the basics of rabies prevention for travelers, the logistics of providing this care in a timely fashion remain a challenge. Unimmunized travelers who are exposed to rabies and other lyssaviruses require proper wound care, infiltration of human rabies immune globulin (HRIG), and a series of 4 or 5 doses of rabies vaccine intramuscularly over a 2- to 4-week period. Travelers who receive 3 doses of rabies vaccine before travel need to receive 2 more doses of rabies vaccine, 3 days apart, after a viral exposure. Notably, HRIG and equine RIG are often unavailable in developing countries, although modern cell culture rabies vaccines are increasingly available. Thus, preexposure rabies immunization can facilitate the traveler's access to adequate postexposure rabies prophylaxis.

One limiting factor in the use of preexposure rabies immunization has been the cost of the vaccine in most developed countries. In the United States, rabies vaccine may cost more than $200 per dose, resulting in a cost to the patient in excess of $600 for three 1.0-mL intramuscular injections. As one way of decreasing the cost of preexposure immunization, some practitioners have used a 0.1-mL dose of rabies vaccine administered intradermally.

At approximately $45 per dose in the early 1980s, many people considered the vaccine too expensive. Thus, intradermal rabies immunization began almost as soon as the intramuscular human diploid cell vaccine (HDCV) was manufactured. By reconstituting the 1.0 mL of vaccine in the vial, practitioners could draw up approximately eight 0.1-mL doses. One problem was that the entire vial had to be used within a few hours of reconstituting, meaning that a provider had to either be in a very busy clinic or line up groups of people, such as families, for rabies immunization at the same time.

Early studies of the immune response to intradermal rabies vaccine, using HDCV and later other rabies vaccines, were uniformly encouraging. Virtually 100% of vaccinees seroconverted. A 1982 statement by the US Advisory Committee on Immunization Practices (ACIP) reviewed data on >1,500 vaccinees and declared, "It appears that, with this vaccine, the 0.1-mL intradermal (ID) regimen is an acceptable alternative to the currently approved 1.0-mL intramuscular (IM) regimen for preexposure prophylaxis." They called upon manufacturers to produce a product with appropriate packaging and labeling.

In 1986, the Merieux Institute (now Sanofi Pasteur) received approval to market a 0.1-mL dose in an individual syringe. Sharing reconstituted vials of 1.0 mL between patients remained off-label. Although the new product solved one logistical problem of providing individual travelers with an ID dose, the cost of the prepackaged ID dose was 75% of the full 1.0-mL IM dose.

Perspectives sections are written as editorial discussions aiming to add depth and clinical perspective to the official recommendations contained in the book. The views and opinions expressed in this section are those of the author and do not necessarily represent the official position of CDC.

As ID rabies immunization was being implemented, a death from rabies in an American Peace Corps volunteer in Kenya brought the enthusiasm for ID immunization to a temporary halt. The 23-year-old female volunteer died of rabies after a bite from a stray puppy that she had adopted. She had received 3 doses of ID rabies vaccine in Kenya, finishing 6 months before the bite. She did not suspect that the dog had rabies, even though it died shortly after biting her. As a result, she did not seek postexposure boosters. The Peace Corps medical personnel wondered why the recent ID immunization had not been effective. Serum drawn at the onset of her symptoms revealed she did not have an adequate antibody response. Concerned that she may have had an atypical response to immunization, they tested serum specimens from 11 other Peace Corps volunteers in Kenya who had been immunized at the same time. To their surprise, 9 (82%) of 11 also had an inadequate immunologic response. As a control group, Peace Corps volunteers who had received rabies ID preexposure immunization in Nepal and Morocco were also tested, and 31 (39%) of 79 had an inadequate antibody response.

Studies were undertaken to confirm the potency of the vaccine lot, maintenance of the cold chain, the method of administration, and the effect of concomitant medication. None of these factors proved to be an entirely adequate explanation. For example, chloroquine taken as an antimalarial medication during ID rabies immunization reduced the levels of antibody induced. However, the seroconversion rate of chloroquine was still adequate, and the volunteers in Morocco and Nepal were not taking chloroquine. After the investigation, it was recommended that people using ID preexposure immunization should complete the course before starting chloroquine and traveling abroad, or else use the IM regimen.

The ACIP continued to endorse the concept of ID preexposure rabies immunization in a 1999 statement on rabies prevention. However, 3 lots of a prepackaged rabies ID vaccine were recalled during 2000 for having a potency that fell below the specification level before the expiration date. In 2001, the ID rabies vaccine was withdrawn from the market. Since then, authorities in the United States have not recommended sharing 1.0-mL vials for ID rabies immunization, as the manufacturer has not applied for the appropriate packaging and labeling to the Food and Drug Administration (FDA). This lack of endorsement of ID preexposure immunization has frustrated some travel medicine professionals.

Based on recent data, the World Health Organization has recommended the use of ID preexposure rabies immunization as an alternative to IM immunization. In a recent study of 420 Australian travelers given a modified ID rabies preexposure immunization (2 doses on day 0, 2 doses on day 7, and 1 dose on day 21–28), a seroconversion rate of 98.3% was documented. Although a potential savings might accrue from use of only 0.5 mL of vaccine total, this does not alleviate the point of identifying several travelers in a few hours or using multiple doses from a single-use vial and would not provide any temporal benefit due to the 3- to 4-week interval needed for vaccination before departure.

Neither ACIP nor FDA are likely to endorse the use of 1.0-mL vials of rabies vaccine for multiple-dose ID use unless the manufacturer requests that indication. Until then, the use of ID rabies vaccine will remain off-label in the United States. The current status of ID rabies immunization in the United States reflects a regulatory situation and ACIP opinion and is not a comment on the effectiveness of ID rabies preexposure immunization for travelers elsewhere.

BIBLIOGRAPHY

1. Bernard KW, Fishbein DB, Miller KD, Parker RA, Waterman S, Sumner JW, et al. Pre-exposure rabies immunization with human diploid cell vaccine: decreased antibody responses in persons immunized in developing countries. Am J Trop Med Hyg. 1985 May;34(3):633–47.

2. CDC. Recommendation of the Immunization Practices Advisory Committee (ACIP). Supplementary statement on pre-exposure rabies prophylaxis by the intradermal route. MMWR Morb Mortal Wkly Rep. 1982 Jun 4;31(21):279–80, 85.

3. Mills DJ, Lau CL, Fearnley EJ, Weinstein P. The immunogenicity of a modified intradermal pre-exposure rabies vaccination schedule—a case series of 420 travelers. J Travel Med. 2011 Sep–Oct;18(5):327–32.

RICKETTSIAL (SPOTTED & TYPHUS FEVERS) & RELATED INFECTIONS (ANAPLASMOSIS & EHRLICHIOSIS)

Marina E. Eremeeva, Gregory A. Dasch

INFECTIOUS AGENT

Rickettsial infections are caused by a variety of obligate intracellular, gram-negative bacteria from the genera *Rickettsia*, *Orientia*, *Ehrlichia*, *Neorickettsia*, *Neoehrlichia*, and *Anaplasma*, belonging to the Alphaproteobacteria (Table 3-18). *Rickettsia* were classically divided into the typhus group and spotted fever group (SFG), although the genus has been subdivided further based on phylogenetic analysis. *Orientia* spp. make up the scrub typhus group.

TRANSMISSION

Most rickettsial pathogens are transmitted by ectoparasites such as fleas, lice, mites, and ticks during feeding or by scratching crushed arthropods or infectious feces into the skin. Inhaling dust or inoculating conjunctiva with infectious material may also cause infection. The specific vectors that transmit each form of rickettsiae are listed in Table 3-18. Transmission of some rickettsial diseases after transfusion or organ transplantation is rare but has been reported.

EPIDEMIOLOGY

All age groups are at risk for rickettsial infections during travel to endemic areas. Transmission is increased during outdoor activities in the spring and summer months when ticks and fleas are most active. However, infection can occur throughout the year. Because of the 5- to 14-day incubation period for most rickettsial diseases, tourists may not necessarily experience symptoms during their trip, and onset may coincide with their return home or develop within a week after returning.

The most commonly diagnosed rickettsial diseases in travelers are usually in the spotted fever or typhus groups, but travelers may acquire a wide range of rickettsioses, including emerging and newly recognized species (Table 3-18). Game hunting and traveling to southern Africa from November through April are risk factors for African tick-bite fever in travelers, which is the most frequently reported travel-associated rickettsiosis. However, Mediterranean spotted fever infections occur over an even larger region and can be quite severe.

Rickettsialpox, transmitted by house-mouse mites, circulates in urban centers in Ukraine, South Africa, Korea, the Balkan states, and the United States. Outbreaks of

Table 3-18. Classification, primary vector, and reservoir occurrence of rickettsiae known to cause disease in humans

ANTIGENIC GROUP	DISEASE	SPECIES	VECTOR	ANIMAL RESERVOIR(S)	GEOGRAPHIC DISTRIBUTION
Anaplasma	Human granulocytic anaplasmosis	Anaplasma phagocytophilum	Tick	Small mammals, rodents, and deer	Primarily United States, worldwide
Ehrlichia	Human monocytic ehrlichiosis	Ehrlichia chaffeensis	Tick	Deer, wild and domestic dogs, domestic ruminants, and rodents	Common in United States, probably worldwide
	Ehrlichiosis	E. muris	Tick	Deer and rodents	North America, Europe, Asia
	Ehrlichiosis	E. ewingii	Tick	Deer, wild and domestic dogs, and rodents	North America, Cameroon, Korea
Neoehrlichia	Human neoehrlichiosis	Neoehrlichia mikurensis	Tick	Rodents	Europe, Asia
Neorickettsia	Sennetsu fever	Neorickettsia sennetsu	Trematode	Fish	Japan, Malaysia, possibly other parts of Asia
Scrub typhus	Scrub typhus	Orientia tsutsugamushi	Larval mite (chigger)	Rodents	Asia-Pacific region from maritime Russia and China to Indonesia and North Australia to Afghanistan
	Scrub typhus	Orientia chuto	Unknown	Unknown	Dubai
Spotted fever	Rickettsiosis	Rickettsia aeschlimannii	Tick	Unknown	South Africa, Morocco, Mediterranean littoral
	African tick-bite fever	R. africae	Tick	Ruminants	Sub-Saharan Africa, West Indies
	Rickettsialpox	R. akari	Mite	House mice, wild rodents	Countries of the former Soviet Union, South Africa, Korea, Turkey, Balkan countries, North and South America
	Queensland tick typhus	R. australis	Tick	Rodents	Australia, Tasmania
	Mediterranean spotted fever or Boutonneuse fever	R. conorii[1]	Tick	Dogs, rodents	Southern Europe, southern and western Asia, Africa, India

Group	Disease	Organism	Vector	Host	Geographic distribution
	Cat flea rickettsiosis	R. felis	Flea	Domestic cats, rodents, opossums	Europe, North and South America, Africa, Asia
	Far Eastern spotted fever	R. heilongjiangensis	Tick	Rodents	Far East of Russia, Northern China, eastern Asia
	Aneruptive fever	R. helvetica	Tick	Rodents	Central and northern Europe, Asia
	Flinders Island spotted fever, Thai tick typhus	R. honei, including strain "marmionii"	Tick	Rodents, reptiles	Australia, Thailand
	Japanese spotted fever	R. japonica	Tick	Rodents	Japan
	Mediterranean spotted fever–like disease	R. massiliae	Tick	Unknown	France, Greece, Spain, Portugal, Switzerland, Sicily, central Africa, and Mali
	Mediterranean spotted fever–like illness	R. monacensis	Tick	Lizards, possibly birds	Europe, North Africa
	Maculatum infection	R. parkeri and related agents	Tick	Rodents	North and South America
	Tickborne lymphadenopathy, Dermacentor-borne necrosis and lymphadenopathy	R. raoultii	Tick	Unknown	Europe, Asia
	Rocky Mountain spotted fever, febre maculosa, São Paulo exanthematic typhus, Minas Gerais exanthematic typhus, Brazilian spotted fever	R. rickettsii	Tick	Rodents	North, Central, and South America
	North Asian tick typhus, Siberian tick typhus	R. sibirica	Tick	Rodents	Russia, China, Mongolia
	Lymphangitis- associated rickettsiosis	R. sibiricamongo-lotimonae	Tick	Rodents	Southern France, Portugal, China, Africa
	Tickborne lymphadenopathy (TIBOLA), Dermacentor-borne necrosis and lymphadenopathy (DEBONEL)	R. slovaca	Tick	Lagomorphs, rodents	Southern and eastern Europe, Asia
Typhus fever	Epidemic typhus, sylvatic typhus	R. prowazekii	Human body louse, flying squirrel ectoparasites, Amblyomma ticks	Humans, flying squirrels	Central Africa, Asia, Central, North, and South America
	Murine typhus	R. typhi	Flea	Rodents	Tropical and subtropical areas worldwide

[1] Includes 4 different subspecies that can be distinguished serologically and by PCR assay and that respectively are the etiologic agents of Boutonneuse fever and Mediterranean tick fever in southern Europe and Africa (R. conorii subsp. conorii), Indian tick typhus in south Asia (R. conorii subsp. indica), Israeli tick typhus in southern Europe and Middle East (R. conorii subsp. israelensis), and Astrakhan spotted fever in the North Caspian region of Russia (R. conorii subsp. caspiae).

rickettsialpox most often occur after contact with infected rodents and their mites, especially during natural die-offs or exterminations of infected rodents that cause the mites to seek out new hosts, including humans. The agent may spill over and occasionally be found in other wild rodent populations.

Scrub typhus is endemic in northern Japan, Southeast Asia, the western Pacific Islands, eastern Australia, China, maritime areas and several parts of south-central Russia, India, and Sri Lanka. More than 1 million cases occur annually. Most travel-acquired cases of scrub typhus occur during visits to rural areas in endemic countries for activities such as camping, hiking, or rafting, but urban cases have also been described.

Fleaborne rickettsioses caused by R. typhi and R. felis are widely distributed, especially throughout the tropics and subtropics and in port cities and coastal regions with rodents. Humans exposed to flea-infested cats, dogs, and peridomestic animals while traveling in endemic regions or entering areas infested with rodents are at most risk for fleaborne rickettsioses. Murine typhus has been reported among travelers returning from Asia, Africa, and the Mediterranean Basin and has also been reported from Hawaii, California, and Texas in the United States.

Epidemic typhus occurs in communities and refugee populations where body lice are prevalent. Outbreaks often occur during the colder months when infested clothing is not laundered. Travelers at most risk for epidemic typhus include those who may work with or visit areas with large homeless populations, impoverished areas, refugee camps, and regions that have recently experienced war or natural disasters. Active foci of endemic typhus are known in the Andes regions of South America and in Burundi and Ethiopia. Sylvatic epidemic typhus cases occur only from direct contact with flying squirrels or their nesting materials and squirrel ecoparasites in the eastern United States. Tick-associated reservoirs of R. prowazekii have been described in Ethiopia, Mexico, and Brazil.

Ehrlichiosis is most commonly reported in the southeastern and south-central United States where the lonestar tick, Amblyomma americanum, and white-tailed deer are commonplace. In Europe and Asia, transmission of monocytic ehrlichiosis appears to be due primarily to Ehrlichia chaffeensis or related organisms, which may also occur in Brazil, Panama, and Africa. E. muris and Neoehrlichia mikurensis are associated with ticks of the Ixodes persulcatus complex and their rodent hosts. These agents cause human infections in the upper Midwestern United States and Europe, respectively, and probably also cause disease in other regions. E. ruminantium and a related agent from the United States have been identified as causes of human infections in South Africa and the southeastern United States. E. canis has been reported to cause human infections in Venezuela.

Human Anaplasma infections are most commonly reported in the United States but can occur more rarely in Europe and Asia. The agent occurs worldwide, corresponding with the ranges of I. persulcatus group ticks. Although nonpathogenic genetic variants are common worldwide in many vertebrate hosts, human pathogenic types are present in rodent and small-mammal reservoirs in North America and in deer (roe and red) and wild boar in Europe.

Sennetsu fever occurs in Japan, Malaysia, and possibly other parts of Asia. This disease can be contracted from eating raw infected fish.

CLINICAL PRESENTATION
Rickettsioses are difficult to specifically diagnose, even by physicians experienced with these diseases. Clinical presentations vary with the causative agent and patient; however, common symptoms that typically develop within 1–2 weeks of infection include fever, headache, malaise, and sometimes nausea and vomiting. Most symptoms associated with acute rickettsial infections are nonspecific. Many rickettsioses are accompanied by a maculopapular, vesicular, or petechial rash or an eschar at the site of the tick bite. African tick-bite fever should be suspected in a patient who presents with fever, headache, myalgia, and an eschar (tache noir) after recent travel to southern Africa. Mediterranean spotted fever should be suspected in patients with rash and fever after recent travel to northern Africa or the Mediterranean littoral. Scrub typhus should be suspected in patients with a fever, headache, and myalgia after recent travel to Asia; eschar, lymphadenopathy, cough, hearing difficulties, and encephalitis may also be

present. Patients with typhus usually present with a severe but nonspecific febrile illness. Ehrlichiosis and anaplasmosis should be suspected in febrile patients with leukopenia and transaminitis with an exposure history. Most symptomatic rickettsial diseases cause moderate illness, but epidemic typhus and Rocky Mountain spotted fever can be severe and may be fatal in 20%–60% of untreated cases.

DIAGNOSIS

Diagnosis is usually based on clinical recognition and serology; the latter requires comparison of acute- to convalescent-phase serology, so is only helpful in retrospect. Etiologic agents can generally only be identified to the genus level by serologic testing. PCR and immunohistochemical analyses may also be helpful. If ehrlichiosis or anaplasmosis is suspected, a buffy coat may be examined to identify characteristic intraleukocytic morulae. Contact the CDC Rickettsial Zoonoses Branch at 404-639-1075 for further information.

TREATMENT

Treatment of patients with possible rickettsioses should be started early and should not await confirmatory testing. Treatment usually involves doxycycline. Chloramphenicol, azithromycin, fluoroquinolones, and rifampin may be alternatives, depending on the scenario. Expert advice should be sought if these alternative agents are being considered.

PREVENTION

No vaccine is available for preventing rickettsial infections. Antibiotics are not recommended for prophylaxis of rickettsial diseases.

Travelers should be instructed to minimize exposure to infectious arthropods (including lice, fleas, ticks, mites) and animal reservoirs, particularly dogs and cats, when traveling in endemic areas. The proper use of insect or tick repellents or insecticides and acaricides, self-examination after visits to vector-infested areas, and wearing protective clothing are ways to reduce risk. These precautions are especially important for people with underlying conditions that may compromise their immune systems, as these people may be more susceptible to severe disease. For more detailed information, see Chapter 2, Protection against Mosquitoes, Ticks, & Other Insects & Arthropods.

CDC website: www.cdc.gov/ticks

BIBLIOGRAPHY

1. Angelakis E, Botelho E, Socolovschi C, Sobas CR, Piketty C, Parola P, et al. Murine typhus as a cause of fever in travelers from Tunisia and Mediterranean areas. J Travel Med. 2010 Sep–Oct;17(5):310–5.
2. Demeester R, Claus M, Hildebrand M, Vlieghe E, Bottieau E. Diversity of life-threatening complications due to Mediterranean spotted fever in returning travelers. J Travel Med. 2010 Mar–Apr;17(2):100–4.
3. Dobler G, Wolfel R. Typhus and other rickettsioses: emerging infections in Germany. Dtsch Arztebl Int. 2009 May;106(20):348–54.
4. Hendershot EF, Sexton DJ. Scrub typhus and rickettsial diseases in international travelers: a review. Curr Infect Dis Rep. 2009 Jan;11(1):66–72.
5. Jensenius M, Davis X, von Sonnenburg F, Schwartz E, Keystone JS, Leder K, et al. Multicenter GeoSentinel analysis of rickettsial diseases in international travelers, 1996–2008. Emerg Infect Dis. 2009 Nov;15(11):1791–8.
6. Leshem E, Meltzer E, Schwartz E. Travel-associated zoonotic bacterial diseases. Curr Opin Infect Dis. 2011 Oct;24(5):457–63.
7. Nachega JB, Bottieau E, Zech F, Van Gompel A. Travel-acquired scrub typhus: emphasis on the differential diagnosis, treatment, and prevention strategies. J Travel Med. 2007 Sep–Oct;14(5):352–5.
8. Raoult D, Parola P, editors. Rickettsial Diseases. New York: Informa Healthcare USA, Inc; 2007.
9. Rar V, Golovljova I. *Anaplasma, Ehrlichia*, and "*Candidatus* Neoehrlichia" bacteria: pathogenicity, biodiversity, and molecular genetic characteristics, a review. Infect Genet Evol. 2011 Dec;11(8):1842–61.
10. Roch N, Epaulard O, Pelloux I, Pavese P, Brion JP, Raoult D, et al. African tick bite fever in elderly patients: 8 cases in French tourists returning from South Africa. Clin Infect Dis. 2008 Aug 1;47(3):e28–35.

RUBELLA

Huong Q. McLean, Susan E. Reef

INFECTIOUS AGENT
Rubella virus (family *Togaviridae*, genus *Rubivirus*).

TRANSMISSION
Person-to-person contact or droplets shed from the respiratory secretions of infected people. Transmission from mother to fetus can also occur, resulting in an infant being born with congenital rubella syndrome.

EPIDEMIOLOGY
Occurs worldwide outside the Americas. In the United States, endemic rubella virus transmission has been eliminated, but it continues to be imported.

CLINICAL PRESENTATION
Average incubation period is 14 days (range, 12–23 days). Usually presents as a nonspecific, maculopapular, generalized rash that lasts ≤3 days with generalized lymphadenopathy. Rash may be preceded by low-grade fever, malaise, anorexia, mild conjunctivitis, runny nose, and sore throat. Asymptomatic rubella virus infections are common. Infection during early pregnancy can lead to miscarriage, fetal death, or severe birth defects known as congenital rubella syndrome.

DIAGNOSIS
Demonstration of specific IgM or significant increase in IgG in acute- and convalescent-phase specimens. RT-PCR can be used to detect virus; viral culture is also acceptable but is time-consuming and expensive.

TREATMENT
Supportive care.

PREVENTION
All travelers age ≥12 months should have evidence of immunity to rubella, as documented by ≥1 dose of rubella-containing vaccine on or after the first birthday, laboratory evidence of immunity, or birth before 1957 (except women who could become pregnant).

CDC website: www.cdc.gov/rubella

BIBLIOGRAPHY
1. CDC. Rubella. In: Atkinson W, Wolfe S, Hamborsky J, editors. Epidemiology and Prevention of Vaccine-Preventable Diseases. 12th ed. Washington, DC: Public Health Foundation; 2012. p. 275–89.
2. Reef SE, Plotkin SA. Rubella vaccine. In: Plotkin SA, Orenstein WA, Offit PA, editors. Vaccines. 6th ed. Philadelphia: Saunders Elsevier; 2012. p. 688–717.
3. Reef SE, Redd SB, Abernathy E, Kutty PK, Icenogle JP. Evidence used to support the achievement and maintenance of elimination of rubella and congenital rubella syndrome in the United States. J Infect Dis. 2011 Sep 1;204(Suppl 2):S593–7.

SALMONELLOSIS (NONTYPHOIDAL)

Maho Imanishi, Shua J. Chai

INFECTIOUS AGENT

Salmonella enterica subspecies *enterica*, a gram-negative, rod-shaped bacillus. Nontyphoidal salmonellosis refers to illnesses caused by all serotypes of *Salmonella* except for Typhi, Paratyphi A, Paratyphi B (tartrate negative), and Paratyphi C.

TRANSMISSION

Usually through the consumption of foods contaminated with animal feces. Transmission can also occur through direct contact with infected animals or their environment.

EPIDEMIOLOGY

Nontyphoidal salmonellae are a leading cause of bacterial diarrhea worldwide; they are estimated to cause 94 million cases of gastroenteritis and 115,000 deaths globally each year. The risk of *Salmonella* infection among travelers returning to the United States varies by region of the world visited. In one analysis, the incidence of laboratory-confirmed infections from 2004 through 2009 was 7.1 cases per 100,000 among travelers to Latin American and Caribbean, 5.8 cases per 100,000 among travelers to Asia, and 25.8 cases per 100,000 among travelers to Africa. The true number of illnesses is much higher, because most ill people do not have a stool specimen tested. Travelers with salmonellosis were most likely to report visiting the following countries: Mexico (38% of travel-associated salmonellosis), India (9%), Jamaica (7%), the Dominican Republic (4%), China (3%), and the Bahamas (2%).

CLINICAL PRESENTATION

The incubation period of nontyphoidal salmonellosis is 6–72 hours, and illness usually occurs within 12–36 hours after exposure. Illness is commonly manifested by acute diarrhea, with sudden onset of headache, abdominal pain, fever, and sometimes vomiting. The illness usually lasts 4–7 days, and most people recover without treatment. Salmonellosis outcomes differ by serotype. Approximately 5% of people develop bacteremia or focal infection (such as meningitis or osteomyelitis). Infections with some serotypes, including Dublin and Choleraesuis, are more likely to result in invasive infections. Rates of invasive infections and death are generally higher among infants, older adults, and people with immunosuppressive conditions (including HIV), hemoglobinopathies, and malignant neoplasms.

DIAGNOSIS

Diagnosis is based on isolation of *Salmonella* organisms. About 90% of isolates are obtained from routine stool culture, but isolates are also obtained from blood, urine, and material from sites of infection. Isolates of salmonellae are needed for serotyping and antimicrobial susceptibility testing.

TREATMENT

Current recommendations are to treat most patients with uncomplicated *Salmonella* infection with supportive therapy and no antimicrobial agents; however, many receive empiric therapy (or take self-treatment) without a stool culture. Antimicrobial therapy is recommended for gastroenteritis caused by *Salmonella* species in people at increased risk of invasive disease (infants aged <3 months, older adults aged ≥60 years, the debilitated or immunosuppressed) and patients with continued high fever or manifestations of extraintestinal infection. Fluoroquinolones are often employed for empiric treatment; azithromycin and rifaximin are also commonly used to treat travelers' diarrhea. Resistance to antimicrobial agents varies by serotype and geographic region. Resistance to older antimicrobial agents (chloramphenicol, ampicillin, and trimethoprim-sulfamethoxazole) has been present for many years, and resistance to both fluoroquinolones and third-generation cephalosporins has been reported.

PREVENTION

No vaccine is available against nontyphoidal *Salmonella* infection. Preventive measures are aimed at avoiding foods at high risk for contamination; frequent handwashing, especially after contacting animals or their environment; and taking additional food and water precautions while traveling (see Chapter 2, Food & Water Precautions).

CDC website: www.cdc.gov/salmonella

BIBLIOGRAPHY

1. American Academy of Pediatrics. *Salmonella* infections. In: Pickering LK, editor. Red Book: 2012 Report of the Committee on Infectious Diseases. 29th ed. Elk Grove Village, IL: American Academy of Pediatrics; 2012. p. 635–40.
2. American Medical Association; American Nurses Association—American Nurses Foundation; CDC; Center for Food Safety and Applied Nutrition, Food and Drug Administration; Food Safety and Inspection Service, US Department of Agriculture. Diagnosis and management of foodborne illnesses: a primer for physicians and other health care professionals. MMWR Recomm Rep. 2004 Apr 16;53(RR-4):1–33.
3. American Public Health Association. Salmonellosis. In: Heymann DL, editor. Control of Communicable Diseases Manual. 19th ed. Washington, DC: American Public Health Association; 2008. p. 534–40.
4. CDC. National *Salmonella* Surveillance Annual Summary, 2009. Atlanta: CDC; 2011 [cited 2012 Sep 21]. Available from: http://www.cdc.gov/ncezid/dfwed/PDFs/salmonella-annual-summary-2009-508c.pdf.
5. Galanis E, Lo Fo Wong DM, Patrick ME, Binsztein N, Cieslik A, Chalermchikit T, et al. Web-based surveillance and global *Salmonella* distribution, 2000–2002. Emerg Infect Dis. 2006 Mar;12(3):381–8.
6. Johnson LR, Gould LH, Dunn JR, Berkelman R, Mahon BE, FoodNet Travel Working Group. *Salmonella* infections associated with international travel: a Foodborne Diseases Active Surveillance Network (FoodNet) study. Foodborne Pathog Dis. 2011 Sep;8(9):1031–7.
7. Jones TF, Ingram LA, Cieslak PR, Vugia DJ, Tobin-D'Angelo M, Hurd S, et al. Salmonellosis outcomes differ substantially by serotype. J Infect Dis. 2008 Jul 1;198(1):109–14.
8. Kendall ME, Crim S, Fullerton K, Han PV, Cronquist AB, Shiferaw B, et al. Travel-associated enteric infections diagnosed after return to the United States, Foodborne Diseases Active Surveillance Network (FoodNet), 2004–2009. Clin Infect Dis. 2012 Jun;54 Suppl 5:S480–7.
9. Majowicz SE, Musto J, Scallan E, Angulo FJ, Kirk M, O'Brien SJ, et al. The global burden of nontyphoidal *Salmonella* gastroenteritis. Clin Infect Dis. 2010 Mar 15;50(6):882–9.
10. Paredes-Paredes M, Flores-Figueroa J, Dupont HL. Advances in the treatment of travelers' diarrhea. Curr Gastroenterol Rep. 2011 Oct;13(5):402–7.
11. Su LH, Chiu CH, Chu C, Ou JT. Antimicrobial resistance in nontyphoid *Salmonella* serotypes: a global challenge. Clin Infect Dis. 2004 Aug 15;39(4):546–51.

SCABIES
Els Mathieu

INFECTIOUS AGENT
The human itch mite, *Sarcoptes scabiei* var. *hominis*.

TRANSMISSION
Through prolonged skin-to-skin contact with a person with conventional scabies or via brief skin-to-skin contact with a person with crusted (Norwegian) scabies (a more severe form of scabies in which a person is infested with a large number of mites). Indirect transmission may occur through contact with objects contaminated by a person with crusted (Norwegian) scabies but is rare if the person has conventional scabies.

EPIDEMIOLOGY
Scabies occurs worldwide. It is transmitted most easily in settings where skin contact is common. Crusted (Norwegian) scabies most commonly occurs among elderly, disabled, debilitated, or immunosuppressed people.

CLINICAL PRESENTATION

Symptoms occur 2–6 weeks after a person is first infested. However, if someone has had scabies before, symptoms appear much sooner (1–4 days after exposure). Conventional scabies is characterized by intense itching, particularly at night, and by a papular or papulovesicular, erythematous rash. Crusted (Norwegian) scabies is characterized by widespread crusts and scales that contain large numbers of mites, although itching may be less than in conventional scabies.

DIAGNOSIS

Generally diagnosed by identifying burrows in a patient with itching and by observing the characteristic rash. Diagnosis can be confirmed by microscopically identifying mites, mite eggs, or scybala (mite feces).

TREATMENT

Permethrin (5%) cream is considered by many to be the drug of choice. Ivermectin is reported to be safe and effective to treat scabies, including crusted (Norwegian) scabies. It is not FDA-approved but should be considered for patients in whom treatment has failed or who cannot tolerate other approved medications.

PREVENTION

Avoid prolonged skin-to-skin contact with people who have conventional scabies and even brief skin-to-skin contact with people who have crusted (Norwegian) scabies. Contact with items such as clothing and bed linens that have been used by an infested person should be avoided, especially if the person has crusted (Norwegian) scabies.

CDC website: www.cdc.gov/parasites/scabies

BIBLIOGRAPHY

1. American Academy of Pediatrics. Scabies. In: Pickering LK, editor. Red Book: 2012 Report of the Committee on Infectious Diseases. 29th ed. Elk Grove Village, IL: American Academy of Pediatrics; 2012. p. 641–3.
2. Chosidow O. Clinical practices. Scabies. N Engl J Med. 2006 Apr 20;354(16):1718–27.
3. Hengge UR, Currie BJ, Jager G, Lupi O, Schwartz RA. Scabies: a ubiquitous neglected skin disease. Lancet Infect Dis. 2006 Dec;6(12):769–79.
4. Heukelbach J, Feldmeier H. Scabies. Lancet. 2006 May 27;367(9524):1767–74.

SCHISTOSOMIASIS
Susan Montgomery

INFECTIOUS AGENT

Schistosomiasis is caused by helminth parasites of the genus Schistosoma. Other helminth infections are discussed in the Helminths, Soil-Transmitted section earlier in this chapter.

TRANSMISSION

Waterborne transmission occurs when larval cercariae, found in contaminated bodies of freshwater, penetrate the skin.

EPIDEMIOLOGY

An estimated 85% of the world's cases of schistosomiasis are in Africa, where prevalence rates can exceed 50% in local populations. Schistosoma mansoni and S. haematobium are distributed throughout Africa; only S. haematobium is found in areas of the Middle East, and S. japonicum is found in Indonesia and parts of China and Southeast Asia (Map 3-12). Two other species can infect humans: S. mekongi, found in Cambodia and Laos, and S. intercalatum, found in parts of Central and West Africa. These 2 species are rarely reported causes of infection. Many countries endemic for schistosomiasis have established control programs, but others have not. Countries where development has led to widespread improvements in sanitation and water safety,

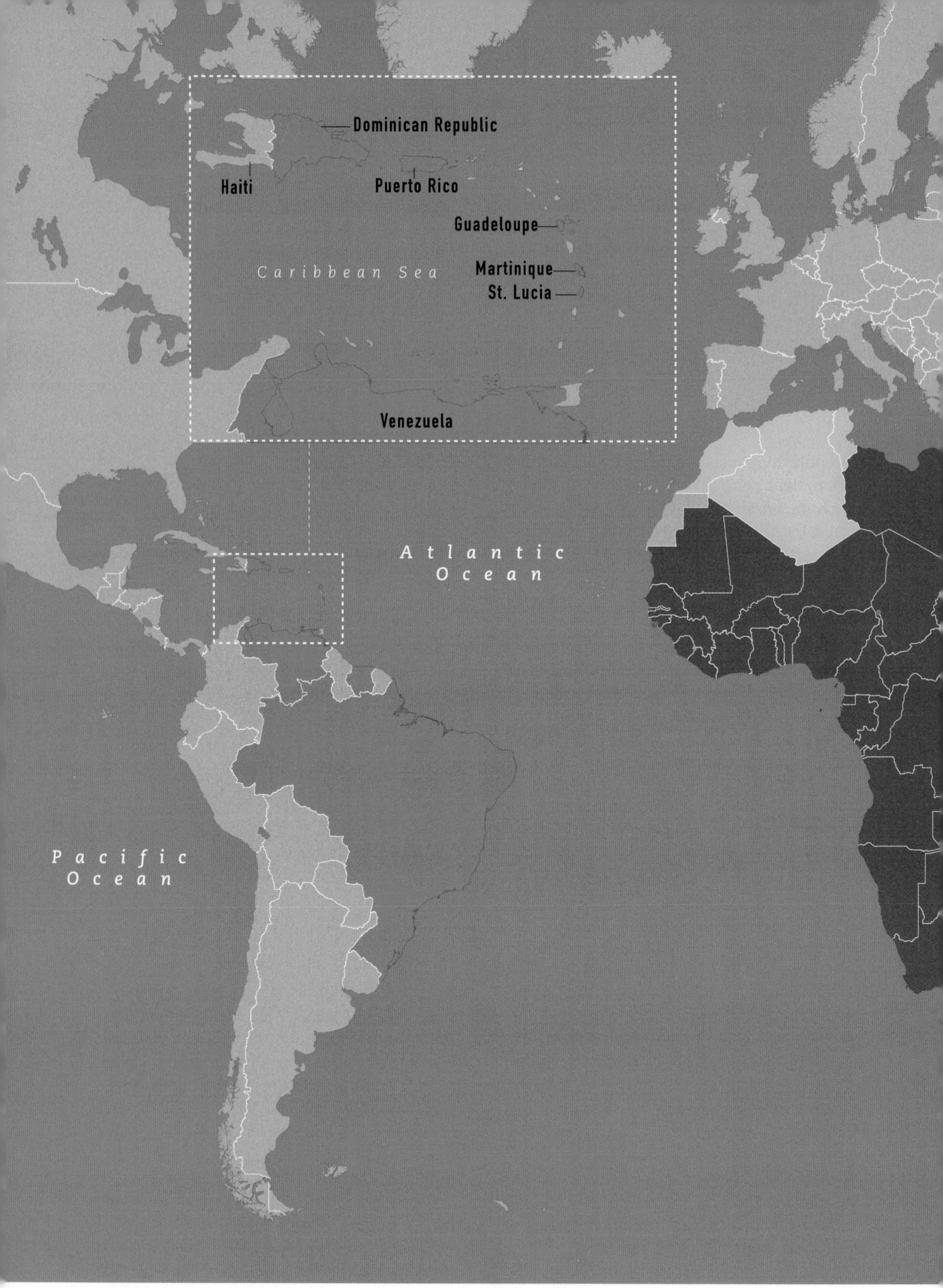

MAP 3-12. GEOGRAPHIC DISTRIBUTION OF SCHISTOSOMIASIS[1]

[1] The distribution of schistosomiasis is very focal; however, surveillance for schistosomiasis is limited in most countries. Therefore, this map shades entire countries where schistosomiasis transmission has been reported.

INFECTIOUS DISEASES RELATED TO TRAVEL

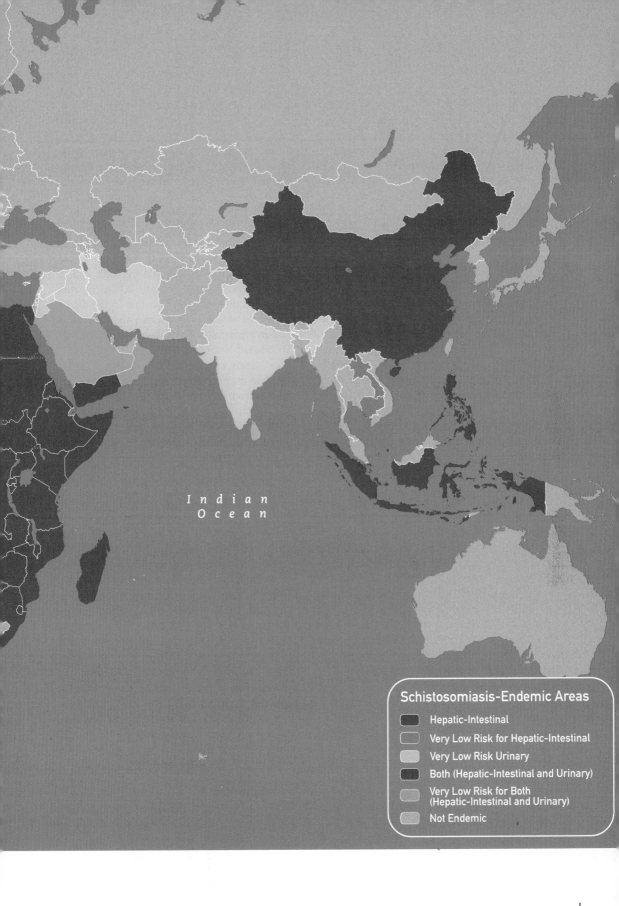

Schistosomiasis-Endemic Areas

- Hepatic-Intestinal
- Very Low Risk for Hepatic-Intestinal
- Very Low Risk Urinary
- Both (Hepatic-Intestinal and Urinary)
- Very Low Risk for Both (Hepatic-Intestinal and Urinary)
- Not Endemic

Indian Ocean

as well as successful schistosomiasis control programs, may have eliminated this disease. However, there are currently no international guidelines for certification of elimination.

All ages are at risk for infection with freshwater exposure in endemic areas. Swimming, bathing, and wading in contaminated freshwater can result in infection. Human schistosomiasis is not acquired by contact with saltwater (oceans or seas). The distribution of schistosomiasis is very focal and determined by the presence of competent snail vectors, inadequate sanitation, and infected humans. The geographic distribution of cases of schistosomiasis acquired by travelers reflects travel and immigration patterns. Most travel-associated cases of schistosomiasis are acquired in sub-Saharan Africa. Sites in Africa frequently visited by travelers are common sites of infection. These sites include rivers and water sources in the Banfora region (Burkina Faso) and areas populated by the Dogon people (Mali); Lake Malawi; Lake Tanganyika; Lake Victoria; the Omo River (Ethiopia); the Zambezi River; and the Nile River. However, as visitors travel to more uncommon sites, it is important to remember that most freshwater surface water sources in Africa are potentially contaminated and can be sources of infection. A local claim that there is no schistosomiasis in a body of freshwater is not necessarily reliable.

The specific snail vectors can be difficult to identify, and infection of snails with human schistosome species must be determined in the laboratory. The types of travelers and expatriates potentially at increased risk for infection include adventure travelers, Peace Corps volunteers, missionaries, soldiers, and ecotourists. Outbreaks of schistosomiasis have occurred among adventure travelers on river trips in Africa.

CLINICAL PRESENTATION

The incubation period is typically 14–84 days for acute schistosomiasis (Katayama syndrome), but chronic infection can remain asymptomatic for years. Penetration of cercariae can be associated with a rash that develops within hours or up to a week after contaminated water exposures. Acute schistosomiasis is characterized by fever, headache, myalgia, diarrhea, and respiratory symptoms. Eosinophilia is present, as well as often painful hepatomegaly or splenomegaly.

The clinical manifestations of chronic schistosomiasis are the result of host immune responses to schistosome eggs. Eggs secreted by adult worm pairs enter the circulation and lodge in organs and cause granulomatous reactions. Eosinophilia may be present. S. mansoni and S. japonicum eggs most commonly lodge in the blood vessels of the liver or intestine and can cause diarrhea, constipation, and blood in the stool. Chronic inflammation can lead to bowel wall ulceration, hyperplasia, and polyposis and, with heavy infections, to periportal liver fibrosis. S. haematobium eggs typically lodge in the urinary tract and can cause dysuria and hematuria. Calcifications in the bladder may appear late in the disease. S. haematobium infection can also cause genital symptoms and has been associated with increased risk of bladder cancer.

Rarely, central nervous system schistosomiasis may develop; this form is thought to result from aberrant migration of adult worms or eggs depositing in the spinal cord or brain. Signs and symptoms are related to ectopic granulomas in the central nervous system and can present as transverse myelitis.

DIAGNOSIS

Diagnosis is made by microscopic identification of parasite eggs in stool (S. mansoni or S. japonicum) or urine (S. haematobium). Serologic tests are useful to diagnose light infections where egg shedding may not be consistent in travelers and in others who have not had schistosomiasis previously. Antibody tests do not distinguish between past and current infection. Test sensitivity and specificity vary, depending on the antigen preparation used and how the test is performed. Consider screening asymptomatic people who may have been exposed during travel and may benefit from treatment.

More detailed information and assistance with diagnosis may be obtained from CDC (www.cdc.gov/parasites/schistosomiasis or CDC Parasitic Diseases Inquiries, 404-718-4745).

TREATMENT

Schistosomiasis is uncommon in the United States, and the inexperienced physician should consult an infectious disease or tropical medicine specialist for diagnosis and treatment. Praziquantel is used to treat schistosomiasis. Praziquantel is most effective against adult forms of the parasite and requires an immune response to the adult worm to be fully effective.

PREVENTION

No vaccine is available. No drugs for preventing infection are available. Preventive measures are primarily avoiding wading, swimming, or other contact with freshwater in disease-endemic countries. Untreated piped water coming directly from freshwater sources may contain cercariae, but filtering with fine-mesh filters, heating bathing water to 122°F (50°C) for 5 minutes, or allowing water to stand for ≥24 hours before exposure can eliminate risk for infection.

Swimming in adequately chlorinated swimming pools is virtually always safe, even in disease-endemic countries. Vigorous towel-drying after accidental exposure to water has been suggested as a way to remove cercariae before they can penetrate, but this may only prevent some infections and should not be recommended as a preventive measure. Topical applications of insect repellents such as DEET can block penetrating cercariae, but the effect depends on the repellent formulation, may be short-lived, and cannot reliably prevent infection.

CDC website: www.cdc.gov/parasites/ schistosomiasis

BIBLIOGRAPHY

1. Bierman WF, Wetsteyn JC, van Gool T. Presentation and diagnosis of imported schistosomiasis: relevance of eosinophilia, microscopy for ova, and serology. J Travel Med. 2005 Jan–Feb;12(1): 9–13.
2. Clerinx J, Van Gompel A. Schistosomiasis in travellers and migrants. Travel Med Infect Dis. 2011 Jan;9(1):6-24.
3. Corachan M. Schistosomiasis and international travel. Clin Infect Dis. 2002 Aug 15;35(4):446–50.
4. Doenhoff MJ, Cioli D, Utzinger J. Praziquantel: mechanisms of action, resistance and new derivatives for schistosomiasis. Curr Opin Infect Dis. 2008 Dec;21(6):659–67.
5. Grobusch MP, Muhlberger N, Jelinek T, Bisoffi Z, Corachan M, Harms G, et al. Imported schistosomiasis in Europe: sentinel surveillance data from TropNetEurop. J Travel Med. 2003 May–Jun;10(3): 164–9.
6. King CH, Sturrock RF, Kariuki HC, Hamburger J. Transmission control for schistosomiasis—why it matters now. Trends Parasitol. 2006 Dec;22(12): 575–82.
7. Meltzer E, Artom G, Marva E, Assous MV, Rahav G, Schwartzt E. Schistosomiasis among travelers: new aspects of an old disease. Emerg Infect Dis. 2006 Nov;12(11):1696–700.
8. Morgan OW, Brunette G, Kapella BK, McAuliffe I, Katongole-Mbidde E, Li W, et al. Schistosomiasis among recreational users of Upper Nile River, Uganda, 2007. Emerg Infect Dis. 2010 May;16(5): 866–8.
9. Nicolls DJ, Weld LH, Schwartz E, Reed C, von Sonnenburg F, Freedman DO, et al. Characteristics of schistosomiasis in travelers reported to the GeoSentinel Surveillance Network 1997–2008. Am J Trop Med Hyg. 2008 Nov;79(5):729–34.
10. Ross AG, Bartley PB, Sleigh AC, Olds GR, Li Y, Williams GM, et al. Schistosomiasis. N Engl J Med. 2002 Apr 18;346(16):1212–20.
11. Ross AG, Vickers D, Olds GR, Shah SM, McManus DP. Katayama syndrome. Lancet Infect Dis. 2007 Mar;7(3):218–24.
12. World Health Organization Expert Committee. Prevention and control of schistosomiasis and soil-transmitted helminthiasis. World Health Organ Tech Rep Ser. 2002;912:1–57.

SEXUALLY TRANSMITTED DISEASES

Kimberly Workowski, Sarah Kidd

INFECTIOUS AGENT

Sexually transmitted diseases (STDs) are the infections and resulting clinical syndromes caused by >25 infectious organisms.

TRANSMISSION

Sexual activity is the predominant mode of transmission, through genital, anal, or oral mucosal contact.

EPIDEMIOLOGY

STDs are among the most common infectious diseases. Annually, an estimated 448 million infections occur worldwide, and 19 million infections occur in the United States. Some STDs are more prevalent in developing countries (chancroid, lymphogranuloma venereum, granuloma inguinale [donovanosis]) or in specific regions (gonorrhea with treatment failure and decreased susceptibility to cephalosporins in East Asia) and may be imported into developed countries by travelers returning from such locales.

Casual sexual relationships occur frequently during travel to foreign countries; 5%–50% of travelers report casual sex with a new partner while abroad. In addition, commercial sex in various destinations, such as Southeast Asia, attracts many foreign travelers. Commercial sex workers in some regions have high rates of STDs, including HIV, and travelers who have sex with them risk acquiring these infections.

Knowledge of the clinical presentation, frequency of infection, and antimicrobial resistance patterns is needed to manage STDs that occur in travelers. Assessing risk for men who have sex with men is important because of the recent increased rates of infectious syphilis, gonorrhea with treatment failure and decreased susceptibility to cephalosporins, and lymphogranuloma venereum in various geographic locations.

CLINICAL PRESENTATION

Many infections may be asymptomatic (chlamydia, gonorrhea), so screening for these infections at anatomic sites of contact and serologic testing for syphilis should be encouraged among travelers who present in clinic concerned they may have acquired an STD. Any traveler who might have been exposed and who develops vaginal, urethral, or rectal discharge, an unexplained rash or genital lesion, or genital or pelvic pain should be advised to cease sexual activity and promptly seek medical evaluation.

Some systemic infections are acquired through sexual transmission (hepatitis A, hepatitis B, hepatitis C, HIV, syphilis). Because many travelers do not volunteer a history of sexual contact during travel, clinicians should inquire about sexual exposures when caring for returned travelers.

DIAGNOSIS

Genital ulcer evaluation should include a serologic test for syphilis, a culture or PCR testing for genital herpes, and a culture for chancroid (if exposure occurred in areas where chancroid is more common, such as Africa, Asia, and Latin America). Lymphadenopathy can accompany genital ulceration with these infections, as well as with lymphogranuloma venereum and donovanosis. Lymphogranuloma venereum should be suspected in a traveler with tender unilateral inguinal or femoral lymphadenopathy or proctocolitis. If painful perianal ulcers are present or mucosal ulcers are detected on anoscopy, a diagnosis of genital herpes or lymphogranuloma venereum should be considered. Genital and lymph node specimens should be tested for *Chlamydia trachomatis* by culture, direct immunofluorescence, or nucleic acid testing. Donovanosis is endemic in India, Papua New Guinea, central Australia, and southern Africa and is diagnosed with a crush tissue preparation from the lesion.

Testing specimens from the anatomic site of exposure with nucleic acid amplification testing or culture can detect *C. trachomatis* and *Neisseria gonorrhoeae*. Culture and antibiotic susceptibility testing should be considered when gonorrhea is suspected, because of geographic differences in antimicrobial susceptibility. Various diagnostic methods are available to identify the cause of an abnormal vaginal discharge, including microscopic evaluation and pH testing of vaginal secretions, DNA probe-based testing, nucleic acid amplification testing, and culture. Anyone who seeks evaluation or treatment for STDs should be screened for HIV infection.

TREATMENT

Evaluation, management, and follow-up of STDs should be based on standard guidelines (CDC and the World Health Organization), and the prevalence of antimicrobial resistance in different geographic areas should be considered. Early detection and treatment are important. STDs can often result in serious and long-term complications, including pelvic inflammatory disease, infertility, stillbirths and neonatal infections, genital cancers, and an increased risk for HIV acquisition and transmission.

PREVENTION

The prevention and control of STDs are based on education, counseling, early identification, and treatment. Specific messages to avoid acquiring or transmitting STDs should be part of the health advice given to travelers. Abstinence or mutual monogamy is the most reliable way to avoid acquiring and transmitting STDs.

For people whose sexual behaviors place them at risk for STDs, correct and consistent use of the male latex condom can reduce the risk of HIV infection and many common STDs, including chlamydia, gonorrhea, and trichomoniasis. Preventing lower genital tract infections might reduce the risk of pelvic inflammatory disease in women. Condoms might protect against genital herpes, syphilis, and chancroid, although data are limited.

Only water-based lubricants (such as K-Y Jelly or glycerin) should be used with latex condoms because oil-based lubricants (such as petroleum jelly, shortening, mineral oil, or massage oil) can weaken latex condoms. Spermicides containing nonoxynol-9 are not recommended for STD/HIV prevention, as nonoxynol-9 can increase the risk of HIV transmission. Contraceptive methods that are not mechanical barriers do not protect against HIV or other STDs.

Prompt evaluation of sexual partners is necessary to prevent reinfection and disrupt transmission of many STDs. Preexposure vaccination is among the most effective methods for preventing some STDs. Two human papillomavirus (HPV) vaccines are available and licensed for girls and women aged 9–26 years to prevent cervical precancers and cancers: the quadrivalent HPV and the bivalent HPV vaccine. The quadrivalent vaccine also prevents genital warts and is recommended for boys and men aged 9–26 years as well as girls and women (see the Human Papillomavirus section in this chapter). Preexposure vaccination against hepatitis A and B is recommended, as these infections can be sexually transmissible. Hepatitis A vaccine is recommended for all unvaccinated injection drug users and sexually active men who have sex with men. Hepatitis B vaccine is recommended for all unvaccinated men who have sex with men, as well as people who have a history of an STD, have had >1 sexual partner in the previous 6 months, use injection drugs, or have a sex partner who uses injection drugs. However, all travelers should be considered candidates for both these vaccines. Travelers, particularly those at high risk for acquiring HIV infection (such as men who have sex with men), may consider discussing preexposure prophylaxis with their health care provider (see www.cdc.gov/hiv/prep).

CDC website: www.cdc.gov/std

BIBLIOGRAPHY

1. Ansart S, Hochedez P, Perez L, Bricaire F, Caumes E. Sexually transmitted diseases diagnosed among travelers returning from the tropics. J Travel Med. 2009 Mar–Apr;16(2):79–83.
2. CDC. Condoms and STDs: factsheet for public health personnel. Atlanta: CDC; 2011 [cited 2012 Sep 21]. Available from: http://www.cdc.gov/condomeffectiveness/latex.htm.
3. Leder K, Tong S, Weld L, Kain KC, Wilder-Smith A, von Sonnenburg F, et al. Illness in travelers visiting friends and relatives: a review of the GeoSentinel Surveillance Network. Clin Infect Dis. 2006 Nov 1;43(9):1185–93.

4. Matteelli A, Carosi G. Sexually transmitted diseases in travelers. Clin Infect Dis. 2001 Apr 1;32(7):1063–7.

5. Peterman TA, Heffelfinger JD, Swint EB, Groseclose SL. The changing epidemiology of syphilis. Sex Transm Dis. 2005 Oct;32(10 Suppl):S4–10.

6. Tapsall JW. *Neisseria gonorrhoeae* and emerging resistance to extended spectrum cephalosporins. Curr Opin Infect Dis. 2009 Feb;22(1):87–91.

7. Tietz A, Davies SC, Moran JS. Guide to sexually transmitted disease resources on the Internet. Clin Infect Dis. 2004 May 1;38(9):1304–10.

8. US Preventive Services Task Force. Behavioral counseling to prevent sexually transmitted infections: US Preventive Services Task Force recommendation statement. Ann Intern Med. 2008 Oct 7;149(7):491–6, W95.

9. Vivancos R, Abubakar I, Hunter PR. Foreign travel, casual sex, and sexually transmitted infections: systematic review and meta-analysis. Int J Infect Dis. 2010 Oct;14(10):e842–51.

10. Ward BJ, Plourde P. Travel and sexually transmitted infections. J Travel Med. 2006 Sep–Oct;13(5):300–17.

11. Ward H, Martin I, Macdonald N, Alexander S, Simms I, Fenton K, et al. Lymphogranuloma venereum in the United Kingdom. Clin Infect Dis. 2007 Jan 1;44(1):26–32.

12. Weinstock H, Berman S, Cates W Jr. Sexually transmitted diseases among American youth: incidence and prevalence estimates, 2000. Perspect Sex Reprod Health. 2004 Jan–Feb;36(1):6–10.

13. Workowski KA, Berman S. Sexually transmitted diseases treatment guidelines, 2010. MMWR Recomm Rep. 2010 Dec 17;59(RR-12):1–110.

14. Workowski KA, Berman SM, Douglas JM, Jr. Emerging antimicrobial resistance in *Neisseria gonorrhoeae*: urgent need to strengthen prevention strategies. Ann Intern Med. 2008 Apr 15;148(8):606–13.

15. World Health Organization. Prevalence and incidence of selected sexually transmitted infections, *Chlamydia trachomatis, Neisseria gonorrhoeae*, syphilis and *Trichomonas vaginalis*: methods and results used by WHO to generate 2005 estimates. Geneva: World Health Organization; 2011. Available from: http://whqlibdoc.who.int/publications/2011/9789241502450_eng.pdf.

Perspectives

SEX & TOURISM

Elissa Meites

TRAVEL AND SEXUAL HEALTH

Whether or not sex is the purpose of a trip, sex with a new partner is common during travel. An estimated 20% of international travelers have sex with a new partner while abroad, and the risk of developing a sexually transmitted disease (STD) may be up to 3 times higher in people who experience casual travel sex. Travelers may be unaware of local information about the high prevalence of HIV and STDs in certain countries. In addition, alcohol or drugs used during travel may lower the threshold for sexual encounters.

Perspectives sections are written as editorial discussions aiming to add depth and clinical perspective to the official recommendations contained in the book. The views and opinions expressed in this section are those of the author and do not necessarily represent the official position of CDC.

The mainstays of sexually transmitted infection prevention (condoms and vaccinations against hepatitis A, hepatitis B, and human papillomavirus), contraception, and other prescription medications may not be subject to US quality control standards in manufacturing, storage, or distribution when obtained in other countries. Condoms that are past their expiration date or that have been stored at extreme temperatures may be less effective at reducing the risk of HIV and STD transmission. Clinicians seeing travelers at high risk for acquiring HIV infection (particularly men who have sex with men) should consider discussing preexposure prophylaxis with them (see www.cdc.gov/HIV/PREP).

All people who have sex with a new partner should consult a physician about recommended screening tests to check for HIV and treatable STDs. Travelers should also be alert to attempts at coercion or fraud from previously unknown partners professing romantic interest, especially in relationships beginning exclusively online. People who have experienced a high-risk sexual encounter should consider taking medications for postexposure prophylaxis of HIV or unintended pregnancy within 72 hours. These and other prescription medications can be costly or difficult to obtain overseas, but US consular officers may be able to assist in locating needed medical services. See Box 3-5 for a summary of sexual health recommendations for travelers.

SEX TOURISM

"Sex tourism" has been defined as travel planned specifically to procure sex. Sex tourism commonly involves male tourists traveling to economically disadvantaged countries to pay for sex with female sex workers. In certain regions, commercial sex work is legal and culturally acceptable. However, travelers should be aware that HIV and STD infections are more common among commercial sex workers. Also, sex tourism helps to support sex trafficking, one of the largest criminal industries in the world, in which victims are forced to perform sex work. Travelers should be familiar with applicable US and local laws and should report known or suspected violations promptly to the authorities. The regional security officer at the local US embassy or foreign law enforcement officials can assist.

SEXUAL ABUSE AND THE LAW

Although commercial sex work may be legal in some countries, sex trafficking, sex with a minor, and child pornography are always criminal activities according to US law and can be prosecuted in the United States even if the behavior occurred abroad. The Trafficking Victims Protection Act makes it illegal to recruit, entice, or obtain a person of any age to engage in commercial sex acts or to benefit from such activities. Federal law also bars US residents from engaging in sexual or pornographic activities with a child aged <18 years anywhere in the world, regardless of local age of consent, or to travel abroad for the purpose of having sex with a minor. In addition, child pornography, including sexual photographs or videos of minors in foreign countries, is illegal in the United States. These crimes are subject to prosecution with penalties of up to 30 years in prison.

Nearly 2 million children around the world are victims of commercial sexual exploitation, and roughly 1 million children are victims of trafficking. Children abused by sex tourists suffer not only sexual abuse but also poverty, homelessness, and physical, emotional, and psychological abuse, as well as health problems including illnesses, addictions, malnourishment, infections, physical injuries, and STDs.

If you suspect child sexual exploitation occurring overseas, you can call the Immigration and Customs Enforcement hotline toll-free at 866-347-2423 or submit the information online at www.ice.gov/exec/forms/hsi-tips/tips.asp. In the United States, the National Center for Missing & Exploited Children's Cybertipline collects reports of child prostitution and other crimes against children (toll-free at 800-843-5678, www.cybertipline.com), and 655 incidents of child sex tourism were reported in 2007. At least 669 Americans have been arrested for child pornography and 67 Americans have been arrested for child sex tourism since 2003, when the PROTECT Act was passed to strengthen the US government's prosecution of crimes related to sex tourism.

Americans and US permanent residents account for an estimated 25% of child sex tourists worldwide and up to 80% in Latin America. These are typically Caucasian men aged ≥40 and have been traced visiting Mexico, Central and South America (Brazil, Colombia, Costa Rica, Dominican Republic), Southeast Asia (Cambodia, India, Laos, Philippines, Thailand), and sometimes Eastern Europe (Lithuania, Russia) and other regions.

To combat child sexual abuse, some international hotels and other tourism services have voluntarily adopted a code of conduct that includes training and reporting suspicious activities. Tourist establishments supporting this initiative to protect children from sex tourism are listed online (www.thecode.org). For more ways you can help, see the US Department of State list of 20 ways to fight human trafficking (www.state.gov/j/tip/id/help).

BOX 3-5. SUMMARY OF SEXUAL HEALTH RECOMMENDATIONS FOR TRAVELERS

Before travel

- Obtain recommended vaccinations, including those that protect against sexually transmitted infections.
- Get recommended screening tests for HIV and treatable STDs.
- Pack sufficient quantities of needed prescription medications and supplies. Check condom expiration dates.
- Review local laws and contact information for medical and law enforcement services.

During travel

- Use good judgment in choosing consensual adult sex partners.
- Latex condoms, when used consistently and correctly, can decrease the risk of HIV and STD transmission.
- If indicated, be prepared to start taking medications for postexposure prophylaxis of HIV or unintended pregnancy within 72 hours after a high-risk sexual encounter.
- Never engage in sex with a minor (<18 years old), child pornography, or trafficking activities, in any country.
- Report suspicious activity to US and local authorities as soon as it occurs.

After travel

- To avoid exposing sex partners at home to STDs, get recommended screening tests for HIV and treatable STDs.

BIBLIOGRAPHY

1. CDC. Interim guidance: preexposure prophylaxis for the prevention of HIV infection in men who have sex with men. MMWR Morb Mortal Wkly Rep. 2011 Jan 28;60(3):65–8.

2. International Labour Organization, International Programme on the Elimination of Child Labour. Every child counts: new global estimates on child labour. Geneva: International Labour Organization; 2002 [cited 2012 Sep 21]. Available from: http://www.ilo.org/ipecinfo/product/download.do?type=document&id=742.

3. Marrazzo JM. Sexual tourism: implications for travelers and the destination culture. Infect Dis Clin North Am. 2005 Mar;19(1):103–20.

4. Pan American Health Organization. Trafficking of women and children for sexual exploitation in the Americas. Washington DC: Women, Health and Development Program, Pan American Health Organization; 2001 [cited 2012 Sep 21]. Available from: http://www.paho.org/English/AD/GE/TraffickingPaper.pdf.

5. Public Health Agency of Canada, Committee to Advise on Tropical Medicine and Travel (CATMAT). Statement on travellers and sexually transmitted infections. Canada Communicable Disease Report [Internet]. 2006 [cited 2012 Sep 21];32(ACS-5). Available from: http://www.phac-aspc.gc.ca/publicat/ccdr-rmtc/06vol32/acs-05/.

6. Smith DK, Grohskopf LA, Black RJ, Auerbach JD, Veronese F, Struble KA, et al. Antiretroviral postexposure prophylaxis after sexual, injection-drug use, or other nonoccupational exposure to HIV in the United States: recommendations from the US Department of Health and Human Services. MMWR Recomm Rep. 2005 Jan 21;54(RR-2):1–20.

7. United Nations Children's Fund (UNICEF). The state of the world's children 2012: children in an urban world. New York: United Nations Children's Fund (UNICEF); 2012 [cited 2012 Sep 21]. Available from: http://www.unicef.org/sowc/files/SOWC_2012-Main_Report_EN_21Dec2011.pdf.

8. US Department of Health and Human Services, Administration for Children and Families. Rescue and restore campaign fact sheets. Washington, DC: Administration for Children and Families; 2012 [cited 2012 Sep 21]. Available from: http://www.acf.hhs.gov/trafficking/about/factsheets.html.

9. US Department of Homeland Security, Immigration and Customs Enforcement. Fact sheet: operation predator—targeting child exploitation and sexual crimes. Washington, DC: Immigration and Customs Enforcement; 2012 [cited 2012 Sep 21]. Available from: http://www.ice.gov/news/library/factsheets/predator.htm.

10. US Department of Justice. The national strategy for child exploitation prevention and interdiction: a report to Congress. Washington, DC: US Department of Justice; 2010 [cited 2012 Sep 21]. Available from: http://www.justice.gov/psc/docs/natstrategyreport.pdf.

11. US Department of State. Internet dating and romance scams. Washington, DC: US Department of State; 2012 [cited 2012 Sep 21]. Available from: http://travel.state.gov/travel/cis_pa_tw/financial_scams/financial_scams_4554.html.

12. Vivancos R, Abubakar I, Hunter PR. Foreign travel, casual sex, and sexually transmitted infections: systematic review and meta-analysis. Int J Infect Dis. 2010 Oct;14(10):e842–51.

13. Workowski KA, Berman S. Sexually transmitted diseases treatment guidelines, 2010. MMWR Recomm Rep. 2010 Dec 17;59(RR-12):1–110.

SHIGELLOSIS
Katherine E. Heiman, Anna Bowen

INFECTIOUS AGENT
Shigellosis is an acute infection of the intestine caused by bacteria in the genus *Shigella*. There are 4 species of *Shigella*: *Shigella dysenteriae*, *S. flexneri*, *S. boydii*, and *S. sonnei* (also referred to as group A, B, C, and D, respectively). Several distinct serotypes are recognized within the first 3 species.

TRANSMISSION
Transmission occurs via the fecal-oral route, through direct person-to-person contact, or indirectly through contaminated food, water, or fomites. As few as 10 organisms can cause infection. Only humans and higher primates carry *Shigella*. In the United States, *S. sonnei* infection is usually transmitted through interpersonal contact, particularly among young children in day care settings. Foodborne outbreaks have been linked to contaminated foods commonly consumed raw, as well as infected food handlers. Outbreaks have also been traced to contaminated drinking water, swimming in contaminated water, and sexual contact between men.

EPIDEMIOLOGY
Worldwide, *Shigella* is estimated to cause 80–165 million cases of disease and 600,000 deaths annually. *Shigella* spp. are endemic in temperate and tropical climates. Transmission of *Shigella* spp. is most likely when hygiene and sanitation are insufficient. Shigellosis is predominantly caused by *S. sonnei* in industrialized countries, whereas *S. flexneri* prevails in the developing world. Infections caused by *S. boydii* are uncommon. *S. dysenteriae* is even more uncommon, but makes up ≥25% of all *Shigella* spp. isolated in sub-Saharan Africa and South Asia. *Shigella* spp. are detected in the stools of 5%–18% of patients with travelers' diarrhea. In a FoodNet study of travel-associated enteric infections diagnosed after return to the United States, *Shigella* was the third most common bacterial pathogen isolated by clinical laboratories (of note, these laboratories do not test for enterotoxigenic *Escherichia coli*, a common cause of travelers' diarrhea).

Most infections caused by *S. dysenteriae* were travel-associated (56%). Many infections caused by *S. boydii* (44%) were acquired while traveling, but infections caused by *S. flexneri* and *S. sonnei* were less often associated with travel (24% and 12%, respectively). Risk of infection caused by *Shigella* spp. is highest for people traveling to Africa, followed by Central America, South America, and Asia.

CLINICAL PRESENTATION
Illness typically begins 12–96 hours after exposure. The symptoms of shigellosis range from mild to severe and typically last 4–7 days. Disease severity varies according to species; serotype *S. dysenteriae* serotype 1 (Sd1) is the agent of epidemic dysentery, while *S. sonnei* is a common cause of milder diarrheal illness. The disease is characterized by watery, bloody, or mucoid diarrhea, fever, stomach cramps, and nausea. Occasionally, patients experience vomiting, seizures (young children), or postinfectious arthritis. Hemolytic uremic syndrome can occur after infection with Sd1.

DIAGNOSIS
Shigellosis is confirmed through culture of a stool specimen or rectal swab. Samples should be processed rapidly because *Shigella* cannot survive for long outside the body. *Shigella* isolates may then be speciated and serotyped and their antimicrobial susceptibilities determined to help guide treatment.

TREATMENT
In healthy people, shigellosis will typically resolve within 4–7 days, even without treatment. Antimicrobial treatment, when given early in the course of illness, can slightly shorten the duration of symptoms and of carriage. The possibility of resistance should be considered for patients in whom treatment is indicated. For shigellosis associated with travel outside the United States, a fluoroquinolone (for adults and, if infection is acquired in regions with high rates of multidrug resistance, children) or ceftriaxone (for children)

may be used empirically until antimicrobial susceptibility data are available. However, resistance to fluoroquinolones and third- and fourth-generation cephalosporins has been reported, particularly among *Shigella* isolates acquired in South and East Asia. Multidrug-resistant strains are especially common among travelers; empiric treatment should be tailored to region of travel.

PREVENTION

No vaccines are available for *Shigella*. The best defense against shigellosis is thorough, frequent handwashing and strict adherence to standard food and water safety precautions (see Chapter 2, Food & Water Precautions).

CDC website: www.cdc.gov/nczved/divisions/dfbmd/diseases/shigellosis

BIBLIOGRAPHY

1. American Academy of Pediatrics. *Shigella* infections. In: Pickering LK, editor. Red Book: 2012 Report of the Committee on Infectious Diseases. 29th ed. Elk Grove Village, IL: American Academy of Pediatrics; 2012. p. 645–7.
2. American Public Health Association. Shigellosis. In: Heymann DL, editor. Control of Communicable Diseases Manual. 19th ed. Washington, DC: American Public Health Association; 2008. p. 556–60.
3. CDC. National *Shigella* surveillance system [annual summaries]. Atlanta: CDC; 2012 [cited 2012 Sep 21]. Available from: http://www.cdc.gov/nationalsurveillance/shigella_surveillance.html.
4. Dutta S, Dutta P, Matsushita S, Bhattacharya SK, Yoshida S. *Shigella dysenteriae* serotype 1, Kolkata, India. Emerg Infect Dis. 2003 Nov;9(11): 1471–4.
5. Folster JP, Pecic G, Bowen A, Rickert R, Carattoli A, Whichard JM. Decreased susceptibility to ciprofloxacin among *Shigella* isolates in the United States, 2006 to 2009. Antimicrob Agents Chemother. 2011 Apr;55(4):1758–60.
6. Gaynor K, Park SY, Kanenaka R, Colindres R, Mintz E, Ram PK, et al. International foodborne outbreak of *Shigella sonnei* infection in airline passengers. Epidemiol Infect. 2009 Mar;137(3): 335–41.
7. Haley CC, Ong KL, Hedberg K, Cieslak PR, Scallan E, Marcus R, et al. Risk factors for sporadic shigellosis, FoodNet 2005. Foodborne Pathog Dis. 2010 Jul;7(7):741–7.
8. Kendall ME, Crim S, Fullerton K, Han PV, Cronquist AB, Shiferaw B, et al. Travel-associated enteric infections diagnosed after return to the United States, Foodborne Diseases Active Surveillance Network (FoodNet), 2004–2009. Clin Infect Dis. 2012 Jun;54 Suppl 5:S480–7.
9. Tajbakhsh M, Garcia Migura L, Rahbar M, Svendsen CA, Mohammadzadeh M, Zali MR, et al. Antimicrobial-resistant *Shigella* infections from Iran: an overlooked problem? J Antimicrob Chemother. 2012 May;67(5):1128–33.
10. von Seidlein L, Kim DR, Ali M, Lee H, Wang X, Thiem VD, et al. A multicentre study of *Shigella* diarrhoea in six Asian countries: disease burden, clinical manifestations, and microbiology. PLoS Med. 2006 Sep;3(9):e353.
11. Zhang W, Luo Y, Li J, Lin L, Ma Y, Hu C, et al. Wide dissemination of multidrug-resistant *Shigella* isolates in China. J Antimicrob Chemother. 2011 Nov;66(11):2527–35.

SMALLPOX & OTHER ORTHOPOXVIRUS-ASSOCIATED INFECTIONS

Mary G. Reynolds

INFECTIOUS AGENT

Smallpox is caused by variola virus, genus *Orthopoxvirus*. Other members of this genus that cause infection in humans are vaccinia virus, monkeypox virus, and cowpox virus.

TRANSMISSION

Smallpox

Person to person, principally respiratory; less commonly through contact with infectious skin lesions or scabs.

Monkeypox

Person to person, principally respiratory; less commonly through contact with infectious skin lesions or scabs. African rodents and primates may harbor the virus and could infect humans, but the reservoir host is unknown.

Vaccinia

Vaccinia virus is the live-virus component of contemporary smallpox vaccines. Rarely, social contacts of people recently vaccinated for smallpox develop infections with vaccinia virus when their skin comes into contact with fluid from the inoculation lesion. Zoonotic infections with vaccinialike viruses have been reported in Brazil and India.

Cowpox

Contact with infected animals; transmission between humans has not been observed.

EPIDEMIOLOGY
Smallpox

Eradicated globally. A single confirmed case of smallpox would be the result of an intentional act (bioterrorism) and would be considered an emergency.

Monkeypox

Endemic in tropical forested regions of West and Central Africa, notably the Congo Basin. Rodents imported from West Africa were the source of a 2003 outbreak of human monkeypox in the United States.

Vaccinia

Infections with wild vaccinialike viruses have been reported among cattle and buffalo herders in India and among dairy workers in southern Brazil.

Cowpox

Human infections with cowpox virus have been reported in Europe and Asia.

CLINICAL PRESENTATION
Smallpox

Infections present with acute onset of fever >101°F (38.3°C), malaise, head and body aches, and sometimes vomiting. This phase is followed by a rash characterized by firm, deep-seated vesicles or pustules in the same stage of development. Clinically, the most common rash illness likely to be confused with smallpox is varicella (chickenpox). A detailed explanation of the clinical signs and symptoms of smallpox can be found at www.bt.cdc.gov/agent/smallpox/overview/disease-facts.asp.

Monkeypox

Clinically identical to smallpox, with fever and widespread vesiculopustular rash involving the palms and soles. One feature distinctive to monkeypox is marked lymphadenopathy.

Vaccinia and Cowpox

Human infections with vaccinia, wild vaccinialike viruses, and cowpox virus are most often self-limited, characterized by localized pustular (and in cowpox, occasionally ulcerative) lesions. Fever and other constitutional symptoms may occur briefly after lesions first appear. Lesions can be painful and can persist for weeks. People who are immunocompromised or who have exfoliative skin conditions (such as eczema or atopic dermatitis) are at higher risk of severe illness or death.

DIAGNOSIS

Orthopoxvirus infection is confirmed by PCR or virus isolation. Physicians can refer to the CDC smallpox website (www.bt.cdc.gov/agent/smallpox/diagnosis) for guidance in the application of a clinical algorithm designed to aid in distinguishing orthopoxvirus infections from other disseminated rash illnesses, namely chickenpox.

TREATMENT

Mainly supportive, to include hydration, nutritional supplementation, and prevention of secondary infections. Vaccinia lesions should remain covered until the scab detaches to diminish chances of spreading virus to other parts of the body or to another person. Physicians managing orthopoxvirus infection in a patient who is at high risk for severe outcome (such as a patient who is immunocompromised or has an underlying skin condition) should consult with CDC to explore investigational treatment options (770-488-7100). Investigational use of antivirals could be considered.

PREVENTION

Smallpox vaccine is not recommended for international travelers. Smallpox vaccination is recommended only for laboratory workers who handle variola virus (the agent of smallpox) or closely related viruses and health care and public health officials who would be designated first responders in the event of an intentional release of variola virus. In addition, members of the US military may be required to receive the vaccine.

For other orthopoxvirus infections, avoid contact with rodents and sick or dead animals, including pets and domestic ruminants (cattle, buffalo). For more information about monkeypox and other orthopoxviruses, contact the CDC Poxvirus Inquiry Line (404-639-4129).

CDC websites: http://emergency.cdc.gov/agent/smallpox and www.cdc.gov/ncidod/monkeypox

BIBLIOGRAPHY

1. Baxby D, Bennett M, Getty B. Human cowpox 1969–93: a review based on 54 cases. Br J Dermatol. 1994 Nov;131(5):598–607.
2. Levine RS, Peterson AT, Yorita KL, Carroll D, Damon IK, Reynolds MG. Ecological niche and geographic distribution of human monkeypox in Africa. PLoS One. 2007; 2(1):e176.
3. Trindade GS, Guedes MI, Drumond BP, Mota BE, Abrahao JS, Lobato ZI, et al. Zoonotic vaccinia virus: clinical and immunological characteristics in a naturally infected patient. Clin Infect Dis. 2009 Feb 1; 48(3):e37–40.

STRONGYLOIDIASIS
LeAnne M. Fox

INFECTIOUS AGENT
An intestinal nematode, *Strongyloides stercoralis*.

TRANSMISSION
Filariform larvae found in infected soil penetrate human skin. Person-to-person transmission is rare but documented.

EPIDEMIOLOGY
Endemic in the tropics and subtropics, and in limited foci in the southeastern United States, Europe, Australia, and Japan. Estimates of global prevalence vary between 3 million and 100 million. Most infections in the United States occur in immigrants, refugees, and military veterans who have lived in endemic areas for long periods of time. Risk for short-term travelers is low, but infections can occur.

CLINICAL PRESENTATION
Most infections are asymptomatic. With acute infections, a localized, pruritic, erythematous papular rash can develop at the site of skin penetration, followed by pulmonary symptoms (a Löffler-like pneumonitis), diarrhea, abdominal pain, and eosinophilia. Migrating larvae in the skin cause larva currens, a serpiginous urticarial rash.

Immunocompromised people, especially those receiving systemic corticosteroids or patients with human T-cell lymphotropic virus type 1 infection, are at risk for hyperinfection or disseminated disease, characterized by abdominal pain, diffuse pulmonary infiltrates, and septicemia or meningitis from enteric gram-negative bacilli. The death rate from untreated disseminated strongyloidiasis is very high. Unexplained eosinophilia may be a presenting sign.

DIAGNOSIS
Rhabditiform larvae on microscopic examination of stool, either directly or by culture on agar plates. Repeated stool examinations or examination of duodenal contents may be necessary. Hyperinfection and disseminated strongyloidiasis are diagnosed by examining stool, sputum, cerebrospinal fluid, and other body fluids and tissues, which typically contain high numbers of larvae. Serologic testing is available through the National Institutes of Health and CDC (www.dpd.cdc.gov/dpdx; 404-718-4745; parasites@cdc.gov).

TREATMENT

Treatment of choice for both chronic and disseminated disease with hyperinfection is ivermectin. The alternative is albendazole, although associated with slightly lower cure rates. Prolonged or repeated treatment may be necessary in patients with hyperinfection and disseminated disease, and relapse can occur.

PREVENTION

No vaccine or preventative drugs are available. Protective measures include wearing shoes when walking in areas where humans may have defecated.

CDC website: www.cdc.gov/parasites/strongyloides

BIBLIOGRAPHY

1. Abramowicz M. Drugs for Parasitic Infections. New Rochelle (NY): The Medical Letter, Inc; 2010.
2. Adedayo O, Grell G, Bellot P. Hyperinfective strongyloidiasis in the medical ward: review of 27 cases in 5 years. South Med J. 2002 Jul;95(7): 711–6.
3. Angheben A, Mistretta M, Gobbo M, Bonafini S, Iacovazzi T, Sepe A, et al. Acute strongyloidiasis in Italian tourists returning from Southeast Asia. J Travel Med. 2011 Mar–Apr;18(2):138–40.
4. Arthur RP, Shelley WB. Larva currens; a distinctive variant of cutaneous larva migrans due to Strongyloides stercoralis. AMA Arch Derm. 1958 Aug;78(2):186–90.
5. Cappello M, Hotez PJ. Disseminated strongyloidiasis. Semin Neurol. 1993 Jun;13(2):169–74.
6. Genta RM, Weesner R, Douce RW, Huitger-O'Connor T, Walzer PD. Strongyloidiasis in US veterans of the Vietnam and other wars. JAMA. 1987 Jul 3;258(1):49–52.
7. Grove DI. Human strongyloidiasis. Adv Parasitol. 1996;38:251–309.
8. Gyorkos TW, Genta RM, Viens P, MacLean JD. Seroepidemiology of Strongyloides infection in the Southeast Asian refugee population in Canada. Am J Epidemiol. 1990 Aug;132(2):257–64.
9. Keiser PB, Nutman TB. Strongyloides stercoralis in the immunocompromised population. Clin Microbiol Rev. 2004 Jan;17(1):208–17.
10. Siddiqui AA, Berk SL. Diagnosis of Strongyloides stercoralis infection. Clin Infect Dis. 2001 Oct 1;33(7):1040–7.
11. Zaha O, Hirata T, Kinjo F, Saito A. Strongyloidiasis—progress in diagnosis and treatment. Intern Med. 2000 Sep;39(9):695–700.

TAENIASIS

Jeffrey L. Jones

INFECTIOUS AGENT

Taenia solium (pork tapeworm) and T. saginata or T. asiatica (beef tapeworm).

TRANSMISSION

Eating raw or undercooked contaminated pork or beef.

EPIDEMIOLOGY

The highest prevalences are in Latin America, Africa, and South and Southeast Asia. Taeniasis has been reported at lower rates in Eastern Europe, Spain, and Portugal.

CLINICAL PRESENTATION

The incubation period is 8–10 weeks for T. solium and 10–14 weeks for T. saginata. Symptoms may include abdominal discomfort, weight loss, anorexia, nausea, insomnia, weakness, perianal pruritus, and nervousness.

DIAGNOSIS

Presence of eggs, proglottids (segments), or tapeworm antigens in the feces or on anal swabs. Differentiation of T. solium from T. saginata and T. asiatica is based on morphology of the scolex and gravid proglottids.

TREATMENT

Praziquantel is the drug of choice. Niclosamide is an alternative but is not as widely available.

BIBLIOGRAPHY

1. Wittner M, White AC Jr, Tanowitz HB. *Taenia* and other tapeworm infections. In: Guerrant RL, Walker DH, Weller PF, editors. Tropical Infectious Diseases: Principles, Pathogens, and Practice. 3rd ed. Philadelphia: Sanders Elsevier; 2011. p. 839-47.

PREVENTION

Avoid undercooked meat.

CDC website: www.cdc.gov/parasites/taeniasis.

TETANUS

Ryan T. Novak

INFECTIOUS AGENT

Clostridium tetani, a spore-forming, anaerobic, gram-positive bacterium.

TRANSMISSION

Contact with nonintact skin, usually via injuries from contaminated objects. "Tetanus-prone" wounds include those contaminated with dirt, feces, or saliva; punctures; burns; crush injuries; or injuries with necrotic tissue.

EPIDEMIOLOGY

Distributed worldwide; more common in agricultural regions, areas where contact with soil or animal excreta is likely, and areas where immunization is inadequate.

CLINICAL PRESENTATION

Incubation period is 10 days (range, 3–21 days). Acute symptoms typically include muscle rigidity and spasms, often in the jaw and neck. Symptoms of less common forms of tetanus (localized or cephalic) can include muscle spasms confined to the injury site, head or face lesions, and flaccid cranial nerve palsies. Progression from these forms to generalized tetanus may occur. Severe tetanus can lead to respiratory failure and death.

DIAGNOSIS

Diagnosis is made clinically; no confirmatory laboratory tests are available.

TREATMENT

Tetanus requires hospitalization, treatment with human tetanus immune globulin (TIG), a tetanus toxoid booster, agents to control muscle spasm, and aggressive wound care and antibiotics. Metronidazole is the most appropriate antibiotic. The wound should be debrided widely and excised if possible.

PREVENTION

Ensure adequate immunity to tetanus by completing the childhood primary vaccine series with tetanus toxoid, a booster dose during adolescence, and at 10-year intervals thereafter during adulthood. For detailed information regarding the tetanus vaccine, visit www.cdc.gov/vaccines/vpd-vac/tetanus. Additional tetanus prophylaxis may be required in wounded patients.

CDC website: www.cdc.gov/vaccines/vpd-vac/tetanus

BIBLIOGRAPHY

1. CDC. Updated recommendations for use of tetanus toxoid, reduced diphtheria toxoid and acellular pertussis (Tdap) vaccine from the Advisory Committee on Immunization Practices, 2010. MMWR Morb Mortal Wkly Rep. 2011 Jan 14;60(1):13–5.

2. Farrar JJ, Yen LM, Cook T, Fairweather N, Binh N, Parry J, et al. Tetanus. J Neurol Neurosurg Psychiatry. 2000 Sep;69(3):292–301.

TICKBORNE ENCEPHALITIS
Marc Fischer, Stephanie J. Yendell, Pierre E. Rollin

INFECTIOUS AGENT

Tickborne encephalitis virus (TBEV) is a single-stranded RNA virus that belongs to the genus *Flavivirus* and is closely related to Powassan virus. TBEV has 3 subtypes: European, Siberian, and Far Eastern.

TRANSMISSION

TBEV is transmitted to humans through the bite of an infected tick of the *Ixodes* species, primarily *I. ricinus* (European subtype) or *I. persulcatus* (Siberian and Far Eastern subtypes). The virus is maintained in discrete areas of deciduous forests. Ticks act as both vector and virus reservoir, and small rodents are the primary amplifying host. Tickborne encephalitis (TBE) can also be acquired by ingesting unpasteurized dairy products (such as milk and cheese) from infected goats, sheep, or cows. TBEV transmission has infrequently been reported through laboratory exposure and slaughtering viremic animals. Direct person-to-person spread of TBEV occurs only rarely, through blood transfusion or breastfeeding.

EPIDEMIOLOGY

TBE is endemic in focal areas of Europe and Asia (from eastern France to northern Japan and from northern Russia to Albania). From 1990 through 2009, an average of 8,500 cases per year (range, 5,352–12,733 cases) were reported from 19 European countries, with a peak in incidence in the late 1990s. Russia has the largest number of reported TBE cases, and western Siberia has the highest incidence of TBE in the world. Other European countries with known endemic areas include Austria, Croatia, Czech Republic, Denmark, Estonia, Finland, France, Germany, Hungary, Italy, Latvia, Lithuania, Norway, Poland, Romania, Slovakia, Slovenia, Sweden, and Switzerland. Asian countries with reported TBE cases or virus activity include China, Japan, Kazakhstan, Kyrgyzstan, Mongolia, and South Korea.

Most cases occur from April through November, with peaks in early and late summer when ticks are active. The incidence and severity of disease are highest in people aged ≥50 years. Most cases occur in areas <2,500 ft (750 m). In the last 30 years, the geographic range of TBEV appears to have expanded to new areas, and the virus has been found at altitudes up to and above 5,000 ft (1,500 m). These trends are likely due to a complex combination of changes in diagnosis and surveillance, human activities and socioeconomic factors, and ecology and climate.

The overall risk of acquiring TBE for an unvaccinated visitor to a highly endemic area during the TBEV transmission season has been estimated at 1 case per 10,000 person-months of exposure. Most TBEV infections result from tick bites acquired in forested areas through activities such as camping; hiking; fishing; bicycling; collecting mushrooms, berries, or flowers; and outdoor occupations such as forestry or military training. The risk is negligible for people who remain in urban or unforested areas and who do not consume unpasteurized dairy products.

Vector tick population density and infection rates in TBEV-endemic foci are highly variable. For example, TBEV infection rates in *I. ricinus* in central Europe vary from <0.1% to approximately 5%, depending on geographic location and time of year, while rates of up to 40% have been reported in *I. persulcatus* in Siberia. The number of TBE cases reported from a country depends on the ecology and geographic distribution of TBEV, the intensity of diagnosis and surveillance, and the vaccine coverage in the population. Therefore, the number of human TBE cases reported from an area may not be a reliable predictor of a traveler's risk for infection.

From 2000 through 2011, 5 cases of TBE among US travelers to Europe and China were reported. TBE is not a nationally notifiable disease in the United States, and additional cases may have occurred. The same ticks that transmit TBEV can also transmit other pathogens, including *Borrelia burgdorferi* (the agent for Lyme disease), *Anaplasma phagocytophilum* (anaplasmosis), and *Babesia* spp. (babesiosis). Therefore, simultaneous infection with multiple organisms is possible.

CLINICAL PRESENTATION

Approximately two-thirds of infections are asymptomatic. The median incubation period for TBE is 8 days (range, 4–28 days). The incubation period for milkborne exposure is usually shorter (3–4 days). Acute neuroinvasive disease is the most commonly recognized clinical manifestation of TBEV infection. However, TBE disease often presents with milder forms of the disease or a biphasic course:

- First phase: nonspecific febrile illness with headache, myalgia, and fatigue. Usually lasts for several days and may be followed by an afebrile and relatively asymptomatic period. Up to two-thirds of patients may recover without any further illness.
- Second phase: central nervous system involvement resulting in aseptic meningitis, encephalitis, or myelitis. Findings include meningeal signs, altered mental status, cognitive dysfunction, ataxia, tremors, cranial nerve palsies, and limb paresis.

Disease severity increases with age. Clinical course and long-term outcome also vary by TBEV subtype:

- The European subtype is associated with milder disease, a case-fatality ratio of <2%, and neurologic sequelae in up to 30% of patients.

- The Far Eastern subtype is often associated with a more severe disease course, including a case-fatality ratio of 20%–40% and higher rates of severe neurologic sequelae.
- The Siberian subtype is more frequently associated with chronic or progressive disease and has a case-fatality ratio of 2%–3%.

DIAGNOSIS

TBE should be suspected in travelers who develop a nonspecific febrile illness that progresses to neuroinvasive disease within 4 weeks of arriving from an endemic area. A history of tick bite may be a clue to this diagnosis; however, approximately 30% of TBE patients do not recall a tick bite.

Serology is typically used for laboratory diagnosis. IgM-capture ELISA performed on serum or cerebrospinal fluid is virtually always positive during the neuroinvasive phase of the illness. Vaccination history, date of onset of symptoms, and information regarding other flaviviruses known to circulate in the geographic area that may cross-react in serologic assays need to be considered when interpreting results. During the first phase of the illness, TBEV or TBEV RNA can sometimes be detected in serum samples by virus isolation or RT-PCR. However, by the time neurologic symptoms are recognized, the virus or viral RNA is usually undetectable. Therefore, virus isolation and RT-PCR should not be used to rule out a diagnosis of TBE. Clinicians should contact their state or local health department, CDC's Viral Special Pathogens Branch (404-639-1115), or CDC's Division of Vector-Borne Diseases (970-221-6400) for assistance with diagnostic testing.

TREATMENT

There is no specific antiviral treatment for TBE; therapy consists of supportive care and management of complications.

PREVENTION
Personal Protection Measures

Travelers should avoid consuming unpasteurized dairy products and use all measures to avoid tick bites (see Chapter 2, Protection against Mosquitoes, Ticks, & Other Insects & Arthropods).

Vaccine

No TBE vaccines are licensed or available in the United States. Two inactivated cell culture-derived TBE vaccines are available in Europe, in adult and pediatric formulations: FSME-IMMUN (Baxter, Austria) and Encepur (Novartis, Germany). The adult formulation of FSME-IMMUN is also licensed in Canada. Two other inactivated TBE vaccines are available in Russia: TBE-Moscow (Chumakov Institute, Russia) and EnceVir (Microgen, Russia). At least one other TBE vaccine is produced in China, but information regarding this vaccine is not available in the English literature.

Immunogenicity studies suggest that the European and Russian vaccines should provide cross-protection against all 3 TBEV subtypes. For both FSME-IMMUN and Encepur, the primary vaccination series consists of 3 doses (Table 3-19). The specific recommended intervals between doses vary by country and vaccine. Although no formal efficacy trials of these vaccines have been conducted, indirect evidence suggests that their efficacy is >95%. Vaccine failures have been reported, particularly in people aged ≥50 years. Regardless of age, the first booster dose should be given 3 years after the primary series. Recommended intervals for subsequent booster doses vary by age; boosters should be given every 5 years for people aged <50 years and every 3 years for those aged ≥50 years.

Because the routine primary vaccination series requires ≥6 months for completion, most travelers to TBE-endemic areas will find

Table 3-19. Tickborne encephalitis (TBE) vaccines licensed in Canada, Europe, and Russia[1]

TRADE NAME (MANUFACTURER, LOCATION)	AGE (Y)	DOSE	ROUTE	PRIMARY SERIES	FIRST BOOSTER (Y)	SUBSEQUENT BOOSTERS (Y)
FSME-IMMUN (Baxter, Austria)	≥16	0.5 mL	IM	3 doses (0, 1–3 mo, 6–15 mo)[2]	3	5[3]
FSME-IMMUN Junior (Baxter, Austria)	1–15	0.25 mL	IM	3 doses (0, 1–3 mo, 6–15 mo)[2]	3	5
Encepur-Adults (Novartis, Germany)	≥17	0.5 mL	IM	3 doses (0, 1–3 mo, 9–12 mo)[4]	3	5[3]
Encepur-Children (Novartis, Germany)	1–11	0.25 mL	IM	3 doses (0, 1–3 mo, 9–12 mo)[4]	3	5
EnceVir (Microgen, Russia)	≥3	0.5 mL	IM	2 doses (0, 5–7 mo)[5]	1	3
TBE-Moscow (Chumakov Institute, Russia)	≥3	0.5 mL	IM	2 doses (0, 1–7 mo)	1	3

[1] No TBE vaccines are licensed or available in the United States. FSME-IMMUN is licensed in Canada and Europe; FSME-IMMUN Junior, Encepur-Adults, and Encepur-Children are licensed in Europe; and EnceVir and TBE-Moscow are licensed in Russia.

[2] If a rapid immune response is required, the second dose can be administered 2 weeks after the first dose.

[3] Booster doses recommended every 3 years for people aged ≥50 years.

[4] An accelerated schedule has been used with 3 doses given on days 0, 7, and 21. After the primary series, the first booster dose is administered at 12–18 months.

[5] For emergency situations, there is a rapid primary series schedule of 0 and 1–2 months.

avoiding tick bites to be more practical than vaccination. However, an accelerated vaccination schedule has been evaluated for both European vaccines, and results in seroconversion rates are similar to those observed with the standard vaccination schedule. Travelers anticipating high-risk exposures, such as working or camping in forested areas or farmland, adventure travel, or living in TBE-endemic countries for an extended period of time, may wish to be vaccinated in Canada or Europe.

CDC website: www.cdc.gov/ncidod/dvrd/spb/mnpages/dispages/TBE.htm

BIBLIOGRAPHY

1. Banzhoff A, Broker M, Zent O. Protection against tick-borne encephalitis (TBE) for people living in and travelling to TBE-endemic areas. Travel Med Infect Dis. 2008 Nov;6(6):331–41.
2. CDC. Tick-borne encephalitis among US travelers to Europe and Asia—2000–2009. MMWR Morb Mortal Wkly Rep. 2010 Mar 26;59(11):335–8.
3. Committee to Advise on Tropical Medicine and Travel (CATMAT). Statement on tick-borne encephalitis. An Advisory Committee Statement (ACS). Can Commun Dis Rep. 2006 Apr 1;32(ACS-3):1–18.
4. Czupryna P, Moniuszko A, Pancewicz SA, Grygorczuk S, Kondrusik M, Zajkowska J. Tick-borne encephalitis in Poland in years 1993–2008—epidemiology and clinical presentation. A retrospective study of 687 patients. Eur J Neurol. 2011 May;18(5):673–9.
5. Donoso Mantke O, Escadafal C, Niedrig M, Pfeffer M, Working Group For Tick-Borne Encephalitis Virus. Tick-borne encephalitis in Europe, 2007 to 2009. Euro Surveill. 2011;16(39).
6. Haglund M, Gunther G. Tick-borne encephalitis—pathogenesis, clinical course and long-term follow-up. Vaccine. 2003 Apr 1;21 Suppl 1:S11–8.
7. Holzmann H. Diagnosis of tick-borne encephalitis. Vaccine. 2003 Apr 1;21 Suppl 1:S36–40.
8. Korenberg EI. Chapter 4. Recent epidemiology of tick-borne encephalitis an effect of climate change? Adv Virus Res. 2009;74:123–44.
9. Lindquist L, Vapalahti O. Tick-borne encephalitis. Lancet. 2008 May 31;371(9627):1861–71.
10. Lu Z, Broker M, Liang G. Tick-borne encephalitis in mainland China. Vector Borne Zoonotic Dis. 2008 Oct;8(5):713–20.
11. Ruzek D, Dobler G, Donoso Mantke O. Tick-borne encephalitis: pathogenesis and clinical implications. Travel Med Infect Dis. 2010 Jul;8(4):223–32.
12. Stefanoff P, Polkowska A, Giambi C, Levy-Bruhl D, O'Flanagan D, Dematte L, et al. Reliable surveillance of tick-borne encephalitis in European countries is necessary to improve the quality of vaccine recommendations. Vaccine. 2011 Feb 1;29(6):1283–8.
13. Suss J. Tick-borne encephalitis 2010: epidemiology, risk areas, and virus strains in Europe and Asia—an overview. Ticks Tick Borne Dis. 2011 Mar;2(1):2–15.
14. World Health Organization. Vaccines against tick-borne encephalitis: WHO position paper. Wkly Epidemiol Rec. 2011 Jun 10;86(24):241–56.

TOXOPLASMOSIS
Jeffrey L. Jones

INFECTIOUS AGENT
Toxoplasma gondii, an intracellular coccidian protozoan parasite.

TRANSMISSION
Ingestion of soil, water, or food contaminated with cat feces, ingestion of undercooked meat, congenital transmission when a woman becomes infected during pregnancy, and contaminated blood transfusion and organ transplantation.

EPIDEMIOLOGY
Risk is higher in developing and tropical countries, especially when people eat undercooked meat, drink untreated water, or are extensively exposed to soil.

CLINICAL PRESENTATION

Incubation period is 5–23 days. Symptoms may include influenzalike symptoms or symptoms of a mononucleosis syndrome with prolonged fever, lymphadenopathy, elevated liver enzymes, lymphocytosis, and weakness. In severely immunocompromised people, severe and even fatal toxoplasmic encephalitis, pneumonitis, and other systemic illnesses can occur, most often from reactivation of a previous infection. Infants with congenital toxoplasmosis are often asymptomatic, but eye disease, neurologic disease, or other systemic symptoms can occur, and learning disabilities, mental retardation, or visual impairments may develop later in life.

DIAGNOSIS

Serologic testing for *T. gondii* antibodies. Eye disease is diagnosed by ocular examination. Diagnosis of toxoplasmic encephalitis in immunocompromised people can be based on typical clinical course and identification of ≥1 mass lesion by CT, MRI, or other radiographic testing. Biopsy may be needed to make a definitive diagnosis.

TREATMENT

Pyrimethamine and sulfadiazine are the mainstays of treatment.

PREVENTION

Food and water precautions (see Chapter 2, Food & Water Precautions). Avoid direct contact with soil or sand. If caring for a cat, change the litter box daily. If pregnant or immunocompromised, avoid changing cat litter if possible, and do not adopt or handle stray cats.

CDC website: www.cdc.gov/parasites/toxoplasmosis

BIBLIOGRAPHY

1. Bottieau E, Clerinx J, Van den Enden E, Van Esbroeck M, Colebunders R, Van Gompel A, et al. Infectious mononucleosis-like syndromes in febrile travelers returning from the tropics. J Travel Med. 2006 Jul–Aug;13(4):191–7.

2. Montoya JG, Liesenfeld O. Toxoplasmosis. Lancet. 2004 Jun 12;363(9425):1965–76.

3. Montoya JG, Remington JS. Management of *Toxoplasma gondii* infection during pregnancy. Clin Infect Dis. 2008 Aug 15;47(4):554–66.

TRYPANOSOMIASIS, AFRICAN (SLEEPING SICKNESS)

Anne Moore

INFECTIOUS AGENT

Two subspecies of the protozoan parasite *Trypanosoma brucei* (*T. b. rhodesiense* and *T. b. gambiense*).

TRANSMISSION

The bite of an infected tsetse fly (*Glossina* spp.). Bloodborne and congenital transmission are rare.

EPIDEMIOLOGY

Endemic in rural sub-Saharan Africa. *T. b. rhodesiense* is found in eastern and southeastern Africa, especially Tanzania, Uganda, Malawi, and Zambia. *T. b. gambiense* is found in central Africa and in limited areas of West Africa, primarily in Democratic Republic of the Congo, Angola, Sudan, Central African Republic, Republic of the Congo, Chad, and northern Uganda. Tsetse flies inhabit rural, densely vegetated areas; travelers to urban areas are not at risk. Flies bite during the day, and fewer than 1% are infected.

CLINICAL PRESENTATION

T. b. rhodesiense

Symptoms generally appear within 1–3 weeks of the infective bite and may include high fever, a chancre at the bite site, skin rash, headache, myalgia, thrombocytopenia, and less commonly, splenomegaly, renal failure, or cardiac dysfunction. Central nervous system involvement can occur within a month of infection and results in mental deterioration and eventually, death.

T. b. gambiense

Nonspecific but may include fever, headache, malaise, myalgia, facial edema, pruritus, lymphadenopathy, and weight loss. Central nervous system involvement occurs after months to years of infection and is characterized by somnolence, severe headache, and a range of neurologic manifestations, including mood disorders, behavior change, focal deficits, and endocrine disorders. The clinical course of disease caused by *T. b. gambiense* is generally less severe than that caused by *T. b. rhodesiense*, but both are fatal if not treated.

DIAGNOSIS

Identification of parasites in specimens of blood, chancre fluid or tissue, lymph node aspirate, or cerebrospinal fluid. Buffy-coat preparations concentrate the parasite. Diagnostic assistance is available through CDC (www.dpd.cdc.gov/dpdx; 404-718-4745; parasites@cdc.gov).

TREATMENT

Infection can usually be cured by a course of antitrypanosomal therapy. Treatment drugs (suramin, melarsoprol, eflornithine) are provided by CDC under investigational protocols. Physicians can consult with CDC for assistance with treatment.

PREVENTION

Avoid tsetse fly bites. Travelers should wear clothing of wrist and ankle length made of medium-weight fabric in neutral colors, as tsetse flies are attracted to bright, dark colors and can bite through lightweight clothing. Permethrin-impregnated clothing and use of DEET repellent may minimally reduce the number of fly bites.

CDC website: www.cdc.gov/parasites/sleepingsickness

BIBLIOGRAPHY

1. Brun R, Blum J, Chappuis F, Burri C. Human African trypanosomiasis. Lancet. 2010 Jan 9;375(9709): 148–59.
2. Simarro PP, Franco JR, Cecchi G, Paone M, Diarra A, Ruiz Postigo JA, et al. Human African trypanosomiasis in non-endemic countries (2000–2010). J Travel Med. 2012 Jan–Feb; 19(1):44–53.

TRYPANOSOMIASIS, AMERICAN (CHAGAS DISEASE)

Susan Montgomery

INFECTIOUS AGENT

The protozoan parasite *Trypanosoma cruzi*.

TRANSMISSION

Typically through feces of the triatomine insect (reduviid bug), may occur when a bug bite is scratched; may also be transmitted through blood transfusion or organ transplantation, from mother to infant, and by consuming contaminated food or beverages.

EPIDEMIOLOGY

Endemic in Mexico and Central and South America. The risk to travelers is extremely low, but they could be at risk if staying in poor-quality housing in endemic areas.

CLINICAL PRESENTATION

Acute illness typically develops ≥1 week after exposure and lasts up to 90 days. A chagoma may develop at the site of infection; for example, the Romaña sign (edema of the eyelid and ocular tissues). Most infected people never develop symptoms but remain infected throughout their lives. Approximately 20%–30% of patients will develop chronic manifestations of Chagas disease after a prolonged period without any clinical disease. Chronic Chagas disease usually affects the heart; clinical signs include conduction system abnormalities, ventricular arrhythmias, and in late-stage disease, congestive cardiomyopathy. Less common chronic gastrointestinal problems may ensue (such as megaesophagus or megacolon). Reactivation disease can occur in immunocompromised patients.

DIAGNOSIS

During the acute phase, parasites may be detectable in fresh preparations of buffy coat or stained peripheral blood specimens. After the acute phase, diagnosis requires 2 or more serologic tests (most commonly, ELISA and the immunofluorescent antibody test).

TREATMENT

Antitrypanosomal drug treatment is always recommended for acute, early congenital, and reactivated *T. cruzi* infection and for chronic *T. cruzi* infection in children aged <18 years old. In adults, treatment is usually recommended. In the United States, treatment drugs (benznidazole and nifurtimox) are provided by CDC under investigational protocols. Contact CDC (chagas@cdc.gov; 404-718-4745) for assistance with clinical management.

PREVENTION

Insect precautions (see Chapter 2, Protection against Mosquitoes, Ticks, & Other Insects & Arthropods) and food and water precautions (see Chapter 2, Food & Water Precautions).

CDC website: www.cdc.gov/parasites/chagas

BIBLIOGRAPHY

1. Bern C. Antitrypanosomal therapy for chronic Chagas' disease. N Engl J Med. 2011 Jun 30;364(26):2527–34.
2. Bern C, Montgomery SP, Herwaldt BL, Rassi A Jr, Marin-Neto JA, Dantas RO, et al. Evaluation and treatment of Chagas disease in the United States: a systematic review. JAMA. 2007 Nov 14;298(18):2171–81.
3. Rassi A Jr, Rassi A, Marin-Neto JA. Chagas disease. Lancet. 2010 Apr 17;375(9723):1388–402.

TUBERCULOSIS

Philip LoBue

INFECTIOUS AGENT

Mycobacterium tuberculosis is a rod-shaped, nonmotile, slow-growing, acid-fast bacterium.

TRANSMISSION

Tuberculosis (TB) transmission occurs when a contagious patient coughs, spreading bacilli through the air. Bovine TB (caused by the closely related *Mycobacterium bovis*) can be transmitted by consuming contaminated, unpasteurized dairy products from infected cattle.

EPIDEMIOLOGY

Globally, nearly 9 million new TB cases and approximately 1.5 million TB-related deaths occur each year. TB occurs throughout the world, but the incidence varies (see Map 3-13). In the United States, the annual incidence is <4 per 100,000 population, but in some countries in sub-Saharan Africa and Asia, the annual incidence is several hundred per 100,000.

Drug-resistant TB is of increasing concern. Multidrug-resistant (MDR) TB is resistant to the 2 most effective drugs, isoniazid and rifampin. Extensively drug-resistant (XDR) TB is resistant to isoniazid and rifampin, any fluoroquinolone, and ≥1 of 3 injectable second-line drugs (amikacin, kanamycin, or capreomycin). MDR TB is less common than drug-susceptible TB, but nearly 440,000 new cases of MDR TB are diagnosed each year, and some countries have proportions of MDR TB as high as 20% (see Map 3-14). MDR and XDR TB are of particular concern among HIV-infected or other immunocompromised people. As of October 2011, XDR TB had been reported in 77 countries (see Map 3-15).

Travelers who anticipate possible prolonged exposure to TB (such as those who would spend time in hospitals, prisons, or homeless shelters) or those who stay for years in an endemic country should have a 2-step tuberculin skin test (TST) or a single interferon-γ release assay (IGRA), either the QuantiFERON TB test (Gold In-Tube version) or T-SPOT.TB test, before leaving the United States (see *Perspectives*: Tuberculin Skin Testing of Travelers, later in this chapter). If the predeparture test result is negative, a single TST or IGRA should be repeated 8–10 weeks after returning from travel. Because people with HIV infection or other immuno-compromising conditions are more likely to have an impaired response to either a skin or blood test, travelers should inform their physicians about such conditions. Except for those with impaired immunity, travelers who have already been infected are less likely to be reinfected.

The risk of TB transmission on an airplane does not appear to be higher than in any other enclosed space. To prevent TB transmission, people who have infectious TB should not travel by commercial airplanes or other commercial conveyances. The World Health Organization (WHO) has issued guidelines for notifying passengers who might have been exposed to TB aboard airplanes. Passengers concerned about possible exposure to TB should see their primary health care provider for evaluation.

Bovine TB (M. *bovis*) is a risk in travelers who consume unpasteurized dairy products in countries where M. *bovis* in cattle is common. Mexico is a common place of infection for US travelers.

CLINICAL PRESENTATION

TB disease can affect any organ but most commonly occurs in the lungs (70%–80%). Common TB symptoms include prolonged cough, fever, decreased appetite, weight loss, night sweats, and coughing up blood (hemoptysis). The most common sites for TB outside the lungs are the lymph nodes, chest-wall lining, bones and joints, brain and spinal cord lining (meningitis), kidneys, bladder, and genitalia.

Infection is manifested by a positive TST or IGRA result, which usually occurs 8–10 weeks after exposure. Overall, only 5%–10% of people progress from infection to disease during their lifetime. In the remainder, the infection remains in a latent state (latent TB infection or LTBI). However, the risk of progression is much higher in immunosuppressed people (8%–10% per year in HIV-infected people not receiving antiretroviral therapy). In recent years, people who are receiving tumor necrosis factor-α inhibitors to treat rheumatoid arthritis and other chronic inflammatory conditions have also been found to be at increased risk for disease progression. LTBI is an asymptomatic condition, and people with LTBI do not transmit TB. Progression to disease can occur weeks to decades after initial infection.

DIAGNOSIS

Diagnosis of TB disease is confirmed by culturing M. *tuberculosis* from sputum or other respiratory specimens for pulmonary TB and from other affected body tissues or fluids for extrapulmonary TB. On average, it takes about 2 weeks to culture and identify M. *tuberculosis*, even with rapid culture techniques. A preliminary diagnosis of TB can be made when acid-fast bacilli are seen on sputum smear or in other body tissues or fluids. However, microscopy cannot distinguish between M. *tuberculosis* and nontuberculous mycobacteria. This is particularly problematic in countries such as the United States where TB incidence is low. Nucleic acid amplification tests are more rapid than culture and specific for M. *tuberculosis*. They are also more sensitive than the acid-fast bacillus smear but less sensitive than culture. A diagnosis of TB disease can be made by using clinical criteria in the absence of microbiologic confirmation.

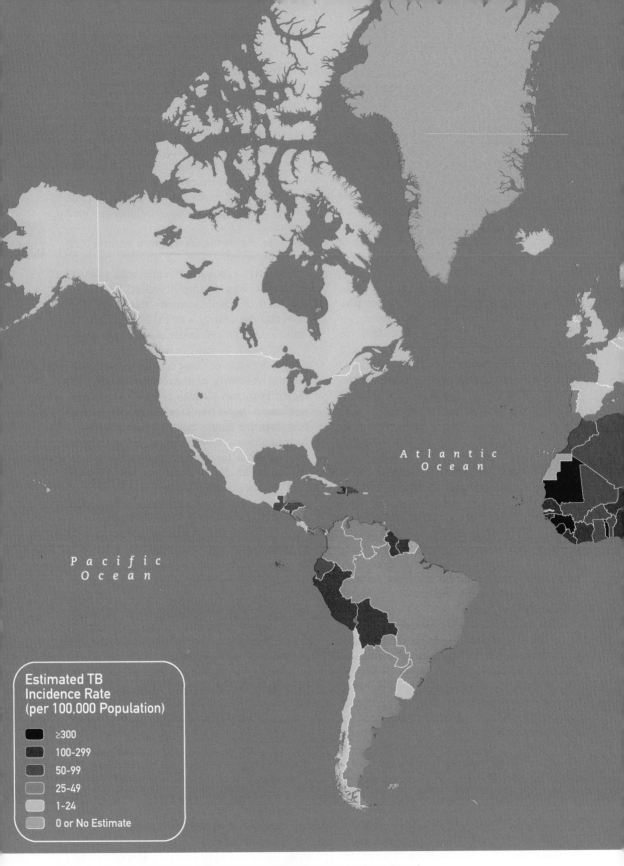

MAP 3-13. ESTIMATED TUBERCULOSIS INCIDENCE RATES, 2010[1]

[1] Data from the World Health Organization's tuberculosis database. Available from: www.who.int/tb/country/data/download/en/index.html. Data accessed July 2012.

Estimated TB Incidence Rate (per 100,000 Population)

- ≥300
- 100–299
- 50–99
- 25–49
- 1–24
- 0 or No Estimate

INFECTIOUS DISEASES RELATED TO TRAVEL

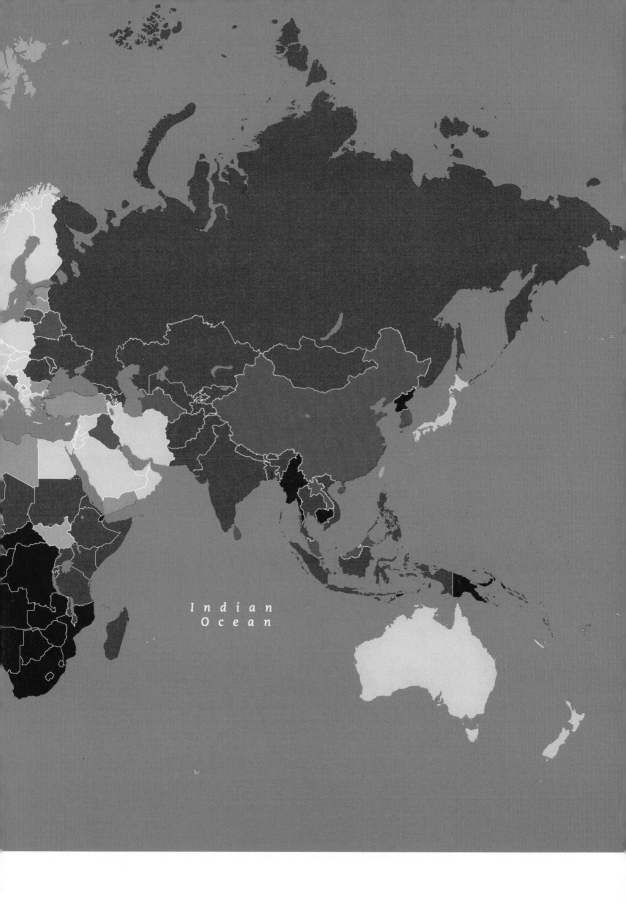

*Indian
Ocean*

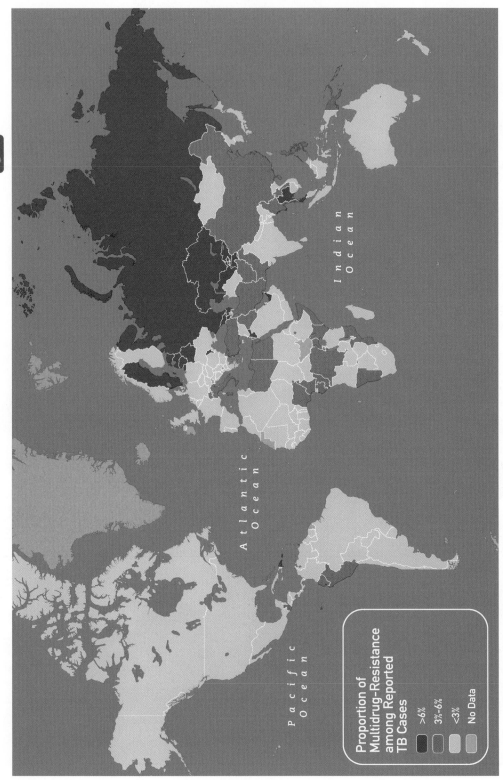

MAP 3-14. PROPORTION OF MULTIDRUG-RESISTANT TUBERCULOSIS AMONG NEW TUBERCULOSIS CASES, 1994–2010[1]

Proportion of Multidrug-Resistance among Reported TB Cases

- >6%
- 3%–6%
- <3%
- No Data

Indian Ocean

Atlantic Ocean

Pacific Ocean

[1] Data from the World Health Organization's tuberculosis database. Available from: www.who.int/tb/country/data/download/en/index.html. Data accessed July 2012.

3

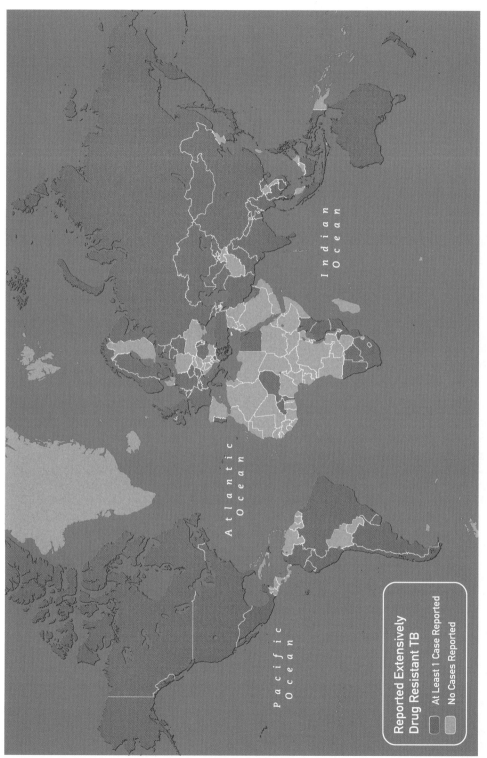

MAP 3-15. DISTRIBUTION OF COUNTRIES AND TERRITORIES REPORTING AT LEAST 1 CASE OF EXTENSIVELY DRUG-RESISTANT TUBERCUOLOSIS[1]

[1] Data from the World Health Organization's tuberculosis database. Available from: www.who.int/tb/country/data/download/en/index.html. Data accessed July 2012.

Reported Extensively
Drug Resistant TB

At Least 1 Case Reported

No Cases Reported

However, laboratory testing should be performed when feasible to confirm the diagnosis and to conduct drug susceptibility testing to guide treatment. LTBI is diagnosed by a positive TST or IGRA.

TREATMENT

People with LTBI can be treated to prevent progression to TB disease. American Thoracic Society (ATS)/CDC guidelines for treatment of LTBI recommend 9 months of isoniazid as the preferred treatment. The combination regimen of isoniazid and rifapentine given as 12 weekly doses using directly observed therapy is recommended as equivalent to 9 months of isoniazid for treating LTBI in otherwise healthy patients aged ≥12 years who are at higher risk of developing active TB, for example after recent exposure to contagious TB. For people who have been exposed to isoniazid-resistant, rifampin-susceptible TB or who cannot tolerate isoniazid, 4 months of rifampin is a reasonable alternative. Travelers who suspect that they have been exposed to TB should inform their health care provider of the possible exposure and receive medical evaluation. CDC and ATS have published guidelines for targeted testing and treatment of LTBI. Recent data from WHO suggest that drug resistance is relatively common in some parts of the world. Travelers who have TST or IGRA conversion associated with international travel should consult experts in infectious diseases or pulmonary medicine.

TB disease is treated with a multiple-drug regimen administered by directly observed therapy for 6–9 months (usually isoniazid, rifampin, ethambutol, and pyrazinamide for 2 months, followed by isoniazid and rifampin for an additional 4 months) if the TB is not MDR TB. MDR TB treatment is more difficult, requiring 4–6 drugs for 18–24 months; it should be managed by an expert in MDR TB. ATS/CDC/Infectious Diseases Society of America have published guidelines on TB treatment.

PREVENTION

Travelers should avoid exposure to TB patients in crowded environments (such as hospitals, prisons, or homeless shelters). Travelers who will be working in hospitals or health care settings where TB patients are likely to be encountered should be advised to consult infection control or occupational health experts about procedures for obtaining personal respiratory protective devices (such as N-95 respirators), along with respirator selection and training.

Based on WHO recommendations, Bacillus Calmette-Guérin (BCG) vaccine is used once at birth in most developing countries to reduce the severe consequences of TB in infants and children. However, BCG vaccine has variable efficacy in preventing the adult forms of TB and interferes with testing for LTBI with the TST. Therefore, BCG is not routinely recommended for use in the United States. Recently, some experts have advocated BCG vaccination for people who are likely to be exposed to MDR or XDR TB patients in settings where the TB infection control measures recommended in the United States are not fully implemented. BCG may offer some protection in this circumstance; however, people who receive BCG vaccination must follow all recommended TB infection control precautions to the extent possible. Additionally, IGRA is preferred over the TST for pre- and post-travel testing in people vaccinated with BCG.

To prevent infections due to *M. bovis*, travelers should also avoid eating or drinking unpasteurized dairy products.

CDC website: www.cdc.gov/tb

BIBLIOGRAPHY

1. American Thoracic Society and CDC. Diagnostic standards and classification of tuberculosis in adults and children. Am J Respir Crit Care Med. 2000 Apr;161(4 Pt 1):1376–95.
2. American Thoracic Society and CDC. Targeted tuberculin testing and treatment of latent tuberculosis infection. Am J Respir Crit Care Med. 2000 Apr;161(4 Pt 2):S221–47.
3. CDC. Recommendations for use of an isoniazid-rifapentine regimen with direct observation to treat latent *Mycobacterium tuberculosis* infection. MMWR Morb Mortal Wkly Rep. 2011 Dec 9;60(48):1650–3.
4. CDC. The role of BCG vaccine in the prevention and control of tuberculosis in the United States. A joint statement by the Advisory Council for the Elimination of Tuberculosis and the Advisory Committee on

Immunization Practices. MMWR Recomm Rep. 1996 Apr 26;45(RR-4):1–18.

5. CDC. Treatment of tuberculosis. MMWR Recomm Rep. 2003 Jun 20;52(RR-11):1–77.

6. CDC. Updated guidelines for using interferon gamma release assays to detect *Mycobacterium tuberculosis* infection, United States. MMWR Recomm Rep. 2010.

7. Jensen PA, Lambert LA, Iademarco MF, Ridzon R. Guidelines for preventing the transmission of *Mycobacterium tuberculosis* in health-care settings, 2005. MMWR Recomm Rep. 2005 Dec 30;54(RR-17):1–141.

8. National Tuberculosis Controllers Association and CDC. Guidelines for the investigation of contacts of persons with infectious tuberculosis. MMWR Recomm Rep. 2005 Dec 16;54(RR-15):1–47.

9. World Health Organization. Anti-tuberculosis drug resistance in the world: fourth global report. Geneva: World Health Organization; 2008 [cited 2012 Sep 21]. Available from: http://www.who.int/tb/features_archive/drsreport_launch_26feb08/en/index.html.

10. World Health Organization. Global tuberculosis control 2011. Geneva: World Health Organization; 2011 [cited 2012 Sep 21]. Available from: http://www.who.int/tb/publications/global_report/en/index.html

11. World Health Organization. Multidrug and extensively drug-resistant TB (M/XDR-TB): 2010 global report on surveillance and response. Geneva: World Health Organization; 2010. Available from: http://www.who.int/tb/features_archive/m_xdrtb_facts/en/index.html.

12. World Health Organization. Tuberculosis and air travel: guidelines for prevention and control. Geneva: World Health Organization; 2008 [cited 2012 Sep 21]. Available from: http://www.who.int/tb/publications/2008/WHO_HTM_TB_2008.399_eng.pdf.

Perspectives

TUBERCULIN SKIN TESTING OF TRAVELERS

Philip LoBue

Screening for asymptomatic tuberculosis (TB) infections should only be carried out among travelers who will be at risk of acquiring TB if they are exposed at their destinations (see the preceding section on Tuberculosis). Screening with a tuberculin skin test (TST) in a very low-risk population of travelers may result in a false-positive test, leading to unnecessary additional screening or unnecessary treatment. Using screening tests in very low-prevalence populations will produce more false positives than true positives.

Therefore, the TST should be considered only for travelers who are spending years in a country with a high risk of TB or for those travelers who will spend any length of time in routine contact with hospital, prison, or homeless shelter populations. The general recommendation is that people at low risk for exposure to TB, which includes most travelers, do not need to be screened before or after travel.

Perspectives sections are written as editorial discussions aiming to add depth and clinical perspective to the official recommendations contained in the book. The views and opinions expressed in this section are those of the author and do not necessarily represent the official position of CDC.

For travelers who anticipate a long stay or contact with a high-risk population, careful pre-travel screening should be carried out, with use of 2-step pre-travel TST screening. For 2-step TSTs, people whose baseline TSTs yield a negative result are retested 1–3 weeks after the initial test; if the second test result is negative, they are considered not infected. If the second test result is positive, they are classified as having had previous TB infection. The 2-step TST is recommended in this population for the following reasons:

- The use of 2-step testing can reduce the number of positive TSTs that would otherwise be misclassified as recent skin test conversions during future periodic screenings.
- Certain people who were infected with *Mycobacterium tuberculosis* years earlier exhibit waning delayed-type hypersensitivity to tuberculin. When they are skin tested years after infection, they might have a false-negative TST result (even though they are truly infected). However, the first TST might stimulate the ability to react to subsequent tests, resulting in a "booster" reaction. When the test is repeated, the reaction might be misinterpreted as a new infection (recent conversion) rather than a boosted reaction.

Two-step testing is important for travelers who will have potential prolonged or substantial TB exposure. Two-step testing before travel will detect boosting and potentially prevent "false conversions"—positive TST results that appear to indicate infection acquired during travel, but which are really the result of previous TB infection. This distinction is particularly important if the traveler is going to a country where extensively drug-resistant TB (XDR TB) is present: it would be critical to know whether the person's skin test had been positive before travel.

If the 2-step pre-travel TST result is negative, the traveler should have a repeat TST 8–10 weeks after returning from the trip or as part of a periodic screening examination for those who remain at high risk. Two-step testing should be considered for the baseline testing of people who report no history of a recent TST and who will receive repeated TSTs as part of ongoing monitoring.

People who have had repeat TSTs must be tested with the same commercial antigen, since switching antigens can also lead to false TST conversions. Two commercial tuberculin skin test antigens are approved by the Food and Drug Administration (FDA) and are commercially available in the United States: Aplisol (JHP Pharmaceuticals) and Tubersol (Sanofi Pasteur).

An alternative to 2-step TST is a single FDA-approved interferon-γ release assay (IGRA), either the QuantiFERON TB test (Gold In-Tube versions) or T-SPOT. TB test. IGRAs, which require a blood draw, are approximately as specific as TST in people who have not been vaccinated with Bacillus Calmette-Guérin (BCG) and are much more specific in BCG-vaccinated populations. For a traveler whose time before departure is short, a single-step TST would be an acceptable alternative if time is insufficient for the 2-step TST and the IGRAs are not available.

In general, it is best not to mix tests. There is approximately 15% discordance between TST and IGRA, usually with the TST positive and the IGRA negative. There are multiple reasons for the discordance, and in any person it is often difficult to be confident about the reason for discordance. However, if the clinician decides to mix tests, it is better to go from TST to IGRA than the other way around, because the likelihood of having a discordant result with the TST negative and the IGRA positive is much lower. Such discordant results may become unavoidable as more medical establishments switch from TSTs to IGRAs.

The use of TSTs among travelers who are visiting friends and relatives in TB-endemic areas should take into account the high rate of TST positivity in people visiting their country of birth. In a study among 53,000 adults in Tennessee, the prevalence of a positive TST among the foreign born was 11 times that among the US born (34% vs 3%). Confirming TST status before travel would prevent the conclusion that a positive TST after travel was due to recent conversion.

BIBLIOGRAPHY

1. Al-Jahdali H, Memish ZA, Menzies D. Tuberculosis in association with travel. Int J Antimicrob Agents. 2003 Feb;21(2):125–30.
2. Cobelens FG, van Deutekom H, Draayer-Jansen IW, Schepp-Beelen AC, van Gerven PJ, van Kessel RP, et al. Risk of infection with *Mycobacterium tuberculosis* in travellers to areas of high tuberculosis endemicity. Lancet. 2000 Aug 5;356(9228):461–5.
3. Haley CA, Cain KP, Yu C, Garman KF, Wells CD, Laserson KF. Risk-based screening for latent tuberculosis infection. South Med J. 2008 Feb;101(2):142–9.
4. Johnston VJ, Grant AD. Tuberculosis in travellers. Travel Med Infect Dis. 2003 Nov;1(4):205–12.
5. Jung P, Banks RH. Tuberculosis risk in US Peace Corps volunteers, 1996 to 2005. J Travel Med. 2008 Mar–Apr;15(2):87–94.
6. Leder K, Tong S, Weld L, Kain KC, Wilder-Smith A, von Sonnenburg F, et al. Illness in travelers visiting friends and relatives: a review of the GeoSentinel Surveillance Network. Clin Infect Dis. 2006 Nov 1;43(9):1185–93.
7. Mancuso JD, Tobler SK, Keep LW. Pseudoepidemics of tuberculin skin test conversions in the US Army after recent deployments. Am J Respir Crit Care Med. 2008 Jun 1;177(11):1285–9.
8. Mazurek M, Jereb J, Vernon A, LoBue P, Goldberg S, Castro K. Updated guidelines for using interferon gamma release assays to detect *Mycobacterium tuberculosis* infection—United States, 2010. MMWR Recomm Rep. 2010 Jun 25;59 (RR-5):1–25.
9. Villarino ME, Burman W, Wang YC, Lundergan L, Catanzaro A, Bock N, et al. Comparable specificity of 2 commercial tuberculin reagents in persons at low risk for tuberculous infection. JAMA. 1999 Jan 13;281(2):169–71.

TYPHOID & PARATYPHOID FEVER
Anna E. Newton, Eric Mintz

INFECTIOUS AGENT

Typhoid fever is a potentially severe and occasionally life-threatening febrile illness caused by the bacterium *Salmonella enterica* serotype Typhi. Paratyphoid fever is a similar illness caused by *S. enterica* serotype Paratyphi A, B (tartrate negative), or C.

TRANSMISSION

Humans are the only source of these bacteria; no animal or environmental reservoirs have been identified. Typhoid and paratyphoid fever are most often acquired through consumption of water or food that has been contaminated by feces of an acutely infected or convalescent person or a chronic, asymptomatic carrier. Transmission through sexual contact, especially among men who have sex with men, has been documented rarely.

EPIDEMIOLOGY

An estimated 22 million cases of typhoid fever and 200,000 related deaths occur worldwide each year; an additional 6 million cases of paratyphoid fever are estimated to occur annually. Each year in the United States, approximately 400 cases of typhoid fever and 100 cases of paratyphoid fever are reported, most in recent travelers. The risk of typhoid fever is highest for travelers to southern Asia (6–30 times higher than for all other destinations). Other areas of risk include East and Southeast Asia, Africa, the Caribbean, and Central and South America. The risk of infection with S. enterica serotype Paratyphi A is also increased among travelers to southern and Southeast Asia. In certain regions, the risk of typhoid fever is decreasing. CDC recently removed pre-travel typhoid vaccination recommendations for 26 destinations; these countries are listed in Johnson et al. in the Bibliography; the most recent pre-travel vaccination guidelines can be found at www.cdc.gov/travel.

Travelers to southern Asia are at highest risk for infection with typhoid and paratyphoid strains that are nalidixic acid–resistant or multidrug-resistant (resistant to ampicillin, chloramphenicol, and trimethoprim-sulfamethoxazole). Travelers who are visiting friends and relatives (VFRs) are at increased risk (see Chapter 8, Immigrants Returning Home to Visit Friends and Relatives [VFRs]). Although the risk of acquiring typhoid or paratyphoid fever increases with the duration of stay, travelers have acquired typhoid fever even during visits of <1 week to countries where the disease is endemic.

CLINICAL PRESENTATION

The incubation period of typhoid and paratyphoid infections is 6–30 days. The onset of illness is insidious, with gradually increasing fatigue and a fever that increases daily from low-grade to as high as 102°F–104°F (38°C–40°C) by the third to fourth day of illness. Headache, malaise, and anorexia are nearly universal. Hepatosplenomegaly can often be detected. A transient, macular rash of rose-colored spots can occasionally be seen on the trunk. Fever is commonly lowest in the morning, reaching a peak in late afternoon or evening. Untreated, the disease can last for a month. The serious complications of typhoid fever generally occur after 2–3 weeks of illness and may include intestinal hemorrhage or perforation, which can be life threatening.

DIAGNOSIS

Infection with typhoid or paratyphoid fever results in a very low-grade septicemia. A single blood culture is positive in only half of cases. Stool culture is not usually positive during the early phase of the disease. Bone marrow culture increases the diagnostic yield to about 80% of cases.

The Widal test is an old serologic assay for detecting IgM and IgG to the O and H antigens of salmonella. The test is unreliable but is widely used in most developing countries because of its low cost. Newer serologic assays for S. enterica serotype Typhi infection are occasionally used in outbreak situations and are somewhat more sensitive and specific than the Widal test, but are not an adequate substitute for blood, stool, or bone marrow culture.

Because there is no definitive serologic test for typhoid or paratyphoid fever, the initial diagnosis often has to be made clinically. The combination of a history of risk for infection and a gradual onset of fever that increases in severity over several days should raise suspicion of typhoid or paratyphoid fever.

TREATMENT

Specific antimicrobial therapy shortens the clinical course of typhoid fever and reduces the risk for death. Empiric treatment in most parts of the world uses a fluoroquinolone, most often ciprofloxacin. However, resistance to fluoroquinolones and nalidixic acid is highest in the Indian subcontinent and increasing in other areas. Injectable third-generation cephalosporins are often the empiric drug of choice when the possibility of fluoroquinolone nonsusceptibility is high. Azithromycin is increasingly used to treat typhoid fever or paratyphoid fever because of the emergence of multidrug-resistant strains.

Patients treated with an antibiotic may still require 3–5 days for fever to subside completely, although the height of the fever decreases each day. Patients may actually feel worse during the several days it takes for the fever to end. If fever does not subside within 5 days, alternative antimicrobial agents or other foci of infection should be considered.

PREVENTION
Food and Water
Safe food and water precautions and frequent handwashing are important in preventing typhoid and paratyphoid fever (see Chapter 2, Food & Water Precautions). Although vaccines are recommended to prevent typhoid fever, they are not 100% effective; therefore, even vaccinated travelers should follow recommended food and water precautions. These precautions are the only prevention method for paratyphoid fever, as no vaccines are available.

Vaccine
Indications for Use
CDC recommends typhoid vaccine for travelers to areas where there is an increased risk of exposure to S. enterica serotype Typhi. Two typhoid vaccines are available in the United States:

- Oral live attenuated vaccine (Vivotif, manufactured from the Ty21a strain of S. enterica serotype Typhi by Crucell/Berna)

- Vi capsular polysaccharide vaccine (ViCPS) (Typhim Vi, manufactured by Sanofi Pasteur) for intramuscular use

Both typhoid vaccines protect 50%–80% of recipients; travelers should be reminded that typhoid immunization is not 100% effective, and typhoid fever could still occur. Available typhoid vaccines offer no protection against S. enterica serotype Paratyphi infection.

Vaccine Administration
Table 3-20 provides information on vaccine dosage, administration, and revaccination. The time required for primary vaccination differs for the 2 vaccines, as do the lower age limits.

Primary vaccination with oral Ty21a vaccine consists of 4 capsules, 1 taken every other day. The capsules should be kept refrigerated (not frozen), and all 4 doses must be taken to achieve maximum efficacy. Each capsule should be taken with cool liquid no warmer than 98.6°F (37°C), approximately 1 hour before a meal. This regimen should be completed 1 week before potential exposure. The vaccine manufacturer recommends that Ty21a not be administered to infants or children aged <6 years.

Primary vaccination with ViCPS consists of one 0.5-mL (25-mg) dose administered intramuscularly. One dose of this vaccine

Table 3-20. Vaccines to prevent typhoid fever

VACCINATION	AGE (Y)	DOSE, MODE OF ADMINISTRATION	NUMBER OF DOSES	DOSING INTERVAL	BOOSTING INTERVAL
Oral, Live, Attenuated Ty21a Vaccine (Vivotif)[1]					
Primary series	≥6	1 capsule,[2] oral	4	48 hours	Not applicable
Booster	≥6	1 capsule,[2] oral	4	48 hours	Every 5 years
Vi Capsular Polysaccharide Vaccine (Typhim Vi)					
Primary series	≥2	0.5 mL, intramuscular	1	Not applicable	Not applicable
Booster	≥2	0.5 mL, intramuscular	1	Not applicable	Every 2 years

[1] The vaccine must be kept refrigerated (35.6°F–46.4°F, 2°C–8°C).
[2] Administer with cool liquid no warmer than 98.6°F (37°C).

should be given ≥2 weeks before expected exposure. The manufacturer does not recommend the vaccine for infants and children aged <2 years.

Vaccine Safety and Adverse Reactions

Adverse reactions to Ty21a vaccine are rare and mainly consist of abdominal discomfort, nausea, vomiting, and rash. ViCPS vaccine is most often associated with headache (16%–20%) and injection-site reactions (7%).

Precautions and Contraindications

No information is available on the safety of these vaccines in pregnancy; it is prudent on theoretical grounds to avoid vaccinating pregnant women. Live attenuated Ty21a vaccine should not be given to immunocompromised travelers, including those infected with HIV. The intramuscular vaccine presents a theoretically safer alternative for this group. The only contraindication to vaccination with ViCPS vaccine is a history of severe local or systemic reactions after a previous dose. Neither of the available vaccines should be given to people with an acute febrile illness.

Theoretical concerns have been raised about the immunogenicity of live, attenuated Ty21a vaccine in people concurrently receiving antimicrobial agents (including antimalarial chemoprophylaxis), viral vaccines, or immune globulin. The growth of the live Ty21a strain is inhibited in vitro by various antibacterial agents, and vaccination with Ty21a should be delayed for >72 hours after the administration of any antibacterial agent. Available data do not suggest that simultaneous administration of oral polio or yellow fever vaccine decreases the immunogenicity of Ty21a. If typhoid vaccination is warranted, it should not be delayed because of administration of viral vaccines. Simultaneous administration of Ty21a and immune globulin does not appear to pose a problem.

CDC website: www.cdc.gov/nczved/divisions/dfbmd/diseases/typhoid_fever

BIBLIOGRAPHY

1. Ackers ML, Puhr ND, Tauxe RV, Mintz ED. Laboratory-based surveillance of *Salmonella* serotype Typhi infections in the United States: antimicrobial resistance on the rise. JAMA. 2000 May 24–31;283(20):2668–73.

2. Beeching NJ, Clarke PD, Kitchin NR, Pirmohamed J, Veitch K, Weber F. Comparison of two combined vaccines against typhoid fever and hepatitis A in healthy adults. Vaccine. 2004 Nov 15;23(1):29–35.

3. CDC. Typhoid immunization: recommendations of the Advisory Committee on Immunization Practices (ACIP). MMWR Recomm Rep. 1994 Dec 9;43(RR-14):1–7.

4. Crump JA, Luby SP, Mintz ED. The global burden of typhoid fever. Bull World Health Organ. 2004 May;82(5):346–53.

5. Effa EE, Bukirwa H. Azithromycin for treating uncomplicated typhoid and paratyphoid fever (enteric fever). Cochrane Database Syst Rev. 2008(4):CD006083.

6. Gupta SK, Medalla F, Omondi MW, Whichard JM, Fields PI, Gerner-Smidt P, et al. Laboratory-based surveillance of paratyphoid fever in the United States: travel and antimicrobial resistance. Clin Infect Dis. 2008 Jun 1;46(11):1656–63.

7. Johnson KJ, Gallagher NM, Mintz ED, Newton AE, Brunette GW, Kozarsky PE. From the CDC: new country-specific recommendations for pre-travel typhoid vaccination. J Travel Med. 2011 Nov–Dec;18(6):430–3.

8. Klugman KP, Gilbertson IT, Koornhof HJ, Robbins JB, Schneerson R, Schulz D, et al. Protective activity of Vi capsular polysaccharide vaccine against typhoid fever. Lancet. 1987 Nov 21;2(8569):1165–9.

9. Kollaritsch H, Que JU, Kunz C, Wiedermann G, Herzog C, Cryz SJ, Jr. Safety and immunogenicity of live oral cholera and typhoid vaccines administered alone or in combination with antimalarial drugs, oral polio vaccine, or yellow fever vaccine. J Infect Dis. 1997 Apr;175(4):871–5.

10. Lynch MF, Blanton EM, Bulens S, Polyak C, Vojdani J, Stevenson J, et al. Typhoid fever in the United States, 1999–2006. JAMA. 2009 Aug 26;302(8):859–65.

11. Parry CM, Hien TT, Dougan G, White NJ, Farrar JJ. Typhoid fever. N Engl J Med. 2002 Nov 28;347(22):1770–82.

12. Simanjuntak CH, Paleologo FP, Punjabi NH, Darmowigoto R, Soeprawoto, Totosudirjo H, et al. Oral immunisation against typhoid fever in Indonesia with Ty21a vaccine. Lancet. 1991 Oct 26;338(8774):1055–9.

13. Steinberg EB, Bishop R, Haber P, Dempsey AF, Hoekstra RM, Nelson JM, et al. Typhoid fever in travelers: who should be targeted for prevention? Clin Infect Dis. 2004 Jul 15;39(2):186–91.

VARICELLA (CHICKENPOX)

Mona Marin, Stephanie R. Bialek

INFECTIOUS AGENT

Varicella-zoster virus, a member of the herpesvirus family. Humans are the only reservoir of the virus, and disease occurs only in humans. After primary infection as varicella (chickenpox), the virus remains dormant in the sensory-nerve ganglia and can reactivate at a later time, causing herpes zoster (shingles).

TRANSMISSION

Varicella-zoster virus is transmitted from person to person by direct contact, inhalation of aerosols from vesicular fluid of skin lesions of varicella or herpes zoster, or from infected respiratory tract secretions that might also be aerosolized. The varicella zoster virus enters the host through the upper respiratory tract or the conjunctiva. The period of communicability is estimated to begin 1–2 days before the onset of rash and ends when all lesions are crusted, typically 4–7 days after onset of rash in immunocompetent people, but this period may be longer in immunocompromised people. People with varicella should be isolated for as long as lesions persist.

In utero infection can also occur as a result of transplacental passage of virus during maternal varicella infection.

EPIDEMIOLOGY

Varicella occurs worldwide. In temperate climates, varicella tends to be a childhood disease, with peak incidence among preschool and school-aged children and during late winter and early spring. In tropical climates, infection tends to occur later during childhood and adolescence, resulting in higher susceptibility among adults than in temperate climates.

Varicella vaccine is routinely used to vaccinate healthy children in only some countries, including the United States, Australia, Canada, Costa Rica, Germany, Greece, Korea, Qatar, Saudi Arabia, Spain, Switzerland, United Arab Emirates, and Uruguay. With the implementation of the varicella vaccination program in the United States, substantial declines have occurred in disease incidence, and although varicella is still endemic, the risk of exposure to varicella zoster virus is higher in most other parts of the world than it is in the United States. Additionally, exposure to herpes zoster poses a risk for varicella in susceptible travelers, although localized herpes zoster is much less infectious than varicella. Travelers at highest risk for severe varicella are infants, immunocompromised people, or pregnant women without evidence of immunity (see criteria for evidence of immunity in "Prevention" below).

CLINICAL PRESENTATION

Varicella is generally a mild disease in children, and most people recover without serious complications. The average incubation period is 14–16 days (range, 10–21 days). Infection is often characterized by a short (1 or 2 days) prodromal period (fever, malaise), although this may be absent in children, and by pruritic rash consisting of crops of macules, papules, and vesicles (typically 250–500 lesions), which appear in ≥3 successive waves and resolve by crusting. Characteristic for varicella is presence of lesions in different stages of development at the same time. Serious complications can occur, most commonly in infants, adolescents, and adults. Complications include secondary bacterial infections of skin lesions, pneumonia, cerebellar ataxia, encephalitis, and hemorrhagic conditions; rarely (about 1 case in 40,000), these complications may result in death.

Modified varicella, also known as breakthrough, can occur in vaccinated people. Breakthrough varicella is usually mild, with <50 lesions, low or no fever, and shorter duration of rash. The rash may be atypical in appearance with fewer vesicles and predominance of maculopapular lesions. Breakthrough varicella is infectious, although less so than varicella in unvaccinated people.

DIAGNOSIS

Varicella is often diagnosed clinically. For laboratory confirmation, skin lesions are the preferred specimen. Vesicular swabs or scrapings and scabs from crusted lesions can be used to identify varicella-zoster virus by PCR or direct fluorescent antibody. In the absence of vesicles or scabs, scrapings of maculopapular lesions can be collected for testing.

Serologic tests may also be used to confirm disease:

- A significant rise in serum varicella IgG from acute- and convalescent-phase samples by any standard serologic assay can confirm a diagnosis retrospectively but may not be reliable in immunocompromised people. Commercially available tests are not sufficiently sensitive to detect antibody following vaccination, and a 4-fold rise in IgG may not occur in vaccinated people.
- Testing for varicella-zoster IgM by using commercial kits is not recommended, because available methods lack sensitivity and specificity; false-positive IgM results are common in the presence of high IgG levels. A capture assay for varicella-zoster IgM is available at CDC; however, there are limitations for IgM testing: a negative IgM result should not be used to rule out the diagnosis, and a positive IgM in the absence of rash should not be used to confirm a diagnosis.

TREATMENT

Treatment with antivirals is not routinely recommended for otherwise healthy children with varicella. Treatment with oral acyclovir should be considered for people at increased risk for moderate to severe disease, such as people aged >12 years, people with chronic cutaneous or pulmonary disorders, people who are receiving long-term salicylate therapy, and people who are receiving short, intermittent, or aerosolized courses of corticosteroids. Intravenous acyclovir is recommended for immunocompromised people, including patients being treated with chronic (or high-dose) corticosteroids, and people with serious, virally mediated complications (such as pneumonia). Therapy initiated within 24 hours of onset maximizes efficacy.

PREVENTION
Vaccine
People traveling or living abroad should ensure that they are immune to varicella.

Evidence of immunity to varicella includes any of the following:

- Documentation of age-appropriate vaccination:
  - > Preschool-aged children aged ≥12 months: 1 dose
  - > School-aged children, adolescents, and adults: 2 doses
- Laboratory evidence of immunity or laboratory confirmation of disease
- Birth in the United States before 1980 (not a criterion for health care personnel, pregnant women, and immunocompromised people)
- A health care provider's diagnosis of varicella or a health care provider's verification of a history of varicella
- A health care provider's diagnosis of herpes zoster or a health care provider's verification of a history of herpes zoster

Varicella vaccine contains live, attenuated varicella-zoster virus. Single-antigen varicella vaccine is licensed for people aged ≥12 months, and the combination measles-mumps-rubella-varicella vaccine (MMRV) is licensed only for children 1–12 years. CDC recommends varicella vaccination for all people aged ≥12 months without evidence of immunity to varicella who do not have contraindications to the vaccine: 1 dose for children aged 1–4 years and 2 doses for people aged ≥4 years. The minimum interval between doses is 3 months for children aged <13 years and 4 weeks for people aged ≥13 years. When evidence of immunity is uncertain, a possible history of varicella is not a contraindication to varicella vaccination. For detailed information regarding the varicella vaccine, visit www.cdc.gov/vaccines/vpd-vac/varicella/default.htm.

POSTEXPOSURE PROPHYLAXIS
Vaccine
Varicella vaccine is recommended for postexposure administration for unvaccinated healthy people aged ≥12 months and without other evidence of immunity, to prevent or modify the disease. The vaccine should be administered as soon as possible within 5 days after exposure to rash, if there are no contraindications to use. Among children, protective efficacy was reported as ≥90% when

vaccination occurred within 3 days of exposure. No data are available regarding a potential benefit of administering a second dose to 1-dose vaccine recipients after exposure. However, administration of the second dose should be considered for these people to bring them up-to-date on vaccination.

Varicella Zoster Immune Globulin

People without evidence of immunity who have contraindications for vaccination and who are at risk for severe varicella and complications are recommended to receive postexposure prophylaxis with varicella zoster immune globulin (VZIG). People at high risk for severe complications include immunocompromised people, pregnant women without evidence of immunity, and some infants.

The VZIG product used in the United States is available under an investigational new drug protocol and can be obtained from the sole authorized US distributor, FFF Enterprises (Temecula, California) toll-free at 800-843-7477 or www.fffenterprises.com.

VZIG provides maximum benefit when administered as soon as possible after exposure but may be effective if administered as late as 10 days after exposure.

If VZIG is not available, CDC recommends that administration of intravenous immune globulin be considered as an alternative (also within 10 days of exposure).

Although there are limited published data on the benefit of acyclovir as postexposure prophylaxis, if VZIG is not available some experts recommend prophylaxis with acyclovir (80 mg/kg/day, administered 4 times per day for 7 days; maximum dose, 800 mg, 4 times per day), beginning 7–10 days after exposure for people without evidence of immunity and with contraindications for varicella vaccination.

CDC website: www.cdc.gov/chickenpox

BIBLIOGRAPHY

1. American Academy of Pediatrics. Varicella-zoster infections. In: Pickering LK, editor. Red Book: 2012 Report of the Committee on Infectious Diseases. 29th ed. Elk Grove Village, IL: American Academy of Pediatrics; 2012. p. 774–89.

2. CDC. FDA approval of an extended period for administering VariZIG for postexposure prophylaxis of varicella. MMWR Morb Mortal Wkly Rep. 2012 Mar 30;61(12):212.

3. Gershon AA, Takahasi M, Seward JF. Varicella vaccine. In: Plotkin SA, Orenstein WA, Offit PA, editors. Vaccines. 6th ed. Philadelphia: Saunders Elsevier; 2012. p. 837–69.

4. Guris D, Jumaan AO, Mascola L, Watson BM, Zhang JX, Chaves SS, et al. Changing varicella epidemiology in active surveillance sites—United States, 1995–2005. J Infect Dis. 2008 Mar 1;197 Suppl 2:S71–5.

5. Harpaz R, Ortega-Sanchez IR, Seward JF. Prevention of herpes zoster: recommendations of the Advisory Committee on Immunization Practices (ACIP). MMWR Recomm Rep. 2008 Jun 6;57(RR-5):1–30.

6. Marin M, Broder KR, Temte JL, Snider DE, Seward JF. Use of combination measles, mumps, rubella, and varicella vaccine: recommendations of the Advisory Committee on Immunization Practices (ACIP). MMWR Recomm Rep. 2010 May 7;59(RR-3):1–12.

7. Marin M, Guris D, Chaves SS, Schmid S, Seward JF. Prevention of varicella: recommendations of the Advisory Committee on Immunization Practices (ACIP). MMWR Recomm Rep. 2007 Jun 22;56 (RR-4):1–40.

8. World Health Organization. Immunization summary: the 2011 edition. Geneva: World Health Organization; 2011 [cited 2012 Sep 21]. Available from: http://www.childinfo.org/files/32775_UNICEF.pdf.

VIRAL HEMORRHAGIC FEVERS

Barbara Knust, Pierre E. Rollin

INFECTIOUS AGENT

Viral hemorrhagic fevers (VHFs) are caused by several families of enveloped RNA viruses: filoviruses (Ebola and Marburg viruses), arenaviruses (Lassa fever, Lujo, Guanarito, Machupo, Junin, Sabia, and Chapare viruses), bunyaviruses (Rift Valley fever [RVF], Crimean-Congo hemorrhagic fever [CCHF], and hantaviruses), and flaviviruses (dengue, yellow fever, Omsk hemorrhagic fever, Kyasanur Forest disease, and Alkhurma viruses); see the Dengue and Yellow Fever sections in this chapter.

TRANSMISSION

Some VHFs are spread person to person through direct contact with symptomatic patients, body fluids, or cadavers or through inadequate infection control in a hospital setting (filoviruses, arenaviruses, CCHF virus). Zoonotic spread may occur from contact with the following:

- Livestock via slaughter or consumption of raw meat from infected animals and, potentially, unpasteurized milk (CCHF, RVF, Alkhurma viruses)
- Bushmeat, likely via slaughter or consumption of infected animals (Ebola, Marburg viruses)
- Rodents via inhalation of or contact with materials contaminated with rodent excreta (arenaviruses, hantaviruses)
- Other reservoir species, such as bats (Ebola, Marburg viruses)

Vectorborne transmission also occurs via mosquito (RVF virus) or tick (CCHF, Omsk, Kyasanur Forest disease, Alkhurma viruses) bites or by crushing infected ticks.

EPIDEMIOLOGY

The viruses that cause VHFs are distributed over much of the globe. Each virus is associated with ≥1 nonhuman host or vector species, restricting the virus and the initial contamination to the areas inhabited by these species. The diseases caused by these viruses are seen in people living in or having visited these areas. Humans are incidental hosts for these enzootic diseases; however, person-to-person transmission of some viruses can result in large human outbreaks. Specific viruses are addressed below.

Ebola and Marburg: Filoviral Diseases

Ebola and Marburg viruses cause hemorrhagic fever in humans and nonhuman primates. Five species of Ebola virus have been identified: Côte d'Ivoire, Sudan, Zaire, Bundibugyo, and Reston. Countries with confirmed human cases of Ebola hemorrhagic fever include Republic of the Congo, Côte d'Ivoire, Democratic Republic of the Congo, Gabon, Sudan, and Uganda. Ebola-Reston virus is believed to be endemic in the Philippines and potentially in neighboring countries but has not been shown to cause human disease. Countries with confirmed human cases of Marburg hemorrhagic fever include Angola, Democratic Republic of the Congo, Kenya, Uganda, and possibly Zimbabwe.

Growing evidence indicates that fruit bats are the natural reservoir for filoviruses. Outbreaks occur when a person becomes infected after exposure to the reservoir species or a secondarily infected nonhuman primate and then transmits the virus to other people in the community. Four cases of Marburg hemorrhagic fever have occurred in travelers visiting caves harboring bats, including Kitum cave in Kenya and a python cave in Maramagambo Forest, Uganda. Miners have also acquired Marburg infection from working in underground mines harboring bats in the Democratic Republic of the Congo and Uganda.

Lassa Fever and Other Arenaviral Diseases

Arenaviruses are transmitted from rodents to humans, except Tacaribe virus, which was found in bats. Most infections are mild, but some result in hemorrhagic fever with high death rates. Old World (Eastern Hemisphere) and New World (Western Hemisphere) viruses cause the following diseases:

- Old World viruses: Lassa virus (Lassa fever) lymphocytic choriomeningitis virus (meningitis, encephalitis, and congenital fetal infection in normal hosts, hemorrhagic fever in organ transplant recipients). Lassa fever occurs in rural West Africa, with hyperendemic areas in Guinea, Liberia, Nigeria, and Sierra Leone. Lujo virus has been recently described in Zambia and the Republic of South Africa during a health care–associated outbreak.
- New World viruses: Junin (Argentine hemorrhagic fever), Machupo (Bolivian hemorrhagic fever), Guanarito (Venezuelan hemorrhagic fever), Sabia (Brazilian hemorrhagic fever), and the recently discovered Chapare virus (a single case in Bolivia).

Reservoir host species are Old World rats and mice (family Muridae, subfamily Murinae) and New World rats and mice (family Muridae, subfamily Sigmodontinae). These rodent types are found worldwide, including Europe, Asia, Africa, and the Americas. Virus is transmitted through inhalation of aerosols from rodent urine, ingestion of rodent-contaminated food, or direct contact of broken skin or mucosa with rodent excreta. Risk of Lassa virus infection is associated with peridomestic rodent exposure. Inappropriate food storage increases the risk for exposure. Health care–associated transmission of Lassa, Lujo, and Machupo viruses has occurred through droplet and contact. One anecdotal report of possible airborne transmission exists. Several cases of Lassa fever have been confirmed in international travelers staying in traditional dwellings in the countryside.

Rift Valley Fever and Other Bunyaviral Diseases

RVF causes fever, hemorrhage, encephalitis, and retinitis in humans, but primarily affects livestock. RVF is endemic to sub-Saharan Africa. Sporadic outbreaks have occurred in humans in Egypt, Madagascar, and Mauritania. Large epidemics occurred in Kenya, Somalia, and Tanzania in 1997–1998 and 2006–2007; Saudi Arabia and Yemen in 2000; Madagascar in 2008; and South Africa, Botswana, Namibia,

and Mauritania in 2010. RVF virus is transmitted by mosquito, percutaneous inoculation, and slaughter or consumption of infected animals.

CCHF is endemic where ticks of the genus *Hyalomma* are found in Africa and Eurasia, including South Africa, the Balkans, the Middle East, Russia, and western China, and is highly endemic in Afghanistan, Iran, Pakistan, and Turkey. CCHF virus is transmitted to humans by infected ticks or direct handling and preparation of fresh carcasses of infected animals, usually domestic livestock. Health care–associated transmission often occurs.

Hantaviruses cause hantavirus pulmonary syndrome (HPS) and hemorrhagic fever with renal syndrome (HFRS). The viruses that cause HPS are present in the New World; those that cause HFRS occur worldwide. The viruses that cause both HPS and HFRS are transmitted to humans through contact with urine, feces, or saliva of infected rodents. Travelers staying in rodent-infested dwellings are at risk for HPS and HFRS. Human-to-human transmission has been reported only with Andes virus in Chile and Argentina.

CLINICAL PRESENTATION

Signs and symptoms vary by disease, but in general, patients with VHF present with abrupt onset of fever, myalgias, and prostration, followed in severe forms by coagulopathy with a petechial rash or ecchymoses and sometimes overt bleeding. Vascular endothelial damage leads to shock and pulmonary edema; liver injury is common. Signs seen with specific viruses include renal failure (HFRS); ecchymoses and bruises (CCHF); hearing loss, anasarca and shock in newborns (Lassa fever); and spontaneous abortion and birth defects (Lassa and lymphocytic choriomeningitis viruses). Because the incubation period may be as long as 21 days, patients may not develop illness until returning from travel; therefore, a thorough travel and exposure history is critical.

DIAGNOSIS

US-based clinicians should notify local health authorities and CDC immediately of any suspected cases of VHF occurring in patients residing in or requiring evacuation to the United States (CDC Viral Special Pathogens

Branch [404-639-1115] during business hours or the CDC Emergency Operations Center [770-488-7100] after hours). CDC also provides consultation for international clinicians and health ministries. Whole blood or serum may be tested for virologic (PCR, antigen detection, virus isolation) and immunologic (IgM, IgG) evidence of infection. Tissue may be tested by immunohistochemistry, PCR, and virus isolation. Postmortem skin biopsies fixed in formalin and blood collected within a few hours after death by cardiac puncture can be used for diagnosis. Samples should be sent for testing to a reference laboratory with biosafety level 3 and 4 capability.

TREATMENT

Ribavirin is effective for treating Lassa fever and other Old World arenaviruses, New World arenaviruses, and potentially CCHF, but it is not approved by the Food and Drug Administration (FDA) for these indications. Convalescent-phase plasma is effective in treating Argentine hemorrhagic fever. Intravenous ribavirin can be obtained for compassionate use through FDA from Valeant Pharmaceuticals (Aliso Viejo, California). Requests should be initiated by the provider through FDA (301-736-3400), with simultaneous notification to Valeant (800-548-5100, extension 5 [domestic telephone] or 949-461-6971 [international telephone]).

PREVENTION

The risk of acquiring VHF is low for international travelers. Travelers at increased risk for exposure include those engaging in animal research, health care workers, and others providing care for patients in the community, particularly where outbreaks of VHF are occurring.

Prevention should focus on avoiding contact with host or vector species in endemic countries. Travelers should not visit locations where an outbreak is occurring, avoid contact with rodents and bats, and avoid livestock in RVF- and CCHF-endemic areas. To prevent vectorborne disease, travelers should use insecticide-treated bed nets and wear insect repellent.

Standard precautions and contact and droplet precautions for suspected VHF case-patients are recommended to avoid transmission. Direct contact should be avoided with corpses of patients suspected of having died of Ebola, Marburg, or Old World arenavirus infection. Contact with or consumption of primates, bats, and other bushmeat should be avoided. Bat-inhabited caves or mines should be avoided. Investigational vaccines exist for Argentine hemorrhagic fever and RVF; however, neither is approved by FDA nor are they commonly available in the United States.

CDC website: www.cdc.gov/ncidod/dvrd/spb/mnpages/dispages/vhf.htm

BIBLIOGRAPHY

1. Bausch DG, Borchert M, Grein T, Roth C, Swanepoel R, Libande ML, et al. Risk factors for Marburg hemorrhagic fever, Democratic Republic of the Congo. Emerg Infect Dis. 2003 Dec;9(12):1531–7.

2. Bausch DG, Ksiazek TG. Viral hemorrhagic fevers including hantavirus pulmonary syndrome in the Americas. Clin Lab Med. 2002 Dec;22(4):981–1020, viii.

3. CDC. Imported case of Marburg hemorrhagic fever—Colorado, 2008. MMWR Morb Mortal Wkly Rep. 2009 Dec 18;58(49):1377–81.

4. Ergonul O, Holbrook MR. Crimean-Congo hemorrhagic fever. In: Guerrant RL, Walker DH, Weller PF, editors. Tropical Infectious Diseases: Principles, Pathogens and Practice. 3rd ed. Philadelphia: Saunders Elsevier; 2011. p. 466–9.

5. Feldmann H, Jones SM, Schnittler HJ, Geisbert T. Therapy and prophylaxis of Ebola virus infections. Curr Opin Investig Drugs. 2005 Aug;6(8):823–30.

6. Geisbert TW, Jahrling PB. Exotic emerging viral diseases: progress and challenges. Nat Med. 2004 Dec;10(12 Suppl):S110–21.

7. Gunther S, Lenz O. Lassa virus. Crit Rev Clin Lab Sci. 2004;41(4):339–90.

8. Heyman P, Vaheri A, Lundkvist A, Avsic-Zupanc T. Hantavirus infections in Europe: from virus carriers to a major public-health problem. Expert Rev Anti Infect Ther. 2009 Mar;7(2):205–17.

9. Madani TA, Al-Mazrou YY, Al-Jeffri MH, Mishkhas AA, Al-Rabeah AM, Turkistani AM, et al. Rift Valley fever epidemic in Saudi Arabia: epidemiological, clinical, and laboratory characteristics. Clin Infect Dis. 2003 Oct 15;37(8):1084–92.

10. Marty AM, Jahrling PB, Geisbert TW. Viral hemorrhagic fevers. Clin Lab Med. 2006 Jun;26(2):345–86, viii.

11. Ozkurt Z, Kiki I, Erol S, Erdem F, Yilmaz N, Parlak M, et al. Crimean-Congo hemorrhagic fever in eastern

Turkey: clinical features, risk factors and efficacy of ribavirin therapy. J Infect. 2006 Mar;52(3):207–15.

12. Peters CJ, Jahrling PB, Khan AS. Patients infected with high-hazard viruses: scientific basis for infection control. Arch Virol Suppl. 1996;11:141–68.

13. Peters CJ, Makino S, Morrill JC. Rift Valley fever. In: Guerrant RL, Walker DH, Weller PF, editors. Tropical Infectious Diseases: Principles, Pathogens and Practice. 3rd ed. Philadelphia: Saunders Elsevier; 2011. p. 462–5.

14. Peters CJ, Zaki SR. Overview of viral hemorrhagic fevers. In: Guerrant RL, Walker DH, Weller PF, editors. Tropical Infectious Diseases: Principles, Pathogens

and Practice. 3rd ed. Philadelphia: Saunders Elsevier; 2011. p. 441–8.

15. Rollin PE, Nichol ST, Zaki S, Ksiazek TG. Arenaviruses and filoviruses. In: Versalovic J, Carroll KC, Funke G, Jorgensen JH, Landry ML, Warnock DW, editors. Manual of Clinical Microbiology. 10th ed. Washington, DC: ASM Press; 2011. p. 1514–29.

16. Wahl-Jensen V, Peters CJ, Jahrling PB, Feldman H, Kuhn JH. Filovirus infections. In: Guerrant RL, Walker DH, Weller PF, editors. Tropical Infectious Diseases: Principles, Pathogens and Practice. 3rd ed. Philadelphia: Saunders Elsevier; 2011. p. 483–91.

YELLOW FEVER
Mark D. Gershman, J. Erin Staples

INFECTIOUS AGENT

Yellow fever virus (YFV) is a single-stranded RNA virus that belongs to the genus *Flavivirus*.

TRANSMISSION

Vectorborne transmission occurs via the bite of an infected mosquito, primarily *Aedes* or *Haemagogus* spp. Nonhuman and human primates are the main reservoirs of the virus, with anthroponotic (human-to-vector-to-human) transmission occurring. There are 3 transmission cycles for yellow fever: sylvatic (jungle), intermediate (savannah), and urban.

- The sylvatic (jungle) cycle involves transmission of the virus between nonhuman primates and mosquito species found in the forest canopy. The virus is transmitted via mosquitoes from monkeys to humans when the humans encroach into the jungle during occupational or recreational activities.
- In Africa, an intermediate (savannah) cycle involves transmission of YFV from tree hole-breeding *Aedes* spp. to humans living or working in jungle border areas. In this cycle, the virus may be transmitted from monkeys to humans or from human to human via these mosquitoes.
- The urban cycle involves transmission of the virus between humans and urban mosquitoes, primarily *Aedes aegypti*.

Humans infected with YFV experience the highest levels of viremia and can transmit the virus to mosquitoes shortly before onset of fever and for the first 3–5 days of illness. Given the high level of viremia, bloodborne transmission theoretically can occur via transfusion or needlesticks.

EPIDEMIOLOGY

Yellow fever occurs in sub-Saharan Africa and tropical South America, where it is endemic and intermittently epidemic (see Tables 3-21 and 3-22 for a list of countries with risk of YFV transmission). Most yellow fever disease in humans is due to sylvatic or intermediate transmission cycles. However, urban yellow fever occurs periodically in Africa and sporadically in the Americas. In Africa, natural immunity accumulates with age, and thus, infants and children are at highest risk for disease. In South America, yellow fever occurs most frequently in unimmunized young men who are exposed to mosquito vectors through their work in forested areas.

RISK FOR TRAVELERS

A traveler's risk for acquiring yellow fever is determined by various factors, including immunization status, location of travel, season, duration of exposure, occupational and recreational activities while traveling, and local rate of virus transmission at the time of travel. Although reported cases of human disease are the principal indicator of disease risk, case reports may be absent because

Table 3-21. Countries with risk of yellow fever virus (YFV) transmission[1]

AFRICA			CENTRAL AND SOUTH AMERICA
Angola	Ethiopia[2]	Nigeria	Argentina[2]
Benin	Gabon	Rwanda	Bolivia[2]
Burkina Faso	The Gambia	Senegal	Brazil[2]
Burundi	Ghana	Sierra	Colombia[2]
Cameroon	Guinea	Leone	Ecuador[2]
Central African Republic	Guinea-	South Sudan	French Guiana
Chad[2]	Bissau	Sudan[2]	Guyana
Congo, Republic of the	Kenya[2]	Togo	Panama[2]
Côte d'Ivoire	Liberia	Uganda	Paraguay
Democratic Republic of	Mali[2]		Peru[2]
the Congo[2]	Mauritania[2]		Suriname
Equatorial Guinea	Niger[2]		Trinidad and Tobago[2]
			Venezuela[2]

[1] Countries or areas where "a risk of yellow fever transmission is present," as defined by the World Health Organization, are countries or areas where "yellow fever has been reported currently or in the past, plus vectors and animal reservoirs currently exist" (see the current country list within the *International Travel and Health* publication (Annex 1) at www.who.int/ith/en/index.html).
[2] These countries are not holoendemic (only a portion of the country has risk of yellow fever transmission). See Maps 3-16 and 3-17 and yellow fever vaccine recommendations (Travel Vaccines & Malaria Information, by Country) for details.

Table 3-22. Countries with low potential for exposure to yellow fever virus (YFV)[1]

AFRICA
Eritrea[2]
São Tomé and Príncipe[3]
Somalia[2]
Tanzania[3]
Zambia[2]

[1] Countries listed in this table are not contained on the official WHO list of countries with risk of YFV transmission (Table 3-21). Therefore, proof of yellow fever vaccination should not be required if traveling from one of these countries to another country with a vaccination entry requirement (unless that country requires proof of yellow fever vaccination from all arriving travelers; see Table 3-25). An exception is South Africa, which requires YF vaccination for people traveling from or transiting through any of the 5 countries with low potential for exposure.
[2] These countries are classified as "low potential for exposure to YFV" in only some areas; the remaining areas of these countries are classified as having no risk of exposure to YFV.
[3] The entire area of these countries is classified as "low potential for exposure to YFV."

of a low level of transmission, a high level of immunity in the population (because of vaccination, for example), or failure of local surveillance systems to detect cases. This "epidemiologic silence" does not equate to absence of risk and should not lead to travel without taking protective measures.

YFV transmission in rural West Africa is seasonal, with an elevated risk during the end of the rainy season and the beginning of the dry season (usually July–October). However, YFV may be episodically transmitted by *Ae. aegypti* even during the dry season in both rural and densely settled urban areas.

The risk for infection in South America is highest during the rainy season (January–May, with a peak incidence in February and March). Given the high level of viremia that may occur in infected humans and the widespread distribution of *Ae. aegypti* in many towns and cities, South America is at risk for a large-scale urban epidemic.

From 1970 through 2011, a total of 9 cases of yellow fever were reported in unvaccinated travelers from the United States and Europe who traveled to West Africa (5 cases) or South America (4 cases). Eight (89%) of these 9 travelers died. There has been only 1 documented case of yellow fever in a vaccinated traveler. This non-fatal case occurred in a traveler from Spain who visited several West African countries in 1988.

The risk of acquiring yellow fever is difficult to predict because of variations in ecologic determinants of virus transmission. For a 2-week stay, the risks for illness and death due to yellow fever for an unvaccinated traveler visiting an endemic area in:

- West Africa are 50 per 100,000 and 10 per 100,000, respectively
- South America are 5 per 100,000 and 1 per 100,000, respectively

These estimates are a rough guideline based on the risk to indigenous populations, often during peak transmission season. Thus, these risk estimates may not accurately reflect the true risk to travelers, who may have a different immunity profile, take precautions against getting bitten by mosquitoes, and have less outdoor exposure.

The risk of acquiring yellow fever in South America is lower than that in Africa,

because the mosquitoes that transmit the virus between monkeys in the forest canopy in South America do not often come in contact with humans. Additionally, there is a relatively high level of immunity in local residents because of vaccine use, which might reduce the risk of transmission.

CLINICAL PRESENTATION

Asymptomatic or clinically inapparent infection is believed to occur in most people infected with YFV. For people who develop symptomatic illness, the incubation period is typically 3–6 days. The initial illness presents as a nonspecific influenzalike syndrome with sudden onset of fever, chills, headache, backache, myalgias, prostration, nausea, and vomiting. Most patients improve after the initial presentation. After a brief remission of hours to a day, approximately 15% of patients progress to a more serious or toxic form of the disease, characterized by jaundice, hemorrhagic symptoms, and eventually shock and multisystem organ failure. The case-fatality ratio for severe cases with hepatorenal dysfunction is 20%–50%.

DIAGNOSIS

The preliminary diagnosis is based on the patient's clinical features, places and dates of travel, and activities. Laboratory diagnosis is best performed by:

- Serologic assays to detect virus-specific IgM and IgG antibodies. Because of cross-reactivity between antibodies raised against other flaviviruses, more specific antibody testing, such as a plaque reduction neutralization test, should be done to confirm the infection.
- Virus isolation or nucleic acid amplification tests performed early in the illness for YFV or yellow fever viral RNA. However, by the time more overt symptoms are recognized, the virus or viral RNA is usually undetectable. Therefore, virus isolation and nucleic acid amplification should not be used for ruling out a diagnosis of yellow fever.

Clinicians should contact their state or local health department or call the CDC Arboviral Diseases Branch at 970-221-6400 for assistance with diagnostic testing for yellow fever infections and for questions about antibody response to vaccination.

TREATMENT

There are no specific medications to treat YFV infections; treatment is directed at symptomatic relief or life-saving interventions. Rest, fluids, and use of analgesics and antipyretics may relieve symptoms of fever and aching. Care should be taken to avoid certain medications, such as aspirin or nonsteroidal anti-inflammatory drugs, which may increase the risk for bleeding. Infected people should be protected from further mosquito exposure (staying indoors or under a mosquito net) during the first few days of illness, so they do not contribute to the transmission cycle.

PREVENTION

Personal Protection Measures

The best way to prevent mosquitoborne diseases, including yellow fever, is to avoid mosquito bites (see Chapter 2, Protection against Mosquitoes, Ticks, & Other Insects & Arthropods).

Vaccine

Yellow fever is preventable by a relatively safe, effective vaccine. All yellow fever vaccines currently manufactured are live-attenuated viral vaccines. Only 1 yellow fever vaccine is licensed for use in the United States (Table 3-23).

Studies comparing the reactogenicity and immunogenicity of various yellow fever vaccines, including those manufactured outside the United States, suggest that there is no substantial difference in the reactogenicity or immune response generated by the various vaccines. Thus, people who receive yellow fever vaccines in other countries should be considered protected against yellow fever.

Indications for Use

Yellow fever vaccine is recommended for people aged ≥9 months who are traveling to or living in areas with risk for YFV transmission in South America and Africa. In addition, some countries require proof of yellow fever vaccination for entry. See the Travel Vaccines & Malaria Information, by Country section at the end of this chapter for more detailed information on the requirements and recommendations for yellow fever vaccination for specific countries.

Because of the risk of serious adverse events that can occur after yellow fever vaccination, clinicians should only vaccinate people who 1) are at risk of exposure to YFV or 2) require proof of vaccination to enter a country. To further minimize the risk of serious adverse events, clinicians should carefully observe the contraindications and consider the precautions to vaccination before administering yellow fever vaccine (Table 3-24). For additional information, refer to the yellow fever vaccine recommendations of the Advisory Committee on Immunization Practices (ACIP) at www.cdc.gov/vaccines/pubs/ACIP-list.htm.

Vaccine Administration

For all eligible people, a single injection of reconstituted vaccine should be administered subcutaneously. The International Health Regulations (IHR) published by the World Health Organization (WHO) require revaccination at 10-year intervals.

Table 3-23. Vaccine to prevent yellow fever

VACCINE	TRADE NAME (MANUFACTURER)	AGE	DOSE	ROUTE	SCHEDULE	BOOSTER
17D yellow fever vaccine	YF-Vax (Sanofi Pasteur)	≥9 months[1]	0.5 mL[2]	SC	1 dose	10 years[3]

Abbreviation: SC, subcutaneous.
[1] Ages 6–8 months and ≥60 years are precautions for use of yellow fever vaccine.
[2] YF-Vax is available in single-dose and multiple-dose (5-dose) vials.
[3] Revaccination every 10 years is recommended for people at continued risk of exposure to yellow fever virus and is required for entry by certain countries under the International Health Regulations of the World Health Organization.

Table 3-24. Contraindications and precautions to yellow fever vaccine administration

CONTRAINDICATIONS	PRECAUTIONS
• Allergy to vaccine component • Age <6 months • Symptomatic HIV infection or CD4 T-lymphocytes <200/mm³ (or <15% of total in children aged <6 years)[1] • Thymus disorder associated with abnormal immune-cell function • Primary immunodeficiencies • Malignant neoplasms • Transplantation • Immunosuppressive and immunomodulatory therapies	• Age 6–8 months • Age ≥60 years • Asymptomatic HIV infection and CD4 T-lymphocytes 200–499/mm³ (or 15%–24% of total in children aged <6 years)[1] • Pregnancy • Breastfeeding

[1] Symptoms of HIV are classified in 1) Adults and Adolescents, Table 1. CDC. 1993 Revised classification system for HIV infection and expanded surveillance case definition for AIDS among adolescents and adults. MMWR Recomm Rep 1992 Dec 18: 41(RR-17). Available from: www.cdc.gov/mmwr/preview/mmwrhtml/00018871.htm and 2) Panel on Antiretroviral Therapy and Medical Management of HIV-Infected Children. Guidelines for the use of antiretroviral agents in pediatric HIV infection. 2010. Available from: http://aidsinfo.nih.gov/ContentFiles/PediatricGuidelines.pdf. p. 20–2.

Vaccine Safety and Adverse Reactions
Common adverse reactions

Reactions to yellow fever vaccine are generally mild; 10%–30% of vaccinees report mild systemic adverse events. Reported events typically include low-grade fever, headache, and myalgias that begin within days after vaccination and last 5–10 days. Approximately 1% of vaccinees temporarily curtail their regular activities because of these reactions.

Severe adverse reactions
Hypersensitivity

Immediate hypersensitivity reactions, characterized by rash, urticaria, bronchospasm, or a combination of these, are uncommon. Anaphylaxis after yellow fever vaccine is reported to occur at a rate of 1.8 cases per 100,000 doses administered.

Yellow fever vaccine–associated neurologic disease (YEL-AND)

YEL-AND represents a conglomerate of different clinical syndromes, including meningoencephalitis, Guillain-Barré syndrome, acute disseminated encephalomyelitis, and rarely, bulbar and Bell palsies. Historically, YEL-AND was seen primarily among infants as encephalitis, but more recent reports have been among people of all ages.

The onset of illness for documented cases is 3–28 days after vaccination, and almost all cases were in first-time vaccine recipients. YEL-AND is rarely fatal. The incidence of YEL-AND in the United States is 0.8 per 100,000 doses administered. The rate is higher in people aged ≥60 years, with a rate of 1.6 per 100,000 doses in people aged 60–69 years and 2.3 per 100,000 doses in people aged ≥70 years.

Yellow fever vaccine–associated viscerotropic disease (YEL-AVD)

YEL-AVD is a severe illness similar to wild-type disease, with vaccine virus proliferating in multiple organs and often leading to multisystem organ failure and death. Since the initial cases of YEL-AVD were published in 2001, >60 confirmed and suspected cases have been reported throughout the world.

YEL-AVD has been reported to occur only after the first dose of yellow fever vaccine; there have been no reports of YEL-AVD following booster doses. The median time from YF vaccination until symptom onset for YEL-AVD cases was 4 days (range, 0–8 days).

The case-fatality ratio for all reported YEL-AVD cases worldwide is 63%. The incidence of YEL-AVD in the United States is 0.4 cases per 100,000 doses of vaccine administered. The rate is higher for people aged ≥60 years, with a rate of 1.0 per 100,000 doses in people aged 60–69 years and 2.3 per 100,000 doses in people aged ≥70 years.

Contraindications

Infants younger than 6 months

Yellow fever vaccine is contraindicated for infants aged <6 months. This contraindication was instituted in the late 1960s in response to a high rate of YEL-AND documented in vaccinated young infants (50–400 per 100,000). The mechanism of increased neurovirulence in infants is unknown but may be due to the immaturity of the blood-brain barrier, higher or more prolonged viremia, or immune system immaturity.

Hypersensitivity

Yellow fever vaccine is contraindicated for people with a history of hypersensitivity to any of the vaccine components, including eggs, egg products, chicken proteins, or gelatin. The stopper used in vials of vaccine also contains dry natural latex rubber, which may cause an allergic reaction.

If vaccination of a person with a questionable history of hypersensitivity to one of the vaccine components is considered essential because of a high risk for acquiring yellow fever, skin testing, as described in the vaccine package insert, should be performed under close medical supervision. If a person has a positive skin test to the vaccine or has severe egg sensitivity and the vaccination is recommended, desensitization, as described in the package insert, can be performed under direct supervision of a physician experienced in the management of anaphylaxis.

Altered immune status
Thymus disorder

Yellow fever vaccine is contraindicated for people with a thymus disorder that is associated with abnormal immune cell function, such as thymoma or myasthenia gravis. If travel to a yellow fever–endemic area cannot be avoided in a person with such a thymus disorder, a medical waiver should be provided and counseling on protective measures against mosquito bites should be emphasized. Because there is no evidence of immune dysfunction or increased risk of yellow fever vaccine–associated serious adverse events in people who have undergone incidental surgical removal of their thymus or have had indirect radiation therapy in the distant past, these people can be given yellow fever vaccine if recommended or required.

HIV infection

Yellow fever vaccine is contraindicated for people with AIDS or other clinical manifestations of HIV, including people with CD4 T-lymphocyte values <200/mm³ or <15% of total lymphocytes for children aged <6 years. This recommendation is based on a theoretical increased risk of encephalitis in this population (see HIV infection under the following section, Precautions).

If travel to a yellow fever–endemic area cannot be avoided by a person with severe immune suppression based on CD4 counts (<200/mm³ or <15% total for children aged <6 years) or symptomatic HIV, a medical waiver should be provided, and counseling on protective measures against mosquito bites should be emphasized. See the following section, Precautions, for other HIV-infected people not meeting the above criteria.

Immunodeficiencies (other than thymus disorder or HIV infection)

Yellow fever vaccine is contraindicated for people with primary immunodeficiencies, malignant neoplasms, and transplantation. While there are no data on the use of yellow fever vaccine in these people, they presumably are at increased risk for yellow fever vaccine–associated serious adverse events (see the section on Immunocompromised Travelers in Chapter 8).

If someone with an immunodeficiency cannot avoid travel to a yellow fever–endemic area, a medical waiver should be provided, and counseling on protective measures against mosquito bites should be emphasized.

Immunosuppressive and immunomodulatory therapies

Yellow fever vaccine is contraindicated for people whose immunologic response is either suppressed or modulated by current or recent radiation therapies or drugs. Drugs with known immunosuppressive or immunomodulatory properties include, but are not limited to, high-dose systemic corticosteroids, alkylating drugs, antimetabolites, tumor necrosis factor-α inhibitors (such as etanercept), interleukin-1 and interleukin-6 blocking agents (such as anakinra and tocilizumab), or other monoclonal antibodies targeting immune cells (such as rituximab or alemtuzumab; see Table 8-4 in Chapter 8, Immunocompromised Travelers for a longer list of immunosuppressive biologic agents). There are no specific data on the use of yellow fever vaccine in people receiving these therapies. However, these people are presumed to be at increased risk for yellow fever vaccine–associated serious adverse events, and the use of live attenuated vaccines is contraindicated in the package insert for most of these therapies (see Chapter 8, Immunocompromised Travelers).

Live viral vaccines should be deferred in people who have discontinued these therapies until immune function has improved. If travel to a yellow fever–endemic area cannot be avoided for someone receiving immunosuppressive or immunomodulatory therapies, a medical waiver should be provided and counseling on protective measures against mosquito bites should be emphasized.

Family members of people with altered immune status, who themselves have no contraindications, can receive yellow fever vaccine.

Precautions
Infants aged 6–8 months
Age 6–8 months is a precaution for yellow fever vaccination. Two cases of YEL-AND have been reported among infants aged 6–8 months. In infants <6 months of age, the rates of YEL-AND are elevated (50–400 per 100,000). By 9 months of age, risk for YEL-AND is believed to be substantially lower. ACIP generally recommends that, whenever possible, travel to yellow fever-endemic countries should be postponed or avoided for children aged 6–8 months. If travel is unavoidable, the decision of whether to vaccinate these infants needs to balance the risks of YFV exposure with the risk for adverse events after vaccination.

Adults 60 years of age or older
Age ≥60 years is a precaution for yellow fever vaccination, particularly if this is the first dose of the yellow fever vaccine given. A recent analysis of adverse events passively reported to the Vaccine Adverse Events Reporting System (VAERS) from 2000 through 2006 indicates that people aged ≥60 years are at increased risk for any serious adverse event after vaccination, compared with younger people. The rate of serious adverse events in people aged ≥60 years was 8.3 per 100,000 doses distributed, compared with 4.7 per 100,000 for all vaccine recipients. The risk of YEL-AND and YEL-AVD is also increased in this age group, at 1.8 and 1.4 per 100,000 doses, respectively, compared with 0.8 and 0.4 per 100,000 for all vaccine recipients. Given that YEL-AVD has been reported exclusively, and YEL-AND almost exclusively, in primary vaccine recipients, more caution should be exercised with older travelers who may be receiving yellow fever vaccine for the first time. If travel is unavoidable, the decision to vaccinate travelers aged ≥60 years needs to weigh the risks and benefits of the vaccination in the context of their destination-specific risk for exposure to YFV.

HIV infection
Asymptomatic HIV infection with CD4 T-lymphocyte values 200–499/mm³ or 15%–24% of total lymphocytes for children aged <6 years is a precaution for yellow fever vaccination (see also the discussion of HIV infection in the Contraindications section above). Large prospective, randomized trials have not been performed to adequately address the safety and efficacy of yellow fever vaccine among this group. Several retrospective and prospective studies including >500 people infected with HIV have reported no serious adverse events among patients considered moderately immunosuppressed based on their CD4 counts. However, HIV infection has been associated with a reduced immunologic response to a number of inactivated and live attenuated vaccines, including yellow fever vaccine. The mechanisms for the diminished immune response in HIV-infected people are uncertain but appear to be correlated with HIV RNA levels and CD4 T-cell counts.

Because vaccinating asymptomatic HIV-infected people might be less effective than vaccinating people not infected with HIV, measuring their neutralizing antibody response to vaccination should be considered before travel. Contact the state health department or the CDC Arboviral Diseases Branch (970-221-6400) to discuss serologic testing.

If an asymptomatic HIV-infected person with moderate immune suppression (CD4 T-lymphocyte values 200–499/mm³ or 15%–24% of total lymphocytes for children aged <6 years) is traveling to a yellow fever–endemic area, vaccination may be considered. Vaccinated people should be monitored closely after vaccination for evidence of adverse events, and the state health department or CDC should be notified if an adverse event occurs. However, if international travel requirements—not risk of yellow fever—are the only reason to vaccinate an HIV-infected person, the person should be excused from immunization and issued a medical waiver to fulfill health regulations.

If an asymptomatic HIV-infected person has no evidence of immune suppression based on CD4 counts (CD4 T-lymphocyte values ≥500/mm³ or ≥25% of total lymphocytes for children aged <6 years), yellow fever vaccine can be administered if recommended.

Pregnancy

Pregnancy is a precaution for yellow fever vaccine administration. The safety of yellow fever vaccination during pregnancy has not been studied in a large prospective trial. However, a recent study of women who were vaccinated with yellow fever vaccine early in their pregnancies found no major malformations in their infants. A slight increased risk was noted for minor, mostly skin, malformations in infants. A higher rate of spontaneous abortions in pregnant women receiving the vaccine was reported but not substantiated. The proportion of women vaccinated during pregnancy who develop YFV-specific IgG antibodies is variable depending on the study (39% or 98%) and may be correlated with the trimester in which they received the vaccine. Because pregnancy may affect immunologic function, serologic testing can be considered to document a protective immune response to the vaccine.

If travel is unavoidable and the vaccination risks are felt to outweigh the risks of YFV exposure, pregnant women should be excused from immunization and issued a medical waiver to fulfill health regulations. Pregnant women who must travel to areas where YFV exposure is likely should be vaccinated. Although there are no specific data, ACIP recommends that a woman wait 4 weeks after receiving the yellow fever vaccine before conceiving.

Breastfeeding

Breastfeeding is a precaution for yellow fever vaccine administration. Three YEL-AND cases have been reported in exclusively breastfed infants whose mothers were vaccinated with yellow fever vaccine. All 3 infants were aged <1 month at the time of exposure. Further research is needed to document the risk of potential vaccine exposure through breastfeeding. Until more information is available, yellow fever vaccine should be avoided in breastfeeding women. However, when travel of nursing mothers to a yellow fever–endemic area cannot be avoided or postponed, these women should be vaccinated.

Other Considerations

Chronic medical conditions that may be associated with varying degrees of immune deficit include, but are not limited to, chronic renal disease, chronic liver disease (including hepatitis C), and diabetes mellitus. Because no information is available regarding possible increased adverse events or decreased vaccine efficacy after administration of yellow fever vaccine to patients with these diseases, caution should be used if considering vaccination of such patients. Factors to consider in assessing patients' general level of immune competence include disease severity, duration, clinical stability, complications, and comorbidities.

Simultaneous Administration of Other Vaccines and Drugs

Determination of whether to administer yellow fever vaccine and other immunobiologics simultaneously (administration on the same day but at a different injection site) should be made on the basis of convenience to the traveler in completing the desired vaccinations before travel and on information regarding potential immune interference. No evidence exists that inactivated vaccines interfere with the immune response to yellow fever vaccine. Therefore, inactivated vaccines can be administered either simultaneously or at any time before or after yellow fever vaccination. ACIP recommends that yellow fever vaccine be given at the same time as other live-virus vaccines. Otherwise, the clinician should wait 30 days between vaccinations, as the immune response to one live-virus vaccine might be impaired if administered within 30 days of another live-virus vaccine. A recent study involving the simultaneous administration of yellow fever and measles-mumps-rubella (MMR) vaccines in children found a decrease in the immune response against yellow fever, mumps, and rubella when the vaccines were given on the same day versus 30 days apart. Additional studies are needed to confirm these findings, but they suggest that if possible, yellow fever and MMR should be given 30 days apart. Because of the different routes of administration, oral Ty21a typhoid vaccine can be administered simultaneously or at any interval before or after yellow fever vaccine.

INTERNATIONAL CERTIFICATE OF VACCINATION OR PROPHYLAXIS (ICVP)

The IHR allow countries to require proof of yellow fever vaccination as a condition of entry for travelers arriving from certain countries, even if only in transit, to prevent importation and indigenous transmission of YFV. Some countries require evidence of vaccination from all entering travelers, which includes direct travel from the United States (Table 3-25). Travelers who arrive in a country with a yellow fever vaccination entry requirement without proof of yellow fever vaccination may be quarantined for up to 6 days, refused entry, or vaccinated on site. A traveler who has a specific contraindication to yellow fever vaccine and who cannot avoid travel to a country requiring vaccination should request a waiver from a physician before embarking on travel (see the Medical Waivers [Exemptions] section below).

Authorization to Provide Vaccinations and to Validate the ICVP

Under the revised IHR (2005), effective December 15, 2007, all state parties (countries) are required to issue a new ICVP. This is intended to replace the former International Certificate of Vaccination against Yellow Fever (ICV). People who received a yellow fever vaccination after December 15, 2007, must provide proof of vaccination on the new ICVP. If the person received the vaccine before December 15, 2007, the original ICV card is still valid, provided that the vaccination was given <10 years previously. Vaccinees should receive a completed ICVP (Figure 3-1), validated (stamped and signed) with the stamp of the center where the vaccine was given (see below). An ICVP must be complete in every detail; if incomplete or inaccurate, it is not valid. Failure to secure validations can

Table 3-25. Countries that require proof of yellow fever vaccination from all arriving travelers[1]

Angola	Ghana
Benin	Guinea-Bissau
Burkina Faso	Liberia
Burundi	Mali
Cameroon	Niger
Central African Republic	Rwanda
Congo, Republic of the	São Tomé and Príncipe
Côte d'Ivoire	Sierra Leone
Democratic Republic of the Congo	Togo
French Guiana	
Gabon	

[1] Country requirements for yellow fever vaccination are subject to change at any time; therefore, CDC encourages travelers to check with the destination country's embassy or consulate before departure.

INTERNATIONAL CERTIFICATE OF VACCINATION OR PROPHYLAXIS Certificat international de vaccination ou de prophylaxie					

This is to certify that
Nous certifions que _(name – nom)_ _____ _(date of birth – né(e) le)_ _____ _(sex – de sexe)_ _____ _(nationality – et de nationalité)_ _____

whose signature follows
(national identification document, if applicable – document d'identification nationale, le cas échéant) dont la signature suit _____

has on the date indicated been vaccinated or received prophylaxis against in accordance with the International Health Regulations.
a été vacciné(e) ou a reçu une prophylaxie à la date indiquée _(name of disease or condition – nom de la maladie ou de l'affection)_ conformément au Règlement sanitaire international.

Vaccine or prophylaxis Vaccin ou agent prophylactique	Date	Signature and professional status of supervising clinician Signature et titre du professionel de santé responsable	Manufacturer and batch no. of vaccine or prophylaxis Fabricant du vaccin ou de l'agent prophlactique et numéro du lot	Certificate valid from: until: Certificat valable à partir du : jusqu'au :	Official stamp of the administering center Cachet officiel du centre habilité

FIGURE 3-1. EXAMPLE INTERNATIONAL CERTIFICATE OF VACCINATION OR PROPHYLAXIS (ICVP)

(1) Name should appear exactly as on the patient's passport.

(2, 5, 7) All dates should be entered with the day in numerals, followed by the month in letters, then the year. For example: in the above example, the patient's date of birth is 22 March 1960.

(3) This space is for the patient's signature.

(4) For a yellow fever vaccination, 'Yellow Fever' should be written in both spaces. Should the ICVP be used for a required vaccination or prophylaxis against another disease or condition (following an amendment to the International Health Regulations or by recommendation of WHO), that disease or condition should be written in this space. Other vaccinations may be listed on the other side.

(5) The date on which the vaccination is given should be entered as shown above.

(6) A handwritten signature of the clinician—either the stamp holder or another health care provider authorized by the stamp holder—administering or supervising the administration of the vaccine (or prophylaxis) should appear in this box. A signature stamp is not acceptable.

(7) The certificate of yellow fever vaccination is valid for 10 years, beginning 10 days after the date of primary vaccination. The ending date for a valid vaccination recorded on the ICVP is 1 calendar day prior to the calendar day on which the vaccine became valid. For example, a vaccination given on 15 June 2012 will be valid on 25 June 2012 and will expire on 24 June 2022. In the case of revaccination, the certificate of yellow fever vaccination is valid immediately if documentation exists on an ICVP demonstrating that the previous yellow fever vaccination was given within the last 10 years.

(8) The Uniform Stamp of the vaccinating center should appear in this box.

cause a traveler to be quarantined, denied entry, or possibly revaccinated at the point of entry to a country. Revaccination at the point of entry is not a recommended option for the traveler.

Clinics may purchase ICVPs, CDC 731 (formerly PHS 731), from the US Government Printing Office (http://bookstore.gpo.gov/, 866-512-1800). This certificate of vaccination is valid for a period of 10 years, beginning 10 days after the date of vaccination. When a booster dose of the vaccine is given within this 10-year period, the certificate is considered valid from the date of revaccination.

People Authorized to Sign the ICVP and Designated Yellow Fever Vaccination Centers

The ICVP must be signed by a medical provider, who may be a licensed physician or a health care worker designated by the physician, supervising the administration of the vaccine (Figure 3-1). A signature stamp is not acceptable. Yellow fever vaccination must be given at a certified center in possession of an official "uniform stamp," which can be used to validate the ICVP.

State health departments are responsible for designating nonfederal yellow fever vaccination centers and issuing uniform stamps to clinicians. Information about the location and hours of yellow fever vaccination centers may be obtained by visiting CDC's website at wwwnc.cdc.gov/travel/yellow-fever-vaccination-clinics-search.aspx.

Medical Waivers (Exemptions)

Some countries do not require an ICVP for infants younger than a certain age (<6 months, <9 months, or <1 year of age, depending on the country). Age requirements for vaccination for individual countries can be found in the Travel Vaccines & Malaria Information, by Country section at the end of this chapter. For medical contraindications, a clinician who has decided to issue a waiver should fill out and sign the Medical Contraindications to Vaccination section of the ICVP (Figure 3-2). The clinician should also do the following:

- Give the traveler a signed and dated exemption letter on the physician's letterhead stationery, clearly stating the contraindications to vaccination and bearing the stamp used by the yellow fever vaccination center to validate the ICVP.

- Inform the traveler of any increased risk for yellow fever infection associated with lack of vaccination and how to minimize this risk by avoiding mosquito bites.

Reasons other than medical contraindications are not acceptable for exemption from vaccination. The traveler should be advised that issuance of a waiver does not guarantee its acceptance by the destination country. On arrival at the destination, the traveler may be faced with quarantine, refusal of entry, or vaccination on site. To improve the likelihood that the waiver will be accepted at the destination country, clinicians can suggest that the traveler take the following additional measures before beginning travel:

- Obtain specific and authoritative advice from the embassy or consulate of the destination country or countries.
- Request documentation of requirements for waivers from embassies or consulates and retain these, along with the completed Medical Contraindication to Vaccination section of the ICVP.

MEDICAL CONTRAINDICATION TO VACCINATION
Contre-indication médicale à la vaccination

This is to certify that immunization against
Je soussigné(e) certifie que la vaccination contre

_____ for
(Name of disease – Nom de la maladie)   pour

_____ is medically
(Name of traveler – Nom du voyageur)   est médicalement

contraindicated because of the following conditions:
contre-indiquée pour les raisons suivantes :

_____
_____
_____

_____
(Signature and address of physician)
(Signature et adresse du médecin)

FIGURE 3-2. MEDICAL CONTRAINDICATION TO VACCINATION SECTION OF THE INTERNATIONAL CERTIFICATE OF VACCINATION OR PROPHYLAXIS (ICVP)

REQUIREMENTS VERSUS RECOMMENDATIONS

Country entry requirements for proof of yellow fever vaccination under the IHR differ from CDC's recommendations. Yellow fever vaccine entry requirements are established by countries to prevent the importation and transmission of YFV and are allowed under the IHR. Travelers must comply with these to enter the country, unless they have been issued a medical waiver. Certain countries require vaccination from travelers arriving from all countries (Table 3-25), while some countries require vaccination only for travelers coming from "a country with risk of yellow fever transmission" (see Travel Vaccines & Malaria Information, by Country at the end of this chapter). WHO defines those areas "with risk of yellow fever transmission" as countries or areas where yellow fever has been reported currently or in the past, plus where vectors and animal reservoirs exist. Country requirements are subject to change at any time; therefore, CDC encourages travelers to check with the relevant embassy or consulate before departure.

The information in the section on yellow fever vaccine recommendations is advice given by CDC to prevent yellow fever infections among travelers. Recommendations are subject to change at any time because of changes in YFV circulation; therefore, CDC encourages travelers to check the destination pages for up-to-date vaccine information and to check for relevant travel notices on the CDC website before departure (www.cdc.gov/travel).

RECENT CHANGES TO YELLOW FEVER RISK CLASSIFICATION

In 2010, CDC, WHO, and other yellow fever experts completed a comprehensive review of available data and revised the criteria and global maps designating the risk of YFV transmission. The new criteria established 4 categories of risk for YFV transmission that apply to all geographic areas: endemic, transitional, low potential for exposure, and no risk.

Yellow fever vaccination is recommended for travel to endemic and transitional areas. Although vaccination is generally not recommended for travel to areas with low potential for exposure, it might be considered for a small subset of travelers whose itinerary could place them at increased risk for exposure to YFV (such as prolonged travel, heavy exposure to mosquitoes, or inability to avoid mosquito bites).

Based on the revised criteria for yellow fever risk classification, the current maps (Maps 3-16 and 3-17) and country-specific information (see Travel Vaccines & Malaria Information, by Country at the end of this chapter) designate 3 levels of yellow fever vaccine recommendations: recommended, generally not recommended, and not recommended. **Note: The revised yellow fever Maps 3-16 and 3-17 depict areas where yellow fever vaccination is recommended rather than yellow fever risk.**

Countries that only contain areas with low potential for exposure to YFV (Table 3-22) are not included on the official WHO list of countries with risk of YFV transmission (Table 3-21). Therefore, proof of yellow fever vaccination should not be required if traveling from a country with low potential for exposure to YFV to a country with a vaccination entry requirement (unless that country requires proof of yellow fever vaccination from all arriving travelers; see Table 3-25). An exception is South Africa, which since the end of 2011 has required yellow fever vaccination for people traveling from or transiting through any of the 5 countries with low potential for exposure, in addition to those with risk of YFV transmission.

VACCINATION FOR TRAVEL ON MILITARY ORDERS

Because military requirements may exceed those indicated in this publication, any person who plans to travel on military orders (civilians and military personnel) should contact the nearest military medical facility to determine the requirements for his or her trip (see also Chapter 8, Special Considerations for US Military Deployments).

CDC website: www.cdc.gov/yellowfever

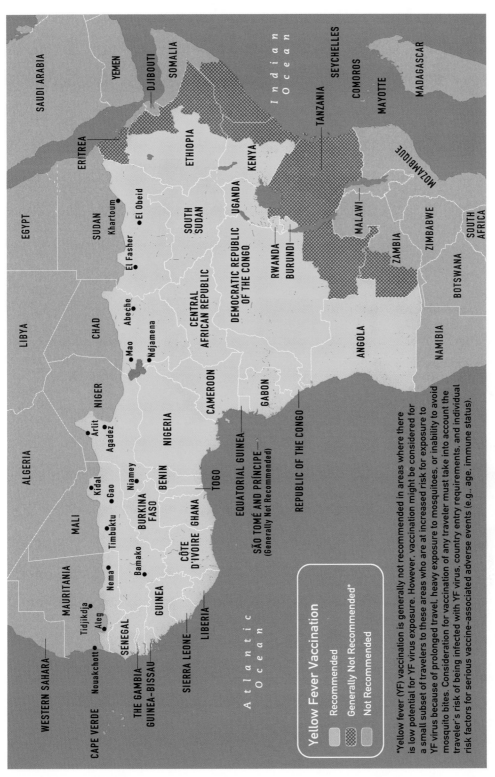

MAP 3-16. YELLOW FEVER VACCINE RECOMMENDATIONS IN AFRICA[1]

Yellow Fever Vaccination

Recommended

Generally Not Recommended*

Not Recommended

*Yellow fever (YF) vaccination is generally not recommended in areas where there is low potential for YF virus exposure. However, vaccination might be considered for a small subset of travelers to these areas who are at increased risk for exposure to YF virus because of prolonged travel, heavy exposure to mosquitoes, or inability to avoid mosquito bites. Consideration for vaccination of any traveler must take into account the traveler's risk of being infected with YF virus, country entry requirements, and individual risk factors for serious vaccine-associated adverse events (e.g., age, immune status).

1 Current as of September 2012. This map, which aligns with recommendations also published by the World Health Organization (WHO), is an updated version of the 2010 map created by the Informal WHO Working Group on the Geographic Risk of Yellow Fever.

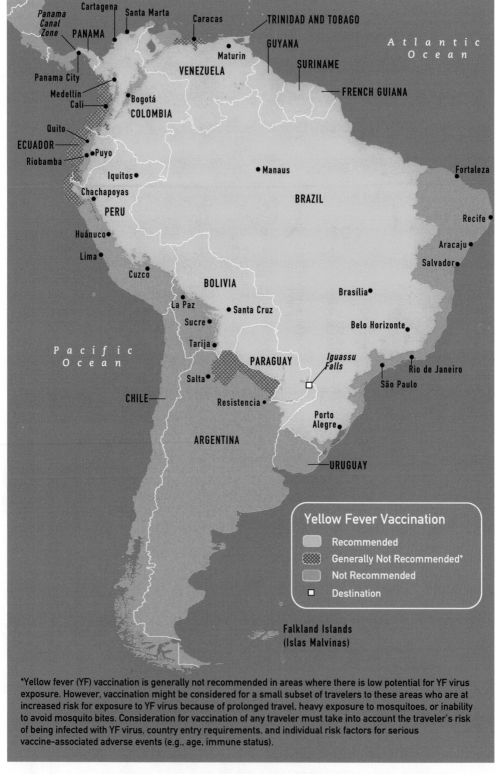

Yellow Fever Vaccination

- Recommended
- Generally Not Recommended*
- Not Recommended
- □ Destination

*Yellow fever (YF) vaccination is generally not recommended in areas where there is low potential for YF virus exposure. However, vaccination might be considered for a small subset of travelers to these areas who are at increased risk for exposure to YF virus because of prolonged travel, heavy exposure to mosquitoes, or inability to avoid mosquito bites. Consideration for vaccination of any traveler must take into account the traveler's risk of being infected with YF virus, country entry requirements, and individual risk factors for serious vaccine-associated adverse events (e.g., age, immune status).

MAP 3-17. YELLOW FEVER VACCINE RECOMMENDATIONS IN THE AMERICAS[1]

[1] Current as of September 2012. This map, which aligns with recommendations also published by the World Health Organization (WHO), is an updated version of the 2010 map created by the Informal WHO Working Group on the Geographic Risk of Yellow Fever.

BIBLIOGRAPHY

1. Barwick R. History of thymoma and yellow fever vaccination. Lancet. 2004 Sep 11–17;364(9438):936.

2. Cavalcanti DP, Salomao MA, Lopez-Camelo J, Pessoto MA. Early exposure to yellow fever vaccine during pregnancy. Trop Med Int Health. 2007 Jul;12(7): 833–7.

3. CDC. General recommendations on immunization—recommendations of the Advisory Committee on Immunization Practices (ACIP). MMWR Recomm Rep. 2011 Jan 28;60(2):1–64.

4. CDC. Transmission of yellow fever vaccine virus through breast-feeding—Brazil, 2009. MMWR Morb Mortal Wkly Rep. 2010 Feb 12;59(5):130–2.

5. Hayes EB. Acute viscerotropic disease following vaccination against yellow fever. Trans R Soc Trop Med Hyg. 2007 Oct;101(10):967–71.

6. Jentes ES, Poumerol G, Gershman MD, Hill DR, Lemarchand J, Lewis RF, et al. The revised global yellow fever risk map and recommendations for vaccination, 2010: consensus of the Informal WHO Working Group on Geographic Risk for Yellow Fever. Lancet Infect Dis. 2011 Aug;11(8):622–32.

7. Lindsey NP, Schroeder BA, Miller ER, Braun MM, Hinckley AF, Marano N, et al. Adverse event reports following yellow fever vaccination. Vaccine. 2008 Nov 11;26(48):6077–82.

8. McMahon AW, Eidex RB, Marfin AA, Russell M, Sejvar JJ, Markoff L, et al. Neurologic disease associated with 17D-204 yellow fever vaccination: a report of 15 cases. Vaccine. 2007 Feb 26;25(10):1727–34.

9. Monath TP, Cetron MS. Prevention of yellow fever in people traveling to the tropics. Clin Infect Dis. 2002 May 15;34(10):1369–78.

10. Monath TP, Gershman M, Staples JE, Barrett ADT. Yellow fever vaccine. In: Plotkin SA, Orenstein WA, Offit PA, editors. Vaccines. 6th ed. Philadelphia: Saunders Elsevier; 2012. p. 870–968.

11. Nascimento Silva JR, Camacho LA, Siqueira MM, Freire Mde S, Castro YP, Maia Mde L, et al. Mutual interference on the immune response to yellow fever vaccine and a combined vaccine against measles, mumps and rubella. Vaccine. 2011 Aug 26;29(37):6327–34.

12. Nasidi A, Monath TP, Vandenberg J, Tomori O, Calisher CH, Hurtgen X, et al. Yellow fever vaccination and pregnancy: a four-year prospective study. Trans R Soc Trop Med Hyg. 1993 May–Jun;87(3):337–9.

13. Nishioka SD, Nunes-Araujo FRF, Pires WP, Silva FA, Costa HL. Yellow fever vaccination during pregnancy and spontaneous abortion: a case-control study. Trop Med Int Health. 1998 Jan;3(1):29–33.

14. Staples JE, Gershman M, Fischer M. Yellow fever vaccine: recommendations of the Advisory Committee on Immunization Practices (ACIP). MMWR Recomm Rep. 2010 Jul 30;59(RR-7):1–27.

15. Suzano CES, Amaral E, Sato HK, Papaiordanou PM, Campinas Group on Yellow Fever Vaccination. The effects of yellow fever immunization (17DD) inadvertently used in early pregnancy during a mass campaign in Brazil. Vaccine. 2006 Feb 27;24(9):1421–6.

16. Whittembury A, Ramirez G, Hernandez H, Ropero AM, Waterman S, Ticona M, et al. Viscerotropic disease following yellow fever vaccination in Peru. Vaccine. 2009 Oct 9;27(43):5974–81.

17. World Health Organization. International Health Regulations, 2005. 2008 [cited 2010 Oct 19]. Available from: http://whqlibdoc.who.int/publications/2008/9789241580410_eng.pdf.

3

A HISTORY OF YELLOW FEVER VACCINATION REQUIREMENTS

Mark D. Gershman

The history of yellow fever vaccination requirements is best understood in the larger context of the history of international measures to prevent the spread of infectious diseases. The first international disease control measures were instituted in Europe in the 14th century in an attempt to prevent the spread of bubonic plague. Over the years, subsequent control measures were next directed at cholera. The lack of agreement between countries on the most effective means of disease prevention and lack of consistency in quarantine regulations eventually led to a series of International Sanitary Conferences.

The first International Sanitary Conference was held in Paris in 1851, and others were held periodically until 1944. Several international health organizations, including the Health Organization of the League of Nations, were established to oversee the various international regulations on disease control. The onset of World War II in 1939 severely disrupted the international public health functions of these agencies. The United Nations Relief and Rehabilitation Administration (UNRRA) was created by the Allies in 1943 to provide economic assistance to war-ravaged European nations, assist refugees, and conduct public health functions. (The UNRRA is unrelated to the more familiar United Nations organization, founded in 1945.) The public health responsibilities included the oversight of international quarantine activities, particularly those delineated in the updated International Sanitary Conventions of 1944, which contained yellow fever control measures. Specific provisions for national governments included quarantining a traveler from an endemic area who did not possess a valid vaccination certificate. This provision, which directed countries how to deal with unvaccinated travelers who may have been exposed to yellow fever virus, was the precursor to formal yellow fever vaccination requirements.

In order to fully carry out the provisions of the Sanitary Conventions of 1944, areas where yellow fever was endemic had to be determined. The conventions delegated this responsibility to the UNRRA, which appointed the Expert Commission on Quarantine. This commission created the first official map of yellow fever–endemic areas in 1945. Soon after the end of World War II, the responsibilities of the UNRRA were assumed by the newly formed World Health Organization (WHO), which appointed the Yellow Fever Panel. In 1949, the Yellow Fever Panel modified the original UNRRA map and issued its first report, which recommended that "measures may be applied permanently against arrivals from endemic areas."

The International Sanitary Regulations (ISR), drafted by WHO to replace the previous International Sanitary Conventions, were adopted by the World Health Assembly in 1951. The ISR stipulated that "vaccination against yellow fever shall be required of any person leaving an infected local area on an international voyage and proceeding to a yellow fever receptive area." Although only alluded to in previous International Sanitary Conventions, this was the first regulatory language that overtly mandated yellow fever vaccination requirements for country entry. The ISR were modified and renamed the International Health Regulations (IHR) in 1969; the IHR were completely revised in 2005, the most current iteration. The text regarding yellow fever vaccination requirements has been gradually modified. The IHR (2005) stipulate, "Vaccination against yellow fever may be required of any traveler leaving an area where the Organization has determined that a risk of yellow fever transmission is present."

In 1960, WHO started to publish annually a listing of all the national yellow fever vaccination requirements in the booklet *Vaccination Certificate Requirements for International Travel*. This booklet gradually evolved into the current book *International Travel and Health*, which is also published annually and lists country-specific vaccination requirements. To keep its list current, WHO sends a questionnaire to all member countries yearly requesting any updates to their vaccination requirements. CDC publishes these same country requirements.

BIBLIOGRAPHY

1. Strode GK, editor. Yellow Fever. 1st ed. New York: McGraw Hill; 1951.
2. Wilder-Smith A, Martinez L, Rietveld A, Duclos P, Hardiman M, Gollogly L. World Health Organization and *International Travel and Health*. Travel Med Infect Dis. 2007 May;5(3):147–9.
3. World Health Organization. International Health Regulations (1969): 1st annotated edition. Geneva: World Health Organization; 1971.
4. World Health Organization. International Health Regulations (2005): 2nd edition. Geneva: World Health Organization; 2008 [cited 2012 Sep 21]. Available from: http://whqlibdoc.who.int/publications/2008/9789241580410_eng.pdf.
5. World Health Organization. International Sanitary Regulations: 2nd annotated edition. Geneva: World Health Organization; 1961.

YERSINIOSIS

L. Hannah Gould

INFECTIOUS AGENT

Facultative anaerobic gram-negative coccobacilli in the genus *Yersinia* (most commonly *Yersinia enterocolitica* serogroups O:3; O:5,27; O:8; and O:9).

TRANSMISSION

Consuming or handling contaminated food (most commonly raw or undercooked pork products), unpasteurized or inadequately pasteurized milk, or untreated water; or by direct or indirect contact with animals.

EPIDEMIOLOGY

Most common in northern Europe (particularly Scandinavia), Japan, and Canada. Risk is higher in cooler months in temperate climates. The incidence among travelers to developing countries is generally low. People with high iron levels are at higher risk of infection and severe disease.

CLINICAL PRESENTATION

Incubation period is 4–6 days (range, 1–14 days). Symptoms include fever, abdominal pain (may mimic appendicitis), and diarrhea (may be bloody and can persist for several weeks). Necrotizing enterocolitis has been described in young infants. Reactive arthritis affecting the wrists, knees, and ankles can occur, usually 1 month after the initial diarrhea episode, resolving after 1–6 months. Erythema nodosum can also occur, manifesting as painful, raised red or purple lesions along the trunk and legs, usually resolving spontaneously within 1 month.

DIAGNOSIS

Isolation of the organism from stool, blood, bile, wound, throat swab, mesenteric lymph node, cerebrospinal fluid, or peritoneal fluid. If yersiniosis is suspected, the clinical laboratory should be notified and instructed to culture on CIN agar.

TREATMENT

Antibiotic treatment should be given for severe cases. Y. *enterocolitica* isolates are usually susceptible to trimethoprim-sulfamethoxazole, aminoglycosides, third-generation cephalosporins, fluoroquinolones, and tetracyclines; they are typically resistant to first-generation cephalosporins and most penicillins. Antimicrobial therapy has no effect on postinfectious sequelae.

PREVENTION

Avoid raw or undercooked pork products, unpasteurized milk products, and untreated water (see Chapter 2, Food & Water Precautions).

CDC website: www.cdc.gov/nczved/divisions/dfbmd/diseases/yersinia

BIBLIOGRAPHY

1. Cover TL, Aber RC. *Yersinia enterocolitica.* N Engl J Med. 1989 Jul 6;321(1):16–24.
2. Perdikogianni C, Galanakis E, Michalakis M, Giannoussi E, Maraki S, Tselentis Y, et al. *Yersinia enterocolitica* infection mimicking surgical conditions. Pediatr Surg Int. 2006 Jul;22(7):589–92.
3. Swaminathan A, Torresi J, Schlagenhauf P, Thursky K, Wilder-Smith A, Connor BA, et al. A global study of pathogens and host risk factors associated with infectious gastrointestinal disease in returned international travellers. J Infect. 2009 Jul;59(1):19–27.

Travel Vaccines & Malaria Information, by Country

Mark D. Gershman, Emily S. Jentes, Katherine J. Johnson (YELLOW FEVER)

Kathrine R. Tan, Paul M. Arguin, Stefanie F. Steele (MALARIA)

Stefanie Erskine, C. Virginia Lee (OTHER VACCINES)

The following pages present country-specific information on yellow fever vaccine requirements and recommendations, malaria transmission information and prophylaxis recommendations, and general recommendations for other vaccines to consider during the pre-travel consultation. Reference maps of 13 countries and 10 country-specific maps of malaria transmission areas are included to aid in interpreting the recommendations. The information was accurate at the time of publication; however, this information is subject to change at any time as a result of changes in disease transmission or, in the case of yellow fever, changing country entry requirements. Updated information, reflecting changes since publication, can be found in the online version of this book (www.cdc.gov/yellowbook) and on the CDC Travelers' Health website (www.cdc.gov/travel).

Yellow Fever

Country-specific yellow fever vaccination recommendations were changed substantially after the 2010 edition of *CDC Health Information for International Travel*; however, they have remained essentially the same since the 2012 edition. From 2008 through 2010, CDC, the World Health Organization (WHO), and other yellow fever and travel medicine experts reviewed available data and revised the criteria and maps that describe the risk of yellow fever virus (YFV) transmission. Based on the review, updated recommendations were made for Argentina, Brazil, Colombia, Democratic Republic of the Congo, Ecuador, Eritrea, Ethiopia, Kenya, Panama, Paraguay, Peru, São Tomé and Príncipe, Somalia, Tanzania, Trinidad and Tobago, Venezuela, and Zambia.

The review process also resulted in the creation of 3 categories of recommendations regarding yellow fever vaccination. See Table 3-26 for definitions of these recommendation categories. *Note: The format of the yellow fever maps (Maps 3-16 and 3-17) depicts country-specific vaccination recommendations rather than yellow fever risk.*

Ultimately, the clinician's decision whether or not to vaccinate any traveler must take into account the traveler's risk of being infected with YFV, country entry requirements, and individual risk factors for serious adverse events after yellow fever vaccination (such as age and immune status). For a thorough discussion of yellow fever and guidance for appropriate vaccination, see the Yellow Fever section earlier in this chapter.

Malaria

The recommendations for malaria prevention include estimates of malaria risk to US travelers. These estimates are based on numbers of malaria cases reported in US travelers and the estimated volume of travel to these countries. In some instances, the risk may be low because the actual intensity of transmission is low in that country. In other instances, significant malaria transmission may occur only in small focal areas of the country where US travelers seldom go. Thus, even though the risk for the average traveler to that country may be low, the risk for the rare traveler going to the areas with higher transmission intensity will be higher. For some countries rarely visited by US travelers, insufficient information exists to make a risk estimate. Information about malaria species present in each country is based on the best available data from multiple sources.

Several medications are available for malaria chemoprophylaxis. When deciding on which drug to use, clinicians should consider the specific itinerary, length of trip, cost of the drugs, previous adverse reactions to antimalarials, drug allergies, and medical history.

For a thorough discussion of malaria and guidance for appropriate prophylaxis, see the Malaria section earlier in this chapter.

Other Vaccines to Consider

As with all parts of the pre-travel consultation, vaccine recommendations need to be individualized after a comprehensive risk assessment, taking into account both the traveler and the trip. The list of vaccines for each country under "Other Vaccines To Consider" is meant to outline those that the clinician should consider during the pre-travel consultation; the listed vaccines are not absolute recommendations. Refer to the corresponding disease sections earlier in this chapter for more in-depth discussions.

In the list you may see any combination of the following entries:

- **Routine vaccines:** Recommended for all travelers. These vaccines include age-specific routine vaccines, such as measles-mumps-rubella (MMR), tetanus-diphtheria-pertussis (Td/Tdap), poliovirus, varicella, and seasonal influenza. Refer to the age-appropriate immunization schedule at www.cdc.gov/vaccines/schedules for further details.
- **Hepatitis A:** Routinely recommended for US children; recommended for travelers to countries with high or intermediate hepatitis A endemicity; may be considered for all travelers.
- **Hepatitis B:** Routinely recommended for US children, health care workers, and for people of any age with high-risk behaviors; recommended for travelers to countries with high or intermediate prevalence of chronic hepatitis B. Vaccination may be considered for all international travelers, regardless of destination, depending on the traveler's behavioral risk as determined by the provider and traveler.
- **Typhoid:** Recommended for travelers to areas with increased risk of exposure, especially in smaller cities, villages, or rural areas and for more adventurous eaters.
- **Adult polio:** Recommended for adults as a one-time booster or to complete a primary series if traveling to countries with endemic polio, reestablished transmission, or recently imported cases, or to countries at risk because of their proximity to these areas.
- **Meningococcal:** Routinely recommended for certain ages and risk groups in the United States. Recommended for travelers to the meningitis belt of Africa during the dry season (December–June) and in other countries during an outbreak. The recommendation for vaccination may also be limited to certain regions of a country; see Map 3-11 for details. Required for travelers to Saudi Arabia for the Hajj pilgrimage.
- **Japanese encephalitis:** Recommended for travelers staying for ≥1 month in endemic areas during the Japanese encephalitis virus transmission season and should be considered for those staying for <1 month who are at increased risk because of their activities or itineraries (such as prolonged outdoor exposure in rural areas or staying in accommodations without air conditioning, screens, or bed nets).
- **Rabies:** Preexposure rabies vaccine may be recommended for certain international travelers based on the prevalence of rabies in the country to be visited, the availability of appropriate antirabies biologics, intended activities, and duration of stay. Refer to corresponding footnotes for additional details.

Table 3-26. Categories of recommendations for yellow fever vaccination

YELLOW FEVER VACCINATION CATEGORY	RATIONALE FOR RECOMMENDATION
Recommended	Vaccination recommended for all travelers ≥9 months of age to areas with endemic or transitional yellow fever risk, as determined by persistent or periodic YFV transmission.
Generally not recommended	Vaccination generally not recommended in areas where the potential for YFV exposure is low, as determined by absence of reports of human yellow fever and past evidence suggestive of only low levels of YFV transmission. However, vaccination might be considered for a small subset of travelers who are at increased risk for exposure to YFV because of prolonged travel, heavy exposure to mosquitoes, or inability to avoid mosquito bites.
Not recommended	Vaccination not recommended in areas where there is no risk of YFV transmission, as determined by absence of past or present evidence of YFV circulation in the area or environmental conditions not conducive to YFV transmission.

Abbreviation: YFV, yellow fever virus.

Country-Specific Information

AFGHANISTAN
Yellow Fever
Requirements: Required if traveling from a country with risk of YFV transmission.[1]
Recommendations: None.

Malaria
Areas with malaria: April–December in all areas <2,500 m (8,202 ft).
Estimated relative risk of malaria for US travelers: High.[3]
Drug resistance[4]: Chloroquine.
Malaria species: *P. vivax* 80%–90%, *P. falciparum* 10%–20%.
Recommended chemoprophylaxis: Atovaquone-proguanil, doxycycline, or mefloquine.

Other Vaccines To Consider
Routine, hepatitis A & B, typhoid, adult polio booster, and rabies.[6]

ALBANIA
Yellow Fever
Requirements: Required if traveling from a country with risk of YFV transmission and ≥1 year of age.[1]
Recommendations: None.

Malaria
No malaria transmission.

Other Vaccines To Consider
Routine, hepatitis A & B, and rabies.[8]

ALGERIA
Yellow Fever
Requirements: Required if traveling from a country with risk of YFV transmission and ≥1 year of age and for travelers who have been in transit >12 hours in an airport located in a country with risk of YFV transmission.[1]
Recommendations: None.

Malaria
No malaria transmission.

Other Vaccines To Consider
Routine, hepatitis A & B, typhoid, and rabies.[6]

AMERICAN SAMOA (US)
Yellow Fever
No requirements or recommendations.

Malaria
No malaria transmission.

Other Vaccines To Consider
Routine, hepatitis A & B, and typhoid.

ANDORRA
Yellow Fever
No requirements or recommendations.

Malaria
No malaria transmission.

Other Vaccines To Consider
Routine, hepatitis B, and rabies.[9]

ANGOLA
Yellow Fever
Requirements: Required upon arrival from all countries if traveler is ≥1 year of age.
Recommendations: *Recommended* for all travelers ≥9 months of age.

Malaria
Areas with malaria: All.
Estimated relative risk of malaria for US travelers: Moderate.
Drug resistance[4]: Chloroquine.
Malaria species: *P. falciparum* 90%, *P. ovale* 5%, *P. vivax* 5%.
Recommended chemoprophylaxis: Atovaquone-proguanil, doxycycline, or mefloquine.

Other Vaccines To Consider
Routine, hepatitis A & B, typhoid, adult polio booster, and rabies.[6]

ANGUILLA (UK)
Yellow Fever
Requirements: Required if traveling from a country with risk of YFV transmission and ≥1 year of age and for travelers who have been in transit in an airport located in a country with risk of YFV transmission.[1]
Recommendations: None.

Malaria
No malaria transmission.

Other Vaccines To Consider
Routine, hepatitis A & B, typhoid, and rabies.[9]

*All footnotes are located on page 404.

ANTARCTICA
Yellow Fever
No requirements or recommendations.

Malaria
No malaria transmission.

Other Vaccines To Consider
Routine and hepatitis B.

ANTIGUA AND BARBUDA
Yellow Fever
Requirements: Required if traveling from a country with risk of YFV transmission and ≥1 year of age.[1]
Recommendations: None.

Malaria
No malaria transmission.

Other Vaccines To Consider
Routine, hepatitis A & B, typhoid, and rabies.[9]

ARGENTINA (See Map 3-18.)
Yellow Fever
Requirements: None.
Recommendations:
Recommended for all travelers ≥9 months of age who are going to areas <2,300 m in elevation[2] in northern and northeastern forested areas of Argentina bordering Brazil and Paraguay (see Map 3-17). Travelers to designated departments in the following provinces should be vaccinated: Corrientes (Berón de Astrada, Capital, General Alvear, General Paz, Itatí, Ituzaingó, Paso de los Libres, San Cosme, San Martín, San Miguel, Santo Tomé) and Misiones (all departments). Vaccination is also recommended for travelers visiting Iguassu Falls.
Generally not recommended for travelers whose itinerary is limited to areas <2,300 m in elevation[2] in the designated departments of the following provinces: Chaco (Bermejo), Formosa (all departments), Jujuy (Ledesma, San Pedro, Santa Bárbara, Valle Grande), and Salta (Anta, General José de San Martín, Oran, Rivadavia) (see Map 3-17).
Not recommended for travelers whose itineraries are limited to areas >2,300 m in elevation[2] and all provinces and departments not listed above.

Malaria
Areas with malaria: Rural areas of northern Jujuy and Salta Province (along Bolivian border). Rare cases reported in the city of Puerto Iguazú in Misiones Province. No transmission at Iguassu Falls.

Estimated relative risk of malaria for US travelers: Very low.
Drug resistance[4]: None.
Malaria species: *P. vivax* 100%.
Recommended chemoprophylaxis:
Jujuy and Salta provinces: Atovaquone-proguanil, chloroquine, doxycycline, mefloquine, or primaquine.[5]
Misiones province: Mosquito avoidance only.

Other Vaccines To Consider
Routine, hepatitis A & B, typhoid, and rabies.[7]

ARMENIA
Yellow Fever
No requirements or recommendations.

Malaria
No malaria transmission.

Other Vaccines To Consider
Routine, hepatitis A & B, and rabies.[6]

ARUBA
Yellow Fever
Requirements: Required if traveling from a country with risk of YFV transmission and ≥6 months of age.[1]
Recommendations: None.

Malaria
No malaria transmission.

Other Vaccines To Consider
Routine, hepatitis A & B, typhoid, and rabies.[9]

AUSTRALIA
Yellow Fever
Requirements: Required for all people ≥1 year of age who enter Australia within 6 days of having stayed overnight or longer in a country with risk of YFV transmission,[1] including São Tomé and Príncipe, Somalia, and Tanzania, but excluding Galápagos Islands in Ecuador and limited to Misiones Province in Argentina.
Recommendations: None.

Malaria
No malaria transmission.

Other Vaccines To Consider
Routine, hepatitis B, and rabies.[9]

AUSTRIA
Yellow Fever
No requirements or recommendations.

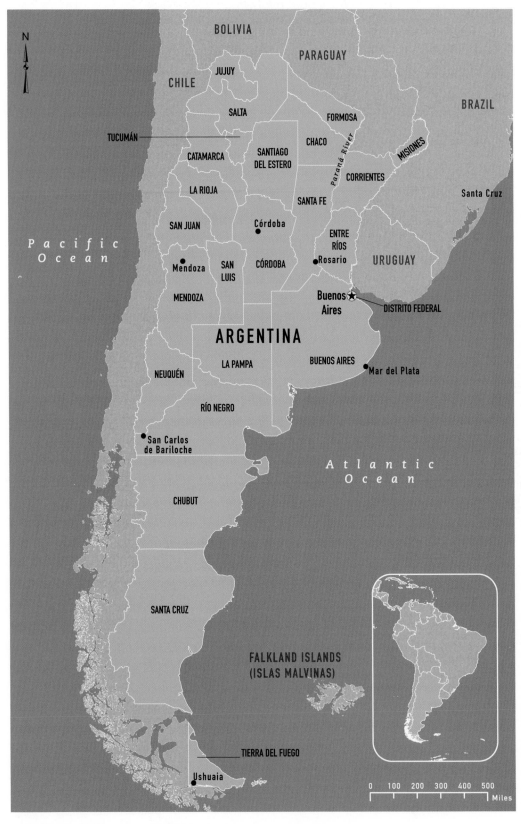

MAP 3-18. ARGENTINA REFERENCE MAP

Malaria
No malaria transmission.

Other Vaccines To Consider
Routine, hepatitis B, and rabies.[8]

AZERBAIJAN
Yellow Fever
No requirements or recommendations.

Malaria
Areas with malaria: May–October in rural areas <1,500 m (4,921 ft). None in Baku.
Estimated relative risk of malaria for US travelers: Very low.
Drug resistance[4]: None.
Malaria species: *P. vivax* 100%.
Recommended chemoprophylaxis: Mosquito avoidance only.

Other Vaccines To Consider
Routine, hepatitis A & B, and rabies.[6]

AZORES (PORTUGAL)
Yellow Fever
No requirements or recommendations.

Malaria
No malaria transmission.

Other Vaccines To Consider
Routine, hepatitis B, and rabies.[9]

BAHAMAS, THE
Yellow Fever
Requirements: Required if traveling from a country with risk of YFV transmission and ≥1 year of age and for travelers who have been in transit >12 hours in an airport located in a country with risk of YFV transmission.[1]
Recommendations: None.

Malaria
No malaria transmission.

Other Vaccines To Consider
Routine, hepatitis A & B, typhoid, and rabies.[9]

BAHRAIN
Yellow Fever
Requirements: Required if traveling from a country with risk of YFV transmission and ≥1 year of age.[1]
Recommendations: None.

Malaria
No malaria transmission.

Other Vaccines To Consider
Routine, hepatitis A & B, typhoid, and rabies.[7]

BANGLADESH
Yellow Fever
Requirements: Required if traveling from a country with risk of YFV transmission and ≥1 year of age.[1]
Recommendations: None.

Malaria
Areas with malaria: All areas, except in the city of Dhaka.
Estimated relative risk of malaria for US travelers: Low.
Drug resistance[4]: Chloroquine.
Malaria species: More than half *P. falciparum*, remainder *P. vivax*.
Recommended chemoprophylaxis: Atovaquone-proguanil, doxycycline, or mefloquine.

Other Vaccines To Consider
Routine, hepatitis A & B, typhoid, Japanese encephalitis, and rabies.[6]

BARBADOS
Yellow Fever
Requirements: Required if ≥1 year of age and traveling from a country with risk of YFV transmission (except Guyana and Trinidad and Tobago) and for travelers who have been in transit >12 hours in an airport located in a country with risk of YFV transmission.[1]
Recommendations: None.

Malaria
No malaria transmission.

Other Vaccines To Consider
Routine, hepatitis A & B, typhoid, and rabies.[9]

BELARUS
Yellow Fever
No requirements or recommendations.

Malaria
No malaria transmission.

Other Vaccines To Consider
Routine, hepatitis A & B, and rabies.[7]

BELGIUM
Yellow Fever
No requirements or recommendations.

*All footnotes are located on page 404.

Malaria
No malaria transmission.

Other Vaccines To Consider
Routine, hepatitis B, and rabies.[9]

BELIZE
Yellow Fever
Requirements: Required if traveling from a country with risk of YFV transmission and ≥1 year of age.[1]
Recommendations: None.

Malaria
Areas with malaria: All areas, especially the districts of Cayo, Stann Creek, and Toledo. None in Belize City and islands frequented by tourists.
Estimated relative risk of malaria for US travelers: Low.
Drug resistance[4]: None.
Malaria species: *P. vivax* 95%, *P. falciparum* 5%.
Recommended chemoprophylaxis: Districts of Cayo, Stann Creek, and Toledo: Atovaquone-proguanil, chloroquine, doxycycline, mefloquine, or primaquine.[5] All other areas with malaria: Mosquito avoidance only.

Other Vaccines To Consider
Routine, hepatitis A & B, typhoid, and rabies.[6]

BENIN
Yellow Fever
Requirements: Required upon arrival from all countries if traveler is ≥1 year of age.
Recommendations: *Recommended* for all travelers ≥9 months of age.

Malaria
Areas with malaria: All.
Estimated relative risk of malaria for US travelers: High.
Drug resistance[4]: Chloroquine.
Malaria species: *P. falciparum* 85%, *P. ovale* 5%–10%, *P. vivax* rare.
Recommended chemoprophylaxis: Atovaquone-proguanil, doxycycline, or mefloquine.

Other Vaccines To Consider
Routine, hepatitis A & B, typhoid, adult polio booster, meningococcal, and rabies.[6]

BERMUDA (UK)
Yellow Fever
No requirements or recommendations.

Malaria
No malaria transmission.

Other Vaccines To Consider
Routine, hepatitis A & B, typhoid, and rabies.[9]

BHUTAN
Yellow Fever
Requirements: Required if traveling from a country with risk of YFV transmission and for travelers who have been in transit in an airport located in a country with risk of YFV transmission.[1]
Recommendations: None.

Malaria
Areas with malaria: All rural areas <1,700 m (5,577 ft), especially the southern belt districts along the border with India: Chirang, Geylegphug, Samchi, Samdrup Jongkhar, and Shemgang.
Estimated relative risk of malaria for US travelers: Very low.
Drug resistance[4]: Chloroquine.
Malaria species: *P. falciparum* 60%, *P. vivax* 40%.
Recommended chemoprophylaxis: Atovaquone-proguanil, doxycycline, or mefloquine.

Other Vaccines To Consider
Routine, hepatitis A & B, typhoid, Japanese encephalitis, and rabies.[6]

BOLIVIA (See Maps 3-19 and 3-20.)
Yellow Fever
Requirements: Required for travelers ≥1 year of age arriving from countries with risk of YFV transmission.[1]
Recommendations:
Recommended for all travelers ≥9 months of age traveling to the following areas <2,300 m in elevation[2] and east of the Andes Mountains: the entire departments of Beni, Pando, Santa Cruz, and designated areas (see Map 3-17) of Chuquisaca, Cochabamba, La Paz, and Tarija departments.
Not recommended for travelers whose itineraries are limited to areas >2,300 m in elevation[2] and all areas not listed above, including the cities of La Paz and Sucre.

*All footnotes are located on page 404.

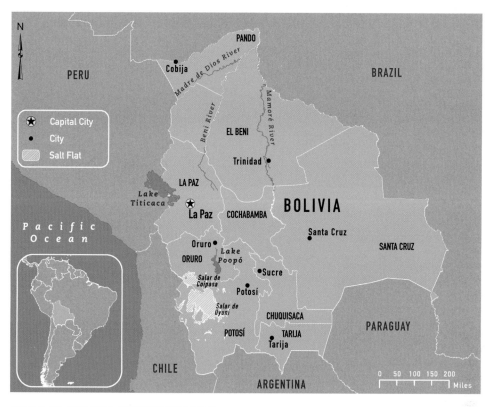

MAP 3-19. BOLIVIA REFERENCE MAP

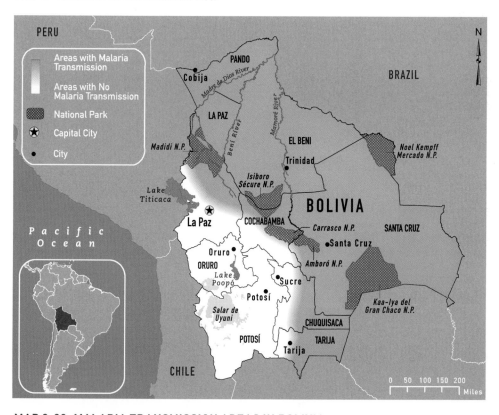

MAP 3-20. MALARIA TRANSMISSION AREAS IN BOLIVIA

Malaria

Areas with malaria: All areas <2,500 m (8,202 ft). None in the city of La Paz.
Estimated relative risk of malaria for US travelers: Low.
Drug resistance[4]: Chloroquine.
Malaria species: *P. vivax* 93%, *P. falciparum* 7%.
Recommended chemoprophylaxis: Atovaquone-proguanil, doxycycline, mefloquine, or primaquine.[5]

Other Vaccines To Consider

Routine, hepatitis A & B, typhoid, and rabies.[6]

BOSNIA AND HERZEGOVINA

Yellow Fever

No requirements or recommendations.

Malaria

No malaria transmission.

Other Vaccines To Consider

Routine, hepatitis A & B, and rabies.[7]

BOTSWANA (See Map 3-21.)

Yellow Fever

Requirements: Required for travelers ≥1 year of age arriving from or having passed through countries with risk of YFV transmission and for travelers who have been in transit >12 hours in an airport located in a country with risk of YFV transmission.[1]
Recommendations: None.

Malaria

Areas with malaria: Present in the following districts: Central and North West (including Chobe National Park). None in the cities of Francistown and Gaborone.
Estimated relative risk of malaria for US travelers: Very low.

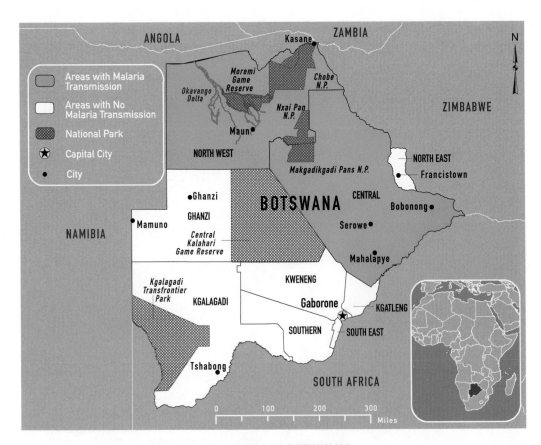

MAP 3-21. MALARIA TRANSMISSION AREAS IN BOTSWANA

*All footnotes are located on page 404.

Drug resistance[4]: Chloroquine.
Malaria species: *P. falciparum* 90%, *P. vivax* 5%, *P. ovale* 5%.
Recommended chemoprophylaxis:
Atovaquone-proguanil, doxycycline, or mefloquine.

Other Vaccines To Consider
Routine, hepatitis A & B, typhoid, and rabies.[6]

BRAZIL (See Maps 3-22 and 3-23.)
Yellow Fever
Requirements: None.
Recommendations:
Recommended for all travelers ≥9 months of age going to the following areas: the entire states of Acre, Amapá, Amazones, Distrito Federal (including the capital city of Brasília), Goiás, Maranhão, Mato Grosso, Mato Grosso do Sul, Minas Gerais, Pará, Rondônia, Roraima, Tocantins, and designated areas (see Map 3-17) of the following states: Bahia, Paraná, Piauí, Rio Grande do Sul, Santa Catarina, and São Paulo (state). Vaccination is also recommended for travelers visiting Iguassu Falls. Note that in 2011, the Brazil Ministry of Health expanded the list of municipalities for which yellow fever vaccination is recommended in the 4 southeastern states of São Paulo, Paraná, Santa Catarina, and Rio Grande do Sul.
Not recommended for travelers whose itineraries are limited to areas not listed above, including the cities of Fortaleza, Recife, Rio de Janeiro, Salvador, and São Paulo (see Map 3-17).

Malaria
Areas with malaria: States of Acre, Amapá, Amazonas, Mato Grosso, Maranhaõ, Para, Rondonia, Roraima, and Tocantins. Also present in urban areas, including cities such as Belem, Boa Vista, Macapa, Manaus, Maraba, Porto Velho, and Santarem. No transmission at Iguassu Falls.
Estimated relative risk of malaria for US travelers: Low.
Drug resistance[4]: Chloroquine.
Malaria species: *P. vivax* 85%, *P. falciparum* 15%.
Recommended chemoprophylaxis:
Atovaquone-proguanil, doxycycline, or mefloquine.

Other Vaccines To Consider
Routine, hepatitis A & B, typhoid, and rabies.[7]

BRITISH INDIAN OCEAN TERRITORY, INCLUDES DIEGO GARCIA (UK)
Yellow Fever
No requirements or recommendations.

Malaria
No malaria transmission.

Other Vaccines To Consider
Routine, hepatitis A & B, and typhoid.

BRUNEI
Yellow Fever
Requirements: Required for travelers ≥1 year of age arriving from countries with risk of YFV transmission and for travelers who have been in transit >12 hours in an airport located in a country with risk of YFV transmission.[1]
Recommendations: None.

Malaria
No malaria transmission.

Other Vaccines To Consider
Routine, hepatitis A & B, typhoid, Japanese encephalitis, and rabies.[6]

BULGARIA
Yellow Fever
No requirements or recommendations.

Malaria
No malaria transmission.

Other Vaccines To Consider
Routine, hepatitis A & B, and rabies.[7]

BURKINA FASO
Yellow Fever
Requirements: Required upon arrival from all countries if traveler is ≥1 year of age.
Recommendations: *Recommended* for all travelers ≥9 months of age.

Malaria
Areas with malaria: All.
Estimated relative risk of malaria for US travelers: High.
Drug resistance[4]: Chloroquine.
Malaria species: *P. falciparum* 80%, *P. ovale* 5%–10%, *P. vivax* rare.
Recommended chemoprophylaxis:
Atovaquone-proguanil, doxycycline, or mefloquine.

Other Vaccines To Consider
Routine, hepatitis A & B, typhoid, adult polio booster, meningococcal, and rabies.[6]

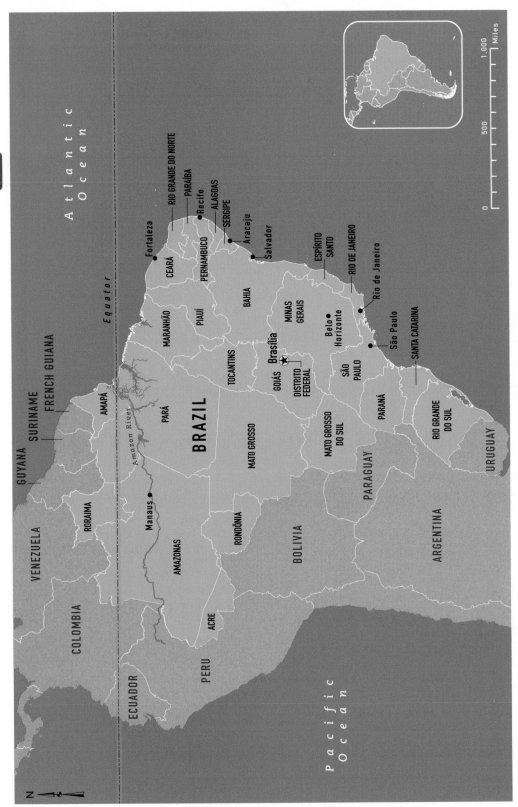

MAP 3-22. BRAZIL REFERENCE MAP

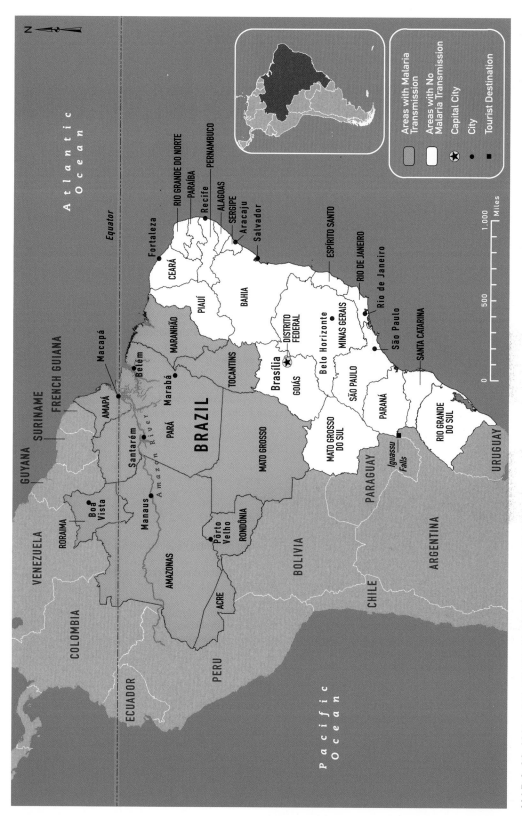

MAP 3-23. MALARIA TRANSMISSION AREAS IN BRAZIL

Areas with Malaria Transmission
Areas with No Malaria Transmission
Capital City
City
Tourist Destination

BURMA (MYANMAR)

Yellow Fever

Requirements: Required if ≥1 year of age and traveling from a country with risk of YFV transmission and for travelers who have been in transit >12 hours in an airport located in a country with risk of YFV transmission.[1] Required also for nationals and residents of Burma (Myanmar) departing for a country with risk of YFV transmission.

Recommendations: None.

Malaria

Areas with malaria: Present at altitudes <1,000 m (3,281 ft). None in the cities of Mandalay and Rangoon (Yangoon).
Estimated relative risk of malaria for US travelers: Moderate.
Drug resistance[4]: Chloroquine and mefloquine.
Malaria species: *P. falciparum* 90%, remainder *P. malariae, P. ovale,* and *P. vivax.*
Recommended chemoprophylaxis:
In the provinces of Bago, Kachin, Kayah, Kayin, Shan, and Tanintharyi: Atovaquone-proguanil or doxycycline.
All other areas with malaria: Atovaquone-proguanil, doxycycline, or mefloquine.

Other Vaccines To Consider

Routine, hepatitis A & B, typhoid, Japanese encephalitis, and rabies.[6]

BURUNDI

Yellow Fever

Requirements: Required upon arrival from all countries if traveler is ≥1 year of age.
Recommendations: *Recommended* for all travelers ≥9 months of age.

Malaria

Areas with malaria: All.
Estimated relative risk of malaria for US travelers: Moderate.
Drug resistance[4]: Chloroquine.
Malaria species: *P. falciparum* 86%, remainder *P. malariae, P. ovale,* and *P. vivax.*
Recommended chemoprophylaxis:
Atovaquone-proguanil, doxycycline, or mefloquine.

Other Vaccines To Consider

Routine, hepatitis A & B, typhoid, adult polio booster, and rabies.[6]

CAMBODIA

Yellow Fever

Requirements: Required if traveling from a country with risk of YFV transmission and ≥1 year of age and for travelers who have been in transit >12 hours in an airport located in a country with risk of YFV transmission.[1]
Recommendations: None.

Malaria

Areas with malaria: Present throughout the country, including Siem Reap city. Rare cases in Phnom Penh. None at the temple complex at Angkor Wat and around Lake Tonle Sap.
Estimated relative risk of malaria for US travelers: Low.
Drug resistance[4]: Chloroquine and mefloquine.
Malaria species: *P. falciparum* 86%, *P. vivax* 12%, *P. malariae* 2%.
Recommended chemoprophylaxis:
In the provinces of Banteay Meanchey, Battambang, Kampot, Koh Kong, Odder Meanchey, Pailin, Preah Vihear, Pursat, and Siem Reap bordering Thailand: Atovaquone-proguanil or doxycycline.
All other areas with malaria: Atovaquone-proguanil, doxycycline, or mefloquine.

Other Vaccines To Consider

Routine, hepatitis A & B, typhoid, Japanese encephalitis, and rabies.[6]

CAMEROON

Yellow Fever

Requirements: Required upon arrival from all countries if traveler is ≥1 year of age.
Recommendations: *Recommended* for all travelers ≥9 months of age.

Malaria

Areas with malaria: All.
Estimated relative risk of malaria for US travelers: High.
Drug resistance[4]: Chloroquine.
Malaria species: *P. falciparum* 85%, *P. ovale* 5%–10%, *P. vivax* rare.
Recommended chemoprophylaxis:
Atovaquone-proguanil, doxycycline, or mefloquine.

*All footnotes are located on page 404.

Other Vaccines To Consider
Routine, hepatitis A & B, typhoid, adult polio booster, meningococcal, and rabies.[6]

CANADA

Yellow Fever
No requirements or recommendations.

Malaria
No malaria transmission.

Other Vaccines To Consider
Routine, hepatitis B, and rabies.[8]

CANARY ISLANDS (SPAIN)

Yellow Fever
No requirements or recommendations.

Malaria
No malaria transmission.

Other Vaccines To Consider
Routine, hepatitis B, and rabies.[9]

CAPE VERDE

Yellow Fever
Requirements: Required if traveling from a country with risk of YFV transmission and ≥1 year of age.[1]
Recommendations: None.

Malaria
Areas with malaria: Limited cases in São Tiago Island.
Estimated relative risk of malaria for US travelers: Very low.
Drug resistance[4]: Chloroquine.
Malaria species: Primarily *P. falciparum*.
Recommended chemoprophylaxis: Mosquito avoidance only.

Other Vaccines To Consider
Routine, hepatitis A & B, typhoid, and rabies.[9]

CAYMAN ISLANDS (UK)

Yellow Fever
No requirements or recommendations.

Malaria
No malaria transmission.

Other Vaccines To Consider
Routine, hepatitis A & B, typhoid, and rabies.[9]

CENTRAL AFRICAN REPUBLIC

Yellow Fever
Requirements: Required upon arrival from all countries if traveler is ≥9 months of age.
Recommendations: *Recommended* for all travelers ≥9 months of age.

Malaria
Areas with malaria: All.
Estimated relative risk of malaria for US travelers: High.
Drug resistance[4]: Chloroquine.
Malaria species: *P. falciparum* 85%; *P. malariae*, *P. ovale*, and *P. vivax* 15% combined.
Recommended chemoprophylaxis: Atovaquone-proguanil, doxycycline, or mefloquine.

Other Vaccines To Consider
Routine, hepatitis A & B, typhoid, adult polio booster, meningococcal, and rabies.[6]

CHAD

Yellow Fever
Requirements: Required if traveling from a country with risk of YFV transmission.[1]
Recommendations:
Recommended for all travelers ≥9 months of age traveling to areas south of the Sahara Desert (see Map 3-16).
Not recommended for travelers whose itineraries are limited to areas in the Sahara Desert (see Map 3-16).

Malaria
Areas with malaria: All.
Estimated relative risk of malaria for US travelers: High.
Drug resistance[4]: Chloroquine.
Malaria species: *P. falciparum* 85%; *P. malariae*, *P. ovale*, and *P. vivax* 15% combined.
Recommended chemoprophylaxis: Atovaquone-proguanil, doxycycline, or mefloquine.

Other Vaccines To Consider
Routine, hepatitis A & B, typhoid, adult polio booster, meningococcal, and rabies.[6]

CHILE

Yellow Fever
No requirements or recommendations.

Malaria
No malaria transmission.

Other Vaccines To Consider
Routine, hepatitis A & B, typhoid, and rabies.[9]

CHINA (See Map 3-24.)
Yellow Fever
Requirements: Required if traveling from a country with risk of YFV transmission and ≥9 months of age and for travelers who have been in transit in an airport located in a country with risk of YFV transmission.[1]
Recommendations: None.

Malaria
Areas with malaria: Present year round in rural parts of Anhui, Guizhou, Hainan, Henan, Hubei, and Yunnan Provinces. Rare cases occur in other rural parts of the country <1,500 m (4,921 ft) May–December. None in urban areas. Some major river cruises may go through malaria-endemic areas in Anhui and Hubei Provinces.
Estimated relative risk of malaria for US travelers: Low.
Drug resistance[4]: Chloroquine and mefloquine.
Malaria species: Primarily *P. vivax*; *P. falciparum* in select locations.
Recommended chemoprophylaxis:
Along China-Burma (Myanmar) border in the western part of Yunnan Province: Atovaquone-proguanil or doxycycline.
Hainan and other parts of Yunnan Province: Atovaquone-proguanil, doxycycline, or mefloquine.
Anhui, Guizhou, Henan, and Hubei provinces: Atovaquone-proguanil, chloroquine, doxycycline, mefloquine, or primaquine.[5]
All other areas with malaria, including river cruises that pass through malaria-endemic provinces: Mosquito avoidance only.

Other Vaccines To Consider
Routine, hepatitis A & B, typhoid, adult polio booster, Japanese encephalitis, and rabies.[6]

CHRISTMAS ISLAND (AUSTRALIA)
Yellow Fever
Requirements: Required for all people ≥1 year of age who enter Australia within 6 days of having stayed overnight or longer in a country with risk of YFV transmission,[1] including São Tomé and Príncipe, Somalia, and Tanzania, but excluding Galápagos Islands in Ecuador and limited to Misiones Province in Argentina.
Recommendations: None.

Malaria
No malaria transmission.

Other Vaccines To Consider
Routine, hepatitis A & B, and typhoid.

COCOS (KEELING) ISLANDS (AUSTRALIA)
Yellow Fever
Requirements: Required for all people ≥1 year of age who enter Australia within 6 days of having stayed overnight or longer in a country with risk of YFV transmission,[1] including São Tomé and Príncipe, Somalia, and Tanzania, but excluding Galápagos Islands in Ecuador and limited to Misiones Province in Argentina.
Recommendations: None.

Malaria
No malaria transmission.

Other Vaccines To Consider
Routine, hepatitis A & B, and typhoid.

COLOMBIA (See Maps 3-25 and 3-26.)
Yellow Fever
Requirements: None.
Recommendations:
Recommended for all travelers ≥9 months of age traveling to areas <2,300 m in elevation[2] in the following departments (see Map 3-17): Amazonas, Antioquia, Arauca, Atlántico, Bolivar, Boyacá, Caldas, Caquetá, Casanare, Cauca, Cesar, Choco (only the municipalities of Acandí, Juradó, Riosucio, and Unguía), Códoba, Cundinamarca, Guainía, Guaviare, Huila, La Guajira (only the municipalities of Albania, Barrancas, Dibulla, Distracción, El Molino, Fonseca, Hatonuevo, La Jagua del Pilar, Maicao, Manaure, Riohacha, San Juan del Cesar, Urumita, and Villanueva), Magdalena, Meta, Norte de Santander, Putumayo, Quindio, Risaralda, San Andrés and Providencia, Santander, Sucre, Tolima, Vaupés, and Vichada.
Generally not recommended for travelers whose itinerary is limited to areas <2,300 m in elevation[2] and west of the Andes mountains: the departments of Cauca, Nariño, Valle de Cauca, and central and southern Choco, and the cities of Barranquilla, Cali, Cartagena, and Medellín (see Map 3-17).
Not recommended for travelers whose itineraries are limited to all areas >2,300 m

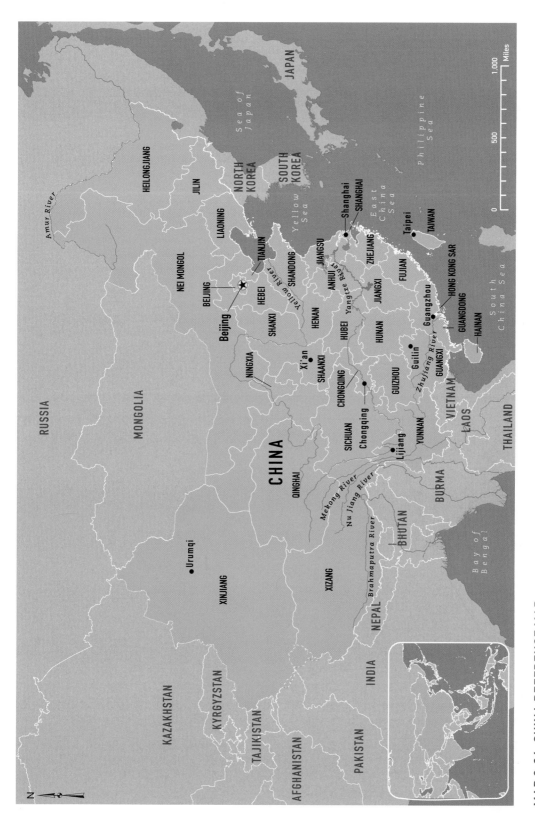

MAP 3-24. CHINA REFERENCE MAP

in elevation,[2] including the city of Bogotá, and also the municipality of Uribia in the La Guajira department.

Malaria

Areas with malaria: All areas <1,700 m (5,577 ft). None in Bogotá and Cartagena.
Estimated relative risk of malaria for US travelers: Low.
Drug resistance[4]: Chloroquine.
Malaria species: *P. falciparum* 35%–40%, *P. vivax* 60%–65%.
Recommended chemoprophylaxis: Atovaquone-proguanil, doxycycline, or mefloquine.

Other Vaccines To Consider

Routine, hepatitis A & B, typhoid, and rabies.[7]

COMOROS

Yellow Fever

No requirements or recommendations.

Malaria

Areas with malaria: All.

Estimated relative risk of malaria for US travelers: No data.
Drug resistance[4]: Chloroquine.
Malaria species: Primarily *P. falciparum*.
Recommended chemoprophylaxis: Atovaquone-proguanil, doxycycline, or mefloquine.

Other Vaccines To Consider

Routine, hepatitis A & B, typhoid, and rabies.[9]

CONGO, REPUBLIC OF THE (CONGO-BRAZZAVILLE)

Yellow Fever

Requirements: Required upon arrival from all countries for travelers ≥1 year of age.
Recommendations: *Recommended* for all travelers ≥9 months of age.

Malaria

Areas with malaria: All.
Estimated relative risk of malaria for US travelers: High.
Drug resistance[4]: Chloroquine.

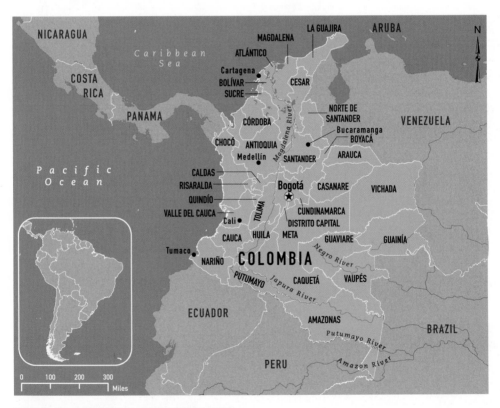

MAP 3-25. COLOMBIA REFERENCE MAP

*All footnotes are located on page 404.

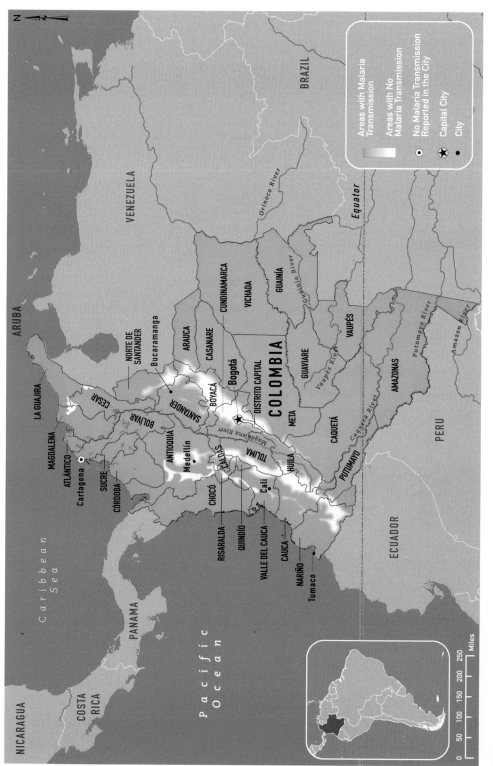

MAP 3-26. MALARIA TRANSMISSION AREAS IN COLOMBIA

Malaria species: *P. falciparum* 90%, *P. ovale* 5%–10%, *P. vivax* rare.
Recommended chemoprophylaxis: Atovaquone-proguanil, doxycycline, or mefloquine.

Other Vaccines To Consider
Routine, hepatitis A & B, typhoid, adult polio booster, and rabies.[6]

COOK ISLANDS (NEW ZEALAND)
Yellow Fever
No requirements or recommendations.

Malaria
No malaria transmission.

Other Vaccines To Consider
Routine, hepatitis A & B, and typhoid.

COSTA RICA (See Map 3-27.)
Yellow Fever
Requirements: Required for travelers ≥9 months of age arriving from countries with risk of YFV transmission (with the exception

of Argentina, Panama, and Trinidad and Tobago) and for travelers who have been in transit >12 hours in an airport located in a country with risk of YFV transmission.[1]
Recommendations: None.

Malaria
Areas with malaria: Rare cases in Limón Province.
Estimated relative risk of malaria for US travelers: Very low.
Drug resistance[4]: None.
Malaria species: Predominantly *P. vivax*.
Recommended chemoprophylaxis: Mosquito avoidance only.

Other Vaccines To Consider
Routine, hepatitis A & B, typhoid, and rabies.[8]

CÔTE D'IVOIRE (IVORY COAST)
Yellow Fever
Requirements: Required upon arrival from all countries for travelers ≥1 year of age.

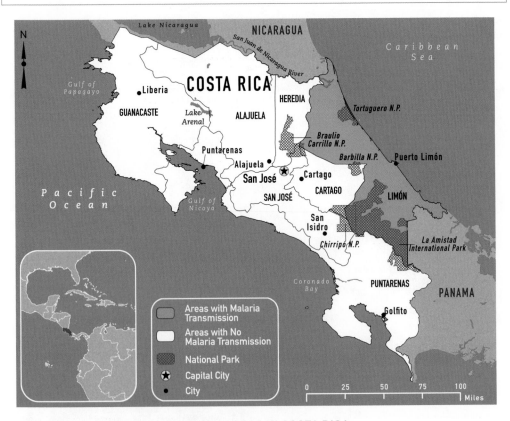

MAP 3-27. MALARIA TRANSMISSION AREAS IN COSTA RICA

*All footnotes are located on page 404.

Recommendations: *Recommended* for all travelers ≥9 months of age.

Malaria
Areas with malaria: All.
Estimated relative risk of malaria for US travelers: High.
Drug resistance[4]**:** Chloroquine.
Malaria species: *P. falciparum* 85%, *P. ovale* 5%–10%, *P. vivax* rare.
Recommended chemoprophylaxis: Atovaquone-proguanil, doxycycline, or mefloquine.

Other Vaccines To Consider
Routine, hepatitis A & B, typhoid, meningococcal, and rabies.[6]

CROATIA
Yellow Fever
No requirements or recommendations.

Malaria
No malaria transmission.

Other Vaccines To Consider
Routine, hepatitis A & B, and rabies.[6]

CUBA
Yellow Fever
No requirements or recommendations.

Malaria
No malaria transmission.

Other Vaccines To Consider
Routine, hepatitis A & B, typhoid, and rabies.[6]

CYPRUS
Yellow Fever
No requirements or recommendations.

Malaria
No malaria transmission.

Other Vaccines To Consider
Routine, hepatitis A & B, and rabies.[9]

CZECH REPUBLIC
Yellow Fever
No requirements or recommendations.

Malaria
No malaria transmission.

Other Vaccines To Consider
Routine, hepatitis A & B, and rabies.[9]

DEMOCRATIC REPUBLIC OF THE CONGO (CONGO-KINSHASA)
Yellow Fever
Requirements: Required upon arrival from all countries for travelers ≥1 year of age.
Recommendations:
Recommended for all travelers ≥9 months of age, except as mentioned below.
Generally not recommended for travelers whose itinerary is limited to Katanga Province.

Malaria
Areas with malaria: All.
Estimated relative risk of malaria for US travelers: Moderate.
Drug resistance[4]**:** Chloroquine.
Malaria species: *P. falciparum* 90%, *P. ovale* 5%, *P. vivax* rare.
Recommended chemoprophylaxis: Atovaquone-proguanil, doxycycline, or mefloquine.

Other Vaccines To Consider
Routine, hepatitis A & B, typhoid, adult polio booster, and rabies.[6]

DENMARK
Yellow Fever
No requirements or recommendations.

Malaria
No malaria transmission.

Other Vaccines To Consider
Routine, hepatitis B, and rabies.[8]

DJIBOUTI
Yellow Fever
Requirements: Required if traveling from a country with risk of YFV transmission and ≥1 year of age.[1]
Recommendations: None.

Malaria
Areas with malaria: All.
Estimated relative risk of malaria for US travelers: No data.
Drug resistance[4]**:** Chloroquine.
Malaria species: *P. falciparum* 90%, *P. vivax* 5%–10%.
Recommended chemoprophylaxis: Atovaquone-proguanil, doxycycline, or mefloquine.

Other Vaccines To Consider
Routine, hepatitis A & B, typhoid, and rabies.[6]

DOMINICA
Yellow Fever
Requirements: Required if traveling from a country with risk of YFV transmission and ≥1 year of age and for travelers who have been in transit >12 hours in an airport located in a country with risk of YFV transmission.[1]
Recommendations: None.

Malaria
No malaria transmission.

Other Vaccines To Consider
Routine, hepatitis A & B, typhoid, and rabies.[9]

DOMINICAN REPUBLIC
Yellow Fever
No requirements or recommendations.

Malaria
Areas with malaria: All areas (including resort areas), except none in the cities of Santiago and Santo Domingo.
Estimated relative risk of malaria for US travelers: Low.

Drug resistance[4]: None.
Malaria species: *P. falciparum* 100%.
Recommended chemoprophylaxis: Atovaquone-proguanil, chloroquine, doxycycline, or mefloquine.

Other Vaccines To Consider
Routine, hepatitis A & B, typhoid, and rabies.[6]

EASTER ISLAND (CHILE)
Yellow Fever
No requirements or recommendations.

Malaria
No malaria transmission.

Other Vaccines To Consider
Routine, hepatitis A & B, and typhoid.

ECUADOR, INCLUDING THE GALÁPAGOS ISLANDS (See Maps 3-28 and 3-29.)
Yellow Fever
Requirements: Required for travelers ≥1 year of age arriving from a country with risk of

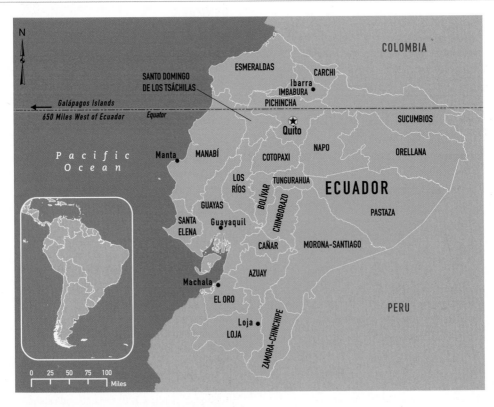

MAP 3-28. ECUADOR REFERENCE MAP

*All footnotes are located on page 404.

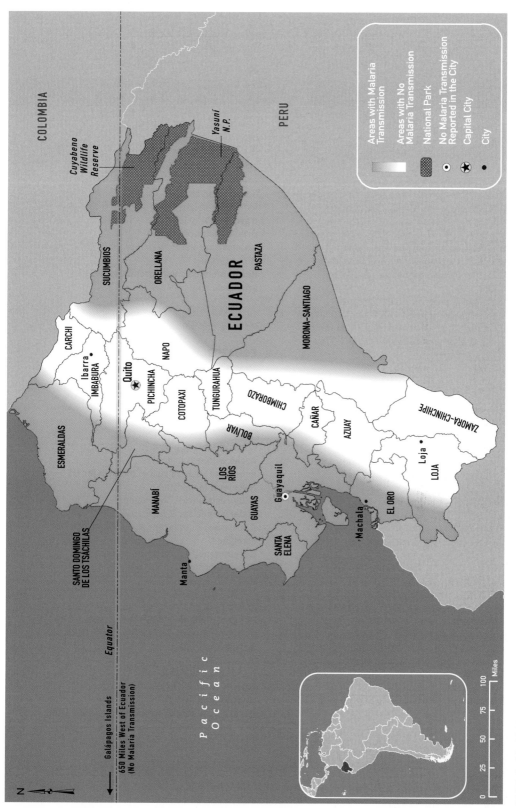

MAP 3-29. MALARIA TRANSMISSION AREAS IN ECUADOR

Areas with Malaria Transmission

Areas with No Malaria Transmission

National Park

No Malaria Transmission Reported in the City

Capital City

City

COLOMBIA

PERU

Cuyabeno Wildlife Reserve

Yasuní N.P.

ECUADOR

SUCUMBÍOS

ORELLANA

PASTAZA

MORONA-SANTIAGO

CARCHI

IMBABURA

Ibarra

Quito

PICHINCHA

NAPO

COTOPAXI

TUNGURAHUA

CHIMBORAZO

BOLÍVAR

CAÑAR

AZUAY

ZAMORA-CHINCHIPE

Loja

LOJA

ESMERALDAS

LOS RÍOS

Guayaquil

GUAYAS

MANABÍ

SANTA ELENA

EL ORO

Machala

Manta

SANTO DOMINGO DE LOS TSÁCHILAS

Equator

Galápagos Islands

650 Miles West of Ecuador (No Malaria Transmission)

Pacific Ocean

N

0   25   50   75   100
Miles

YFV transmission.[1] Nationals and residents of Ecuador are required to possess certificates of vaccination on their departure to an area with risk of YFV transmission.

Recommendations:
Recommended for all travelers ≥9 months of age traveling to areas <2,300 m in elevation[2] in the following provinces east of the Andes Mountains: Morona-Santiago, Napo, Orellana, Pastaza, Sucumbios, and Zamora-Chinchipe (see Map 3-17).

Generally not recommended for travelers whose itinerary is limited to areas <2,300 m in elevation[2] in the following provinces west of the Andes mountains: Esmeraldas, Guayas, Los Rios, Manabi, and designated areas of Azuay, Bolivar, Canar, Carchi, Chimborazo, Cotopaxi, El Oro, Imbabura, Loja, Pichincha, and Tungurahua (see Map 3-17).

Not recommended for travelers whose itineraries are limited to all areas >2,300 m in elevation,[2] the cities of Guayaquil and Quito, or the Galápagos Islands (see Map 3-17).

Malaria
Areas with malaria: All areas <1,500 m (4,921 ft). Not present in the cities of Guayaquil and Quito or the Galápagos Islands.
Estimated relative risk of malaria for US travelers: Low.
Drug resistance[4]: Chloroquine.
Malaria species: *P. vivax* 90%, *P. falciparum* 10%.
Recommended chemoprophylaxis: Atovaquone-proguanil, doxycycline, mefloquine, or primaquine.[5]

Other Vaccines To Consider
Routine, hepatitis A & B, typhoid, and rabies.[7]

EGYPT
Yellow Fever
Requirements: Required if traveling from countries with risk of YFV transmission and ≥1 year of age.[1] All travelers arriving from Sudan are required to have a vaccination certificate or a location certificate issued by a Sudanese official center that states that they have not been in Sudan south of 15°N within the previous 6 days.
Recommendations: None.

Malaria
No malaria transmission.

Other Vaccines To Consider
Routine, hepatitis A & B, typhoid, and rabies.[6]

EL SALVADOR
Yellow Fever
Requirements: Required if traveling from a country with risk of YFV transmission and between 1 and 60 years of age.[1]
Recommendations: None.

Malaria
Areas with malaria: Rare cases along Guatemalan border.
Estimated relative risk of malaria for US travelers: Very low.
Drug resistance[4]: None.
Malaria species: *P. vivax* 99%, *P. falciparum* <1%.
Recommended chemoprophylaxis: Mosquito avoidance only.

Other Vaccines To Consider
Routine, hepatitis A & B, typhoid, and rabies.[6]

EQUATORIAL GUINEA
Yellow Fever
Requirements: Required if traveling from a country with risk of YFV transmission.[1]
Recommendations: ***Recommended*** for all travelers ≥9 months of age.

Malaria
Areas with malaria: All.
Estimated relative risk of malaria for US travelers: Moderate.
Drug resistance[4]: Chloroquine.
Malaria species: *P. falciparum* 85%; *P. malariae*, *P. ovale*, and *P. vivax* 15% combined.
Recommended chemoprophylaxis: Atovaquone-proguanil, doxycycline, or mefloquine.

Other Vaccines To Consider
Routine, hepatitis A & B, typhoid, and rabies.[6]

ERITREA
Yellow Fever
Requirements: Required if traveling from a country with risk of YFV transmission.[1]
Recommendations:
Generally not recommended for travelers going to the following states: Anseba, Debub, Gash Barka, Mae Kel, and Semenawi Keih Bahri.

*All footnotes are located on page 404.

Not recommended for all areas not listed above, including the Dahlak Archipelago (see Map 3-16).

Malaria
Areas with malaria: All areas <2,200 m (7,218 ft). None in Asmara.
Estimated relative risk of malaria for US travelers: No data.
Drug resistance[4]: Chloroquine.
Malaria species: *P. falciparum* 85%, *P. vivax* 10%–15%, *P. ovale* rare.
Recommended chemoprophylaxis: Atovaquone-proguanil, doxycycline, or mefloquine.

Other Vaccines To Consider
Routine, hepatitis A & B, typhoid, meningococcal, and rabies.[6]

ESTONIA
Yellow Fever
No requirements or recommendations.

Malaria
No malaria transmission.

Other Vaccines To Consider
Routine, hepatitis A & B, and rabies.[7]

ETHIOPIA (See Map 3-30.)
Yellow Fever
Requirements: Required if traveling from a country with risk of YFV transmission and ≥1 year of age.[1]
Recommendations:
Recommended for all travelers ≥9 months of age, except as mentioned below.
Generally not recommended for travelers whose itinerary is limited to the Afar and Somali Provinces (see Map 3-16).

Malaria
Areas with malaria: All areas <2,500 m (8,202 ft), except none in city of Addis Ababa.
Estimated relative risk of malaria for US travelers: Moderate.
Drug resistance[4]: Chloroquine.
Malaria species: *P. falciparum* 60%–70%, *P. vivax* 30%–40%, *P. malariae* and *P. ovale* rare.
Recommended chemoprophylaxis: Atovaquone-proguanil, doxycycline, or mefloquine.

Other Vaccines To Consider
Routine, hepatitis A & B, typhoid, meningococcal, and rabies.[6]

FALKLAND ISLANDS (ISLAS MALVINAS)
Yellow Fever
No requirements or recommendations.

Malaria
No malaria transmission.

Other Vaccines To Consider
Routine, hepatitis A & B, and typhoid.

FAROE ISLANDS (DENMARK)
Yellow Fever
No requirements or recommendations.

Malaria
No malaria transmission.

Other Vaccines To Consider
Routine, hepatitis B, and rabies.[9]

FIJI
Yellow Fever
Requirements: Required if traveling from a country with risk of YFV transmission and ≥1 year of age and for travelers who have been in transit >12 hours in an airport located in a country with risk of YFV transmission.[1]
Recommendations: None.

Malaria
No malaria transmission.

Other Vaccines To Consider
Routine, hepatitis A & B, and typhoid.

FINLAND
Yellow Fever
No requirements or recommendations.

Malaria
No malaria transmission.

Other Vaccines To Consider
Routine, hepatitis B, and rabies.[8]

FRANCE
Yellow Fever
No requirements or recommendations.

Malaria
No malaria transmission.

Other Vaccines To Consider
Routine, hepatitis B, and rabies.[9]

FRENCH GUIANA

Yellow Fever

Requirements: Required upon arrival from all countries for travelers ≥1 year of age.
Recommendations: *Recommended* for all travelers ≥9 months of age.

Malaria

Areas with malaria: All areas, except none in the city of Cayenne or Devil's Island (Ile du Diable).
Estimated relative risk of malaria for US travelers: Moderate.
Drug resistance[4]: Chloroquine.
Malaria species: *P. falciparum* <50%, remainder *P. vivax*, *P. malariae* rare.
Recommended chemoprophylaxis: Atovaquone-proguanil, doxycycline, or mefloquine.

Other Vaccines To Consider

Routine, hepatitis A & B, typhoid, and rabies.[6]

FRENCH POLYNESIA, INCLUDING THE ISLAND GROUPS OF SOCIETY ISLANDS (TAHITI, MOOREA, AND BORA-BORA), MARQUESAS ISLANDS (HIVA OA AND UA HUKA), AND AUSTRAL ISLANDS (TUBUAI AND RURUTU)

Yellow Fever

No requirements or recommendations.

Malaria

No malaria transmission.

Other Vaccines To Consider

Routine, hepatitis A & B, and typhoid.

GABON

Yellow Fever

Requirements: Required upon arrival from all countries for travelers ≥1 year of age.
Recommendations: *Recommended* for all travelers ≥9 months of age.

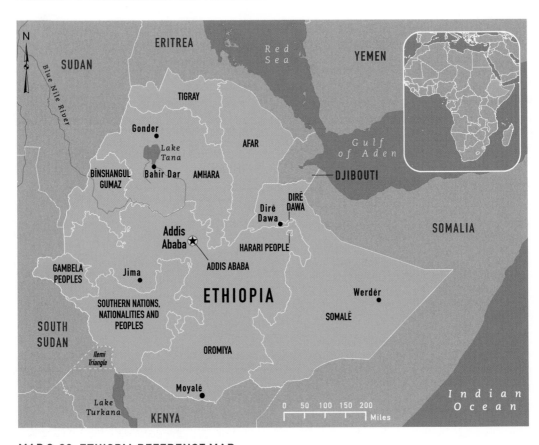

MAP 3-30. ETHIOPIA REFERENCE MAP

*All footnotes are located on page 404.

3

Malaria
Areas with malaria: All.
Estimated relative risk of malaria for US travelers: Moderate.
Drug resistance[4]: Chloroquine.
Malaria species: *P. falciparum* 90%; remainder *P. malariae, P. ovale,* and *P. vivax.*
Recommended chemoprophylaxis: Atovaquone-proguanil, doxycycline, or mefloquine.

Other Vaccines To Consider
Routine, hepatitis A & B, typhoid, and rabies.[6]

GAMBIA, THE
Yellow Fever
Requirements: Required if traveling from a country with risk of YFV transmission and ≥1 year of age.[1]
Recommendations: *Recommended* for all travelers ≥9 months of age.

Malaria
Areas with malaria: All.
Estimated relative risk of malaria for US travelers: High.
Drug resistance[4]: Chloroquine.
Malaria species: *P. falciparum* ≥85%, *P. ovale* 5%–10%, *P. malariae* and *P. vivax* rare.
Recommended chemoprophylaxis: Atovaquone-proguanil, doxycycline, or mefloquine.

Other Vaccines To Consider
Routine, hepatitis A & B, typhoid, meningococcal, and rabies.[6]

GEORGIA
Yellow Fever
No requirements or recommendations.

Malaria
No malaria transmission.

Other Vaccines To Consider
Routine, hepatitis A & B, and rabies.[6]

GERMANY

Yellow Fever
No requirements or recommendations.

Malaria
No malaria transmission.

Other Vaccines To Consider
Routine, hepatitis B, and rabies.[9]

GHANA
Yellow Fever
Requirements: Required upon arrival for all travelers ≥9 months of age.
Recommendations: *Recommended* for all travelers ≥9 months of age.

Malaria
Areas with malaria: All.
Estimated relative risk of malaria for US travelers: High.
Drug resistance[4]: Chloroquine.
Malaria species: *P. falciparum* 90%, *P. ovale* 5%–10%, *P. vivax* rare.
Recommended chemoprophylaxis: Atovaquone-proguanil, doxycycline, or mefloquine.

Other Vaccines To Consider
Routine, hepatitis A & B, typhoid, meningococcal, and rabies.[6]

GIBRALTAR (UK)
Yellow Fever
No requirements or recommendations.

Malaria
No malaria transmission.

Other Vaccines To Consider
Routine, hepatitis B, and rabies.[9]

GREECE
Yellow Fever
No requirements or recommendations.

Malaria
No malaria transmission.

Other Vaccines To Consider
Routine, hepatitis B, and rabies.[9]

GREENLAND (DENMARK)
Yellow Fever
No requirements or recommendations.

Malaria
No malaria transmission.

Other Vaccines To Consider
Routine, hepatitis B, and rabies.[8]

GRENADA
Yellow Fever
Requirements: Required if traveling from a country with risk of YFV transmission and

≥1 year of age and for travelers who have been in transit >12 hours in an airport located in a country with risk of YFV transmission.[1]
Recommendations: None.

Malaria
No malaria transmission.

Other Vaccines To Consider
Routine, hepatitis A & B, typhoid, and rabies.[6]

GUADELOUPE, INCLUDING SAINT-BARTHÉLEMY AND SAINT MARTIN (FRANCE)

Yellow Fever
Requirements: Required if traveling from a country with risk of YFV transmission and ≥1 year of age.[1]
Recommendations: None.

Malaria
No malaria transmission.

Other Vaccines To Consider
Routine, hepatitis A & B, typhoid, and rabies.[9]

GUAM (US)

Yellow Fever
No requirements or recommendations.

Malaria
No malaria transmission.

Other Vaccines To Consider
Routine, hepatitis A & B, and typhoid.

GUATEMALA

Yellow Fever
Requirements: Required if traveling from a country with risk of YFV transmission and ≥1 year of age.[1]
Recommendations: None.

Malaria
Areas with malaria: Rural areas only at altitudes <1,500 m (4,921 ft). None in Antigua, Guatemala City, or Lake Atitlán.
Estimated relative risk of malaria for US travelers: Low.
Drug resistance[4]: None.
Malaria species: *P. vivax* 97%, *P. falciparum* 3%.
Recommended chemoprophylaxis: Atovaquone-proguanil, chloroquine, doxycycline, mefloquine, or primaquine.[5]

Other Vaccines To Consider
Routine, hepatitis A & B, typhoid, and rabies.[6]

GUINEA

Yellow Fever
Requirements: Required if traveling from a country with risk of YFV transmission and ≥1 year of age.[1]
Recommendations: *Recommended* for all travelers ≥9 months of age.

Malaria
Areas with malaria: All.
Estimated relative risk of malaria for US travelers: High.
Drug resistance[4]: Chloroquine.
Malaria species: *P. falciparum* 85%, *P. ovale* 5%–10%, *P. vivax* rare.
Recommended chemoprophylaxis: Atovaquone-proguanil, doxycycline, or mefloquine.

Other Vaccines To Consider
Routine, hepatitis A & B, typhoid, meningococcal, and rabies.[6]

GUINEA-BISSAU

Yellow Fever
Requirements: Required upon arrival from all countries for travelers ≥1 year of age.
Recommendations: *Recommended* for all travelers ≥9 months of age.

Malaria
Areas with malaria: All.
Estimated relative risk of malaria for US travelers: No data.
Drug resistance[4]: Chloroquine.
Malaria species: *P. falciparum* 85%, *P. ovale* 5%–10%, *P. vivax* rare.
Recommended chemoprophylaxis: Atovaquone-proguanil, doxycycline, or mefloquine.

Other Vaccines To Consider
Routine, hepatitis A & B, typhoid, meningococcal, and rabies.[6]

GUYANA

Yellow Fever
Requirements: Required for travelers ≥1 year of age arriving from a country with risk of YFV transmission,[1] with the exception of Argentina, Paraguay, Suriname, and Trinidad and Tobago.
Recommendations: *Recommended* for all travelers ≥9 months of age.

Malaria
Areas with malaria: All areas <900 m (2,953 ft). Rare cases in the cities of Amsterdam and Georgetown.

*All footnotes are located on page 404.

Estimated relative risk of malaria for US travelers: Moderate.
Drug resistance[4]: Chloroquine.
Malaria species: *P. falciparum* 50%, *P. vivax* 50%.
Recommended chemoprophylaxis:
Areas with malaria except cities of Amsterdam and Georgetown: Atovaquone-proguanil, doxycycline, or mefloquine.
Cities of Georgetown and Amsterdam: Mosquito avoidance only.

Other Vaccines To Consider
Routine, hepatitis A & B, typhoid, and rabies.[6]

HAITI
Yellow Fever
Requirements: Required if traveling from a country with risk of YFV transmission.[1]
Recommendations: None.

Malaria
Areas with malaria: All (including Port Labadee).
Estimated relative risk of malaria for US travelers: High.
Drug resistance[4]: None.
Malaria species: *P. falciparum* 99%,
P. malariae rare.
Recommended chemoprophylaxis:
Atovaquone-proguanil, chloroquine, doxycycline, or mefloquine.

Other Vaccines To Consider
Routine, hepatitis A & B, typhoid, and rabies.[6]

HONDURAS
Yellow Fever
Requirements: Required for travelers ≥1 year of age coming from countries with risk of YFV transmission (with the exception of Panama) and for travelers who have been in transit >12 hours in an airport located in a country with risk of YFV transmission.[1]
Recommendations: None.

Malaria
Areas with malaria: Present throughout the country and in Roatán and other Bay Islands. None in San Pedro Sula and Tegucigalpa.
Estimated relative risk of malaria for US travelers: Moderate.
Drug resistance[4]: None.
Malaria species: *P. vivax* 93%, *P. falciparum* 7%.
Recommended chemoprophylaxis:
Atovaquone-proguanil, chloroquine, doxycycline, mefloquine, or primaquine.[5]

Other Vaccines To Consider
Routine, hepatitis A & B, typhoid, and rabies.[6]

HONG KONG SAR (CHINA)
Yellow Fever
No requirements or recommendations.

Malaria
No malaria transmission.

Other Vaccines To Consider
Routine, hepatitis A & B, typhoid, and rabies.[9]

HUNGARY
Yellow Fever
No requirements or recommendations.

Malaria
No malaria transmission.

Other Vaccines To Consider
Routine, hepatitis A & B, and rabies.[7]

ICELAND
Yellow Fever
No requirements or recommendations.

Malaria
No malaria transmission.

Other Vaccines To Consider
Routine, hepatitis B, and rabies.[8]

INDIA (See Map 3-31.)
Yellow Fever
Requirements: Any traveler (except infants <9 months old) arriving by air or sea without a certificate is detained in isolation for up to 6 days if that person—
1) arrives within 6 days of departure from an area with risk of YFV transmission,
2) has been in such an area in transit (except those passengers and members of flight crews who, while in transit through an airport in an area with risk of YFV transmission, remained in the airport during their entire stay and the health officer agrees to such an exemption),
3) arrives on a ship that started from or touched at any port in an area with risk of YFV transmission up to 30 days before its arrival in India, unless such a ship has been disinsected in accordance with the procedure recommended by WHO, or
4) arrives on an aircraft that has been in an area with risk of YFV transmission and has not been disinsected in accordance with the

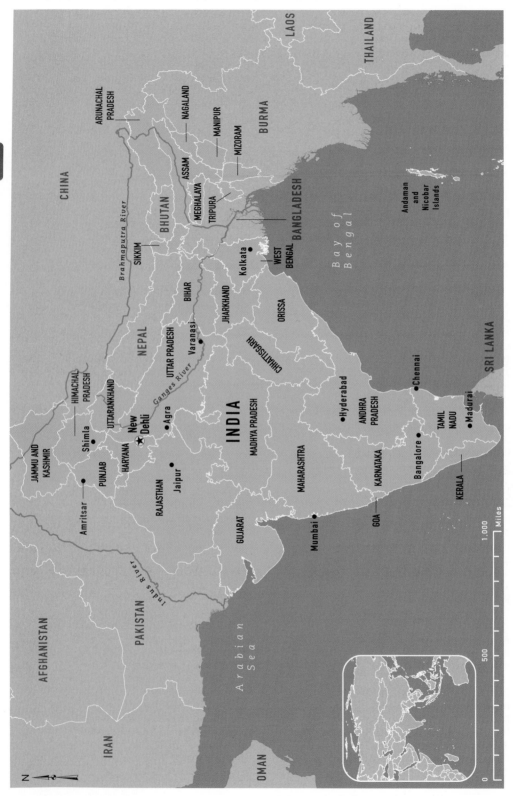

MAP 3-31. INDIA REFERENCE MAP

INFECTIOUS DISEASES RELATED TO TRAVEL

Indian Aircraft Public Health Rules, 1954, or as recommended by WHO.
The following are regarded as countries and areas with risk of YFV transmission:

Africa: Angola, Benin, Burkina Faso, Burundi, Cameroon, Central African Republic, Chad, Congo, Côte d'Ivoire, Democratic Republic of the Congo, Equatorial Guinea, Ethiopia, Gabon, The Gambia, Ghana, Guinea, Guinea-Bissau, Kenya, Liberia, Mali, Niger, Nigeria, Rwanda, Senegal, Sierra Leone, Sudan, Togo, and Uganda.

Americas: Bolivia, Brazil, Colombia, Ecuador, French Guiana, Guyana, Panama, Peru, Suriname, Trinidad and Tobago, and Venezuela.

Note: When a case of yellow fever is reported from any country, that country is regarded by the government of India as a country with risk of yellow fever transmission and is added to the above list.
Recommendations: None.

Malaria

Areas with malaria: All areas throughout the country, including cities of Bombay (Mumbai) and Delhi, except none in areas >2,000 m (6,561 ft) in Himachal Pradesh, Jammu and Kashmir, and Sikkim.
Estimated relative risk of malaria for US travelers: Moderate.
Drug resistance[4]: Chloroquine.
Malaria species: *P. vivax* 50%, *P. falciparum* >40%, *P. malariae* and *P. ovale* rare.
Recommended chemoprophylaxis: Atovaquone-proguanil, doxycycline, or mefloquine.

Other Vaccines To Consider
Routine, hepatitis A & B, typhoid, adult polio booster, Japanese encephalitis, and rabies.[6]

INDONESIA
Yellow Fever
Requirements: Required if traveling from a country with risk of YFV transmission and ≥9 months of age.[1]
Recommendations: None.

Malaria
Areas with malaria: Rural areas of Kalimantan (Borneo), Nusa Tenggara Barat (includes the island of Lombok), Sulawesi, and Sumatra. All areas of eastern Indonesia (provinces of Maluku, Maluku Utara, Nusa Tenggara Timur, Papua, and Papua Barat). None in cities of Jakarta, Ubud, or resort

areas of Bali and Java. Low transmission in rural areas of Java including Ujung Kulong, Sukalumi, and Pangandaran.
Estimated relative risk of malaria for US travelers: Moderate.
Drug resistance[4]: Chloroquine (*P. falciparum* and *P. vivax*).
Malaria species: *P. falciparum* 66%, remainder primarily *P. vivax*.
Recommended chemoprophylaxis: Atovaquone-proguanil, doxycycline, or mefloquine.

Other Vaccines To Consider
Routine, hepatitis A & B, typhoid, Japanese encephalitis, and rabies.[6]

IRAN
Yellow Fever
Requirements: Required if traveling from a country with risk of YFV transmission.[1]
Recommendations: None.

Malaria
Areas with malaria: Rural areas of Fars Province, Sistan-Baluchestan Province and southern, tropical parts of Hormozgan and Kerman Provinces.
Estimated relative risk of malaria for US travelers: Very low.
Drug resistance[4]: Chloroquine.
Malaria species: *P. vivax* 88%, *P. falciparum* 12%.
Recommended chemoprophylaxis: Atovaquone-proguanil, doxycycline, or mefloquine.

Other Vaccines To Consider
Routine, hepatitis A & B, typhoid, adult polio booster, and rabies.[6]

IRAQ
Yellow Fever
Requirements: Required if traveling from a country with risk of YFV transmission.[1]
Recommendations: None.

Malaria
No malaria transmission.

Other Vaccines To Consider
Routine, hepatitis A & B, typhoid, and rabies.[6]

IRELAND
Yellow Fever
No requirements or recommendations.

Malaria
No malaria transmission.

Other Vaccines To Consider
Routine, hepatitis B, and rabies.[9]

ISRAEL

Yellow Fever
No requirements or recommendations.

Malaria
No malaria transmission.

Other Vaccines To Consider
Routine, hepatitis A & B, and rabies.[7]

ITALY, INCLUDING HOLY SEE (VATICAN CITY)

Yellow Fever
No requirements or recommendations.

Malaria
No malaria transmission.

Other Vaccines To Consider
Routine, hepatitis B, and rabies.[8]

JAMAICA

Yellow Fever
Requirements: Required if traveling from a country with risk of YFV transmission and ≥1 year of age and for travelers who have been in transit in an airport located in a country with risk of YFV transmission.[1]
Recommendations: None.

Malaria
No malaria transmission.

Other Vaccines To Consider
Routine, hepatitis A & B, typhoid, and rabies.[9]

JAPAN

Yellow Fever
No requirements or recommendations.

Malaria
No malaria transmission.

Other Vaccines To Consider
Routine, hepatitis B, Japanese encephalitis, and rabies.[9]

JORDAN

Yellow Fever
Requirements: Required if traveling from a country with risk of YFV transmission and ≥1 year of age.[1]
Recommendations: None.

Malaria
No malaria transmission.

Other Vaccines To Consider
Routine, hepatitis A & B, typhoid, and rabies.[6]

KAZAKHSTAN

Yellow Fever
Requirements: Required if traveling from a country with risk of YFV transmission.[1]
Recommendations: None.

Malaria
No malaria transmission.

Other Vaccines To Consider
Routine, hepatitis A & B, typhoid, and rabies.[6]

KENYA (See Map 3-32.)

Yellow Fever
Requirements: Required if traveling from a country with risk of YFV transmission and ≥1 year of age.[1]
Recommendations:
Recommended for all travelers ≥9 months of age, except as mentioned below.
Generally not recommended for travelers whose itinerary is limited to the following areas: the entire North Eastern Province; the states of Kilifi, Kwale, Lamu, Malindi, and Tanariver in the Coastal Province; and the cities of Mombasa and Nairobi (see Map 3-16).

Malaria
Areas with malaria: Present in all areas (including game parks) <2,500 m (8,202 ft). None in the highly urbanized, central part of the city of Nairobi.
Estimated relative risk of malaria for US travelers: Moderate.
Drug resistance[4]: Chloroquine.
Malaria species: *P. falciparum* 85%, *P. vivax* 5%–10%, *P. ovale* up to 5%.

*All footnotes are located on page 404.

Recommended chemoprophylaxis: Atovaquone-proguanil, doxycycline, or mefloquine.

Other Vaccines To Consider

Routine, hepatitis A & B, typhoid, meningococcal, and rabies.[6]

KIRIBATI (FORMERLY GILBERT ISLANDS), INCLUDES TARAWA, TABUAERAN (FANNING ISLAND), AND BANABA (OCEAN ISLAND)

Yellow Fever

Requirements: Required if traveling from a country with risk of YFV transmission and ≥1 year of age.[1]

Recommendations: None.

Malaria

No malaria transmission.

Other Vaccines To Consider

Routine, hepatitis A & B, and typhoid.

KOSOVO

Yellow Fever

Requirements: This country has not stated its yellow fever vaccination certificate requirements.

Recommendations: None.

Malaria

No malaria transmission.

Other Vaccines To Consider

Routine, hepatitis A & B, and rabies.[7]

KUWAIT

Yellow Fever

No requirements or recommendations.

Malaria

No malaria transmission.

Other Vaccines To Consider

Routine, hepatitis A & B, typhoid, and rabies.[7]

KYRGYZSTAN

Yellow Fever

Requirements: Required for travelers ≥1 year of age arriving from countries with risk of YFV transmission and for travelers who have been in transit for >12 hours in an airport located in a country with risk of YFV transmission.[1]

Recommendations: None.

Malaria

No malaria transmission.

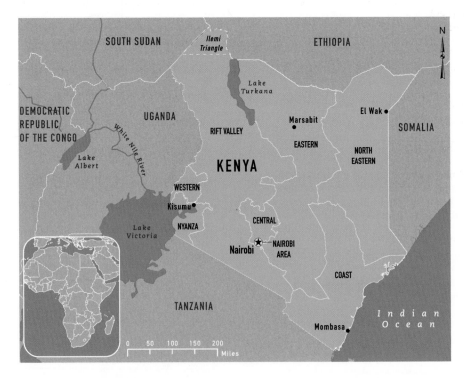

MAP 3-32. KENYA REFERENCE MAP

Other Vaccines To Consider
Routine, hepatitis A & B, typhoid, and rabies.[6]

LAOS
Yellow Fever
Requirements: Required if traveling from a country with risk of YFV transmission.[1]
Recommendations: None.

Malaria
Areas with malaria: All, except none in the city of Vientiane.
Estimated relative risk of malaria for US travelers: Very low.
Drug resistance[4]: Chloroquine and mefloquine.
Malaria species: *P. falciparum* 95%, *P. vivax* 4%, *P. malariae* and *P. ovale* 1% combined.
Recommended chemoprophylaxis:
Along the Laos-Burma (Myanmar) border in the provinces of Bokeo and Louang Namtha and along the Laos-Thailand border in the province of Champasak and Saravan: Atovaquone-proguanil or doxycycline.
All other areas with malaria: Atovaquone-proguanil, doxycycline, or mefloquine.

Other Vaccines To Consider
Routine, hepatitis A & B, typhoid, Japanese encephalitis, and rabies.[6]

LATVIA
Yellow Fever
No requirements or recommendations.

Malaria
No malaria transmission.

Other Vaccines To Consider
Routine, hepatitis A & B, and rabies.[7]

LEBANON
Yellow Fever
Requirements: Required if traveling from a country with risk of YFV transmission and ≥6 months of age.[1]
Recommendations: None.

Malaria
No malaria transmission.

Other Vaccines To Consider
Routine, hepatitis A & B, typhoid, and rabies.[6]

LESOTHO
Yellow Fever
Requirements: Required if traveling from a country with risk of YFV transmission and ≥9 months of age and for travelers who have been in transit for >12 hours in an airport located in a country with risk of YFV transmission.[1]
Recommendations: None.

Malaria
No malaria transmission.

Other Vaccines To Consider
Routine, hepatitis A & B, typhoid, and rabies.[6]

LIBERIA
Yellow Fever
Requirements: Required upon arrival from all countries and ≥1 year of age.
Recommendations: *Recommended* for all travelers ≥9 months of age.

Malaria
Areas with malaria: All.
Estimated relative risk of malaria for US travelers: High.
Drug resistance[4]: Chloroquine.
Malaria species: *P. falciparum* 85%, *P. ovale* 5%–10%, *P. vivax* rare.
Recommended chemoprophylaxis: Atovaquone-proguanil, doxycycline, or mefloquine.

Other Vaccines To Consider
Routine, hepatitis A & B, typhoid, and rabies.[6]

LIBYA
Yellow Fever
Requirements: Required if traveling from a country with risk of YFV transmission.[1]
Recommendations: None.

Malaria
No malaria transmission.

Other Vaccines To Consider
Routine, hepatitis A & B, typhoid, and rabies.[6]

LIECHTENSTEIN
Yellow Fever
No requirements or recommendations.

Malaria
No malaria transmission.

*All footnotes are located on page 404.

Other Vaccines To Consider
Routine, hepatitis B, and rabies.[9]

LITHUANIA
Yellow Fever
No requirements or recommendations.

Malaria
No malaria transmission.

Other Vaccines To Consider
Routine, hepatitis A & B, and rabies.[7]

LUXEMBOURG
Yellow Fever
No requirements or recommendations.

Malaria
No malaria transmission.

Other Vaccines To Consider
Routine, hepatitis B, and rabies.[9]

MACAU SAR (CHINA)
Yellow Fever
No requirements or recommendations.

Malaria
No malaria transmission.

Other Vaccines To Consider
Routine, hepatitis A & B, typhoid, and rabies.[9]

MACEDONIA
Yellow Fever
No requirements or recommendations.

Malaria
No malaria transmission.

Other Vaccines To Consider
Routine, hepatitis A & B, and rabies.[7]

MADAGASCAR
Yellow Fever
Requirements: Required if traveling from a country with risk of YFV transmission.[1]
Recommendations: None.

Malaria
Areas with malaria: All.
Estimated relative risk of malaria for US travelers: Moderate.
Drug resistance[4]: Chloroquine.
Malaria species: *P. falciparum* 85%, *P. vivax* 5%–10%, *P. ovale* 5%.

Recommended chemoprophylaxis: Atovaquone-proguanil, doxycycline, or mefloquine.

Other Vaccines To Consider
Routine, hepatitis A & B, typhoid, and rabies.[6]

MADEIRA ISLANDS (PORTUGAL)
Yellow Fever
No requirements or recommendations.

Malaria
No malaria transmission.

Other Vaccines To Consider
Routine, hepatitis B, and rabies.[9]

MALAWI
Yellow Fever
Requirements: Required if traveling from a country with risk of YFV transmission and ≥1 year of age and for travelers who have been in transit for >12 hours in an airport located in a country with risk of YFV transmission.[1]
Recommendations: None.

Malaria
Areas with malaria: All.
Estimated relative risk of malaria for US travelers: Moderate.
Drug resistance[4]: Chloroquine.
Malaria species: *P. falciparum* 90%; *P. malariae*, *P. ovale*, and *P. vivax* 10% combined.
Recommended chemoprophylaxis: Atovaquone-proguanil, doxycycline, or mefloquine.

Other Vaccines To Consider
Routine, hepatitis A & B, typhoid, and rabies.[6]

MALAYSIA
Yellow Fever
Requirements: Required for travelers ≥1 year of age arriving from countries with risk of YFV transmission and for travelers who have been in transit for >12 hours in an airport located in a country with risk of YFV transmission.[1]
Recommendations: None.

Malaria
Areas with malaria: Present in rural areas of Malaysian Borneo (Sabah and Sarawak Provinces) and to a lesser extent in rural areas of Peninsular Malaysia.
Estimated relative risk of malaria for US travelers: Low.

Drug resistance[4]: Chloroquine.
Malaria species: *P. falciparum* 40%; *P. vivax* 50%; remainder *P. Knowlesi, P. malariae*, and *P. ovale. P. knowlesi* reported to cause 28% of cases in Sarawak and known to cause cases in both Malaysian Borneo and Peninsular Malaysia.
Recommended chemoprophylaxis: Atovaquone-proguanil, doxycycline, or mefloquine.

Other Vaccines To Consider
Routine, hepatitis A & B, typhoid, Japanese encephalitis, and rabies.[7]

MALDIVES
Yellow Fever
Requirements: Required if traveling from a country with risk of YFV transmission and ≥1 year of age.[1]
Recommendations: None.

Malaria
No malaria transmission.

Other Vaccines To Consider
Routine, hepatitis A & B, and typhoid.

MALI
Yellow Fever
Requirements: Required upon arrival from all countries and ≥1 year of age.
Recommendations:
Recommended for all travelers ≥9 months of age going to areas south of the Sahara Desert (see Map 3-16).
Not recommended for travelers whose itineraries are limited to areas in the Sahara Desert (see Map 3-16).

Malaria
Areas with malaria: All.
Estimated relative risk of malaria for US travelers: High.
Drug resistance[4]: Chloroquine.
Malaria species: *P. falciparum* 85%, *P. ovale* 5%–10%, *P. vivax* rare.
Recommended chemoprophylaxis: Atovaquone-proguanil, doxycycline, or mefloquine.

Other Vaccines To Consider
Routine, hepatitis A & B, typhoid, adult polio booster, meningococcal, and rabies.[6]

MALTA
Yellow Fever
Requirements: Required if traveling from a country with risk of YFV transmission

and ≥9 months of age.[1] If indicated on epidemiologic grounds, infants <9 months of age are subject to isolation or surveillance if coming from an area with risk of YFV transmission. No certificate of yellow fever vaccination is required for travelers having transited through an airport located in a country with risk of YFV transmission.[1]
Recommendations: None.

Malaria
No malaria transmission.

Other Vaccines To Consider
Routine, hepatitis B, and rabies.[9]

MARSHALL ISLANDS
Yellow Fever
No requirements or recommendations.

Malaria
No malaria transmission.

Other Vaccines To Consider
Routine, hepatitis A & B, and typhoid.

MARTINIQUE (FRANCE)
Yellow Fever
Requirements: Required if traveling from a country with risk of YFV transmission and ≥1 year of age.[1]
Recommendations: None.

Malaria
No malaria transmission.

Other Vaccines To Consider
Routine, hepatitis A & B, typhoid, and rabies.[9]

MAURITANIA
Yellow Fever
Requirements: Required if traveling from a country with risk of YFV transmission and ≥1 year of age.[1]
Recommendations:
Recommended for all travelers ≥9 months of age traveling to areas south of the Sahara Desert (see Map 3-16).
Not recommended for travelers whose itineraries are limited to areas in the Sahara Desert (see Map 3-16).

Malaria
Areas with malaria: Present in southern provinces, including the city of Nouakchott.

*All footnotes are located on page 404.

Estimated relative risk of malaria for US travelers: High.
Drug resistance[4]: Chloroquine.
Malaria species: *P. falciparum* 85%, *P. ovale* 5%–10%, *P. vivax* rare.
Recommended chemoprophylaxis: Atovaquone-proguanil, doxycycline, or mefloquine.

Other Vaccines To Consider
Routine, hepatitis A & B, typhoid, and rabies.[6]

MAURITIUS
Yellow Fever
Requirements: Required if traveling from a country with risk of YFV transmission and ≥1 year of age and for travelers who have been in transit for >12 hours in an airport located in a country with risk of YFV transmission.[1]
Recommendations: None.

Malaria
No malaria transmission.

Other Vaccines To Consider
Routine, hepatitis A & B, typhoid, and rabies.[9]

MAYOTTE (FRANCE)
Yellow Fever
Requirements: Required for travelers ≥1 year of age arriving from countries with risk of YFV transmission.[1]
Recommendations: None.

Malaria
Areas with malaria: All.
Estimated relative risk of malaria for US travelers: No data.
Drug resistance[4]: Chloroquine.
Malaria species: *P. falciparum* 40%–50%, *P. vivax* 35%–40%, *P. ovale* <1%.
Recommended chemoprophylaxis: Atovaquone-proguanil, doxycycline, or mefloquine.

Other Vaccines To Consider
Routine, hepatitis A & B, typhoid, and rabies.[9]

MEXICO (See Map 3-33.)
Yellow Fever
No requirements or recommendations.

Malaria
Areas with malaria: Present in Chihuahua, Chiapas, Durango, Nayarit, Oaxaca, and Sinaloa. Rare cases in Jalisco, Quintana Roo, Sonora, and Tabasco. No malaria along the United States–Mexico border.
Estimated relative risk of malaria for US travelers: Low.

Drug resistance[4]: None.
Malaria species: *P. vivax* 100%.
Recommended chemoprophylaxis:
Areas with malaria, except states of Jalisco, Quintana Roo, Sonora, and Tabasco: Atovaquone-proguanil, chloroquine, doxycycline, mefloquine, or primaquine.[5]
States of Jalisco, Quintana Roo, Sonora, and Tabasco: Mosquito avoidance only.

Other Vaccines To Consider
Routine, hepatitis A & B, typhoid, and rabies.[7]

MICRONESIA, FEDERATED STATES OF; INCLUDES YAP ISLANDS, POHNPEI, CHUUK, AND KOSRAE
Yellow Fever
No requirements or recommendations.

Malaria
No malaria transmission.

Other Vaccines To Consider
Routine, hepatitis A & B, and typhoid.

MOLDOVA
Yellow Fever
No requirements or recommendations.

Malaria
No malaria transmission.

Other Vaccines To Consider
Routine, hepatitis A & B, and rabies.[6]

MONACO
Yellow Fever
No requirements or recommendations.

Malaria
No malaria transmission.

Other Vaccines To Consider
Routine, hepatitis B, and rabies.[9]

MONGOLIA
Yellow Fever
No requirements or recommendations.

Malaria
No malaria transmission.

Other Vaccines To Consider
Routine, hepatitis A & B, typhoid, and rabies.[6]

MONTENEGRO
Yellow Fever
No requirements or recommendations.

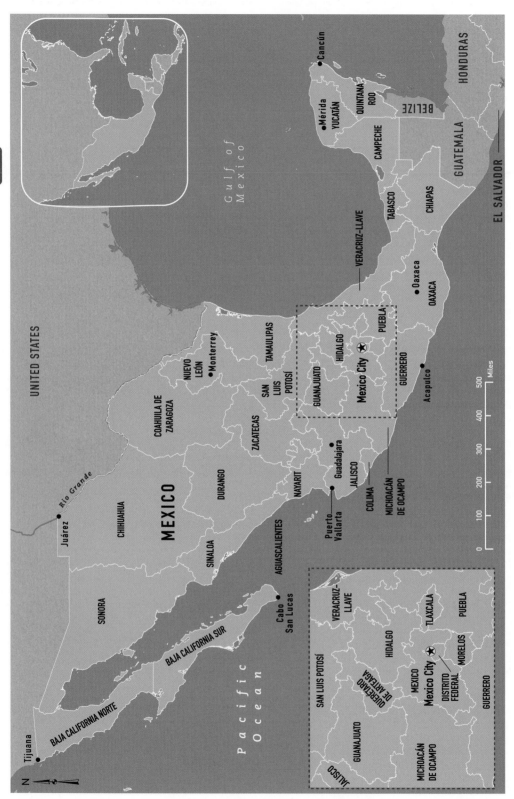

MAP 3-33. MEXICO REFERENCE MAP

Malaria
No malaria transmission.

Other Vaccines To Consider
Routine, hepatitis A & B, and rabies.[7]

MONTSERRAT (UK)
Yellow Fever
Requirements: Required if traveling from a country with risk of YFV transmission and ≥1 year of age.[1]
Recommendations: None.

Malaria
No malaria transmission.

Other Vaccines To Consider
Routine, hepatitis A & B, typhoid, and rabies.[9]

MOROCCO
Yellow Fever
No requirements or recommendations.

Malaria
No malaria transmission.

Other Vaccines To Consider
Routine, hepatitis A & B, typhoid, and rabies.[6]

MOZAMBIQUE
Yellow Fever
Requirements: Required if traveling from a country with risk of YFV transmission and ≥1 year of age.[1]
Recommendations: None.

Malaria
Areas with malaria: All.
Estimated relative risk of malaria for US travelers: Moderate.
Drug resistance[4]: Chloroquine.
Malaria species: *P. falciparum* 90%, *P. malariae*, *P. ovale*, and *P. vivax* rare.
Recommended chemoprophylaxis: Atovaquone-proguanil, doxycycline, or mefloquine.

Other Vaccines To Consider
Routine, hepatitis A & B, typhoid, and rabies.[6]

NAMIBIA (See Map 3-34.)

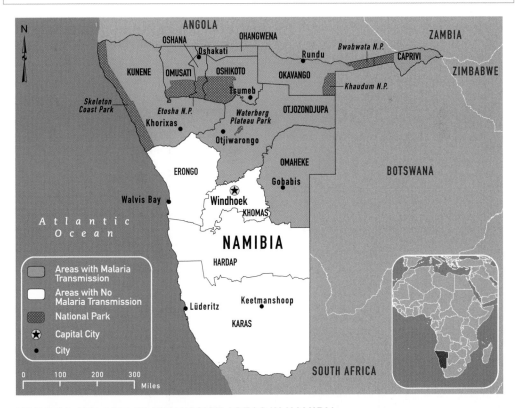

MAP 3-34. MALARIA TRANSMISSION AREAS IN NAMIBIA

*All footnotes are located on page 404.

Yellow Fever
Requirements: Required if traveling from a country with risk of YFV transmission. The countries or parts of countries included in the endemic zones in Africa and South America are regarded as areas with risk of YFV transmission.[1] Travelers on scheduled flights that originated outside the countries with risk of YFV transmission, but who have been in transit through these areas, are not required to possess a certificate provided that they remained at the airport or in the adjacent town during transit. All travelers whose flights originated in countries with risk of YFV transmission or who have been in transit through these countries on unscheduled flights are required to possess a certificate. The certificate is not required for children <1 year of age, but such infants may be subject to surveillance.
Recommendations: None.

Malaria
Areas with malaria: Present in the provinces of Kunene, Ohangwena, Okavango (Kavango), Omaheke, Omusati, Oshana, Oshikoto, and Otjozondjupa and in the Caprivi Strip.
Estimated relative risk of malaria for US travelers: Low.
Drug resistance[4]: Chloroquine.
Malaria species: *P. falciparum* 90%; *P. malariae*, *P. ovale*, and *P. vivax* 10% combined.
Recommended chemoprophylaxis: Atovaquone-proguanil, doxycycline, or mefloquine.

Other Vaccines To Consider
Routine, hepatitis A & B, typhoid, and rabies.[6]

NAURU
Yellow Fever
Requirements: Required if traveling from a country with risk of YFV transmission and ≥1 year of age.[1]
Recommendations: None.

Malaria
No malaria transmission.

Other Vaccines To Consider
Routine, hepatitis A & B, and typhoid.

NEPAL
Yellow Fever
Requirements: Required if traveling from a country with risk of YFV transmission.[1]
Recommendations: None.

Malaria
Areas with malaria: Present throughout the country at altitudes <2,000 m (6,562 ft). None in Kathmandu and on typical Himalayan treks.
Estimated relative risk of malaria for US travelers: No data.
Drug resistance[4]: Chloroquine.
Malaria species: *P. vivax* 85%, *P. falciparum* 15%.
Recommended chemoprophylaxis: Atovaquone-proguanil, doxycycline, or mefloquine.

Other Vaccines To Consider
Routine, hepatitis A & B, typhoid, Japanese encephalitis, and rabies.[6]

NETHERLANDS, THE
Yellow Fever
No requirements or recommendations.

Malaria
No malaria transmission.

Other Vaccines To Consider
Routine, hepatitis B, and rabies.[9]

NETHERLANDS ANTILLES (BONAIRE, CURAÇAO, SABA, SINT EUSTATIUS, AND SINT MAARTEN)
Yellow Fever
Requirements: Required if traveling from a country with risk of YFV transmission and ≥6 months of age.[1]
Recommendations: None.

Malaria
No malaria transmission.

Other Vaccines To Consider
Routine, hepatitis A & B, typhoid, and rabies.[9]

NEW CALEDONIA (FRANCE)
Yellow Fever
Requirements: Required if traveling from a country with risk of YFV transmission and ≥1 year of age.[1] *Note:* In the event of an epidemic threat to the territory, a specific vaccination certificate may be required.
Recommendations: None.

Malaria
No malaria transmission.

Other Vaccines To Consider
Routine, hepatitis A & B, and typhoid.

*All footnotes are located on page 404.

NEW ZEALAND
Yellow Fever
No requirements or recommendations.

Malaria
No malaria transmission.

Other Vaccines To Consider
Routine and hepatitis B.

NICARAGUA
Yellow Fever
Requirements: Required if traveling from a country with risk of YFV transmission and ≥1 year of age.[1]
Recommendations: None.

Malaria
Areas with malaria: Present in districts of Chinandega, Leon, Managua, Matagalpa, Región Autónoma Atlántico Norte (RAAN), and Región Autónoma Atlántico Sur (RAAS).
Estimated relative risk of malaria for US travelers: Low.
Drug resistance[4]: None.
Malaria species: *P. vivax* 90%, *P. falciparum* 10%.
Recommended chemoprophylaxis: Atovaquone-proguanil, chloroquine, doxycycline, mefloquine, or primaquine.[5]

Other Vaccines To Consider
Routine, hepatitis A & B, typhoid, and rabies.[6]

NIGER
Yellow Fever
Requirements: Required upon arrival from all countries if traveler is ≥1 year of age. The government of Niger recommends vaccine for travelers departing Niger.
Recommendations:
Recommended for all travelers ≥9 months of age traveling to areas south of the Sahara Desert (see Map 3-16).
Not recommended for travelers whose itineraries are limited to areas in the Sahara Desert (see Map 3-16).

Malaria
Areas with malaria: All.
Estimated relative risk of malaria for US travelers: High.
Drug resistance[4]: Chloroquine.
Malaria species: *P. falciparum* 85%, *P. ovale* 5%–10%, *P. vivax* rare.
Recommended chemoprophylaxis: Atovaquone-proguanil, doxycycline, or mefloquine.

Other Vaccines To Consider
Routine, hepatitis A & B, typhoid, adult polio booster, meningococcal, and rabies.[6]

NIGERIA
Yellow Fever
Requirements: Required if traveling from a country with risk of YFV transmission and ≥1 year of age.[1]
Recommendations: *Recommended* for all travelers ≥9 months of age.

Malaria
Areas with malaria: All.
Estimated relative risk of malaria for US travelers: High.
Drug resistance[4]: Chloroquine.
Malaria species: *P. falciparum* 85%, *P. ovale* 5%–10%, *P. vivax* rare.
Recommended chemoprophylaxis: Atovaquone-proguanil, doxycycline, or mefloquine.

Other Vaccines To Consider
Routine, hepatitis A & B, typhoid, adult polio booster, meningococcal, and rabies.[6]

NIUE (NEW ZEALAND)
Yellow Fever
Requirements: Required if traveling from a country with risk of YFV transmission and ≥9 months of age.[1]
Recommendations: None.

Malaria
No malaria transmission.

Other Vaccines To Consider
Routine, hepatitis A & B, and typhoid.

NORFOLK ISLAND (AUSTRALIA)
Yellow Fever
Requirements: Required for all people ≥1 year of age who enter Australia within 6 days of having stayed overnight or longer in a country with risk of YFV transmission,[1] including São Tomé and Príncipe, Somalia, and Tanzania, but excluding Galápagos Islands in Ecuador and limited to Misiones Province in Argentina.
Recommendations: None.

Malaria
No malaria transmission.

Other Vaccines To Consider
Routine, hepatitis A & B, and typhoid.

NORTH KOREA
Yellow Fever
Requirements: Required if traveling from a country with risk of YFV transmission and ≥1 year of age.[1]
Recommendations: None.

Malaria
Areas with malaria: Present in southern provinces.
Estimated relative risk of malaria for US travelers: No data.
Drug resistance[4]: None.
Malaria species: Presumed to be 100% *P. vivax*.
Recommended chemoprophylaxis: Atovaquone-proguanil, chloroquine, doxycycline, mefloquine, or primaquine.[5]

Other Vaccines To Consider
Routine, hepatitis A & B, typhoid, Japanese encephalitis, and rabies.[6]

NORTHERN MARIANA ISLANDS (US), INCLUDES SAIPAN, TINIAN, AND ROTA ISLAND
Yellow Fever
No requirements or recommendations.

Malaria
No malaria transmission.

Other Vaccines To Consider
Routine, hepatitis A & B, and typhoid.

NORWAY
Yellow Fever
No requirements or recommendations.

Malaria
No malaria transmission.

Other Vaccines To Consider
Routine, hepatitis B, and rabies.[9]

OMAN
Yellow Fever
Requirements: Required if traveling from a country with risk of YFV transmission and ≥1 year of age.[1]
Recommendations: None.

Malaria
No malaria transmission.

Other Vaccines To Consider
Routine, hepatitis A & B, typhoid, and rabies.[7]

PAKISTAN
Yellow Fever
Requirements: Required for travelers ≥9 months of age arriving from any part of a country where there is a risk of YFV transmission and for travelers who have been in transit for >12 hours in an airport located in a country with risk of YFV transmission.[1]
Recommendations: None.

Malaria
Areas with malaria: All areas (including all cities) <2,500 m (8,202 ft).
Estimated relative risk of malaria for US travelers: Moderate.
Drug resistance[4]: Chloroquine.
Malaria species: *P. falciparum* 30%, *P. vivax* 70%.
Recommended chemoprophylaxis: Atovaquone-proguanil, doxycycline, or mefloquine.

Other Vaccines To Consider
Routine, hepatitis A & B, typhoid, adult polio booster, Japanese encephalitis, and rabies.[6]

PALAU
Yellow Fever
No requirements or recommendations.

Malaria
No malaria transmission.

Other Vaccines To Consider
Routine, hepatitis A & B, and typhoid.

PANAMA (See Map 3-35.)
Yellow Fever
Requirements: Required if traveling from a country with risk of YFV transmission.[1]
Recommendations:
Recommended for all travelers ≥9 months of age traveling to all mainland areas east of the Canal Zone, encompassing the entire *comarcas* (autonomous territories) of Emberá and Kuna Yala, the entire province of Darién, and areas of the provinces of Colón and Panamá that are east of the Canal Zone (see Map 3-17).
Not recommended for travelers whose itineraries are limited to areas west of the Canal Zone, the city of Panama, the Canal Zone itself, the San Blas Islands, and the Balboa Islands (see Map 3-17).

*All footnotes are located on page 404.

Malaria

Areas with malaria: Transmission throughout the country. None in urban areas of Panama City or in the former Canal Zone.

Estimated relative risk of malaria for US travelers: Low.

Drug resistance[4]: Chloroquine (east of the Panama Canal).

Malaria species: *P. vivax* 99%, *P. falciparum* 1%.

Recommended chemoprophylaxis:
Provinces east of the Panama Canal: Atovaquone-proguanil, doxycycline, mefloquine, or primaquine.[5]
Other areas with malaria: Mosquito avoidance only.

Other Vaccines To Consider
Routine, hepatitis A & B, typhoid, and rabies.[8]

PAPUA NEW GUINEA

Yellow Fever

Requirements: Required if traveling from a country with risk of YFV transmission and ≥1 year of age.[1]

Recommendations: None.

Malaria

Areas with malaria: Present throughout the country at altitudes <2,000 m (7,218 ft).

Estimated relative risk of malaria for US travelers: High.

Drug resistance[4]: Chloroquine (both *P. falciparum* and *P. vivax*).

Malaria species: *P. falciparum* 65%–80%, *P. vivax* 10%–30%, remainder *P. malariae* and *P. ovale*.

Recommended chemoprophylaxis:
Atovaquone-proguanil, doxycycline, or mefloquine.

Other Vaccines To Consider
Routine, hepatitis A & B, typhoid, Japanese encephalitis, and rabies.[9]

PARAGUAY (See Map 3-36.)

Yellow Fever

Requirements: Required if traveling from a country with risk of YFV transmission and ≥1 year of age.[1]

Recommendations:
Recommended for all travelers ≥9 months of age, except as mentioned below.

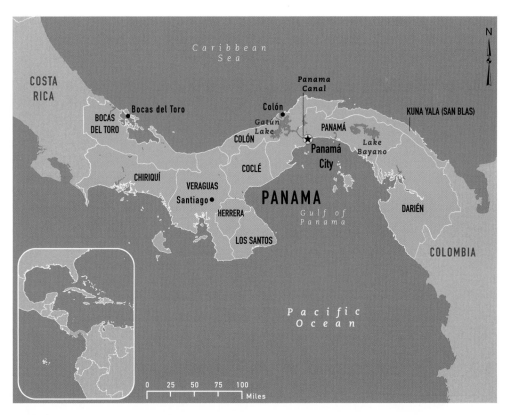

MAP 3-35. PANAMA REFERENCE MAP

Generally not recommended for travelers whose itinerary is limited to the city of Asunción.

Malaria
Areas with malaria: Present in the departments of Alto Paraná, Caaguazú, and Canendiyú.
Estimated relative risk of malaria for US travelers: Very low.
Drug resistance[4]: None.
Malaria species: *P. vivax* 95%, *P. falciparum* 5%.
Recommended chemoprophylaxis: Atovaquone-proguanil, chloroquine, doxycycline, mefloquine, or primaquine.[5]

Other Vaccines To Consider
Routine, hepatitis A & B, typhoid, and rabies.[6]

PERU (See Maps 3-37 and 3-38.)
Yellow Fever
Requirements: None.
Recommendations:
Recommended for all travelers ≥9 months of age going to areas <2,300 m in elevation[2]

in the following: the entire regions of Amazonas, Loreto, Madre de Dios, San Martin, and Ucayali and designated areas (see Map 3-17) of the following regions: far northeastern Ancash; northern Apurimac; northern and northeastern Ayacucho; northern and eastern Cajamarca; northwestern, northern, and northeastern Cusco; far northern Huancavelica; northern, central, and eastern Huanuco; northern and eastern Junin; eastern La Libertad; central and eastern Pasco; eastern Piura; and northern Puno.
Generally not recommended for travelers whose itinerary is limited to the following areas west of the Andes: the entire regions of Lambayeque and Tumbes and the designated areas of west-central Cajamarca and western Piura (see Map 3-17).
Not recommended for travelers whose itineraries are limited to the following areas: all areas >2,300 m in elevation,[2] areas west of the Andes not listed above, the cities of Cuzco and Lima, Machu Picchu, and the Inca Trail (see Map 3-17).

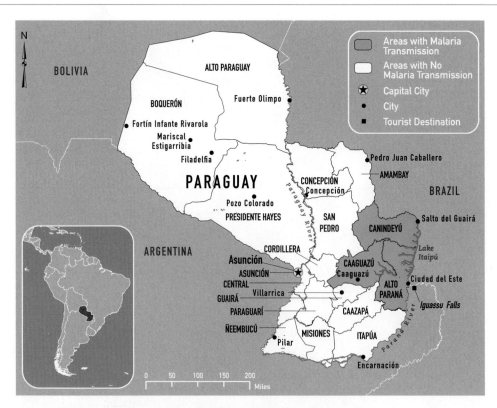

MAP 3-36. MALARIA TRANSMISSION AREAS IN PARAGUAY

*All footnotes are located on page 404.

Malaria

Areas with malaria: All departments <2,000 m (6,561 ft), including the cities of Iquitos and Puerto Maldonado. None in Lima province and coast south of Lima, and none in the cities of Ica and Nazca. None in the highland tourist areas (Cuzco, Machu Picchu, and Lake Titicaca) and southern cities of Arequipa, Moquegua, Puno, and Tacna.

Estimated relative risk of malaria for US travelers: Low.

Drug resistance[4]: Chloroquine.

Malaria species: *P. vivax* 85%, *P. falciparum* 15%.

Recommended chemoprophylaxis: Atovaquone-proguanil, doxycycline, or mefloquine.

Other Vaccines To Consider

Routine, hepatitis A & B, typhoid, and rabies.[7]

PHILIPPINES

Yellow Fever

Requirements: Required if traveling from a country with risk of YFV transmission and ≥1 year of age and for travelers who have been in transit in an airport located in a country with risk of YFV transmission.[1]

Recommendations: None.

Malaria

Areas with malaria: Present in rural areas <600 m (1,969 ft) on the islands of Basilu, Luzon, Mindanao, Mindoro, Palawan, Sulu (Jolo), and Tawi-Tawi. None in urban areas.

Estimated relative risk of malaria for US travelers: Low.

Drug resistance[4]: Chloroquine.

Malaria species: *P. falciparum* 70%–80%, *P. vivax* 20%–30%.

Recommended chemoprophylaxis: Atovaquone-proguanil, doxycycline, or mefloquine.

Other Vaccines To Consider

Routine, hepatitis A & B, typhoid, Japanese encephalitis, and rabies.[6]

PITCAIRN ISLANDS (UK)

Yellow Fever

Requirements: Required if traveling from a country with risk of YFV transmission and ≥1 year of age.[1]

Recommendations: None.

Malaria

No malaria transmission.

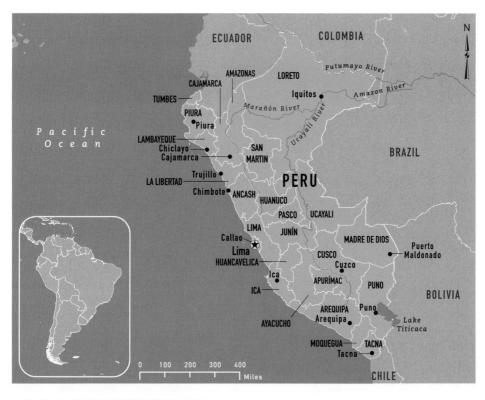

MAP 3-37. PERU REFERENCE MAP

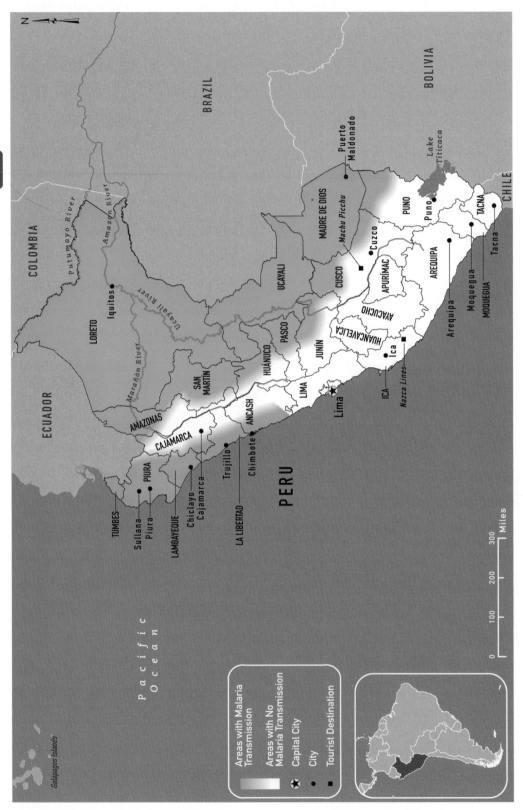

MAP 3-38. MALARIA TRANSMISSION AREAS IN PERU

Other Vaccines To Consider
Routine, hepatitis A & B, and typhoid.

POLAND
Yellow Fever
No requirements or recommendations.

Malaria
No malaria transmission.

Other Vaccines To Consider
Routine, hepatitis A & B, and rabies.[8]

PORTUGAL
Yellow Fever
No requirements or recommendations.

Malaria
No malaria transmission.

Other Vaccines To Consider
Routine, hepatitis B, and rabies.[9]

PUERTO RICO (US)
Yellow Fever
No requirements or recommendations.

Malaria
No malaria transmission.

Other Vaccines To Consider
Routine, hepatitis A & B, typhoid, and rabies.[7]

QATAR
Yellow Fever
No requirements or recommendations.

Malaria
No malaria transmission.

Other Vaccines To Consider
Routine, hepatitis A & B, typhoid, and rabies.[7]

RÉUNION (FRANCE)
Yellow Fever
Requirements: Required if traveling from a country with risk of YFV transmission and ≥1 year of age.[1]
Recommendations: None.

Malaria
No malaria transmission.

Other Vaccines To Consider
Routine, hepatitis A & B, typhoid, and rabies.[9]

ROMANIA
Yellow Fever
No requirements or recommendations.

Malaria
No malaria transmission.

Other Vaccines To Consider
Routine, hepatitis A & B, and rabies.[7]

RUSSIA
Yellow Fever
No requirements or recommendations.

Malaria
No malaria transmission.

Other Vaccines To Consider
Routine, hepatitis A & B, and rabies (see footnote 6 for Caucasus region and footnote 7 for all other areas).

RWANDA
Yellow Fever
Requirements: Required upon arrival from all countries for travelers ≥1 year of age.
Recommendations: *Recommended* for all travelers ≥9 months of age.

Malaria
Areas with malaria: All.
Estimated relative risk of malaria for US travelers: Moderate.
Drug resistance[4]: Chloroquine.
Malaria species: *P. falciparum* 90%, *P. vivax* 5%, *P. ovale* 5%.
Recommended chemoprophylaxis: Atovaquone-proguanil, doxycycline, or mefloquine.

Other Vaccines To Consider
Routine, hepatitis A & B, typhoid, adult polio booster, and rabies.[6]

SAINT HELENA (UK)
Yellow Fever
Requirements: Required if traveling from a country with risk of YFV transmission and ≥1 year of age.[1]
Recommendations: None.

Malaria
No malaria transmission.

Other Vaccines To Consider
Routine, hepatitis A & B, typhoid, and rabies.[9]

*All footnotes are located on page 404.

SAINT KITTS (SAINT CHRISTOPHER) AND NEVIS (UK)
Yellow Fever
Requirements: Required if traveling from a country with risk of YFV transmission and ≥1 year of age and for travelers who have been in transit for >12 hours in an airport located in a country with risk of YFV transmission.[1]
Recommendations: None.

Malaria
No malaria transmission.

Other Vaccines To Consider
Routine, hepatitis A & B, typhoid, and rabies.[9]

SAINT LUCIA
Yellow Fever
Requirements: Required if traveling from a country with risk of YFV transmission and ≥1 year of age.[1]
Recommendations: None.

Malaria
No malaria transmission.

Other Vaccines To Consider
Routine, hepatitis A & B, typhoid, and rabies.[9]

SAINT PIERRE AND MIQUELON (FRANCE)
Yellow Fever
No requirements or recommendations.

Malaria
No malaria transmission.

Other Vaccines To Consider
Routine, hepatitis B, and rabies.[8]

SAINT VINCENT AND THE GRENADINES
Yellow Fever
Requirements: Required if traveling from a country with risk of YFV transmission and ≥1 year of age.[1]
Recommendations: None.

Malaria
No malaria transmission.

Other Vaccines To Consider
Routine, hepatitis A & B, typhoid, and rabies.[9]

SAMOA (FORMERLY WESTERN SAMOA)
Yellow Fever
Requirements: Required if traveling from a country with risk of YFV transmission and ≥1 year of age.[1]
Recommendations: None.

Malaria
No malaria transmission.

Other Vaccines To Consider
Routine, hepatitis A & B, and typhoid.

SAN MARINO
Yellow Fever
No requirements or recommendations.

Malaria
No malaria transmission.

Other Vaccines To Consider
Routine, hepatitis B, and rabies.[9]

SÃO TOMÉ AND PRÍNCIPE
Yellow Fever
Requirements: Required upon arrival from all countries for travelers ≥1 year of age.
Recommendations: *Generally not recommended* for travelers to São Tomé and Príncipe.

Malaria
Areas with malaria: All.
Estimated relative risk of malaria for US travelers: Very low.
Drug resistance[4]: Chloroquine.
Malaria species: *P. falciparum* 85%; remainder *P. malariae, P. ovale*, and *P. vivax*.
Recommended chemoprophylaxis: Atovaquone-proguanil, doxycycline, or mefloquine.

Other Vaccines To Consider
Routine, hepatitis A & B, typhoid, and rabies.[6]

SAUDI ARABIA
Yellow Fever
Requirements: Required if traveling from a country with risk of YFV transmission.[1]
Recommendations: None.

Malaria
Areas with malaria: Present in emirates by border with Yemen, specifically Asir and

Jizan. None in the cities of Jeddah, Mecca, Medina, Riyadh, and Ta'if.
Estimated relative risk of malaria for US travelers: Low.
Drug resistance[4]: Chloroquine.
Malaria species: *P. falciparum* predominantly, remainder *P. vivax.*
Recommended chemoprophylaxis: Atovaquone-proguanil, doxycycline, or mefloquine.

Other Vaccines To Consider
Routine, hepatitis A & B, typhoid, and rabies.[7]

SENEGAL
Yellow Fever
Requirements: Required if traveling from a country with risk of YFV transmission and ≥9 months of age and for travelers who have been in transit in an airport located in a country with risk of YFV transmission.[1]
Recommendations: *Recommended* for all travelers ≥9 months of age.

Malaria
Areas with malaria: All.
Estimated relative risk of malaria for US travelers: High.
Drug resistance[4]: Chloroquine.
Malaria species: *P. falciparum* >85%, *P. ovale* 5%–10%, *P. vivax* rare.
Recommended chemoprophylaxis: Atovaquone-proguanil, doxycycline, or mefloquine.

Other Vaccines To Consider
Routine, hepatitis A & B, typhoid, meningococcal, and rabies.[6]

SERBIA
Yellow Fever
No requirements or recommendations.

Malaria
No malaria transmission.

Other Vaccines To Consider
Routine, hepatitis A & B, and rabies.[7]

SEYCHELLES
Yellow Fever
Requirements: Required if traveling from a country with risk of YFV transmission and ≥1 year of age and for travelers who have been in transit in an airport located in a country with risk of YFV transmission.[1]
Recommendations: None.

Malaria
No malaria transmission.

Other Vaccines To Consider
Routine, hepatitis A & B, typhoid, and rabies.[9]

SIERRA LEONE
Yellow Fever
Requirements: Required upon arrival from all countries.
Recommendations: *Recommended* for all travelers ≥9 months of age.

Malaria
Areas with malaria: All.
Estimated relative risk of malaria for US travelers: High.
Drug resistance[4]: Chloroquine.
Malaria species: *P. falciparum* 85%, *P. ovale* potentially 5%–10%, *P. malariae* and *P. vivax* rare.
Recommended chemoprophylaxis: Atovaquone-proguanil, doxycycline, or mefloquine.

Other Vaccines To Consider
Routine, hepatitis A & B, typhoid, and rabies.[6]

SINGAPORE
Yellow Fever
Requirements: Required for travelers who are ≥1 year of age and who within the preceding 6 days have been in or have transited >12 hours in an airport located in a country with risk of YFV transmission.[1]
Recommendations: None.

Malaria
No malaria transmission.

Other Vaccines To Consider
Routine, hepatitis A & B, typhoid, and rabies.[9]

SLOVAKIA
Yellow Fever
No requirements or recommendations.

Malaria
No malaria transmission.

Other Vaccines To Consider
Routine, hepatitis A & B, and rabies.[9]

SLOVENIA
Yellow Fever
No requirements or recommendations.

Malaria
No malaria transmission.

Other Vaccines To Consider
Routine, hepatitis A & B, and rabies.[7]

SOLOMON ISLANDS
Yellow Fever
Requirements: Required if traveling from a country with risk of YFV transmission.[1]
Recommendations: None.

Malaria
Areas with malaria: All.
Estimated relative risk of malaria for US travelers: High.
Drug resistance[4]: Chloroquine.
Malaria species: *P. falciparum* 60%, *P. vivax* 35%–40%, *P. ovale* <1%.
Recommended chemoprophylaxis: Atovaquone-proguanil, doxycycline, or mefloquine.

Other Vaccines To Consider
Routine, hepatitis A & B, and typhoid.

SOMALIA
Yellow Fever
Requirements: Required if traveling from a country with risk of YFV transmission.[1]
Recommendations:
Generally not recommended for travelers going to the following regions: Bakool, Banaadir, Bay, Galguduud, Gedo, Hiiraan, Lower Jubabada, Lower Shabelle, Middle Jubabada, and Middle Shabelle (see Map 3-16).
Not recommended for all other areas not listed above.

Malaria
Areas with malaria: All.
Estimated relative risk of malaria for US travelers: High.
Drug resistance[4]: Chloroquine.
Malaria species: *P. falciparum* 90%, *P. vivax* 5%–10%, *P. malariae* and *P. ovale* rare.
Recommended chemoprophylaxis: Atovaquone-proguanil, doxycycline, or mefloquine.

Other Vaccines To Consider
Routine, hepatitis A & B, typhoid, and rabies.[6]

SOUTH AFRICA (See Map 3-39.)
Yellow Fever
Requirements: Required for travelers ≥1 year of age arriving from countries with risk of YFV transmission and from Eritrea, São Tomé and Príncipe, Somalia, the United Republic of Tanzania, and Zambia.[1] Vaccine is also required if the traveler has been in transit in an airport located in a country with risk of YFV transmission.[1]
Recommendations: None.

Malaria
Areas with malaria: Present in northeastern KwaZulu-Natal Province as far south as the Tugela River, Limpopo (Northern) Province, and Mpumalanga Province. Present in Kruger National Park.
Estimated relative risk of malaria for US travelers: Low.
Drug resistance[4]: Chloroquine.
Malaria species: *P. falciparum* 90%, *P. vivax* 5%, *P. ovale* 5%.
Recommended chemoprophylaxis: Atovaquone-proguanil, doxycycline, or mefloquine.

Other Vaccines To Consider
Routine, hepatitis A & B, typhoid, and rabies.[6]

SOUTH GEORGIA AND SOUTH SANDWICH ISLANDS (UK)
Yellow Fever
Requirements: These islands have not stated their yellow fever vaccination certificate requirements.
Recommendations: None.

Malaria
No malaria transmission.

Other Vaccines To Consider
Routine, hepatitis A & B, and typhoid.

SOUTH KOREA
Yellow Fever
No requirements or recommendations.

Malaria
Areas with malaria: Limited to the months of March–December in rural areas in the northern parts of Incheon, Kangwon-do, and Kyônggi-do Provinces, including the demilitarized zone (DMZ).
Estimated relative risk of malaria for US travelers: Low.
Drug resistance[4]: None.
Malaria species: *P. vivax* 100%.

*All footnotes are located on page 404.

Recommended chemoprophylaxis:
Atovaquone-proguanil, chloroquine,
doxycycline, mefloquine, or primaquine.[5]

Other Vaccines To Consider
Routine, hepatitis A & B, typhoid, Japanese
encephalitis, and rabies.[7]

SOUTH SUDAN, REPUBLIC OF
Yellow Fever
Requirements: This country has not stated
its yellow fever vaccination certificate
requirements.
Recommendations: *Recommended* for all
travelers ≥9 months of age.

Malaria
Areas with malaria: All.
**Estimated relative risk of malaria for US
travelers:** High.
Drug resistance[4]: Chloroquine.
Malaria species: *P. falciparum* 90%, *P. vivax*
5%–10%, *P. malariae* and *P. ovale* rare.

Recommended chemoprophylaxis: Atovaquone-
proguanil, doxycycline, or mefloquine.

Other Vaccines To Consider
Routine, hepatitis A & B, typhoid, adult polio
booster, meningococcal, and rabies.[6]

SPAIN
Yellow Fever
No requirements or recommendations.

Malaria
No malaria transmission.

Other Vaccines To Consider
Routine, hepatitis B, and rabies.[9]

SRI LANKA
Yellow Fever
Requirements: Required if traveling from a
country with risk of YFV transmission and
≥1 year of age.[1]
Recommendations: None.

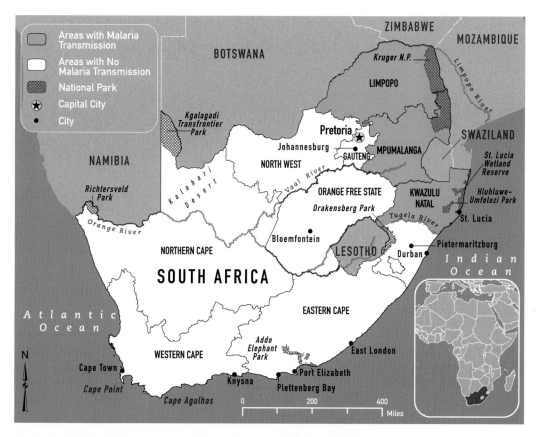

MAP 3-39. MALARIA TRANSMISSION AREAS IN SOUTH AFRICA

Malaria

Areas with malaria: All areas, except none in the districts of Colombo, Galle, Gampaha, Kalutara, Matara, and Nuwara Eliya.
Estimated relative risk of malaria for US travelers: Very low.
Drug resistance[4]: Chloroquine.
Malaria species: *P. vivax* 85%, *P. falciparum* 15%.
Recommended chemoprophylaxis: Atovaquone-proguanil, doxycycline, or mefloquine.

Other Vaccines To Consider

Routine, hepatitis A & B, typhoid, Japanese encephalitis, and rabies.[6]

SUDAN

Yellow Fever

Requirements: Required if traveling from a country with risk of YFV transmission and ≥9 months of age.[1] A certificate may be required for travelers departing Sudan.
Recommendations:
Recommended for all travelers ≥9 months of age traveling to areas south of the Sahara Desert (see Map 3-16).
Not recommended for travelers whose itineraries are limited to areas in the Sahara Desert and the city of Khartoum (see Map 3-16).

Malaria

Areas with malaria: All.
Estimated relative risk of malaria for US travelers: High.
Drug resistance[4]: Chloroquine.
Malaria species: *P. falciparum* 90%, *P. vivax* 5%–10%, *P. malariae* and *P. ovale* rare.
Recommended chemoprophylaxis: Atovaquone-proguanil, doxycycline, or mefloquine.

Other Vaccines To Consider

Routine, hepatitis A & B, typhoid, adult polio booster, meningococcal, and rabies.[6]

SURINAME

Yellow Fever

Requirements: Required if traveling from a country with risk of YFV transmission and ≥1 year of age.[1]
Recommendations: *Recommended* for all travelers ≥9 months of age.

Malaria

Areas with malaria: Present in provinces of Brokopondo and Sipaliwini. Rare cases in Paramaribo.
Estimated relative risk of malaria for US travelers: Moderate.
Drug resistance[4]: Chloroquine.
Malaria species: *P. falciparum* 70%, *P. vivax* 15%–20%.
Recommended chemoprophylaxis: All areas except Paramaribo: Atovaquone-proguanil, doxycycline, or mefloquine. Paramaribo: Mosquito avoidance only.

Other Vaccines To Consider

Routine, hepatitis A & B, typhoid, and rabies.[6]

SWAZILAND

Yellow Fever

Requirements: Required if traveling from a country with risk of YFV transmission.[1]
Recommendations: None.

Malaria

Areas with malaria: Present in eastern areas bordering Mozambique and South Africa, including all of Lubombo district and the eastern half of Hhohho, Manzini, and Shiselweni districts.
Estimated relative risk of malaria for US travelers: Very low.
Drug resistance[4]: Chloroquine.
Malaria species: *P. falciparum* 90%, *P. vivax* 5%, *P. ovale* 5%.
Recommended chemoprophylaxis: Atovaquone-proguanil, doxycycline, or mefloquine.

Other Vaccines To Consider

Routine, hepatitis A & B, typhoid, and rabies.[6]

SWEDEN

Yellow Fever

No requirements or recommendations.

Malaria

No malaria transmission.

Other Vaccines To Consider

Routine, hepatitis B, and rabies.[9]

SWITZERLAND

Yellow Fever

No requirements or recommendations.

Malaria

No malaria transmission.

*All footnotes are located on page 404.

Other Vaccines To Consider
Routine, hepatitis B, and rabies.[9]

SYRIA
Yellow Fever
Requirements: Required if traveling from a country with risk of YFV transmission and ≥6 months of age and for travelers who have been in transit for >12 hours in an airport located in a country with risk of YFV transmission.[1]
Recommendations: None.

Malaria
No malaria transmission.

Other Vaccines To Consider
Routine, hepatitis A & B, typhoid, and rabies.[6]

TAIWAN
Yellow Fever
No requirements or recommendations.

Malaria
No malaria transmission.

Other Vaccines To Consider
Routine, hepatitis A & B, Japanese encephalitis, and rabies.[9]

TAJIKISTAN
Yellow Fever
No requirements or recommendations.

Malaria
Areas with malaria: All areas <2,000 m (6,561 ft).
Estimated relative risk of malaria for US travelers: Very low.
Drug resistance[4]: Chloroquine.
Malaria species: *P. vivax* 90%, *P. falciparum* 10%.
Recommended chemoprophylaxis: Atovaquone-proguanil, doxycycline, mefloquine, or primaquine.[5]

Other Vaccines To Consider
Routine, hepatitis A & B, typhoid, adult polio booster, and rabies.[6]

TANZANIA
Yellow Fever
Requirements: Required if traveling from a country with risk of YFV transmission and ≥1 year of age.[1]
Recommendations: *Generally not recommended* for travelers to Tanzania.

Malaria
Areas with malaria: All areas <1,800 m (5,906 ft).
Estimated relative risk of malaria for US travelers: Moderate.
Drug resistance[4]: Chloroquine.
Malaria species: *P. falciparum* >85%, *P. ovale* >10%, *P. malariae* and *P. vivax* rare.
Recommended chemoprophylaxis: Atovaquone-proguanil, doxycycline, or mefloquine.

Other Vaccines To Consider
Routine, hepatitis A & B, typhoid, adult polio booster, and rabies.[6]

THAILAND
Yellow Fever
Requirements: Required if traveling from a country with risk of YFV transmission and ≥1 year of age and for travelers who have been in transit in an airport located in a country with risk of YFV transmission.[1]
Recommendations: None.

Malaria
Areas with malaria: Rural, forested areas that border Burma (Myanmar), Cambodia, and Laos. Rural, forested areas in districts of Phang Nga and Phuket. None in the cities of Bangkok, Chiang Mai, Chiang Rai, Koh Phangan, Koh Samui, Pattaya, Phang Nga, and Phuket.
Estimated relative risk of malaria for US travelers: Low.
Drug resistance[4]: Chloroquine and mefloquine.
Malaria species: *P. falciparum* 50% (up to 75% in some areas), *P. vivax* 50% (up to 60% in some areas), remainder *P. ovale*.
Recommended chemoprophylaxis: Atovaquone-proguanil or doxycycline.

Other Vaccines To Consider
Routine, hepatitis A & B, typhoid, Japanese encephalitis, and rabies.[7]

TIMOR-LESTE
Yellow Fever
Requirements: Required if traveling from a country with risk of YFV transmission and ≥1 year of age.[1]
Recommendations: None.

Malaria
Areas with malaria: All.
Estimated relative risk of malaria for US travelers: No data.

Drug resistance[4]: Chloroquine.
Malaria Species: *P. falciparum* 50%, *P. vivax* 50%, *P. ovale* <1%, *P. malariae* <1%.
Recommended chemoprophylaxis: Atovaquone-proguanil, doxycycline, or mefloquine.

Other Vaccines To Consider
Routine, hepatitis A & B, typhoid, Japanese encephalitis, and rabies.[6]

TOGO
Yellow Fever
Requirements: Required upon arrival from all countries for travelers ≥1 year of age.
Recommendations: *Recommended* for all travelers ≥9 months of age.

Malaria
Areas with malaria: All.
Estimated relative risk of malaria for US travelers: High.
Drug resistance[4]: Chloroquine.
Malaria species: *P. falciparum* 85%, *P. ovale* 5%–10%, remainder *P. vivax*.
Recommended chemoprophylaxis: Atovaquone-proguanil, doxycycline, or mefloquine.

Other Vaccines To Consider
Routine, hepatitis A & B, typhoid, meningococcal, and rabies.[6]

TOKELAU (NEW ZEALAND)
Yellow Fever
No requirements or recommendations.

Malaria
No malaria transmission.

Other Vaccines To Consider
Routine, hepatitis A & B, and typhoid.

TONGA
Yellow Fever
No requirements or recommendations.

Malaria
No malaria transmission.

Other Vaccines To Consider
Routine, hepatitis A & B, and typhoid.

TRINIDAD AND TOBAGO
Yellow Fever
Requirements: Required if traveling from a country with risk of YFV transmission and ≥1 year of age.[1]

Recommendations:
Recommended for all travelers ≥9 months of age traveling to the island of Trinidad, except as mentioned below.
Generally not recommended for travelers whose itinerary is limited to the urban areas of Port of Spain, cruise ship passengers who do not disembark from the ship, and airplane passengers in transit.
Not recommended for travelers whose itineraries are limited to the island of Tobago.

Malaria
No malaria transmission.

Other Vaccines To Consider
Routine, hepatitis A & B, typhoid, and rabies.[9]

TUNISIA
Yellow Fever
Requirements: Required if traveling from a country with risk of YFV transmission and ≥1 year of age.[1]
Recommendations: None.

Malaria
No malaria transmission.

Other Vaccines To Consider
Routine, hepatitis A & B, typhoid, and rabies.[6]

TURKEY
Yellow Fever
No requirements or recommendations.

Malaria
Areas with malaria: Present in southeastern part of the country. None on the Incerlik US Air Force Base or on typical cruise itineraries.
Estimated relative risk of malaria for US travelers: Very low.
Drug resistance[4]: None.
Malaria species: *P. vivax* predominantly, *P. falciparum* sporadically.
Recommended chemoprophylaxis: Atovaquone-proguanil, chloroquine, doxycycline, mefloquine, or primaquine.[5]

Other Vaccines To Consider
Routine, hepatitis A & B, typhoid, and rabies.[6]

TURKMENISTAN
Yellow Fever
No requirements or recommendations.

*All footnotes are located on page 404.

Malaria
No malaria transmission.

Other Vaccines To Consider
Routine, hepatitis A & B, typhoid, adult polio booster, and rabies.[6]

TURKS AND CAICOS ISLANDS (UK)
Yellow Fever
Requirements: Required if traveling from a country with risk of YFV transmission and ≥1 year of age.[1]
Recommendations: None.

Malaria
No malaria transmission.

Other Vaccines To Consider
Routine, hepatitis A & B, typhoid, and rabies.[9]

TUVALU
Yellow Fever
No requirements or recommendations.

Malaria
No malaria transmission.

Other Vaccines To Consider
Routine, hepatitis A & B, and typhoid.

UGANDA
Yellow Fever
Requirements: Required if traveling from a country with risk of YFV transmission and ≥1 year of age.[1]
Recommendations: *Recommended* for all travelers ≥9 months of age.

Malaria
Areas with malaria: All.
Estimated relative risk of malaria for US travelers: High.
Drug resistance[4]: Chloroquine.
Malaria species: *P. falciparum* >85%; remainder *P. malariae*, *P. ovale*, and *P. vivax*.
Recommended chemoprophylaxis: Atovaquone-proguanil, doxycycline, or mefloquine.

Other Vaccines To Consider
Routine, hepatitis A & B, typhoid, adult polio booster, meningococcal, and rabies.[6]

UKRAINE
Yellow Fever
No requirements or recommendations.

Malaria
No malaria transmission.

Other Vaccines To Consider
Routine, hepatitis A & B, and rabies.[7]

UNITED ARAB EMIRATES
Yellow Fever
No requirements or recommendations.

Malaria
No malaria transmission.

Other Vaccines To Consider
Routine, hepatitis A & B, typhoid, and rabies.[7]

UNITED KINGDOM, WITH CHANNEL ISLANDS AND ISLE OF MAN
Yellow Fever
No requirements or recommendations.

Malaria
No malaria transmission.

Other Vaccines To Consider
Routine, hepatitis B, and rabies.[9]

UNITED STATES
Yellow Fever
No requirements or recommendations.

Malaria
No malaria transmission.

Other Vaccines To Consider
Routine, hepatitis B, and rabies.[8]

URUGUAY
Yellow Fever
Requirements: Required if traveling from a country with risk of YFV transmission.[1]
Recommendations: None.

Malaria
No malaria transmission.

Other Vaccines To Consider
Routine, hepatitis A & B, typhoid, and rabies.[9]

UZBEKISTAN
Yellow Fever
No requirements or recommendations.

Malaria
No malaria transmission.

Other Vaccines To Consider
Routine, hepatitis A & B, typhoid, adult polio booster, and rabies.[6]

VANUATU
Yellow Fever
No requirements or recommendations.

Malaria
Areas with malaria: All.
Estimated relative risk of malaria for US travelers: Moderate.
Drug resistance[4]: Chloroquine.
Malaria species: *P. falciparum* 60%, *P. vivax* 35%–40%, *P. ovale* <1%.
Recommended chemoprophylaxis: Atovaquone-proguanil, doxycycline, or mefloquine.

Other Vaccines To Consider
Routine, hepatitis A & B, and typhoid.

VENEZUELA (See Map 3-40.)
Yellow Fever
Requirements: None.

Recommendations:
Recommended for all travelers ≥9 months of age, except as mentioned below.
Generally not recommended for travelers whose itinerary is limited to the following areas: the states of Aragua, Carabobo, Miranda, Vargas, and Yaracuy, and the Distrito Federal (see Map 3-17).
Not recommended for travelers whose itineraries are limited to the following areas: the states of Falcón and Lara, the peninsular section of Paez Municipality in Zulia Province, Margarita Island, and the cities of Caracas and Valencia (see Map 3-17).

Malaria
Areas with malaria: Rural areas of the following states: Amazonas, Anzoátegui, Apure, Bolivar, Delta Amacuro, Monagas, Sucre, and Zulia. Present in Angel Falls. None in city of Caracas and Margarita Island.
Estimated relative risk of malaria for US travelers: Low.
Drug resistance[4]: Chloroquine.
Malaria species: *P. vivax* 83%, *P. falciparum* 17%.

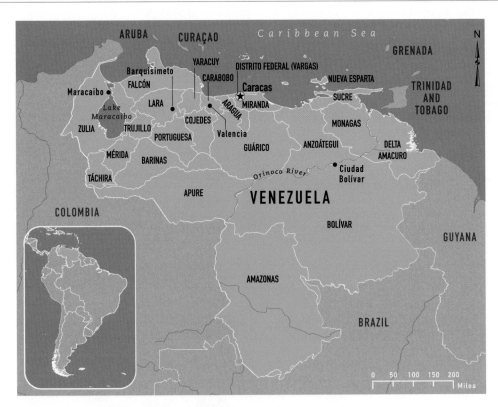

MAP 3-40. VENEZUELA REFERENCE MAP

*All footnotes are located on page 404.

Recommended chemoprophylaxis:
Atovaquone-proguanil, doxycycline, or
mefloquine.

Other Vaccines To Consider
Routine, hepatitis A & B, typhoid, and rabies.[6]

VIETNAM
Yellow Fever
Requirements: Required if traveling from a
country with risk of YFV transmission and
≥1 year of age.[1]
Recommendations: None.

Malaria
Areas with malaria: Rural areas only, except
none in the Red River Delta. Rare cases in the
Mekong Delta. None in Da Nang, Haiphong,
Hanoi, Ho Chi Minh City (Saigon), Nha Trang,
and Qui Nhon.
**Estimated relative risk of malaria for US
travelers:** Low.
Drug resistance[4]: Chloroquine and
mefloquine.
Malaria species: *P. falciparum* 50%–90%,
remainder *P. vivax*.
Recommended chemoprophylaxis:
Southern part of the country in the provinces
of Dac Lac, Gia Lai, Khanh Hoa, Kon Tum,
Lam Dong, Ninh Thuan, Song Be, Tay Ninh:
Atovaquone-proguanil or doxycycline.
Other areas with malaria except Mekong
Delta: Atovaquone-proguanil, doxycycline, or
mefloquine.
Mekong Delta: Mosquito avoidance only.

Other Vaccines To Consider
Routine, hepatitis A & B, typhoid, Japanese
encephalitis, and rabies.[6]

VIRGIN ISLANDS, BRITISH
Yellow Fever
No requirements or recommendations.

Malaria
No malaria transmission.

Other Vaccines To Consider
Routine, hepatitis A & B, typhoid,
and rabies.[9]

VIRGIN ISLANDS, US
Yellow Fever
No requirements or recommendations.

Malaria
No malaria transmission.

Other Vaccines To Consider
Routine, hepatitis A & B, typhoid, and rabies.[9]

WAKE ISLAND, US
Yellow Fever
No requirements or recommendations.

Malaria
No malaria transmission.

Other Vaccines To Consider
Routine, hepatitis A & B, and typhoid.

WALLIS AND FUTUNA ISLANDS (FRANCE)
Yellow Fever
Requirements: These islands have not stated
their yellow fever vaccination certificate
requirements.
Recommendations: None.

Malaria
No malaria transmission.

Other Vaccines To Consider
Routine, hepatitis A & B, and typhoid.

WESTERN SAHARA
Yellow Fever
Requirements: This territory has not stated
its yellow fever vaccination certificate
requirements.
Recommendations: None.

Malaria
Areas with malaria: Rare cases.
**Estimated relative risk of malaria for US
travelers:** No data.
Drug resistance[4]: Chloroquine.
Malaria species: Unknown.
Recommended chemoprophylaxis: Mosquito
avoidance only.

Other Vaccines To Consider
Routine, hepatitis A & B, typhoid, and rabies.[6]

YEMEN
Yellow Fever
Requirements: Required if traveling from a
country with risk of YFV transmission and
≥1 year of age.[1]
Recommendations: None.

Malaria
Areas with malaria: All areas <2,000 m
(6,561 ft). None in Sana'a.
**Estimated relative risk of malaria for US
travelers:** Low.
Drug resistance[4]: Chloroquine.

Malaria species: *P. falciparum* 95%; *P. malariae*, *P. vivax*, and *P. ovale* 5% combined.
Recommended chemoprophylaxis: Atovaquone-proguanil, doxycycline, or mefloquine.

Other Vaccines To Consider
Routine, hepatitis A & B, typhoid, and rabies.[6]

ZAMBIA
Yellow Fever
Requirements: Required if traveling from a country with risk of YFV transmission and ≥9 months of age.[1] Vaccine is also required if the traveler has been in transit for >12 hours in the airport of a country with risk of YFV transmission.
Recommendations:
Generally not recommended for travelers going to the North West and Western Provinces.
Not recommended in all other areas not listed above.

Malaria
Areas with malaria: All.
Estimated relative risk of malaria for US travelers: Moderate.
Drug resistance[4]: Chloroquine.

Malaria species: *P. falciparum* >90%, *P. vivax* up to 5%, *P. ovale* up to 5%.
Recommended chemoprophylaxis: Atovaquone-proguanil, doxycycline, or mefloquine.

Other Vaccines To Consider
Routine, hepatitis A & B, typhoid, adult polio booster, and rabies.[6]

ZIMBABWE
Yellow Fever
Requirements: Required if traveling from a country with risk of YFV transmission.[1]
Recommendations: None.

Malaria
Areas with malaria: All.
Estimated relative risk of malaria for US travelers: Moderate.
Drug resistance[4]: Chloroquine.
Malaria species: *P. falciparum* >90%, *P. vivax* up to 5%, *P. ovale* up to 5%.
Recommended chemoprophylaxis: Atovaquone-proguanil, doxycycline, or mefloquine.

Other Vaccines To Consider
Routine, hepatitis A & B, typhoid, and rabies.[6]

FOOTNOTES:

Yellow Fever
[1] The official WHO list of countries with risk of YFV transmission can be found in Table 3-21. Proof of yellow fever vaccination should be required only if traveling from a country on the WHO list, unless otherwise specified. The following countries, containing only areas with low potential for exposure to YFV, are not on the WHO list: Eritrea, São Tomé and Príncipe, Somalia, Tanzania, Zambia.
[2] An elevation of 2,300 m is equivalent to 7,546 ft.

Malaria
[3] This risk estimate is based largely on cases occurring in US military personnel who travel for extended periods of time with unique itineraries that likely do not reflect the risk for the average US traveler.
[4] Refers to *P. falciparum* malaria unless otherwise noted.
[5] Primaquine can cause hemolytic anemia in people with glucose-6-phosphate dehydrogenase (G6PD) deficiency. Patients must be screened for G6PD deficiency before starting primaquine.

Rabies
[6] Canine rabies and bat lyssavirus present. Rabies also present in other mammals. Vaccine recommended for the following groups:
  • Travelers involved in outdoor and other activities that might bring them into direct contact with dogs, bats, and other mammals (such as campers, hikers, bikers, adventure travelers, and cavers).
  • Those with occupational risks (such as veterinarians, wildlife professionals, researchers).
  • Long-term travelers and expatriates.
  • Children are considered at higher risk; consider lower threshold for vaccination.
[7] Bat lyssavirus and rabies in other mammalian carnivores present. Canine rabies present but not a significant concern to travelers. Vaccine is recommended only for the following groups:
  • Travelers involved in outdoor and other activities in remote areas that might bring them into direct contact with dogs, bats, and other mammals (such as adventure travelers and cavers).
  • Those with occupational risks (such as veterinarians, wildlife professionals, researchers).
  • Long-term travelers and expatriates visiting remote areas.
  • Children are considered at higher risk; consider lower threshold for vaccination.
[8] Bat lyssavirus and rabies in other mammalian carnivores present. Canine rabies is not present. Vaccine is recommended only for the following groups:
  • Travelers involved in outdoor and other activities in remote areas that might bring them into direct contact with bats and other mammals (such as adventure travelers and cavers).
  • Those with occupational risks (such as wildlife professionals and researchers).
[9] Bat lyssavirus present or suspected; canine rabies not present. Vaccine is recommended only for the following groups:
  • Travelers involved in outdoor and other activities in remote areas that might bring them into direct contact with bats (such as adventure travelers and cavers).
  • Those with occupational risks (such as wildlife professionals and researchers).

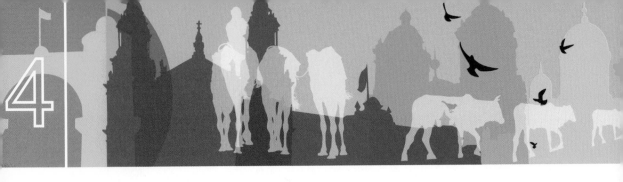

Select Destinations

RATIONALE FOR SELECT DESTINATIONS
David R. Shlim

The quality of travel health advice is based on trying to reduce risks for the traveler in a particular destination. Our ability to counsel travelers is improved when we have visited a particular destination ourselves, or at least are familiar with typical itineraries and the specifics of health risks. However, our own travel experiences rarely encompass all the destinations that our clients plan to visit. Thus, this chapter of the Yellow Book was created to allow experts who have lived in or have frequently visited particular destinations to share their insider's knowledge of these places.

Each of these sections should be considered a personal perspective on the area discussed. They are editorial in nature, containing the author's expressed opinions, and aim to present topics for consideration; they should not necessarily be taken as a prescription for pre-travel care. Preventive recommendations that are covered elsewhere in the book are usually not repeated in these chapters, other than to address controversies or to emphasize important points.

The destination sections have proved to be one of the most popular features of the Yellow Book. The goals of these sections are to help a travel health provider feel more comfortable giving advice about specific destinations that he or she may have never visited, and to provide a level of detail about the attractions and health risks at select destinations that has not been provided elsewhere in this book.

AFRICA

EAST AFRICA: SAFARIS
Karl Neumann

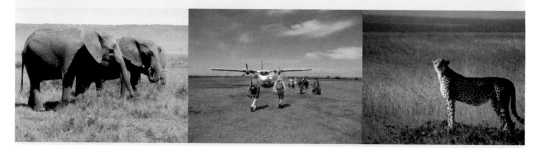

DESTINATION OVERVIEW

Arguably the ultimate in adventure travel, an African safari is also an easily doable family vacation, an experience of a lifetime for people of all ages, and with a little research, not much more difficult to arrange than a week at a Caribbean resort. While the centerpiece of safari-going remains viewing majestic animals in their natural habitats, many tour operators now include programs on local culture, history, geology, and ecosystems and encourage travelers to get to know the people not merely as subjects of photos. Safaris can also be differentiated by the topography, vegetation, and bird life of the region. There are safaris for families, honeymooners, and people with similar interests (serious photography, for example). Many safaris accept children as young as 6 years and have special age-appropriate programs for children and adolescents aged 6–16 years.

Animals can be viewed from open trucks, air-conditioned vans, private aircraft, hot air balloons, or while hiking (where animals are friendly). Trips need not be strenuous. Accommodations range from crawl-in tents to portable, air-conditioned, walk-in tents with full bathrooms. There are even luxurious 5-star lodges with floodlit water holes to view animals at night. Lunch in the wilderness varies from prepackaged sandwiches eaten sitting on a tree stump to 3-course meals served on tables covered with linen cloths and matching napkins. Some safaris include side trips to exotic places—to see or climb Mount Kilimanjaro, visit Zanzibar, or view Victoria Falls, for example.

Travelers on their first safari often choose game parks in Kenya and Tanzania, in East Africa. The most famous game park in Kenya is the Masai Mara National Reserve, which, in effect, is the northern continuation of the Serengeti National Park game reserve in Tanzania, together forming the home of perhaps the grandest and most complete collection of the large wild animals for which Africa is famous. The Serengeti is the starting point of the annual migration of about 2 million wildebeest and several hundred thousand zebras as they search for pasture and water. Tanzania also has the Ngorongoro Crater, a 100-square mile depression (caldera) formed when a giant volcano, perhaps the size of Mount Kilimanjaro, exploded and collapsed on itself millions of years ago. The crater has most of the same animals as the Masai Mara reserve. The major East African game parks are shown on Map 4-1.

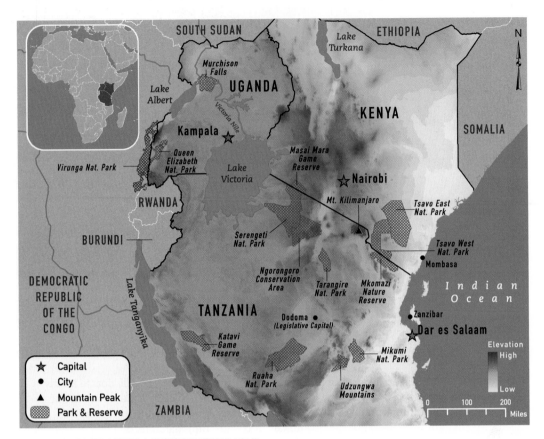

MAP 4-1. EAST AFRICA DESTINATION MAP

Travelers should research the optimum time of the year for their safari. The wildebeest migration in the Serengeti is a seasonal event, for example, although the precise time of the migration may vary from year to year. Some parks have a dry season, offering better views of the animals, as the vegetation is sparser. And many areas of Africa have times of the year that are more comfortable for visitors, with cooler weather, less humidity, and less chance of rain.

HEALTH ISSUES

Health and safety issues that safari-goers are likely to encounter are mostly predictable and largely avoidable. The best insurance for carefree trips is a pre-travel consultation with a travel health provider, choosing an experienced and sophisticated tour operator, and taking along a small, personalized medical kit (see Chapter 2, Travel Health Kits).

Experienced tour operators generally require that clients buy medical evacuation insurance, supply clients with ample literature relating to local conditions, and employ knowledgeable guides who carry first aid kits and communication equipment to summon help, if necessary (see Chapter 2, Travel Insurance, Travel Health Insurance, & Medical Evacuation Insurance).

Health advice must be itinerary- and game park–specific. Immunizations and preventive medications necessary for one park may not be necessary for others. Parks may be long distances apart and located in countries with different health standards and dissimilar climates and various altitudes.

Generally, proper preparations, common sense precautions, the short duration of most trips (usually ≤2 weeks), experienced guides, and leaving the driving to others make safaris relatively low-risk undertakings for travelers of all ages.

Food and Water

Travelers' diarrhea appears to be the most common ailment, and most cases are mild. Sensible food and water selections may reduce the incidence (see Chapter 2, Food & Water Precautions). Illness may occur even on deluxe trips. Carrying medication for self-treatment is generally recommended (see Chapter 2, Travelers' Diarrhea).

Animals

Wild animals are unpredictable. Travelers should follow oral and written instructions provided by safari operators. Animal-related injuries are extremely rare and are usually the result of disregarding rules, such as approaching animals too closely to feed or photograph them.

Rabies exists throughout Africa. While most cases result from bites from dogs, all mammals are susceptible and could transmit the virus. Wounds from mammals should be considered a risk for rabies exposure unless proven otherwise. Licks can also result in rabies, if the virus enters through minor breaks in the skin. In addition to rabies, bats may also transmit other diseases to humans, such as viral hemorrhagic fevers. Travelers should be encouraged to avoid entering caves where bats are known to be present. Recent cases of Marburg fever have occurred in travelers who visited a python cave in western Uganda.

Malaria

Malaria transmission occurs in most game parks. Most infections are caused by *Plasmodium falciparum*, and all *P. falciparum* in sub-Saharan Africa should be considered to be chloroquine-resistant. Safari activities often include sleeping in tents and observing animals at dusk or after dark, sometimes near water holes, all increasing the risk of being bitten by malaria-carrying mosquitoes. Taking preventive medication and using personal protection techniques—wearing long-sleeved shirts and pants, using insect repellents, and sleeping under permethrin-impregnated mosquito netting—are essential.

Yellow Fever

Yellow fever vaccination is recommended for much of East Africa (see Chapter 3, Travel Vaccines & Malaria Information, by Country). In 2010, the World Health Organization and CDC reclassified a portion of East Africa to "low potential for exposure" to yellow fever virus and consequently downgraded the vaccination recommendation for these areas to "generally not recommended." This recommendation limits the need for vaccination to a small subset of travelers who are at increased risk for exposure to yellow fever virus (such as prolonged travel, heavy exposure to mosquitoes, or inability to avoid mosquito bites). These areas of East Africa where vaccine is generally not recommended include, but are not limited to, eastern Kenya, the cities of Nairobi and Mombasa, and all of Tanzania (see Chapter 3, Travel Vaccines & Malaria Information, by Country).

Some countries require a valid yellow fever vaccination certificate as a condition of entry. Moreover, some safaris include >1 country. Travelers must check the requirements of each country on their itinerary, including countries they only transit en route to their destination. Some countries may require the certificate even if there is no yellow fever in the country travelers are leaving or entering.

Other Health Risks

Tryp, dengue, filariasis, oncho, leish, myasis

African trypanosomiasis (sleeping sickness), a disease only rarely seen among travelers, is transmitted by day-biting tsetse flies (*Glossina*). Wearing light-colored clothing (and avoiding wearing blue) seems to deter the flies. Insect repellents are only partially effective. Symptoms include fever, eschar at the site of the bite, headache, and signs of central nervous system involvement. Several cases of trypanosomiasis (*rhodesiense*) have recently been reported in European tourists visiting the Masai Mara National Reserve in Kenya and wildlife reserves in Tanzania.

Dengue, filariasis, leishmaniasis, and onchocerciasis (river blindness) are other diseases carried by insects that occur in East Africa, but they rarely affect travelers. Swimming in freshwater ponds, lakes, and rivers can result in schistosomiasis (bilharzia), a parasite found in freshwater snails and transmitted by exposure to water. All freshwater sources should be considered contaminated. Swimming in the ocean or well-chlorinated pools is safe.

Myiasis and tungiasis are rare skin diseases among travelers. Myiasis is caused by fly larvae penetrating the skin and causing a boil-like lesion with a central aperture. Eggs are usually laid on clothing left to dry outdoors, and the larvae enter the skin when the clothing is worn. Clothing should be dried indoors or ironed before wearing. Tungiasis is caused by direct penetration of skin by sand fleas, causing small, painful nodules, often on the foot adjacent to toenails. Prevention includes wearing closed-toed footwear and not walking barefoot.

Symptoms of many diseases acquired in Africa may surface weeks and occasionally months after exposure, sometimes long after the traveler has returned home. Urge patients to report any history of international travel if they become ill after a trip.

Other Safety Risks

Although being a crime victim is an unusual occurrence for those on safari, robbery, muggings, and carjacking may occur in major urban centers, notably Nairobi and Mombasa. Street muggings during the day and night are common. The rates of fatal motor vehicle accidents in sub-Saharan Africa are among the highest in the world. Within game parks, serious motor vehicle accidents are rare, as the poor roads discourage speeding. However, travel in rural areas between parks is high risk, especially after dark. If at all possible, nighttime driving in sub-Saharan Africa should be avoided.

BIBLIOGRAPHY

1. Gautret P, Schlagenhauf P, Gaudart J, Castelli F, Brouqui P, von Sonnenburg F, et al. Multicenter EuroTravNet/GeoSentinel study of travel-related infectious diseases in Europe. Emerg Infect Dis. 2009 Nov;15(11):1783–90.
2. Meltzer E, Artom G, Marva E, Assous MV, Rahav G, Schwartzt E. Schistosomiasis among travelers: new aspects of an old disease. Emerg Infect Dis. 2006 Nov;12(11):1696–700.
3. Sinha A, Grace C, Alston WK, Westenfeld F, Maguire JH. African trypanosomiasis in two travelers from the United States. Clin Infect Dis. 1999 Oct;29(4):840–4.
4. Thrower Y, Goodyer LI. Application of insect repellents by travelers to malaria endemic areas. J Travel Med. 2006 Jul–Aug;13(4):198–202.
5. Trypanosomiasis (Sleeping sickness and Chagas disease). In: Field VK, Ford L, Hill DR, editors. Health Information for Overseas Travel. London: National Travel Health Network and Centre; 2010. p. 329–30.
6. United Nations office at Nairobi. Security in Kenya. Nairobi: United Nations office at Nairobi; 2012 [cited 2012 Sep 25]. Available from: http://dcs.unon.org/index.php?option=com_content&view=article&id=127&Itemid=177&lang=en.
7. World Health Organization. Global status report on road safety: time for action. Geneva: World Health Organization; 2009 [cited Sep 25]. Available from: http://www.who.int/violence_injury_prevention/road_safety_status/2009/en.

TANZANIA: KILIMANJARO

Kevin C. Kain

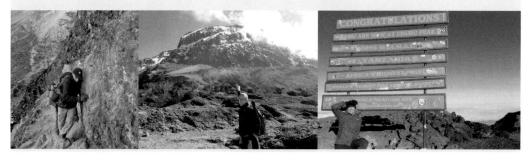

DESTINATION OVERVIEW

As the highest mountain in Africa and one of the largest freestanding volcanoes in the world, Kilimanjaro remains a revered and classic image of East Africa. Its snow-capped peak rising 19,341 ft (5,895 m) above the tropical African savanna is an irresistible draw for trekkers, particularly since no technical climbing is required to reach the summit. Kilimanjaro is one of the "seven summits" representing the highest peaks on each continent. However, because it does not involve technical climbing, the difficulties are often misjudged. Climbing Kilimanjaro is a serious undertaking, requiring serious preparation. Despite being higher than classic trekking destinations in Nepal, such as Kala Pattar (18,450 ft; 5,625 m) or Everest base camp (17,598 ft; 5,364 m), typical ascent rates on Kilimanjaro are considerably faster (4–6 days vs 8–12 days).

The classic route up Kilimanjaro is the Marangu route (64 km), usually sold as a "5 day, 4 night" trip. Marangu is frequently nicknamed the "Coca-Cola" route, since accommodation and food are provided in bunkhouses and the trail is wide and relatively easy compared with other routes. There are at least 9 alternative routes (Map 4-2), including the stunningly beautiful Machame route (the so-called "whiskey" route, since the days are generally longer, with tougher climbs). This author can vouch for the dramatic rugged beauty of this hike. Machame and other routes involve camping but are usually sold as 6- to 9-day packages, providing more opportunity to acclimatize and greater chances to successfully summit. Kilimanjaro can be climbed throughout the year (March–April are often the wettest months), but the weather is unpredictable, and the climber must be prepared for extreme weather and rain at any time of the year.

Climbing Kilimanjaro is a dream for many who visit Africa. However, a large number of travelers are ill-prepared, ascend too quickly, and consequently fail to summit. With due preparation and more reasonable ascent rates, climbing "Kili" is an aspiration that can be successfully and safely accomplished by many.

HEALTH ISSUES

The main medical issues for those attempting Kilimanjaro include the prevention and treatment of altitude illness and the potential for drug interactions between medications used for altitude illness and antimalarial or antidiarrheal agents commonly used by travelers to Tanzania.

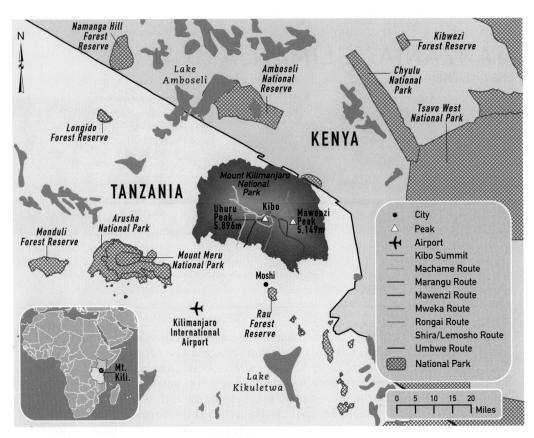

MAP 4-2. KILIMANJARO DESTINATION MAP

Altitude and Acute Mountain Sickness (AMS)

Diamox

Altitude illness is a problem on Kilimanjaro and a major contributor to the reason that only 50% of those attempting the standard 4- to 5-day Marangu route reach the crater rim, known as Gilman's Point (18,652 ft; 5,685 m), and as few as 10% reach the summit, known as Uhuru (Freedom) Peak (19,341 ft; 5,895 m). Prevalence rates of AMS were 75%–77% in recent studies of 4- and 5-day ascents on the Marangu route. Those using acetazolamide were significantly less likely to develop AMS on the 5-day ascents.

Every hiker on Kilimanjaro should receive pre-travel advice on AMS, be able to recognize symptoms, and know how to prevent and treat it. People with certain underlying medical conditions, including pregnancy, cardiac and lung disease, and ocular and neurologic conditions, may be more susceptible to altitude-associated problems or may be taking medications that may interact with altitude medications, and should consult a travel health provider with knowledge of altitude illness before travel.

Enjoying the experience and successfully reaching the summit can be enhanced by allowing more time to acclimatize:

> If Ngorongoro crater is part of the planned combined itinerary, try to spend the last few nights of the safari here, because its elevation (7,500 ft; 2,286 m) will aid acclimatization for the Kilimanjaro trek.
> It is strongly encouraged to add at least an extra day or two to the ascent of Kilimanjaro, regardless of the route, but especially on routes normally promoted as 4- to 6-day trips.

> If possible before attempting Kilimanjaro, acclimatize by hiking nearby Mount Meru (14,978 ft; 4,565 m) or Mount Kenya (to Point Lenana, 16,355 ft; 4,895 m). A number of combined climbing trips for Mount Kenya and Kilimanjaro are now offered commercially.

For those with a past history of susceptibility to AMS and for those in whom adequate acclimatization is not possible (most "Kili" clients), the use of medications such as acetazolamide to prevent altitude illness is recommended. Acetazolamide accelerates acclimatization, is effective in preventing (beginning the day before ascent) and treating AMS, and is safe in children.

For those who are intolerant or allergic to acetazolamide, dexamethasone is an alternative for prevention of AMS, but there are cautions involved in using dexamethasone for ascent. Consideration should be given to carrying a treatment course of dexamethasone for high-altitude cerebral edema (HACE). Travelers with symptoms of altitude illness must not continue to ascend and need to descend if symptoms are worsening at the same altitude. A flexible itinerary and having an extra guide who can accompany any member of the group down the mountain if he or she becomes ill are considerations. See Chapter 2, Altitude Illness for more information about prevention and treatment of altitude illness.

Malaria

Kilimanjaro is unique in that its tropical malaria-endemic location means that many trekkers will be on antimalarial drugs and may need to continue them after their climb, particularly if they are also visiting game parks and staying overnight at altitudes <1,800 m (5,906 ft). Malaria chemoprophylaxis is recommended for Tanzania (even if only for a short trip). If a traveler flew directly into Kilimanjaro International Airport (2,932 ft; 894 m) and went the same day to an altitude above 1,800 m, there would be no risk of malaria. However, most people will be on safari or traveling before or after their Kilimanjaro trip, and therefore will be on prophylaxis.

Kilimanjaro is also a unique destination in that high altitude will affect everyone, and possible interactions should be considered between drugs commonly used for chemoprophylaxis or treatment of AMS, high-altitude pulmonary edema, or high-altitude cerebral edema, such as acetazolamide, dexamethasone, and nifedipine. Fortunately, there are no reported clinically significant drug interactions between common malaria chemoprophylaxis agents (atovaquone-proguanil, doxycycline, or mefloquine) and acetazolamide or dexamethasone used to prevent or treat AMS. Nifedipine is metabolized by the CYP3A4 enzyme and concurrent use of CYP3A4 inhibitors, such as doxycycline, could lead to elevated plasma levels of nifedipine and potentially lower blood pressure. Therefore, it would not be advised to take nifedipine for altitude illness prophylaxis concurrently with doxycycline.

Treatment of Travelers' Diarrhea

There are no reported drug interactions between acetazolamide and the fluoroquinolones (ciprofloxacin, levofloxacin) or macrolides (azithromycin) commonly used to treat travelers' diarrhea. There is a potential increased risk of tendon rupture when dexamethasone is used with fluoroquinolones. Avoid concurrent use of macrolides and nifedipine.

Remote Travel

Treks on Kilimanjaro are physically demanding and require a good level of fitness and preparation for the elements. Kilimanjaro weather is characterized by extremes: be prepared for tropical heat, heavy rains, and bitter cold. Keep gear, especially one's sleeping bag, in waterproof bags. Travelers should have adequate health insurance, including medical evacuation insurance. Travelers are advised to make sure their medical care and medical evacuation policy will cover any potential costs for a rescue or evacuation from the top of the mountain.

Carry a first aid kit that includes bandages, tape, blister kit, antibacterial and antifungal cream, antibiotics for travelers' diarrhea, antimalarials, antiemetics, antihistamines, analgesics, cold and flu medications, throat lozenges, and altitude medications.

BIBLIOGRAPHY

1. Barry PW, Pollard AJ. Altitude illness. BMJ. 2003 Apr 26;326(7395):915–9.
2. Bartsch P, Gibbs JS. Effect of altitude on the heart and the lungs. Circulation. 2007 Nov 6;116(19):2191–202.
3. Basnyat B, Gertsch JH, Holck PS, Johnson EW, Luks AM, Donham BP, et al. Acetazolamide 125 mg BD is not significantly different from 375 mg BD in the prevention of acute mountain sickness: the prophylactic acetazolamide dosage comparison for efficacy (PACE) trial. High Alt Med Biol. 2006 Spring;7(1):17–27.
4. Baumgartner RW, Siegel AM, Hackett PH. Going high with preexisting neurological conditions. High Alt Med Biol. 2007 Summer;8(2):108–16.
5. Davies AJ, Kalson NS, Stokes S, Earl MD, Whitehead AG, Frost H, et al. Determinants of summiting success and acute mountain sickness on Mt Kilimanjaro (5895 m). Wilderness Environ Med. 2009 Winter;20(4):311–7.
6. Hackett PH, Roach RC. High-altitude illness. N Engl J Med. 2001 Jul 12;345(2):107–14.
7. Imray C, Booth A, Wright A, Bradwell A. Acute altitude illnesses. BMJ. 2011;343:d4943.
8. Jean D, Leal C, Kriemler S, Meijer H, Moore LG. Medical recommendations for women going to altitude. High Alt Med Biol. 2005 Spring;6(1):22–31.
9. Karinen H, Peltonen J, Tikkanen H. Prevalence of acute mountain sickness among Finnish trekkers on Mount Kilimanjaro, Tanzania: an observational study. High Alt Med Biol. 2008 Winter;9(4):301–6.
10. Luks AM, Swenson ER. Medication and dosage considerations in the prophylaxis and treatment of high-altitude illness. Chest. 2008 Mar;133(3):744–55.
11. Luks AM, Swenson ER. Travel to high altitude with pre-existing lung disease. Eur Respir J. 2007 Apr;29(4):770–92.
12. Mader TH, Tabin G. Going to high altitude with preexisting ocular conditions. High Alt Med Biol. 2003 Winter;4(4):419–30.
13. Strom BL, Schinnar R, Apter AJ, Margolis DJ, Lautenbach E, Hennessy S, et al. Absence of cross-reactivity between sulfonamide antibiotics and sulfonamide nonantibiotics. N Engl J Med. 2003 Oct 23;349(17):1628–35.

SOUTH AFRICA

Gary W. Brunette

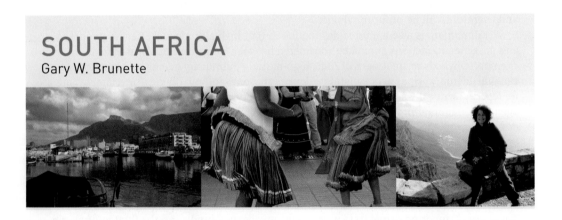

DESTINATION OVERVIEW

South Africa has been called "a world in one country." This refers, in part, to the diversity in the geography, which includes lush subtropical regions, old hardwood forests, sweeping Highveld vistas, and the deep desert of the Kalahari; the splendor of the animal species found throughout the country and protected in expansive game reserves; the diverse origins of the locals (from Africa, Europe, India, and Southeast Asia); the cultural, artistic, and culinary variety; and access to the conveniences of a developed infrastructure amid the challenges of Africa.

South Africa has experienced a surge in tourism in the last 2 decades, with visitors from within the African continent, as well as those from Europe and North America. Business travelers typically head to the commercial centers of Johannesburg, Cape Town, and Durban. Tourists may be attracted by the game reserves, the largest of which is Kruger National Park, located along the Mozambique border in the northeast. Kwa-Zulu Natal has a number of game parks (Hluhluwe-Umfolozi and Saint Lucia) set inland from Durban, and the Eastern Cape has parks (Addo Elephant Park and Shamwari) easily accessed from Port Elizabeth on the southern coast. Many smaller luxury reserves have emerged to cater to the high-end traveler. Visitors may be attracted to itineraries that include a trip from Cape Town along the south coast through the small scenic towns of Knysna and Plettenberg Bay; a tour of the old gold-mining towns in Mpumalanga, many of which are in near-original condition; spectacular drives and fascinating tours of the old wineries along the wine routes in the Western Cape; or visits to the southernmost point of Africa at Cape Agulhas or Cape Point, where the Indian and Atlantic Oceans meet in a roar of foam.

South Africa is also a common destination of humanitarian workers, missionaries, and students. A sizable number of South Africans live outside the country and would be considered VFRs (visiting friends and relatives) when returning to the country for a visit.

While there is a wide range of living standards in South Africa, most visitors experience standards comparable to those in developed countries. A smaller number of visitors may go to less developed areas, either the lower-income townships outside most towns and cities or to rural areas. Hikers, adventure-seekers, and missionaries will experience a wider range of living standards. Similarly, the quality and availability of health care are variable. Middle- and upper-income South Africans live in low-risk environments, have a standard of health comparable to that of North Americans, and have access to world-class medical facilities. Poorer South Africans live in areas with few amenities, are exposed to a wide range of diseases, and have limited access to adequate health care.

HEALTH ISSUES

Vaccine-Preventable Diseases

All travelers to South Africa should be up-to-date with their routine vaccinations. Infectious diseases such as measles and mumps are endemic in the region. In addition, travelers should obtain vaccinations for hepatitis A and B and typhoid.

Yellow Fever Vaccine Requirements   *legal requirement*

As of May 2012, South Africa requires a valid International Certificate of Vaccination or Prophylaxis documenting yellow fever vaccination ≥10 days before arrival in South Africa for all travelers aged ≥1 year who are traveling from or transiting through a country with risk of yellow fever virus transmission, regardless of the amount of time spent at the airport. This requirement also applies to the following countries with low potential for exposure to yellow fever virus: Eritrea, São Tomé and Principe, Somalia, Tanzania, and Zambia. Travelers not meeting this requirement can be refused entry to South Africa or be quarantined for up to 6 days. Unvaccinated travelers with a valid medical waiver should be allowed entry.

South Africa's policy is undergoing review and could change at any time. Travelers going to or transiting through South Africa are advised to seek the most current information by consulting the CDC Travelers' Health website (www.cdc.gov/travel), and also the website of the US Embassy in South Africa (Pretoria) and the Embassy of South Africa in Washington, DC.

HIV and Sexually Transmitted Diseases

South Africa has the largest estimated number of people living with HIV of any other country in the world. The prevalence of HIV infection is approximately 18% among people aged 15–49 years, and the prevalence among sex workers is even higher. Other sexually transmitted diseases are also present at high rates in this population. Travelers should be made aware of these risks and advised to wear condoms if they participate in sexual activities with local residents.

Vectorborne Diseases

Malaria transmission only occurs in the northeast of the country in the Mpumalanga and Limpopo Provinces (including Kruger National Park) and in Kwa-Zulu Natal north of the Tugela River (see Map 3-39). *Plasmodium falciparum* is the predominant species and is universally resistant to chloroquine. Visitors to these areas should be on a malaria chemoprophylaxis regimen and should be advised about mosquito precautions. Malaria in the northeastern game reserves is seasonal; the highest transmission occurs from October through May, peaking from February to early May. The risk to visiting travelers is low. A study conducted in 1999 estimated a case rate of 4.5 cases per 10,000 visitors in April, a high-transmission month. The South African Department of Health recommends malaria chemoprophylaxis for all travelers visiting from September through May and mosquito-avoidance measures for the rest of the year. CDC recommends chemoprophylaxis at all times of the year (see Chapter 3, Travel Vaccines & Malaria Information, by Country).

Tick-bite fever caused by rickettsial species is common in South Africa. The disease is characterized by an eschar at the bite site, regional adenopathy, and a maculopapular to petechial rash. Hikers and campers in rural areas who are exposed to ticks are especially at risk. Measures should be taken to prevent tick bites (see Chapter 2, Protection against Mosquitoes, Ticks, & Other Insects & Arthropods). Travelers who are taking doxycycline for malaria chemoprophylaxis may have some protection against tick-bite fever, but no studies exist to support or refute this viewpoint. Taking doxycycline only as prophylaxis for tick-bite fever (as opposed to taking it for malaria chemoprophylaxis) is not recommended.

Waterborne Diseases

Schistosomiasis, a common parasite throughout Africa, may be present in any body of freshwater, such as lakes, streams, and ponds. Travelers should avoid swimming in fresh, unchlorinated water.

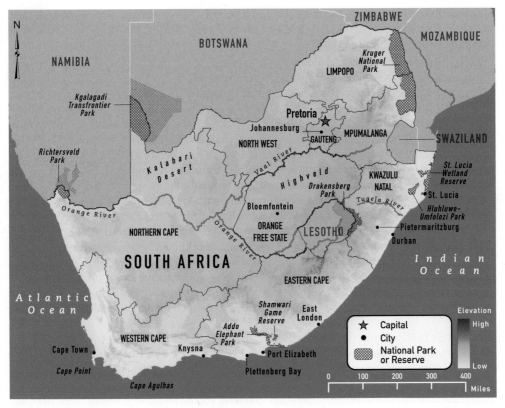

MAP 4-3. SOUTH AFRICA DESTINATION MAP

Animal Avoidance

While most travelers avoid wild animals in game reserves, rabies is common in dogs and other mammals throughout the country. Travelers are unable to tell if a suspected animal is rabid and should avoid all contact with animals. Any bite or scratch from an animal should be washed with soap and water immediately and be evaluated as soon as possible by a clinician. Postexposure prophylaxis and medical care for rabies exposures can be obtained in South Africa. Rabies vaccine is available in South Africa, and human rabies immune globulin is available in major urban medical centers.

Safety and Security

South Africa has struggled with a rise in violent crime, which includes armed robberies, carjackings, home invasions, and rape. Most of these incidents occur in poor areas and, as such, most visitors will not be affected. However, awareness of personal safety and security should be stressed to all visitors. Travelers should rely on local guidance about the security precautions to take in specific areas.

Although South Africa has a modern road system, drivers should be alert for dangerous driving practices, stray animals, and poor roads in remote rural areas.

BIBLIOGRAPHY

1. Blumberg LH, de Frey A, Frean J, Mendelson M. The 2010 FIFA World Cup: communicable disease risks and advice for visitors to South Africa. J Travel Med. 2010 May–Jun;17(3):150–2.
2. Durrheim DN, Braack LE, Waner S, Gammon S. Risk of malaria in visitors to the Kruger National Park, South Africa. J Travel Med. 1998 Dec;5(4):173–7.

The Americas & The Caribbean

ARGENTINA/BRAZIL: IGUASSU FALLS
David O. Freedman

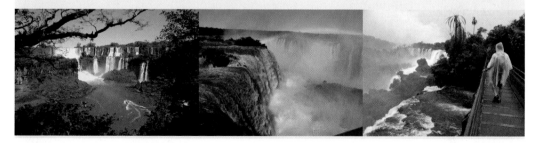

DESTINATION OVERVIEW

Iguassu Falls (*Iguaçu* in Portuguese, the language of Brazil; *Iguazú* in Spanish, the language of Argentina) in the Atlantic rainforest region of South America straddles the border of the southern Brazilian state of Paraná and the northern Argentine province of Misiones.

Brazil, occupying most of eastern South America, is immense and varies from tropical plains and jungle at the equator to cooler uplands in the south. Brazil is a developing nation in the lower half of the world's economies, but the highly industrialized south, which includes São Paulo, is affluent, with modern infrastructure. Argentina is located in the southern part of South America, between the Andes Mountains and the Atlantic Ocean. Except for a tiny northernmost fringe, which is tropical, all of Argentina is temperate, characterized by a cool, dry climate in the south and a more moderate climate in the central portion of the country. Argentina is a developing nation but is in the upper half of the world's economies. In addition, Paraguay is only a few miles away from the falls, so many people travel into Paraguay during the same trip. Most visitors to the falls stay in either the city of Foz do Iguaçu, Paraná, or in Puerto Iguazú, Misiones, each about 12 miles from the falls and each a well-developed city of 60,000 people. However, there is one sizeable hotel right at the falls in each of the separate national parks on either side of the border. This UNESCO World Heritage site also protects an astounding diversity of tropical wildlife. There are airports called Iguassu Falls in both countries, but travelers can fly to the Brazilian airport (IGU) only from Brazil, Lima, or Montevideo and to the Argentinean airport (IGR) only from Argentina.

Higher than Niagara Falls, Iguassu is rivaled only by southern Africa's Victoria Falls, which are higher but narrower. Iguassu Falls is a waterfall system consisting of 275 falls along 1.67 miles (2.67 km) of the Iguassu River, varying from 210 to 270 ft (64 to 82 m) in height. The main feature, the Devil's Throat, is a U-shaped cliff, 490 by 2,300 ft (149 by 701 m), which marks the border between Argentina and Brazil. Two-thirds of the falls are on the Argentine side of the gorge, giving the Brazilian side the best view. However, one cannot directly approach the falls from the Brazilian side. Travelers visiting the Argentine side are able to pass over and under the actual falls on a series of catwalks and trails. The bridge connecting the 2 sides of the river is a number of miles away and crosses the Brazil-Argentina border.

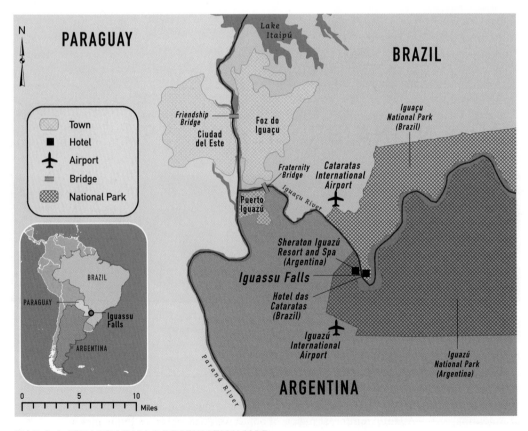

MAP 4-4. IGUASSU FALLS DESTINATION MAP

US travelers require a visa, which must be obtained in advance, to enter Brazil. Many organized day trips do not stop at the Brazilian immigration post, and this seems to be tolerated. However, a US citizen in Brazil without a visa in his or her passport may face arrest or imprisonment if stopped for any reason by authorities during the short visit. US travelers staying on the Brazilian side on a single-entry Brazilian visa can reenter Brazil after a day trip to Argentina. US travelers do not require a visa to enter Argentina. Ideally, one should visit both sides, but most people do not, because their stay is too short to deal with the somewhat complicated logistical issues.

HEALTH ISSUES

The infrastructure in tourist accommodations around Iguassu Falls is good, and most travelers are tourists staying only for a short time. Travelers visiting the usual accommodation and dining facilities are at modest risk for enterically transmitted diseases. Travelers should carry an antibiotic to self-treat travelers' diarrhea. Hepatitis A and B vaccines are recommended for all travelers and typhoid vaccine only for those with adventurous dietary habits or who plan to eat away from usual tourist locations.

Yellow Fever
Yellow fever virus circulates in monkeys and mosquitoes in the forested regions along the Iguassu and Paraná rivers. All travelers, even those on a typical 1- to 2-day itinerary, should be vaccinated. Although requirements may change, at present neither Brazil nor Argentina requires that any travelers have an International Certificate of Vaccination or Prophylaxis for yellow fever.

Malaria
No malaria transmission occurs at the falls and in surrounding areas. In assessing the malaria risk for travelers and recommended preventive measures, the entire itinerary, style of travel, and location of accommodations need to be taken into consideration. Typical travelers on fixed itineraries and staying at the hotels at the falls or in upscale accommodation in the adjacent towns would not be considered at risk for malaria. If the itinerary includes travel to other areas of Brazil, Argentina, or Paraguay where malaria is present, travel health providers should consult the country-specific information in Chapter 3, Travel Vaccines & Malaria Information, by Country and Map 3-23.

Rabies
Both domestic animal and bat rabies are risks in parts of Brazil, but no cases in mammals or humans have been reported around Iguassu Falls. Preexposure vaccine is not necessary for typical travelers, but travelers should be educated about seeking appropriate medical care for any bite injuries or bat exposures that occur.

Leishmaniasis
This protozoan disease, transmitted by sandflies, occurs in Brazil and is most common in the Amazonian and northeast regions, but is present in Paraná and has seen a recent increase in Misiones, Argentina. Cases have not been described in visitors to Iguassu Falls.

Chagas Disease (American Trypanosomiasis)
Risk to travelers is unknown but is thought to be negligible. Few travelers stay in houses constructed of mud, adobe brick, or palm thatch, where the vectors live.

Dengue
Dengue occurs in urban and rural areas in the Iguassu Falls region. Daytime insect precautions will reduce risk.

Schistosomiasis

Schistosomiasis, transmitted in freshwater lakes and rivers, is a public health problem in many states in Brazil. Historically, rare cases have been reported from the Iguassu area, but no recent data are available. Cautious travelers should avoid freshwater exposure while visiting the area.

BIBLIOGRAPHY

1. Jentes ES, Poumerol G, Gershman MD, Hill DR, Lemarchand J, Lewis RF, et al. The revised global yellow fever risk map and recommendations for vaccination, 2010: consensus of the Informal WHO Working Group on Geographic Risk for Yellow Fever. Lancet Infect Dis. 2011 Aug;11(8):622–32.
2. Malaria Atlas Project. The spatial limits of *Plasmodium vivax* malaria transmission map in 2009 in Argentina. 2010 [cited 2012 Sep 25]. Available from: http://www.map.ox.ac.uk/browse-resources/transmission-limits/Pv_limits/ARG/.
3. Padula P, Martinez VP, Bellomo C, Maidana S, San Juan J, Tagliaferri P, et al. Pathogenic hantaviruses, northeastern Argentina and eastern Paraguay. Emerg Infect Dis. 2007 Aug;13(8):1211–4.
4. Salomon OD, Acardi SA, Liotta DJ, Fernandez MS, Lestani E, Lopez D, et al. Epidemiological aspects of cutaneous leishmaniasis in the Iguazu Falls area of Argentina. Acta Trop. 2009 Jan;109(1):5–11.
5. Vezzani D, Carbajo AE. *Aedes aegypti, Aedes albopictus,* and dengue in Argentina: current knowledge and future directions. Mem Inst Oswaldo Cruz. 2008 Feb;103(1):66–74.

GUATEMALA & BELIZE
Ava W. Navin, Emily S. Jentes

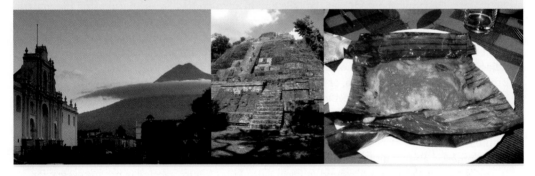

DESTINATION OVERVIEW

Guatemala, known as the Land of Eternal Spring for the temperate climate and lush foliage of its highlands, is located in Central America, with Mexico to the north, Belize to the east, and Honduras and El Salvador to the south and east. In an area the size of Tennessee, Guatemala offers a wide variety of topography: from active volcanoes to the black sand beach and mangrove swamp of Monterrico and the cloud forest reserve of the Biotopo del Quetzal. The visitor to the bustling market town of Chichicastenango in the highlands (6,447 ft; 1,965 m) will need preparation different from that for the visitor to the Mayan temples of Tikal in the hot lowlands of the Petén (500 ft; 150 m). Belize, an equally beautiful tropical paradise, is roughly the size of the state of Massachusetts. Northern Belize is characterized by coastal plains with pockets of dense forest, whereas the west and south are predominantly coastal plains or savannas and low mountains, respectively. To the east, Belize's coastline with the Caribbean Sea boasts sandy white beaches, numerous islands, and the second-longest barrier reef in the world.

Tourists interested in the Ruta Maya often visit sites in both Guatemala and Belize. Temples and ball courts, the remnants of the Mayan civilization that flourished in the Yucatán 1,000 years ago, have been reclaimed from the jungle. In Belize, the Mayan ruins of Xunantunich (Cayo District), Caracol (Cayo District), and Lamanai (Orange Walk District), among others, provide impressive excavated examples of the cities and leave the visitors wondering what else might be hidden underneath the trees and hills.

The colonial capital of Antigua Guatemala (5,029 ft; 1,533 m), a UNESCO World Heritage site, was founded in 1543 by Spanish conquistadors and destroyed by an earthquake in 1773. The ruins of the cathedral, government buildings, and monasteries provide a hint of colonial grandeur. Holy Week, the week in the Christian calendar that precedes Easter, is an especially popular time to visit Antigua, when the images from the churches are carried through the streets in colorful processions.

Travelers visiting Belize's inland regions will enjoy a variety of adventure activities, including climbing the ruins, zip-lining through jungle canopies, cave tubing, hiking, and canoeing. However, most visitors to Belize are drawn to the sandy white beaches and to the barrier reefs off the coast, which boast some of the best scuba diving in the Caribbean. Near Ambergris Caye, the Hol Chan Marine Reserve and the Great Blue Hole (a UNESCO World Heritage site) are popular sites for both scuba divers and snorkelers, who will be delighted by the variety of fish, eels, and coral living in the clear blue-green water.

Guatemala's tremendous geographic variety extends to its linguistic richness: in addition to Spanish, 21 distinct Mayan languages and many more dialects are spoken. In rural areas, Spanish is more often a second language, and Mayan customs and rituals are still observed. Guatemala, especially Antigua, is noted for immersion language schools; students can live with a family while they attend classes. Belize is similarly linguistically diverse. Although the official language of Belize is English, Belizean Creole, Spanish, Mayan languages, and Plautdietsch (a variety of German spoken by Mennonite settlers) are also spoken.

HEALTH ISSUES

Immunizations

All travelers should always be up-to-date on routine vaccinations. Hepatitis A and B vaccines are recommended for visitors to both countries. Typhoid vaccination is also recommended for all travelers. Countries in Central America have been the source of many cases of typhoid fever that continue to be imported into the United States.

Rabies vaccination should be considered for travelers who will be involved in outdoor activities, such as bicycling, camping, or hiking, especially in rural areas, or who will have occupational exposure to animals. It is particularly recommended for long-term travelers such as missionaries and their children. Although yellow fever is not a disease risk in Guatemala or Belize, the governments of both countries require travelers arriving from countries where there is yellow fever virus transmission to present proof of yellow fever vaccination.

Malaria

Malaria is found throughout Belize, except for Belize City and islands frequented by tourists. In Guatemala, malaria is found only in rural areas at altitudes <4,921 ft (1,500 m); therefore, the specific destination is important to know. Travelers who plan to visit only the capital and highlands in Guatemala do not need malaria chemoprophylaxis. Travelers who mention plans to scuba dive or visit Mayan ruins, though, will be at risk for malaria. Some clinicians feel that primaquine is the preferred antimalarial drug (only after G6PD testing and never to be used in pregnant women) because of the amount of *Plasmodium vivax*, although chloroquine, atovaquone-proguanil, doxycycline, and mefloquine can also be prescribed.

Other Vectorborne Diseases   *Dengue   Leish* (handwritten)

Mosquito and insect precautions are important for travelers to Central America to protect themselves from vectorborne diseases (see Chapter 2, Protection against Mosquitoes, Ticks, & Other Insects & Arthropods). All of Central America is endemic for dengue. GeoSentinel Surveillance Network data show that dengue is the most common cause of febrile illness in travelers returning from this area. Cutaneous leishmaniasis has been reported in travelers to these countries as well. Cutaneous larva migrans, caused by skin infection with dog or cat hookworm larva, can occur on any part of the body but is frequently related to walking barefoot on contaminated beaches, so footwear may be protective. Filariasis, onchocerciasis (river blindness), and American trypanosomiasis (Chagas disease) are other diseases carried by insects that have occurred in these areas, mostly in rural areas and mostly in the indigenous populations.

Travelers' Diarrhea

Diarrhea in travelers is common throughout both Guatemala and Belize and is the most common complaint in returning travelers who seek medical attention at GeoSentinel clinics. Travelers should be reminded of precautions for safe food and water and carry an antibiotic for self-treatment (see the Food & Water Precautions and Travelers' Diarrhea sections in Chapter 2).

Other Health and Safety Risks
Safety and Security

For much of the last 30 years, Guatemala's geologic instability was paralleled by its political unrest. Since a peace accord was signed in 1996, safety concerns are more likely to stem from economic conditions and drug-related violence. Although petty crime such as burglary and

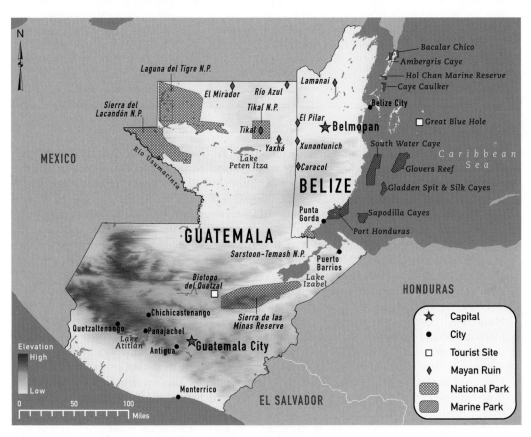

MAP 4-5. GUATEMALA AND BELIZE DESTINATION MAP

pickpocketing can be a problem in Belize, safety concerns more often involve road, boating, and diving accidents. Visitors to both countries are advised to travel in groups and stay on the main roads.

International Adoptions

Guatemala at one time was second only to China as a source country for international adoptions; 4,728 children were adopted by US families in 2007. In early 2008, after allegations of fraud and exploitation, adoptions were suspended until the country's procedures could be made compliant with the Hague Convention on Intercountry Adoption. The National Council for Adoptions (CNA), established to oversee adoptions of Guatemalan children, published new procedures in July 2010 to implement the December 2007 adoption law. Until the system is reformed, the US Department of State does not approve adoptions from Guatemala, and the adoption numbers have declined to as low as 32 in 2011. Concerns about child trafficking have led to suspicion and occasional hostility toward foreigners seen with Guatemalan children. The Department of State advises visitors to avoid close contact with children, especially in rural areas.

Medical Tourism

Travel to obtain medical care has increased in popularity in recent years, and Guatemala, which boasts specialists trained in the United States, has benefited from this trend. Popular procedures sought by medical tourists to this region include cosmetic and bariatric surgery, fertility treatments, and dental procedures. The Internet abounds with sites that promote medical tourism and offer help with transportation, accommodations, and language issues. A government initiative called "International Health City" (*Ciudad Salud Internacional*) has been established under the Tourism and Health Commission to promote medical tourism at a number of health facilities in Guatemala City, including private hospitals, diagnostic centers, clinics, spas, and laboratories. For guidelines for travelers seeking care abroad, see Chapter 2, Medical Tourism.

BIBLIOGRAPHY

1. Central Intelligence Agency. World Factbook: Guatemala. Washington, DC: Central Intelligence Agency; 2012 [updated Sep 12; cited 2012 Sep 25]. Available from: https://www.cia.gov/library/publications/the-world-factbook/geos/gt.html.
2. Lynch MF, Blanton EM, Bulens S, Polyak C, Vojdani J, Stevenson J, et al. Typhoid fever in the United States, 1999–2006. JAMA. 2009 Aug 26;302(8):859–65.
3. Miller L, Chan W, Comfort K, Tirella L. Health of children adopted from Guatemala: comparison of orphanage and foster care. Pediatrics. 2005 Jun;115(6):e710–7.
4. Pan American Health Organization. Country profile, Guatemala. Washington, DC: Pan American Health Organization; 2012 [cited 2012 Sep 25]. Available from: http://new.paho.org/hq/index.php?option=com_content&view=article&id=3223&Itemid=2408.
5. UNICEF. At a glance: Guatemala. Geneva: UNICEF; 2012 [cited 2012 Sep 25]. Available from: http://www.unicef.org/infobycountry/guatemala.html.
6. US Department of State. Guatemala. Washington, DC: US Department of State [cited 2012 Sep 25]. Available from: http://www.state.gov/p/wha/ci/gt/.

JAMAICA

Clive M. Brown

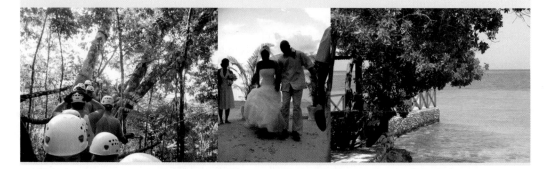

This section discusses specific health risks in Jamaica. For a general discussion of health risks in other Caribbean destinations, visit *The Caribbean* on the CDC website at wwwnc.cdc.gov/travel/yellowbook/2014/chapter-4-select-destinations/the-caribbean.htm.

DESTINATION OVERVIEW

Jamaica (called *Xaymaca*, "the land of wood and water," by the Arawak Indians who originally inhabited the island) is situated in the Caribbean Sea, about 90 miles south of Cuba. Introduced to Spain and Europe by Christopher Columbus in 1494, Jamaica was colonized by Britain in 1655. Port Royal became the most important commercial center in the English colonies and a strategic British military and naval base. It was reputed to be the wickedest city in the world, most likely because it was also a strategic base for pillage and plunder by pirates such as Henry Morgan and "three-fingered" Jack Rackham. The central two-thirds of the island is mountainous, and the highest point, Blue Mountain Peak, reaches 7,402 ft (2,256 m). The beaches on the flat coastal strip are among the most popular in the Caribbean. Jamaica recorded >3 million tourist arrivals in 2011, and the United States accounted for >60% of stop-over visitors. While you lay back and enjoy the sea breeze and reggae music, here are a few tips to help you stay safe, healthy, and "irie" (having an ultimate positive feeling) while in Jamaica. Yeh Mon!

HEALTH ISSUES

Immunizations

In addition to routine vaccines, typhoid vaccine is recommended for some travelers to Jamaica, especially if they are staying long-term, staying with friends or relatives, or visiting smaller cities, villages, or rural areas where exposure might occur through food or water. Hepatitis A vaccine is recommended for all travelers, and hepatitis B vaccine is recommended especially for long-term travelers who will have close contact with local residents or who could be exposed to blood or injections, including those who will be working in health care.

Malaria

Rare cases of autochthonous malaria transmission have been reported in Kingston, Jamaica, since an outbreak was reported in 2006. The risk for acquiring malaria among US travelers is estimated to be very low.

Dengue

Dengue is endemic in Jamaica. Reports of dengue and severe dengue have increased in recent years. Travelers to Jamaica should take measures to protect themselves from daytime mosquito bites to prevent dengue (see Chapter 2, Protection against Mosquitoes, Ticks, & Other Insects & Arthropods).

Travelers' Diarrhea and Food-Related Diseases

Travelers to Jamaica will want to experience the spicy local fare, choosing from jerked chicken, ackee and salt fish (the national dish), curries (goat, chicken, shrimp, or lobster), escovitch (spicy fried) fish, and much, much more. While enjoying the cuisine, travelers should be reminded to select food and beverages carefully (see Chapter 2, Food & Water Precautions). Travelers' diarrhea is one of the most common travel-related illnesses, and Jamaica has attack rates of 8%–20%. Jamaica is unique among tourist destinations for having a hotel-based surveillance system of illness and injuries in travelers and for doing occasional exit surveys among travelers at its airport to estimate the risk of travelers' diarrhea. Since interventions to prevent and control diarrhea in visitors were implemented, Jamaica reported a 72% reduction in diarrhea in the visitor population from 1996 to 2002.

During 2000, an outbreak of eosinophilic meningitis was reported among travelers to the island associated with the roundworm *Angiostrongylus cantonensis*. The source of infection was likely contaminated salad.

Ackee is a red-skinned fruit with golden flesh. Although ackee is generally safe, it should only be eaten if prepared by a reliable source because if picked unripe, it produces hypoglycin, a toxin that causes a drop in blood sugar, vomiting, and in rare cases, convulsions, coma, and death. In 2011 the Jamaican Health Ministry reported >200 suspected cases and >20 deaths. All the ackee poisoning cases involved ackees cooked at home, and none occurred among visitors.

Physical Concerns for the Traveler
Crime and Drugs

The crime rate is high in Jamaica, particularly in Kingston and Montego Bay. Tourists are typically victims of theft; however, the situation may turn violent when victims resist handing over valuables. Criminals have also targeted Jamaican foreign nationals returning to resettle permanently in Jamaica. Visitors to the island should pay extra attention to their surroundings when traveling, avoid walking alone, avoid secluded places or situations, go out in groups and watch out for each other, exercise special care after dark, and always avoid areas known for high crime rates. Travelers should be reminded that possession or use of marijuana and other illicit drugs is illegal in Jamaica. Each year, many American citizens are arrested and incarcerated for drug-related crimes in Jamaica.

Traffic

Drivers drive on the left in Jamaica, which ranks in the top 10 for estimated traffic death rates in countries frequently traveled by US residents. A USA Today analysis of Department of State data for 2003–2010 found that Jamaica accounted for <1% of road traffic deaths among US travelers.

Natural Disasters

Jamaica lies in the path of Atlantic hurricanes, and it is often subject to flooding with high winds, impassable roads, and unsafe travel conditions. Jamaica has also been subject to

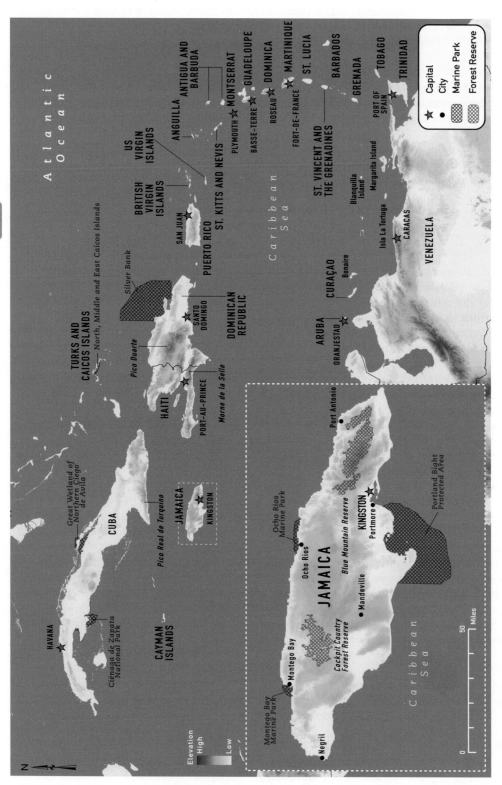

MAP 4-6. JAMAICA DESTINATION MAP[1]

[1] For a general discussion of health risks in other Caribbean destinations, visit *The Caribbean* on the CDC website at wwwnc.cdc.gov/travel/yellowbook/2014/chapter-4-select-destinations/the-caribbean.htm.

major earthquake activity. In 1692, Port Royal was destroyed by an earthquake, seen by some as divine intervention based on its reputation as the wickedest city in the world. In 1907, the city and Port of Kingston was destroyed by an earthquake that caused >800 deaths. The last major destructive earthquake (magnitude 8.0) hit the western end of the island in 1957.

Beaches, Rafting, Diving, and Snorkeling and Mountain Climbing

The average temperature in Jamaica is 81°F (27.1°C) with much warmer temperatures (high 80s to low and mid-90s) from June through November. The coolest temperatures (low 70s) occur in January and February. Because of abundant sunshine, even in the cooler months travelers are at risk for sunburn.

The Jamaican reefs are among the most species-rich in the Caribbean, and some resorts provide diving instruction. In the event of decompression sickness, Jamaica has a decompression facility in Discovery Bay on its north coast near many of the diving areas. Leptospirosis is common in Jamaica; a major outbreak was reported in 2007 after flooding rains.

Hiking overnight to catch the sunrise on the Blue Mountain Peak is a majestic, exhilarating, and exhausting experience. Jamaica has many endemic flowering plant species; >40% of the flowering plants in the Blue Mountains are found nowhere else in the world. Travelers may also encounter wild and endangered animal species. The rise to the peak from the coastal plain is one of the steepest gradients in the world. A mountain trek should not be done within 24 hours of diving to avoid the risk of decompression sickness. For safety, travelers should use known tour operators or hike with guides familiar with the trail. Although Jamaica is warm, the temperature at the peak can be cold, especially between December and June; the coldest temperature is around 40°F (5°C).

BIBLIOGRAPHY

1. Ashley DV, Walters C, Dockery-Brown C, McNab A, Ashley DE. Interventions to prevent and control food-borne diseases associated with a reduction in traveler's diarrhea in tourists to Jamaica. J Travel Med. 2004 Nov–Dec;11(6):364–7.
2. Pan American Health Organization. Dengue. Washington, DC: Pan American Health Organization; 2012 [cited 2012 Sep 26]. Available from: http://new.paho.org/hq/index.php?option=com_content&view=article&id=264&Itemid=363&lang=en.
3. Rawlins SC, Hinds A, Rawlins JM. Malaria and its vectors in the Caribbean: the continuing challenge of the disease forty-five years after eradication from the Islands. West Indian Med J. 2008 Nov;57(5):462–9.
4. Stoller G. Traffic accidents are top killer of US travelers abroad. USA TODAY [Internet]. 2010 [cited 2012 Sep 26]. Available from: http://www.usatoday.com/money/industries/travel/2010-10-21-1Adangerousroads21_ST_N.htm.

MEXICO

Stephen H. Waterman

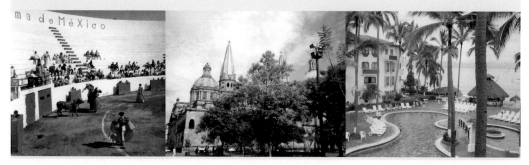

DESTINATION OVERVIEW

Mexico, the second most populous country in Latin America, has a population of >110 million, with 76% living in urban areas. The United States' third-largest trading partner overall and second-largest agricultural trading partner, Mexico is now considered a middle-income country with the world's 14th-largest economy. Mexico has a rich history and proud culture that reflect its pre-Columbian civilizations and Hispanic heritage. With one-fifth the area of the United States (about 3 times the size of Texas), Mexico has diverse geographic features. The Sonoran desert is in the northwest, beautiful beaches are available on both coasts, and forested mountain ranges traverse the western and eastern mainland. Impressive volcanic peaks rise up to 18,000 feet above the high central plateau. The Yucatán Peninsula and southern regions are tropical. The Copper Canyon in the northwestern state of Chihuahua is larger than the US Grand Canyon.

Mexico City is one of the world's largest cities, with a population >20 million. Despite increasing national prosperity, Mexico's large cities contain much poverty. Extensive migration has taken place from the poor rural south to the northern border for jobs in bustling border cities, such as Ciudad Juárez and Tijuana.

Mexico has the most foreign visitors of any Latin American country and is the country most frequently visited by US tourists. Travel to beach resorts such as Acapulco, Cancún, Cozumel, Puerto Vallarta, and Cabo San Lucas, along with cruise ship tours, makes up a large portion of tourist travel to Mexico. Also common are day trips to northern border cities and longer cultural trips to historical and World Heritage sites. Popular pre-Columbian anthropologic destinations include Teotihuacan outside Mexico City, Chichen Itzá in Yucatán, Monte Alban in Oaxaca, and Palenque in Chiapas. Baja California offers whale watching on the Pacific Coast and sports fishing in the Gulf of California.

HEALTH ISSUES

Immunizations

Hepatitis A is still endemic in Mexico, and all susceptible travelers should be immunized for hepatitis A. Hepatitis B vaccine is also recommended. Other vaccines, such as typhoid and rabies, may be considered, especially if visitors, such as field biologists or missionaries, will be traveling extensively to less-developed, nontourist areas.

Travelers' Diarrhea and Foodborne Infections

Travelers' diarrhea is common among visitors to Mexico. In addition to taking food and water precautions, travelers should bring along an antibiotic for empiric self-treatment of diarrhea (see the Food & Water Precautions and Travelers' Diarrhea sections in Chapter 2). Travelers who eat raw dairy products and vegetables are at some risk for more serious foodborne infections, including amebiasis, cysticercosis (especially in rural areas where pigs are raised), brucellosis, *Mycobacterium bovis*, and *Listeria*.

Dengue

Dengue is endemic throughout Mexico, except for the state of Baja California Norte and at higher elevations (for example, it is not present in Mexico City at 7,350 ft [2,240 m]). Large outbreaks of dengue have been reported in recent years, and dengue virus transmission should be considered a risk year-round. Travelers to Mexico should take measures to protect themselves from daytime mosquito bites to prevent dengue (see Chapter 2, Protection against Mosquitoes, Ticks, & Other Insects & Arthropods).

Malaria

Malaria incidence has decreased dramatically in recent decades in Mexico, and only a few cases of *Plasmodium vivax* are reported among US travelers each year. Major resorts are free of malaria, as is the US–Mexico border region. Malaria prophylaxis is recommended only for low-lying areas of Chihuahua, Durango, Sinaloa, and Nayarit in the west and Oaxaca, Chiapas, and Tabasco in the south.

Other Infections

Respiratory Diseases

Influenza virus strains similar to those in the United States circulate in Mexico, as was demonstrated by the emergence of pandemic influenza A H1N1 in North America in the spring of 2009. Coccidioidomycosis, a fungal respiratory disease caused by inhaling spores in the soil, is endemic in northwestern Mexico. Several outbreaks of coccidioidomycosis have been reported among missionary groups from the United States doing construction projects in this region. Histoplasmosis, another fungal respiratory disease agent found in soil, is endemic in other regions of Mexico. As occasional hotel clusters of legionellosis have been reported from Mexico, Legionnaires' disease should be considered in elderly and immunocompromised travelers who develop acute pneumonia.

Parasitic Infections

Cutaneous leishmaniasis, transmitted by sandflies, is found in focal areas of coastal and southern Mexico. The risk is higher for ecotourists and long-term travelers. Vector preventive measures are indicated, including avoiding outdoor activities at night. Travelers to beach areas are at risk for cutaneous larva migrans, a creeping skin eruption most commonly associated with the dog hookworm infection, preventable by wearing shoes and avoiding direct skin contact with sand. Chagas disease is also endemic in Mexico and is sometimes diagnosed in Mexican immigrants to the United States, but no cases have been reported among travelers.

Rabies

All travelers should be warned of the risk of acquiring rabies and educated in how to prevent animal bites. Preexposure rabies vaccination should be considered for those who are likely to come into contact with domestic or wild mammals or those who will be traveling to areas with limited access to medical care.

Rickettsial Disease

In Mexico, rickettsial diseases, febrile rash illnesses transmitted by ticks or fleas, include Rocky Mountain spotted fever, which is potentially fatal unless treated promptly with antibiotics, and fleaborne typhus, which usually causes an illness similar to dengue. Travelers should take precautions to avoid flea and tick bites both indoors and outside. Rocky Mountain spotted fever associated with *Rhipicephalus sanguineus*, the brown dog tick, has been identified recently in northern Mexico in urban and rural areas with large stray dog populations.

Tuberculosis (TB)
Mexico's TB incidence is lower than rates in Asia, Africa, and Eastern Europe but is 5 times that of the United States.

Other Health and Safety Risks
Good health care is available in most sizable Mexican cities, and hotels in tourist resorts usually have well-trained physicians available. Medical tourism has increased in Mexico in recent years. Clinics offering unproven and often dangerous interventions for cancer and other serious illnesses can operate in northern border cities, such as Tijuana, for varying periods before regulatory authorities intervene.

Mexico's highway system and roads have become increasingly modernized over the years. Toll highways are often of high quality. Nevertheless, driving in traffic in cities and at night through the countryside can be dangerous, and motor vehicle accidents are a leading cause of death for visitors. Although travel in Mexico is generally safe and enjoyable, drug-related violence has continued to increase in parts of the country. Department of State advisories should be monitored for alerts in areas where tourists are planning to visit.

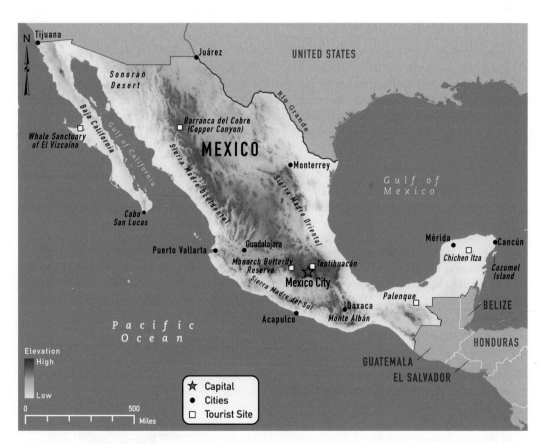

MAP 4-7. MEXICO DESTINATION MAP

Air pollution in Mexico City, while decreased in recent years, can be particularly severe during the dry winter months and can exacerbate asthma and chronic lung and heart conditions. Both healthy travelers from lower elevations and people with lung and heart conditions should cautiously acclimate to Mexico City's altitude.

A population that requires increasing attention is the large numbers of travelers of Mexican birth or descent who return to visit friends and relatives.

BIBLIOGRAPHY

1. CDC. Coccidioidomycosis in travelers returning from Mexico—Pennsylvania, 2000. MMWR Morb Mortal Wkly Rep. 2000 Nov 10;49(44):1004–6.
2. CDC. Dengue hemorrhagic fever—US-Mexico border, 2005. MMWR Morb Mortal Wkly Rep. 2007 Aug 10;56(31):785–9.
3. CDC. Human rabies from exposure to a vampire bat in Mexico— Louisiana, 2010. MMWR Morb Mortal Wkly Rep. 2011 Aug 12;60(31):1050–2.
4. CDC. Preventing and controlling tuberculosis along the US-Mexico border. MMWR Recomm Rep. 2001 Jan 19;50(RR-1):1–27.
5. CDC. Update: novel influenza A (H1N1) virus infection—Mexico, March–May, 2009. MMWR Morb Mortal Wkly Rep. 2009 Jun 5;58(21):585–9.
6. Flores-Figueroa J, Okhuysen PC, von Sonnenburg F, DuPont HL, Libman MD, Keystone JS, et al. Patterns of illness in travelers visiting Mexico and Central America: the GeoSentinel experience. Clin Infect Dis. 2011 Sep;53(6):523–31.
7. Spradling PR, Xing J, Phippard A, Fonseca-Ford M, Montiel S, Guzman NL, et al. Acute viral hepatitis in the United States-Mexico border region: data from the Border Infectious Disease Surveillance (BIDS) project, 2000-2009. J Immigr Minor Health [Internet]. 2012 [cited 2012 Sep 26]. Available from: http://www.springerlink.com/content/1638613t04453x63/.
8. White AC, Atmar RL. Infections in Hispanic immigrants. Clin Infect Dis. 2002 Jun 15;34(12):1627–32.

PERU: CUZCO-MACHU PICCHU

Alan J. Magill

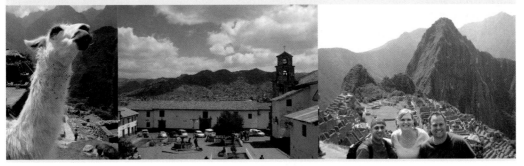

DESTINATION OVERVIEW

Peru is approximately twice the size of the state of Texas, with a population of almost 30 million people. Thousands of tourists are drawn to Peru every year to enjoy the country's magnificent geographic, biologic, and cultural diversity. A primary destination for most travelers is the remarkable Incan ruins of Machu Picchu, named a UNESCO World Heritage site in 1983 and voted one of the New Seven Wonders of the World in 2007. Machu Picchu stands in the middle of a tropical mountain forest, in an extraordinarily beautiful setting. It was probably the most amazing urban creation of the Inca Empire at its height; its giant walls, terraces, and ramps seem as if they have been cut naturally in the continuous rock escarpments. The natural setting, on the eastern slopes of the Andes, is in the upper Amazon Basin, with its rich diversity of flora and fauna.

A typical visit to Peru includes arrival at the capital city of Lima, a megacity the size of the state of Rhode Island, with approximately one-third of Peru's population. Interestingly, many people think Lima is a high-altitude Incan city, but it is actually located on the Pacific coast at sea level. After spending a few days in Lima, one takes an hour-long flight to Cuzco, the gateway to Machu Picchu and a worthwhile destination of its own. Tourists can visit multiple Inca-era ruins and Peruvian mountain villages and markets in the Valle Sagrado (Sacred Valley) before taking the train to Machu Picchu. One of the world's most popular and best-known treks, the Inca Trail, begins classically at kilometer 82 (7,700 ft; 2,600 m) on the Cuzco–Machu Picchu railway. This moderate 26-mile (43-km) trek is usually done in 4 days and 3 nights, and most fit people should be able to complete the hike. Nevertheless it is quite challenging, with 3 high mountain passes; the highest is Warmiwañusca at 13,829 ft (4,215 m), before ending in the ruins of Machu Picchu (7,970 ft; 2,430 m).

Many people also wish to add a tropical rainforest experience to their Cuzco trip and take the 30-minute flight from Cuzco to Puerto Maldonado, 34 miles (55 km) west of the Bolivian border, on the confluence of the Rio Tambopata with the Madre de Dios River, a major tributary of the Amazon River. Most travelers take a boat up the Rio Tambopata to one of several rustic lodges. Visitors wanting to see the Amazon rainforest may also go to Manu National Park in the south, also reached via Cuzco.

Other popular tourist destinations in Peru include the northern Amazon rainforest in Loreto that can be visited by traveling to the lodges around Iquitos or by journeying on the increasingly popular Amazon River cruises that go both upstream and downstream from Iquitos. As elsewhere, ecotourism is a growing activity in Peru. Also, Peru is home to the Cordillera Blanca, a hundred-mile range of spectacular snow-covered peaks that form the backbone of the Andes Mountains in Peru. The Cordillera Blanca boasts 33 peaks >18,040 feet (5,500 meters) and has an international reputation for its spectacular trekking and world-class mountaineering.

HEALTH ISSUES

Important pre-travel information for Peru includes advice on preventing high-altitude illness, the risk for cutaneous leishmaniasis in certain jungle areas, use of yellow fever vaccine in some areas, and the risk of malaria for travelers visiting popular jungle lodges.

Altitude and Acute Mountain Sickness

All travelers to Machu Picchu will arrive and transit through Cuzco, 11,150 ft (3,400 m) above sea level. Most will quickly note shortness of breath on gathering luggage and making their way to local hotels on the hilly streets. Many arriving travelers will find the elevation leads to some degree of acute mountain sickness (AMS), with the initial symptoms of headache, nausea, and loss of appetite beginning 4–8 hours after arrival. The hypoxemia of high altitude can also affect the quality of sleep in the first few nights in Cuzco, causing restless sleep, frequent awakening, and periodic breathing (irregular breathing patterns, often alternating periods of deep breathing and shallow breathing), even in those who appear to be doing well during the day. A few travelers may progress to severe forms of altitude illness, including high-altitude pulmonary edema (HAPE) and high-altitude cerebral edema (HACE). The symptoms of AMS can markedly impair the traveler and prevent enjoyment of the sights of Cuzco.

Surveys have shown that most travelers arrive in Cuzco with limited or no knowledge of AMS or the fact that AMS can be prevented to a large degree by prophylactic use of acetazolamide. **Every traveler to Cuzco should be counseled about AMS pre-travel and be prepared to prevent or self-treat AMS with acetazolamide.** (More information about prevention and treatment of altitude illness can be found in Chapter 2, Altitude Illness.) Locals refer to AMS as *soroche* and will almost always offer the new arrival a cup of hot coca tea (*mate de coca*) when checking in to the hotel. Although many believe *mate de coca* can prevent and treat *soroche*, no data support its use in the prevention or treatment of AMS. Perhaps of concern to some who may experience random drug screening as a condition of employment, people who drink a single cup of coca tea will test positive for cocaine metabolites in standard drug toxicology screens for several days. However, sitting quietly and resting while enjoying a cup of tea is a most civilized activity and a pleasant memory.

New arrivals may also find it helpful to transit directly from Cuzco to the Valle Sagrado of the Rio Urubamba to spend the first few days and nights at a somewhat lower altitude. This spectacular river valley begins 15 miles (24 km) northeast of Cuzco in the town of Pisac (9,751 ft; 2,972 m), known for its colorful Sunday markets, and continues downstream toward the northwest for another 37 miles (60 km) to reach the town of Ollantaytambo (9,160 ft; 2,792 m). One can board the train to Machu Picchu in Ollantaytambo, at the northwest end of the Valle Sagrado, and the not-to-be-missed visit to Cuzco can be made on return from Machu Picchu, when people are better acclimatized. The train follows the Rio Urubamba north and northwest (downstream) to Aguas Calientes (6,690 ft; 2,040 m). Machu Picchu (7,970 ft; 2,430 m) is located on a ridge above the town.

Cutaneous Leishmaniasis

Many areas in the Pacific valleys of the Andes and the Amazon tropical rainforest are endemic for cutaneous leishmaniasis (CL), a parasitic infection transmitted by bites of sand flies (see Chapter 3, Leishmaniasis, Cutaneous). While this disease is widespread in southeastern Peru, the highest risk for travelers seems to be in the Manu Park area in Madre de Dios. In Manu, CL is most often caused by *Leishmania braziliensis*, and there is a risk of both localized ulcerative CL and mucosal leishmaniasis. There is no visceral leishmaniasis in Peru. Travelers should be counseled to be meticulous about vector precautions, as there is no vaccine or chemoprophylaxis to prevent leishmaniasis. Any person with a skin lesion persisting more than a few weeks after return from Peru should be evaluated for CL.

Yellow Fever

Proof of yellow fever vaccination is not required for entry into Peru. Travelers who are limiting travel to the cities of Lima, Cuzco, and Machu Picchu, and the Inca Trail do not need yellow fever vaccination. Peru recommends vaccination for those who intend to visit any jungle areas of the country <2,300 m (7,546 ft). For complete CDC yellow fever vaccination recommendations for Peru, see Chapter 3, Travel Vaccines & Malaria Information, by Country.

Malaria

In general, the risk of malaria in travelers visiting Peru is low. There are, on average, <5 cases reported in the United States each year that were acquired in Peru. Both *Plasmodium vivax* malaria and *P. falciparum* malaria are found in the Peruvian Amazon.

There is no malaria risk for travelers visiting only Lima and vicinity, coastal areas south of Lima, or the popular highland tourist areas (Cuzco, Machu Picchu, and Lake Titicaca). The malaria-endemic areas for most tourists are the neotropical rainforests of the Amazon, with 2 major destinations (see Map 3-38). The city of Iquitos in the northern rainforest is a frequent arrival destination for those traveling to jungle lodges around the city or for boarding river cruise boats for rainforest travel. Malaria transmission occurs in the areas in and around Iquitos. Malaria transmission is seasonal, with peak activity between January and May that correlates with the rainy season and the height of the Amazon River. Chemoprophylaxis is recommended for most travelers.

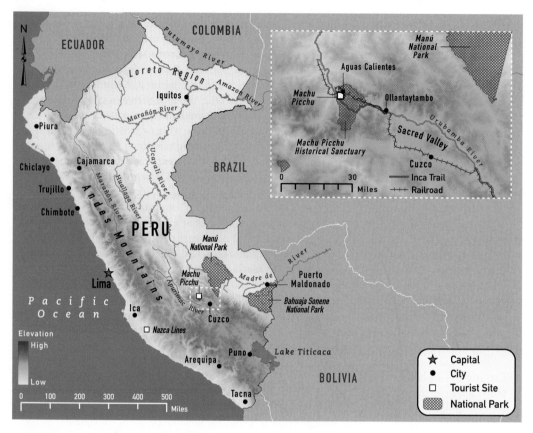

MAP 4-8. PERU DESTINATION MAP

The city of Puerto Maldonado is a 30-minute flight from Cuzco and a popular arrival destination for those visiting the rainforest lodges on the Rio Tambopata. Newly arrived travelers usually transit directly from the airport to the boats that take them up the river to numerous lodges. Peruvian Ministry of Health data document that malaria transmission occurs in Puerto Maldonado. Most cases reported in the region occur in local loggers and gold miners in the forests. Travelers transiting Puerto Maldonado for a short 2- to 3-day visit to lodges on the Rio Tambopata may not need chemoprophylaxis. For those who are staying longer or who are engaging in higher-risk activities and may benefit from chemoprophylaxis, one could consider using daily primaquine in this area of Peru, as the malaria species present is now exclusively *P. vivax*.

Risk for the traveler varies with itinerary, style of travel, and location of accommodations. Malaria in the Peruvian Amazon is unpredictable from season to season; *P. falciparum* epidemics occasionally occur in the Loreto region. When making a decision on whether to recommend chemoprophylaxis or simply mosquito precautions, all these factors and data need to be taken into consideration.

Other Infectious Diseases

Typical travelers' diarrhea is relatively common. Fluoroquinolone-resistant *Campylobacter* gastrointestinal infections are common and should be suspected in anyone with a gastrointestinal illness with fever and systemic symptoms and failure to clinically improve in 12–24 hours after initial empiric fluoroquinolone treatment. Azithromycin is recommended in this setting. Cyclosporiasis, an intestinal illness caused by the parasite *Cyclospora cayetanensis*, is also common in Peru. This diagnosis should be considered in people with watery diarrhea, loss of appetite, weight loss, cramping, and bloating that persist for days to weeks. Treatment is with trimethoprim-sulfamethoxazole.

Dengue is common in the neotropical areas of Peru and the northern coast. Mayaro virus, an alphavirus found in the Amazon Basin and transmitted by mosquitos, causes a denguelike illness. As with other alphaviruses, Mayaro can result in lengthy and debilitating arthralgias. Physicians treating patients with signs and symptoms of a denguelike illness and a recent history of travel to the Amazon should consider Mayaro infection in the differential diagnosis, especially if arthralgia is prominent and prolonged and dominates the clinical picture. Travelers to Peru should take measures to protect themselves from daytime mosquito bites to prevent dengue (see Chapter 2, Protection against Mosquitoes, Ticks, & Other Insects & Arthropods).

BIBLIOGRAPHY

1. Behrens RH, Carroll B, Beran J, Bouchaud O, Hellgren U, Hatz C, et al. The low and declining risk of malaria in travellers to Latin America: is there still an indication for chemoprophylaxis? Malar J. 2007;6:114.
2. Cabada MM, Maldonado F, Quispe W, Serrano E, Mozo K, Gonzales E, et al. Pretravel health advice among international travelers visiting Cuzco, Peru. J Travel Med. 2005 Mar–Apr;12(2):61–5.
3. Mazor SS, Mycyk MB, Wills BK, Brace LD, Gussow L, Erickson T. Coca tea consumption causes positive urine cocaine assay. Eur J Emerg Med. 2006 Dec;13(6):340–1.
4. Merritt AL, Camerlengo A, Meyer C, Mull JD. Mountain sickness knowledge among foreign travelers in Cuzco, Peru. Wilderness Environ Med. 2007 Spring;18(1):26–9.
5. Steinhardt LC, Magill AJ, Arguin PM. Review: Malaria chemoprophylaxis for travelers to Latin America. Am J Trop Med Hyg. 2011 Dec;85(6):1015–24.

Asia

CAMBODIA: ANGKOR WAT

Carol Ciesielski

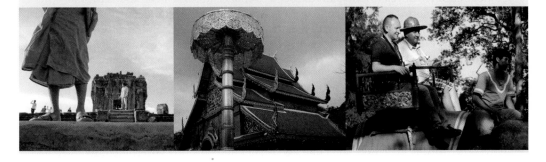

DESTINATION OVERVIEW

Every year, more than a million tourists travel to Siem Reap, Cambodia, the gateway to the ancient Angkor temples, a collection of approximately 100 structures covering 400 km^2

(150 square miles) in the northwestern Cambodia jungle. The Angkor Temple Complex is considered one of the architectural wonders of the world and, in 1992, was designated a World Heritage Site. The temples were built between the 9th and 14th centuries AD, at the height of the Khmer empire. These historical structures are decorated with intricately carved Khmer artwork depicting Hindu and Buddhist themes, providing an archaeological portrayal of the empire that ruled much of Southeast Asia for 5 centuries. After the decline of the Khmer empire, the site was largely abandoned to the surrounding jungle and remained virtually untouched until descriptions of the "lost temples of Cambodia" were published late in the 19th century. Restorations began as international visitors arrived, but the emergence of the Khmer Rouge and the ensuing decades of civil war halted most tourist travel to the site until the late 1990s. As Cambodia has emerged from more than 20 years of political and economic turmoil, the Angkor temples have become one of the most popular tourist destinations in Southeast Asia.

Cambodia is one of the poorest countries in Southeast Asia but is rapidly developing, especially with the tourist boom in its second largest city, Siem Reap. Most visitors arrive in Siem Reap via the short plane ride from Bangkok; however, flights from other Asian cities, including Singapore, Hong Kong, and Ho Chi Minh City, also serve Siem Reap. Overland travel is also possible from Bangkok and Cambodia's capital, Phnom Penh.

Typical itineraries for visiting the Angkor Temple Complex are for 2–4 days. The temples are spread over a large area throughout the surrounding forest. The closest temple to Siem Reap, Angkor Wat, is the most famous. Other popular sites close to Siem Reap include the walled city of Angkor Thom (principally the Bayon), and Ta Prohm. These sites can get crowded, especially around sunrise and sunset. Angkor is best experienced by exploring the temples at a leisurely pace, especially in intense heat, and good walking shoes, adequate hydration, sunscreen, and insect protection are critical. The temples are several kilometers apart, ordinarily requiring some sort of transportation; the most popular are *tuk-tuks* or car taxis.

HEALTH ISSUES

Immunizations

All travelers to Cambodia should be up-to-date with their routine immunizations and should be protected against hepatitis A and B and typhoid fever.

Japanese encephalitis (JE) is considered endemic throughout Cambodia; transmission occurs year-round but peaks during the May to October rainy season. The vaccine is recommended for travelers who plan to spend ≥1 month in rural areas and should be considered for short-term travelers who may be at increased risk for JE virus exposure, such as those who will spend substantial time outdoors in rural or agricultural areas, especially after dusk and during the rainy season. Travelers on a typical 2- to 4-day visit to the close-in Angkor temples, staying in air-conditioned hotels in Siem Reap, are at minimal risk, but mosquito prevention measures should be employed.

Rabies is endemic throughout Cambodia. For most travelers on a short tour of the temples, the risk is minimal. The chief risk is from dog bites, but the many monkeys and other wildlife around Angkor should be avoided. The Pasteur Institute in Phnom Penh can provide rabies vaccine and consultation.

Although yellow fever is not a disease risk in Cambodia, the government requires travelers arriving from countries with a risk of yellow fever virus transmission to present proof of yellow fever vaccination.

Other Health and Safety Risks
Travelers' Diarrhea

Diarrhea and foodborne infections in travelers are common in Cambodia. Avoid water that is not bottled, ice, and food from street vendors. Safe, bottled water is readily available. Travelers should practice safe food and water precautions (see Chapter 2, Food & Water Precautions) and carry an antibiotic for self-treatment (see Chapter 2, Travelers' Diarrhea for self-treatment recommendations).

Dengue

Dengue is endemic throughout Cambodia, with large epidemics every several years. Peak transmission occurs during the rainy season, although cases occur year-round even in non-epidemic years. Travelers to Cambodia should take measures to protect themselves from daytime mosquito bites to prevent dengue (see Chapter 2, Protection against Mosquitoes, Ticks, & Other Insects & Arthropods).

Malaria   *Malarone or Doxy   & Mefl*

The highest risk of malaria infection for the traveler in Cambodia is in forested areas. There is little to no transmission of malaria around Angkor Wat, Tonle Sap Lake around Siem Reap, and Phnom Penh. On a typical 2- to 4-day visit that involves exploring the close-in temples during the day and staying in an air-conditioned hotel in Siem Reap at night, malaria risk is minimal. However, mosquito protection measures should still be employed. Travelers planning to visit the more remote temples deeper in the forest, especially in the early morning and evening, should consider malaria chemoprophylaxis. The recommended chemoprophylaxis regimen for Siem Reap Province is atovaquone-proguanil or doxycycline.

Transportation

Driving in Cambodia is chaotic at best and is a rapidly rising cause of injury and death to passengers and pedestrians. In addition to the ever-growing number of cars and motorcycles,

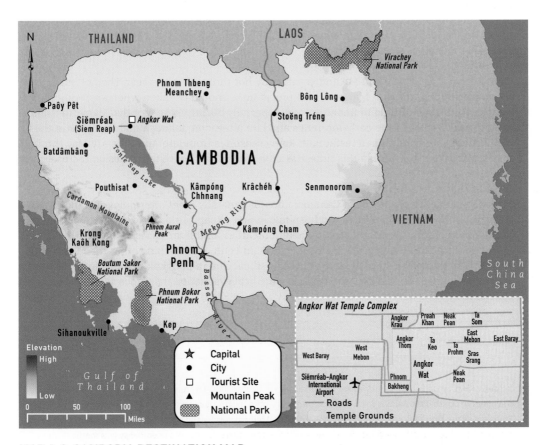

MAP 4-9. CAMBODIA DESTINATION MAP

there is lax enforcement of traffic laws and scant understanding of rules of the road. Travelers should carefully look in every direction before crossing the street in Siem Reap. During the rainy season, road conditions deteriorate rapidly. Most travelers use *tuk-tuks*, which are readily available, or hire cars with a driver guide to tour the temples. The fare should be negotiated at the outset. For those who, in spite of the risk, end up riding on the back of a *tuk-tuk*, wearing a helmet is essential.

Safety

While in Siem Reap, travelers should use common-sense measures such as not walking alone at night. The most common type of theft is "snatch and grab" robbery. Travelers should keep belongings out of sight if traveling via *tuk-tuk* and carry items and bags away from the street side while walking.

Land Mines

Land mines and unexploded ordnance from the decades of conflict are still found in rural areas in Cambodia, including those located in Siem Reap Province. Given the millions of visitors to the Angkor Temples in the past decade, Siem Reap town and the areas around the popular temples appear to be low risk. However, it is wise to exercise caution, especially when venturing out to the more remote temples and forest, by staying on roads and paths and using a guide with knowledge of local hazards. Travelers should not touch anything resembling a mine or unexploded ordnance; if these items are observed, the Cambodia Mine Action Center should be notified.

Counterfeit Drugs

Local pharmacies provide a limited number of prescription and over-the-counter medications, but because the quality of locally obtained medications can vary greatly, travelers should bring an adequate supply of medications. Counterfeit drugs are commonly found and are often indiscernible from authentic medication.

Climate

Siem Reap has a tropical climate and is generally hot throughout the year. The hottest months are March through May, and heat precautions should be taken when exploring the temples from midmorning to midafternoon, especially during these months. Many travelers explore the temples in the early mornings and late afternoon, taking a midday break in the comfort of an air-conditioned restaurant. Rainy season is from late April or early May through October or November. During this time, risk of vectorborne disease transmission increases.

Medical Care

Medical facilities and services in Cambodia do not generally meet international standards. A few internationally run clinics and hospitals in Siem Reap can provide basic medical care and stabilization. Some information on health facilities and pharmacies in Siem Reap can be found on the website for the US Embassy in Phnom Penh. For anything other than basic care and stabilization, most travelers should seek medical care in Bangkok or Singapore. For this reason, travel health insurance that includes medical evacuation insurance should be strongly considered.

BIBLIOGRAPHY

1. Behrens RH, Carroll B, Hellgren U, Visser LG, Siikamaki H, Vestergaard LS, et al. The incidence of malaria in travellers to South-East Asia: is local malaria transmission a useful risk indicator? Malar J. 2010;9:266.
2. Embassy of the United States, Phnom Penh, Cambodia. Medical services in Cambodia. Phnom Penh: US Department of State; 2012 [cited 2012 Sep 26]. Available from: http://cambodia.usembassy.gov/medical_information.html.

3. Ledgerwood J. Landmines in Cambodia. DeKalb, IL: Northern Illinois University [cited 2012 Sep 26]. Available from: http://www.seasite.niu.edu/khmer/Ledgerwood/Landmines.htm.

4. Ly S, Buchy P, Heng NY, Ong S, Chhor N, Bourhy H, et al. Rabies situation in Cambodia. PLoS Negl Trop Dis. 2009;3(9):e511.

5. Rogers WO, Sem R, Tero T, Chim P, Lim P, Muth S, et al. Failure of artesunate-mefloquine combination therapy for uncomplicated *Plasmodium falciparum* malaria in southern Cambodia. Malar J. 2009;8:10.

6. Touch S, Hills S, Sokhal B, Samnang C, Sovann L, Khieu V, et al. Epidemiology and burden of disease from Japanese encephalitis in Cambodia: results from two years of sentinel surveillance. Trop Med Int Health. 2009 Nov;14(11):1365–73.

7. US Department of State. Cambodia country specific information. Washington, DC: US Department of State; 2012 [cited 2012 Sep 26]. Available from: http://www.travel.state.gov/travel/cis_pa_tw/cis/cis_1080.html.

8. World Health Organization. Cambodia. Geneva: World Health Organization; 2012 [cited 2012 Sep 26]. Available from: http://www.who.int/countries/khm/en/.

9. World Health Organization. Cambodia. In: World Malaria Report 2011. Geneva: World Health Organization; 2011 [cited 2012 Sep 26]. p. 98. Available from: http://www.who.int/malaria/publications/country-profiles/profile_khm_en.pdf.

CHINA

Sarah T. Borwein

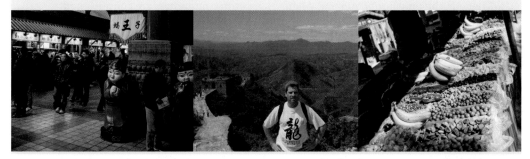

DESTINATION OVERVIEW

China, with >1.3 billion people, is the world's most populous country and the fourth largest geographically, behind Russia, Canada, and the United States. It shares a border with 14 other countries and has approximately 18,000 km of coastline. China is divided into 23 provinces, 5 autonomous regions, and 4 municipalities. This large landmass is home to diverse topography, languages, and customs. The climate varies from tropical in the south to subarctic in the north, with wide variations between regions and seasons. Natural hazards include typhoons along the southern and eastern seaboards, dust storms in the north, floods, earthquakes, and landslides. Six of the 10 deadliest natural disasters in history occurred in China, including the 1556 Shaanxi earthquake, which is thought to have killed >800,000 people, making it the most lethal earthquake in history. Chinese superstition holds that natural disasters foretell the death of a ruler or the end of a dynasty, and indeed Mao Tse Tung died only 6 weeks after the 1976 Tangshan earthquake, the death toll of which was also in the hundreds of thousands. More recently, devastating earthquakes have struck the western provinces of Sichuan in 2008 and Qinghai in 2010. Torrential rain, floods, and landslides plagued large areas of China in the summer of 2010, as well as drought and dust storms in the north.

China has one of the world's oldest continuous civilizations, dating back >5,000 years. It has the world's longest continuously used written language system and is the source of many major inventions, including the "four great inventions of Ancient China": paper, the compass, gunpowder, and printing. Today, China is considerably more advanced (with the ability to put men in space, for example) and wealthier than many other developing countries, yet rural poverty and underdevelopment are still problems, particularly in the western part of the country.

Approximately 700 million Chinese live in rural areas. Urban areas are growing rapidly, however, and China is now home to many of the world's largest megacities. Shanghai and Beijing each have ≥20 million inhabitants, and Chongqing, with a metropolitan population >30 million, is the fastest-growing urban center in the world. Rivers play a central role in China's economy, history, and culture. The Yangtze River basin, stretching 4,000 miles from the Tibetan plateau to the East China Sea near Shanghai, is home to >5% of the world's population.

In 2010, >55 million tourists visited China, and by 2020, China is widely predicted to be both the largest tourist destination and the largest source of tourists to other countries. China's long history and varied natural beauty can be traced in its 41 UNESCO World Heritage sites, from the imperial grandeur of the Forbidden City and the Temple of Heaven, to the marvel of the Great Wall, the Terracotta Warriors in Xi'an, and the spectacular mountainous sanctuaries of the west. Popular itineraries often include Beijing and the Great Wall, Xi'an, and the Yangtze River (see Box 4-1 for information specifically about Yangtze River cruises). Other tourist destinations include the following:

> Shanghai and Hong Kong, with their futuristic architecture and East-meets-West mystique
> Lijiang in the province of Yunnan, where many ethnic minorities are concentrated
> Sichuan province, home to China's iconic symbol, the panda
> Guilin, famous for its uniquely shaped limestone karst mountains that are often featured in Chinese paintings
> Tibet, accessible now by the world's highest railroad directly to Lhasa, with a maximum altitude of 16,640 ft (5,072 m)

BOX 4-1. CRUISING DOWN THE YANGTZE: WHAT TO CONSIDER

The Yangtze River is the third longest river in the world and one of the world's busiest (and most polluted) waterways. Yangtze River cruises are popular with tourists, and there are several heath considerations for this trip:

- At least 1 case of Japanese encephalitis has been documented in a tourist whose 3-week trip to rural and urban China included a Yangtze River cruise, and documented cases are likely to be an underestimate.
- Malaria is not a substantial risk on this itinerary; only insect bite precautions are recommended.
- Schistosomiasis—*Schistosoma japonicum*—exists in the Yangtze River basin. Swimming is ill-advised.
- Motion sickness is rare on Yangtze cruises, since much of it takes place on a calm reservoir. However, susceptible travelers should carry antiemetic medication.
- Excursions off the boat often involve steep climbs, many stairs, and long walking distances and may not be appropriate for physically infirm tourists.
- Air pollution can be a problem on Yangtze River cruises and can cause eye and throat irritation, as well as respiratory problems in susceptible travelers. September and October are said to be the clearest months.
- Most non-Chinese–speaking tourists will prefer a 4- or 5-star "luxury" cruise. First class on a Chinese tourist boat may not meet expectations for cleanliness, and English may not be spoken.
- Food and water precautions apply, even on a luxury boat.

Specialized itineraries are increasingly being offered, including hiking, mountain climbing, village tours, the Silk Road, and other more remote regions. Aside from tourism, increasing numbers of people travel to China to visit friends and relatives, to study, or to adopt children. These groups may be at particularly high risk of illness, because they underestimate their risks, are less likely to seek pre-travel advice, and stay in more local or rural accommodations. People traveling to China to adopt children often worry about the health of the child but neglect their own health.

HEALTH ISSUES

Although China is now the world's second-largest economy, in per capita terms income is still below the world average, with wide disparity in wealth and development between rural and urban, as well as east and west. Health risks vary accordingly.

Immunizations

Routine vaccinations should be up-to-date, including tetanus, diphtheria, measles, mumps, rubella, varicella, influenza, and pneumococcal vaccines, as indicated. In addition, hepatitis A and B and typhoid vaccinations are usually recommended. Since the Xinjiang Uygur Autonomous Region borders Pakistan, a polio-endemic country, adults traveling to this region may consider a booster dose of polio vaccine (IPV). Measles and rubella immunity is particularly important, although a massive vaccination campaign begun in September 2010

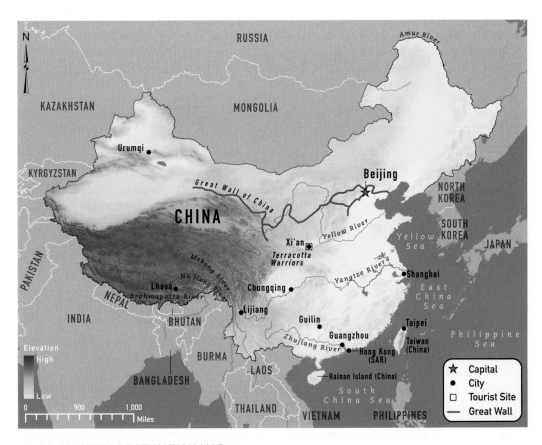

MAP 4-10. CHINA DESTINATION MAP

has decreased the number of reported measles cases, from 131,000 in 2008 to 10,000 in 2011. Nonetheless, a few travelers have made news headlines by triggering outbreaks in their home countries after returning from China. Although limited data exist on rubella in China, it was not part of the national immunization program until 2008, and incidence is believed to be high.

Rabies Vaccine

Rabies is a serious problem in China, as in much of Asia, with >3,000 human deaths per year reported in recent years. Mammal bites in any area of China, including urban areas, must be considered high risk for rabies. As international standard rabies immune globulin is generally unavailable, animal bites are often trip-enders, requiring evacuation to Hong Kong, Bangkok, or home for postexposure prophylaxis. Bites are surprisingly common in tourists. For example, dog bites were the most common dermatologic problem seen after China travel in a recent analysis of data from the GeoSentinel Surveillance Network. Rabies risk and prevention should be discussed in pre-travel consultations, and a strategy for dealing with a possible exposure should be developed. Long-term travelers and expatriates living in China should consider the preexposure vaccination series. Travel health insurance, including medical evacuation insurance, should be encouraged (see Chapter 2, Travel Insurance, Travel Health Insurance, & Medical Evacuation Insurance).

Japanese Encephalitis Vaccine

Japanese encephalitis (JE) occurs in all regions except Qinghai, Xinjiang, and Xizang (Tibet) (see Map 3-8 and Table 3-6). China has greatly reduced the incidence of JE through vaccination, and as of 2008, included JE in its expanded national immunization program; however, the disease remains a threat to unimmunized travelers. Although the JE season varies by region, most cases in local residents are reported from June through October. The risk of JE for most travelers to China is low but varies based on season, destination, duration, and activities. Risk is highest among travelers to rural areas during the transmission season. JE vaccine is recommended for travelers who plan to spend ≥1 month in endemic areas during June through October. It should be considered for shorter-term travelers if they plan to travel to rural areas and will have an increased risk for JE virus exposure based on their activities or itineraries, such as spending substantial time outdoors or staying in accommodations without air conditioning, screens, or bed nets. However, rare sporadic cases have occurred on an unpredictable basis in short-term travelers, including in periurban Beijing and Shanghai.

Malaria *(rare) Vivax - Meflo + Chloro resistance.*

Malaria risk is low for travelers to China, with the exception of those visiting rural parts of southern Yunnan Province or Hainan Island. For these areas, chemoprophylaxis should be considered. Mefloquine resistance in southern Yunnan means that prophylaxis should be given doxycycline or atovaquone-proguanil for travel in this area. For travelers to other regions, the risk is too low to warrant chemoprophylaxis. Rare cases occur in other rural parts of the country at <1,500 m (4,921 ft) from May through December, usually *Plasmodium vivax* infections, and only insect precautions are recommended.

Other Health Risks

Foodborne Illnesses

The risk for travelers' diarrhea appears to be low in deluxe accommodations in China but moderate elsewhere. Usual food and water precautions should apply, and travelers should carry an antibiotic for self-treatment. Since highly quinolone-resistant *Campylobacter* is a problem in China, azithromycin may be a good choice. Tap water is not safe to drink even in major cities. Most hotels provide bottled or boiled water, and bottled water is easily available. In addition, there have been several well-publicized episodes of contamination of food with pesticides and other substances. Travelers should strictly avoid undercooked fish and shellfish and unpasteurized milk.

Sexually Transmitted Diseases

Sexually transmitted diseases, including syphilis, HIV, gonorrhea, and chlamydia, are a growing problem in China, particularly along the booming eastern seaboard. Travel is associated with loosened inhibitions and increased casual sexual liaisons. In addition to risk-reduction counseling, consider hepatitis B vaccination.

Air Pollution

Air pollution is a problem in most major cities in China. There is potential for exacerbation of respiratory conditions, including asthma and chronic obstructive pulmonary disease, and heightened risk for respiratory infections. All travelers should receive influenza vaccine, and susceptible people should also receive pneumococcal vaccination and bring any inhaled medications they may use.

Accidents

Traffic in China is often chaotic, and the rate of accidents, including fatal ones, is among the highest in the world. Driving is on the right side of the road in mainland China but on the left in Hong Kong and Macau. In practice, many people drive down the middle of the road. Child safety seats, rear seat belts, and bicycle or motorcycle helmets are not widely available. Accidents, even minor ones, can create major traffic jams and sometimes turn into violent altercations, particularly when foreigners are involved. China has not signed the convention that created the International Driving Permit, and travelers require a Chinese license to drive in China. For all of these reasons, it is often simpler and safer to hire a local driver than to drive oneself. It is also advisable to avoid driving at night or when weather conditions are bad and not to assume that traffic rules or right-of-way will be respected.

Medical Care in China

Western-style medical facilities that meet international standards are available in Beijing, Shanghai, and Hong Kong. Some hospitals in other cities have "VIP wards" (*gaogan bingfang*), which may have English-speaking staff. The standard of care in such facilities is somewhat unpredictable, and cultural and regulatory differences can cause difficulties for travelers. In rural areas, only rudimentary medical care may be available. Hepatitis B transmission from poorly sterilized medical equipment remains a risk outside major centers.

Ambulances are not staffed with trained paramedics and often have little or no medical equipment. Therefore, injured travelers may need to take taxis or other immediately available vehicles to the nearest major hospital rather than waiting for ambulances to arrive.

Pharmacies often sell prescription medications over the counter. Such medications have sometimes been counterfeit, substandard, or even contaminated. Travelers should carry all their regular medications in sufficient quantity; if more or other medications are required, it is advisable to visit a reputable clinic or hospital.

Some travelers wish to try traditional Chinese medicine and acupuncture. Although most do so uneventfully, there is a risk of bloodborne and skin infections from acupuncture needles, and traditional medicine products may be contaminated with heavy metals or pharmaceutical agents. Acupressure may be preferable to acupuncture.

Travelers are strongly advised to purchase travel health and medical evacuation insurance before travel. Most hospitals will not directly accept foreign medical insurance, however, and patients will often be expected to pay a deposit before care to cover the expected cost of the treatment.

BIBLIOGRAPHY

1. CDC. Measles among adults associated with adoption of children in China—California, Missouri, and Washington, July–August 2006. MMWR Morb Mortal Wkly Rep. 2007 Feb 23;56(7):144–6.

2. Chen XS, Gong XD, Liang GJ, Zhang GC. Epidemiologic trends of sexually transmitted diseases in China. Sex Transm Dis. 2000 Mar;27(3):138–42.

3. Cutfield NJ, Anderson NE, Brickell K, Hueston L, Pikholz C, Roxburgh RH. Japanese encephalitis acquired during travel in China. Intern Med J. 2005 Aug;35(8):497–8.

4. Davis XM, MacDonald S, Borwein S, Freedman DO, Kozarsky PE, von Sonnenburg F, et al. Health risks in travelers to China: the GeoSentinel experience and implications for the 2008 Beijing Olympics. Am J Trop Med Hyg. 2008 Jul;79(1):4–8.

5. Hills SL, Griggs AC, Fischer M. Japanese encephalitis in travelers from non-endemic countries, 1973–2008. Am J Trop Med Hyg. 2010 May;82(5):930–6.

6. Shaw MT, Leggat PA, Borwein S. Travelling to China for the Beijing 2008 Olympic and Paralympic games. Travel Med Infect Dis. 2007 Nov;5(6):365–73.

7. Shlim DR, Solomon T. Japanese encephalitis vaccine for travelers: exploring the limits of risk. Clin Infect Dis. 2002 Jul 15;35(2):183–8.

8. Tang X, Luo M, Zhang S, Fooks AR, Hu R, Tu C. Pivotal role of dogs in rabies transmission, China. Emerg Infect Dis. 2005 Dec;11(12):1970–2.

9. United Nations World Tourism Organization. UNWTO tourism highlights. Madrid: United Nations World Tourism Organization; 2012 [cited 2012 Sep 26]. Available from: http://mkt.unwto.org/en/publication/unwto-tourism-highlights-2012-edition.

10. World Health Organization. Measles bulletin: Western Pacific region. Geneva: World Health Organization; 2010 [cited 2012 Sep 26]. Available from: http://www.wpro.who.int/entity/immunization/documents/docs/MeasBulletinVol4Issue1_F840.pdf.

11. Zhang J, Jin Z, Sun GQ, Zhou T, Ruan S. Analysis of rabies in China: transmission dynamics and control. PloS One. 2011;6(7):e20891.

12. Zhang YZ, Xiong CL, Xiao DL, Jiang RJ, Wang ZX, Zhang LZ, et al. Human rabies in China. Emerg Infect Dis. 2005 Dec;11(12):1983–4.

INDIA
Phyllis E. Kozarsky

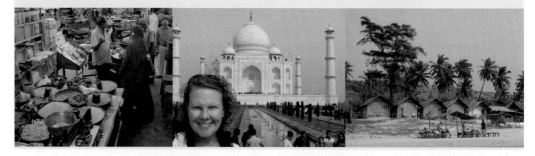

DESTINATION OVERVIEW

India is approximately one-third the size of the United States and has 4 times the population (1.2 billion people). This makes it the second most populous country in the world, behind China. Rich in history, vibrant culture, and diversity, India is the birthplace of 4 world religions: Hinduism, Buddhism, Jainism, and Sikhism. Despite the growth of megacities such as Mumbai and Delhi (both >15 million people), 70% of the population still resides in rural areas, and 60% work in agriculture. Although India is one of the fastest-growing economies in the world, the literacy rate is 74%, and the level of poverty is high. The topography is varied, ranging from tropical beaches to foothills, deserts, and the Himalayan Mountains. The north has a more temperate climate, while the south is more tropical year round. Many travelers prefer India during the winter—November through March, when the temperatures are more agreeable—although some, particularly families with children, must travel during the summer vacation time.

India is becoming more popular for US travelers, and rates of travel from the United States are increasing. International businesses are flourishing in India; tourists are flocking to the temples, beaches, and the Taj Mahal. For some new US residents, India remains their homeland, and they make frequent visits to family and friends.

Because tourists could not possibly visit all the tourist sites in India during a 2-week holiday, they usually select a part of India for any given trip. A typical itinerary in the north of India includes Delhi, Agra, and cities in Rajasthan, such as Jaipur (the "pink" city). Agra is the home of the Taj Mahal, a breathtaking monument to lost love. Along the northern travel circle, one can stop to enjoy the magnificent bird sanctuary at Keoladeo Ghana and the tiger reserve at Ran Thambore. Another frequent stop is Goa and its beaches on the western coast, where swaying coconut palms form the backdrop for great parties and old-time hippies. Mumbai, another common entry point to India, hosts Bollywood, the largest film industry in the world. Kolkata is considered the cultural capital of the country. Bengaluru (Bangalore) in the south-central region has become a worldwide information technology center and has managed to meld the very old and traditional India with a new image of a modern hub. And Varanasi boasts extraordinary experiences along the Ganges. Despite the many and varied itineraries, most health recommendations for travelers to India are similar. The incidences of some illnesses, such as those transmitted by mosquitoes, increase during the monsoon season (May–October) with the high temperatures, heavy rains, and the risk of flooding.

Some of the most important health considerations of travel to India are those for travelers who are visiting friends and relatives (VFRs). These travelers often do not seek pre-travel health advice, since they are returning to their land of origin. Such travelers may stay in rural areas often not visited by tourists or business people, live in homes, and eat and drink with their families and thus are at higher risk of many travel-related illnesses (see Chapter 8, Immigrants Returning Home to Visit Friends and Relatives [VFRs]).

HEALTH ISSUES

Immunizations

All travelers to India should be up-to-date with their routine immunizations and are advised to consider hepatitis B vaccine. Particularly important is making sure that the traveler is immune to measles. Although India has not had a case of wild poliovirus since early 2011 and is therefore considered to have interrupted transmission, a polio booster (IPV) is recommended for all adult travelers to India, if the childhood series was completed (www.polioeradication.org) (see Chapter 3, Poliomyelitis, for information on travelers who have not completed the childhood series).

Hepatitis A Vaccine

All travelers to India should be protected against hepatitis A. Although some assume that those born in India would have been exposed to hepatitis A in childhood and thus be immune, this may no longer be true, particularly for younger people. Providers should consider serologic testing for hepatitis A IgG in VFR travelers, or they should be immunized.

Typhoid Vaccine

The incidence of typhoid in US citizens traveling to the Indian subcontinent has been reported to be ≥18 times higher than from any other geographic region. It is the country from which most travel-related typhoid is imported, and thus, even for short-term travel, a typhoid vaccine should be recommended. More compelling for those who are hesitant is the fact that typhoid fever acquired in India is becoming increasingly resistant to quinolone antibiotics, sometimes requiring parenteral therapy.

Japanese Encephalitis Vaccine

Although there has never been a published case of a traveler acquiring Japanese encephalitis (JE) in India, the disease is present in many parts of the country. Risk is highest during the monsoon season from May through October; however, the season may be extended or year-round in some areas, especially in the south. Vaccination is not recommended for the typical 2-week trip most travelers take to see the major tourist sites in urban areas. However, vaccination is recommended for travelers who plan to spend ≥1 month in endemic areas during the JE virus transmission season and should be considered for short-term travelers if they plan to travel outside an urban area and have an increased risk for JE virus exposures (see Chapter 3, Japanese Encephalitis). Publicized outbreaks in recent years have not been in typical tourist destinations.

Rabies Vaccine

India has the highest burden of rabies in the world, with estimates of 15,000–20,000 human cases per year. Dogs roam in packs in many areas of the country. Unfortunately, human rabies immune globulin is not readily available in India. If a traveler does not have preexposure rabies vaccination, a bite may result in having to leave the country for postexposure prophylaxis. Even so, a preexposure series is not recommended for all travelers to India. Cost is a consideration for many. Long-term travelers, expatriates, missionaries, and volunteers may want to obtain preexposure immunization for themselves and their children. Travelers may want to purchase a medical evacuation insurance policy that will cover travel for recommended rabies postexposure prophylaxis.

Malaria

Although the intensity of malaria may be related to the season, unlike other countries in Asia, malaria is holoendemic in India (except at altitudes >2,000 m [6,561 ft]) and occurs in both rural and urban areas. Rates of *Plasmodium falciparum* have increased in the last 2 decades, and thus chemoprophylaxis is recommended for all destinations. For short-term travelers spending 1–2 days in Delhi in the winter, insect precautions alone may be sufficient to prevent malaria. Travelers should be reminded that malaria-transmitting mosquitoes primarily bite between dusk and dawn.

Other Infections

General

More recently in India, new strains of bacteria that are resistant to most antibiotics have been carried by travelers to many other countries, including the United States. For example, resistance to carbapenem antibiotics is conferred by enzymes such as New Delhi metallo-β-lactamase-1, which makes it more difficult to treat problems such as skin and bloodstream infections.

Dengue

Dengue is endemic in all of India, although it is poorly reported at the local and national levels, and large outbreaks have occurred. The incidence is highest during the wet summer season, which includes the monsoon season (September–October). Travelers to India should take measures to protect themselves from daytime mosquito bites to prevent dengue (see Chapter 2, Protection against Mosquitoes, Ticks, & Other Insects & Arthropods).

Chikungunya

During the last several years there have been outbreaks of chikungunya, which, like dengue, is transmitted by day-biting mosquitoes. Symptoms are similar to those of dengue and malaria, although often with severe and persistent arthralgia.

4

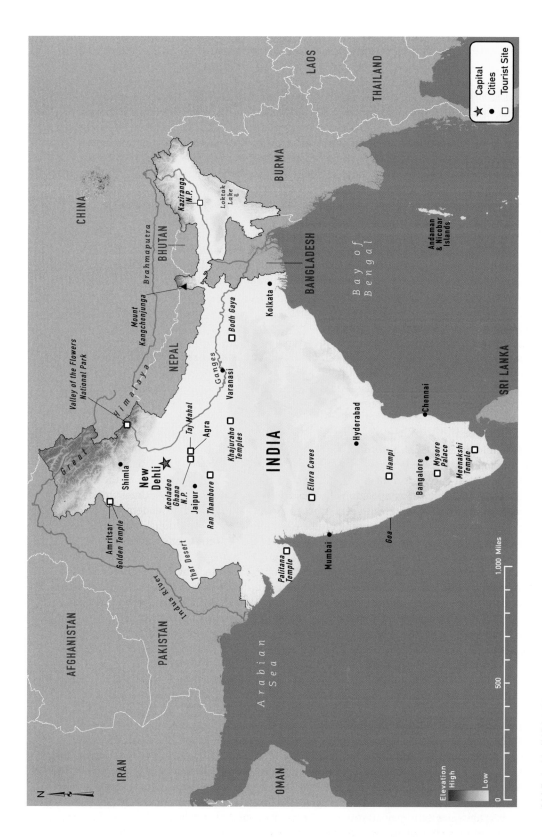

MAP 4-11. INDIA DESTINATION MAP

Hepatitis E

Hepatitis E is being recognized more frequently in travelers to India. A traveler who develops symptomatic hepatitis, despite being immunized against hepatitis A, will likely have hepatitis E.

Animal Bites and Wounds

In addition to rabies, other diseases can be transmitted by animal bites and wounds. Cellulitis, fasciitis, and wound infections may result from scratches or bites of any animal. Herpes B virus is carried by Old World monkeys and may be transmitted by active macaques that are kept as pets, inhabit many of the temples, and scatter themselves in many tourist gathering places. Monkeys can be aggressive and often approach travelers seeking food. When visiting temple areas that have monkeys, travelers should not carry any food in their hands, pockets, or bags. It is important to stress to travelers that monkeys and other animals should not be approached or handled at all. If travelers are bitten, they should seek medical care.

Travelers' Diarrhea

The risk for travelers' diarrhea is moderate to high in India, with an estimated 30%–50% risk during a 2-week journey. Travelers should practice safe food and water precautions (see Chapter 2, Food & Water Precautions) and carry an antibiotic for empiric self-treatment of diarrhea (see Chapter 2, Travelers' Diarrhea).

Tuberculosis

Tuberculosis (TB) is a major problem in India: 26% of all TB cases worldwide occur there. Unfortunately, >2% of these cases are estimated to be multidrug-resistant, and a smaller number are extensively drug-resistant. Travelers who plan to work in medical settings or in crowded institutions (such as prisons or homeless shelters) should speak to their health care providers about measures for prevention and testing for exposure after travel.

Miscellaneous

Arrival in India for the first time may be shocking to travelers who have never ventured into the developing world. The crowds, the intense colors, heat, and smells are striking and invade all the senses at once. It is difficult to enjoy the beauty without being touched by the enormity of the poverty. The close juxtaposition of the old and new is noteworthy. At times this can be overwhelming for travelers. Health care is quite variable in India and dependent on the location.

Transportation in India remains problematic. While traveling through India, travelers should be advised to carry food and beverages with them in the event of delays, almost inevitable no matter the mode of transport. Traveling by train can be harrowing, particularly having to force one's way through the crowd and onto the train. Travelers should make sure to keep passports and valuables safe while in a crowd. Roadways are some of the most hazardous in the world. Animals, rickshaws, motor scooters, people, bicycles, trucks, and overcrowded buses compete for space in an unregulated free-for-all. Rural, nighttime driving should be discouraged, even when a paid driver has been hired. Air pollution is a problem in the major cities, so those with chronic lung disease or asthma may consider spending time outdoors when there is less traffic or staying in facilities outside major cities.

Medical tourism is a growing industry in India. Many newer medical facilities have recently opened for travelers desiring cardiac, orthopedic, dental, or plastic surgery or transplantations at a substantially lower cost than in the United States. The benefits and hazards require careful examination (see Chapter 2, Medical Tourism).

In general, travelers feel safe while in India. Peddlers and promoters are aggressive with tourists, however, and may require a firm "no." Travelers may want to avoid making eye contact with a peddler or his goods, or they may risk having someone follow them down the street trying to sell them something. The stress of negotiating one's way through India makes this destination a place where having a close traveling companion is important.

It is always wise to pay attention to Department of State advisories in case of issues that arise at some borders or occasional increases in religious tensions or terrorist activities.

BIBLIOGRAPHY

1. Bacaner N, Stauffer B, Boulware DR, Walker PF, Keystone JS. Travel medicine considerations for North American immigrants visiting friends and relatives. JAMA. 2004 Jun 16;291(23):2856–64.
2. Baggett HC, Graham S, Kozarsky PE, Gallagher N, Blumensaadt S, Bateman J, et al. Pretravel health preparation among US residents traveling to India to VFRs: importance of ethnicity in defining VFRs. J Travel Med. 2009 Mar–Apr;16(2):112–8.
3. Connor BA, Schwartz E. Typhoid and paratyphoid fever in travellers. Lancet Infect Dis. 2005 Oct;5(10): 623–8.
4. Das K, Jain A, Gupta S, Kapoor S, Gupta RK, Chakravorty A, et al. The changing epidemiological pattern of hepatitis A in an urban population of India: emergence of a trend similar to the European countries. Eur J Epidemiol. 2000 Jun;16(6):507–10.
5. Kumarasamy KK, Toleman MA, Walsh TR, Bagaria J, Butt F, Balakrishnan R, et al. Emergence of a new antibiotic resistance mechanism in India, Pakistan, and the UK: a molecular, biological, and epidemiological study. Lancet Infect Dis. 2010 Sep;10(9):597–602.
6. Leder K, Tong S, Weld L, Kain KC, Wilder-Smith A, von Sonnenburg F, et al. Illness in travelers visiting friends and relatives: a review of the GeoSentinel Surveillance Network. Clin Infect Dis. 2006 Nov 1;43(9):1185–93.
7. Steinberg EB, Bishop R, Haber P, Dempsey AF, Hoekstra RM, Nelson JM, et al. Typhoid fever in travelers: who should be targeted for prevention? Clin Infect Dis. 2004 Jul 15;39(2):186–91.

NEPAL
David R. Shlim

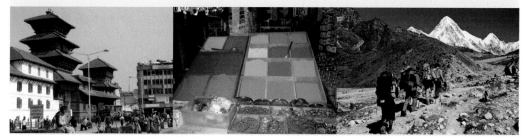

DESTINATION OVERVIEW

Nepal is a country of >28 million people that stretches for 500 miles (805 km) along the Himalayan mountains that form the border of Nepal and Tibet. The topography rises from low plains with an altitude of 200 ft (70 m) to the highest point in the world at 29,029 ft (8,848 m), the summit of Mount Everest. Approximately 30% of tourists come to Nepal to trek into the mountains, while others come to experience the culture and stunning natural beauty. Kathmandu is the capital city, with a population of well over a million people. It sits in a lush valley at 4,344 ft (1,324 m) in altitude. Nepal's latitude of 28° North (the same as Florida) means that the nonmountainous areas are temperate year round. Most of the annual rainfall comes during the monsoon season (June through September). The main tourist seasons are in the spring (March to May) and fall (October and November). The winter months, December through February, are pleasant in the lowlands but can be too cold to make trekking enjoyable in the high mountains.

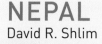

Hicking March-May
+Oct-Nov

There are 3 main trekking areas: the Mount Everest region east of Kathmandu, the Annapurna region to the west, and the Langtang region north of Kathmandu. Trekkers into the Mount Everest region routinely sleep at altitudes of 14,000–16,000 ft (4,267–4,876 m) and hike to altitudes >18,000 ft (5,486 m). This prolonged exposure to very high altitudes means that tourists must be knowledgeable about the risks of altitude illness and may need to carry specific medications to prevent and treat the problem (see Chapter 2, Altitude Illness). Most trekkers into the Mount Everest region arrive there by flying to a tiny airstrip at Lukla at 9,383 ft (2,860 m). The following day they reach Namche Bazaar at 11,290 ft (3,440 m). Acetazolamide prophylaxis can substantially decrease the chances of developing acute mountain sickness in Namche.

In the Annapurna region, short-term trekkers may choose to hike to viewpoints in the foothills without reaching any high altitudes. Others may undertake a longer trek around the Annapurna massif, going over a 17,769-ft (5,416-m) pass (the Thorung La). Roads have been constructed up the 2 major valleys of this trek, shortening the overall trekking distance and changing the nature of the experience (cars and motorcycles may be encountered along the trek). The total exposure to high altitude is less in this region than in the Everest region. The Langtang region has a high point of 14,000 ft (4,200 m).

In addition to trekking, Nepal has some of the best rafting and kayaking rivers in the world. Jungle lodges in Chitwan National Park allow tourists to view a wide range of wildlife, including tigers, rhinoceroses, bears, and crocodiles, and a huge variety of exotic birds. It is also possible to travel by road to comfortable lodges in the foothills that afford panoramic views of the Himalayas.

HEALTH ISSUES

Immunizations

Travelers to Nepal are at high risk for enterically transmitted diseases. Hepatitis A vaccine and typhoid vaccine are the 2 most important immunizations. The risk of typhoid fever and paratyphoid fever among travelers to Nepal is among the highest in the world, and the prevalence of fluoroquinolone resistance is high.

Japanese encephalitis (JE) is endemic in Nepal, with highest disease risk occurring in the Terai region during and immediately after the monsoon season (June through October). JE has been identified in local residents of the Kathmandu Valley, but no cases of JE acquired in Nepal have been reported in tourists or expatriates. JE vaccine is not routinely recommended for those trekking in higher altitude areas or spending short periods in Kathmandu or Pokhara en route to such treks (see Chapter 3, Japanese Encephalitis).

Malaria

Malaria is not a risk for most travelers to Nepal. There is no transmission of malaria in Kathmandu or Pokhara, the 2 main cities in Nepal. All the main trekking routes in Nepal are free of malaria transmission. Chitwan National Park is a popular tourist destination for wildlife viewing in the Terai. Although the Nepalese Ministry of Health and other regional organizations regard the Terai to be a malaria transmission area, this author, in 30 years of treating travelers in Nepal, has not seen a single case of malaria in a traveler to Chitwan, including foreign workers living in the park.

Other Health and Safety Risks
Gastrointestinal Issues

Cyclospora cayetanensis is an intestinal protozoal pathogen that is highly endemic in Nepal. The risk for infection is distinctly seasonal: transmission occurs almost exclusively from May through October, with a peak in June and July. Because this is outside the main tourist seasons, the primary effect is on expatriates who stay through the monsoon. In addition to watery diarrhea, profound anorexia and fatigue are the hallmark symptoms of *Cyclospora* infection. The treatment of choice is trimethoprim-sulfamethoxazole; no highly effective alternatives have been identified.

Since many tourists are heading to remote areas that do not have medical care available, they should be provided with medications for self-treatment. Travelers' diarrhea is a risk, and the risk in the spring trekking season (March through May) is double that in the fall trekking season (October and November). All trekkers should have an antibiotic such as ciprofloxacin for empiric treatment of bacterial diarrhea. *Campylobacter* causes as much as 20% of the bacterial diarrhea in Nepal, and up to 70% of the *Campylobacter* isolates are resistant to fluoroquinolones. Although ciprofloxacin remains an excellent choice for empiric treatment of bacterial diarrhea, azithromycin is a good alternative and should be used if the diarrhea does not respond to ciprofloxacin.

– Hepatitis E virus is endemic in Nepal, and several cases each year are diagnosed in tourists or expatriates. There is no vaccine commercially available against hepatitis E.

Respiratory Issues

The Kathmandu Valley often has air pollution. People with chronic respiratory diseases, such as asthma and chronic obstructive pulmonary disease, may suffer exacerbations in Kathmandu, particularly after a viral upper respiratory infection. Exacerbation of chronic respiratory disease has not been a problem for tourists outside Kathmandu.

Viral upper respiratory infections are extremely common, and the percentage of these that lead to bacterial sinusitis or bronchitis is high. Trekkers should consider carrying an antibiotic, such as azithromycin, to empirically treat a respiratory infection that lasts >7 days

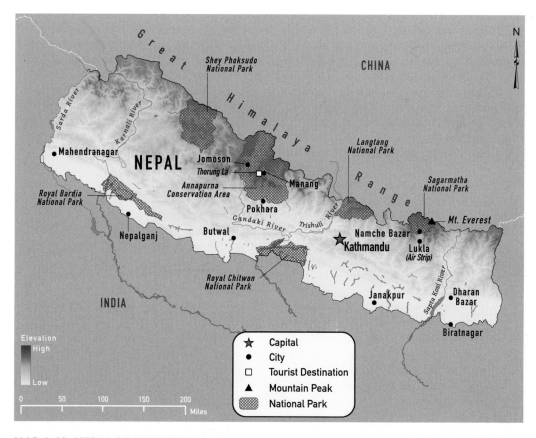

MAP 4-12. NEPAL DESTINATION MAP

with no sign of improvement. More treks may have been ruined by prolonged respiratory infection than by gastrointestinal illness.

Rabies

Rabies is highly endemic among dogs in Nepal, but in recent years there are fewer stray dogs in Kathmandu. Half of all tourist exposures to a possibly rabid animal occur near Swayambunath, a beautiful hilltop shrine also known as the monkey temple. Tourists should be advised to be extra cautious with dogs and monkeys in this area. The monkeys can be aggressive if approached and can jump on a person's back if they smell food in a backpack. Clinics in Kathmandu that specialize in the care of foreigners almost always have complete postexposure rabies prophylaxis, including human rabies immune globulin. Trekkers who are bitten in the mountains should be able to return to Kathmandu within an average of 5 days.

Evacuation and Medical Care

Helicopter evacuation from most areas is readily available. Communication has improved from remote areas because of satellite and cellular telephones, and private helicopter companies accept credit cards and are eager to perform evacuations for profit. Evacuation can often take place on the same day as the request, if weather permits. Helicopter rescue is usually limited to morning hours because of afternoon winds in the mountains. Helicopter rescue is billed at $2,500 per hour, with an average total cost of $7,500.

Two main clinics in Kathmandu specialize in the care of foreigners in Nepal. Contact information is available on the International Society of Travel Medicine website (www.istm. org). Hospital facilities have improved steadily over the years, and general and orthopedic emergency surgery are reliable and available in Kathmandu. The closest evacuation point for definitive care is Bangkok.

The Political Situation

The political situation in Nepal has been in transition since 1990, when a mainly peaceful democratic revolution led to a multiparty parliamentary system under a constitutional monarch. Frustration with the rate of progress in rural areas led to a Maoist insurrection and 10 years of low-grade but violent civil war. A peace agreement was reached and the monarchy abolished in 2008, but an effective government has yet to remain in place. The main effect on tourists can be disruptions to their schedule by demonstrations and strikes, but none of the political tension has been aimed at foreigners; Nepal remains a safe destination to visit. However, visitors should monitor the political situation while planning their journey.

BIBLIOGRAPHY

1. Cave W, Pandey P, Osrin D, Shlim DR. Chemoprophylaxis use and the risk of malaria in travelers to Nepal. J Travel Med. 2003 Mar–Apr;10(2):100–5.
2. Hoge CW, Shlim DR, Echeverria P, Rajah R, Herrmann JE, Cross JH. Epidemiology of diarrhea among expatriate residents living in a highly endemic environment. JAMA. 1996 Feb 21;275(7):533–8.
3. Schwartz E, Shlim DR, Eaton M, Jenks N, Houston R. The effect of oral and parenteral typhoid vaccination on the rate of infection with *Salmonella typhi* and *Salmonella paratyphi* A among foreigners in Nepal. Arch Intern Med. 1990 Feb;150(2):349–51.

THAILAND
Gabrielle A. Benenson

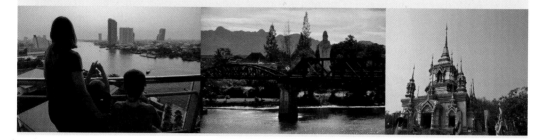

DESTINATION OVERVIEW

Thailand, known as "the Land of Smiles" is a popular travel destination because of its warm and welcoming reception of tourists and expatriates, beautiful beaches, delicious cuisine, excellent shopping, fabulous golf courses, exciting nightlife, and exotic adventure opportunities. Many travelers also visit Thailand for business, and the country is quickly becoming a regional business hub. The Thai language is a melodic, tonal language that can be difficult to learn. Luckily, most popular destinations in Thailand feature Thai people who speak English and road signs, maps, and tourist guides that provide information in English and Thai.

With close to 67 million people, divided into 76 political provinces, Thailand is a geographically diverse country a little smaller than the state of Texas. Thailand's geography includes:

> Sandy beaches and rocky shores along its 2,000-mile coastline and >1,400 islands
> Central plains made up of extensive rice fields along the Chao Phraya River
> Mountainous areas in northern, western, and eastern Thailand
> The dry Khorat Plateau in northeastern Thailand.

Because Thailand is so close to the equator, the climate is tropical and often hot and humid. Flooding is always a possibility in Thailand, and various regions are prone to flash floods. Monsoon rains fall from May through July and can last until cooler, drier weather comes in November, making the North American winter a popular time of year to visit Thailand. Thailand's central location and major international airport in Bangkok make it an easy access point for other destinations in Asia.

Approximately 9.5 million people live in the capital city of Bangkok, a major metropolis and center of commerce. Bangkok is a mix of old and new— skyscrapers and waterways, bustling city streets full of people, vendors, dogs, uneven sidewalks, and lots of traffic, in contrast to the fast, quiet, and cool modern monorail and subway systems. Tourists visit historic sites of glittering grandeur such as the Grand Palace to catch a glimpse of the Emerald Buddha or one of Bangkok's 400 Buddhist temples. The main artery of Bangkok is the Chao Phraya River and its canals, which provide access to tourist sites, boat tours, the floating market, and restaurants and lend justification to Bangkok's nickname, "Venice of the East." Bangkok is a paradise of culinary delights, from local fare at a sidewalk noodle stand to a fancy 4-star meal in a restaurant. Rounding off a visit to Bangkok, many tourists will enjoy the pleasures of Thai nightlife, which includes a variety of bars and pubs, dance clubs, drag shows, and the famous red light districts of Soi Cowboy and Patpong.

Visitors to Thailand will also likely visit Chiang Mai, in northern Thailand. The city, surrounded by a moat and defensive wall, has >300 temples, a popular night bazaar for great shopping, and easy access to the handicraft villages, elephant nature parks, and outdoor adventures that are popular in the region.

A popular reason to visit Thailand is for rest and relaxation on sandy beaches along the coast or on one of the many islands. Beach destinations include plenty of opportunities for snorkeling, scuba diving, windsurfing, sailing, swimming, and dining on fresh seafood. A growing number of tourists seek out such relaxation opportunities as part of their recovery from medical or dental procedures. Over the years, medical tourism to Thailand has increased, as the costs for treatment are much lower and the quality of care is good (see Chapter 2, Medical Tourism). In 2005, an estimated 1 million foreigners were treated in Thailand. Thailand's Bumrungrad Hospital charges only $16,000 for a heart bypass operation performed by a US-trained, board-certified physician. The same operation costs >$56,000 in the United States.

Thailand has a large expatriate community and has also become a popular destination for Western retirees. In 2008, over 98,000 Westerners were estimated to be living in Thailand. The warm climate and low cost of living make Thailand an attractive place to live.

HEALTH ISSUES

Immunizations

All travelers should be up-to-date on their routine vaccinations. In addition, most travelers to Thailand should also be vaccinated against hepatitis A and hepatitis B. Typhoid vaccine should be considered.

Japanese Encephalitis Vaccine

Japanese encephalitis (JE) is endemic throughout Thailand. Transmission occurs year-round, with seasonal epidemics from May through October in the northern provinces. JE vaccine is recommended for travelers who plan to visit Thailand for ≥1 month and should be considered for those visiting for a shorter period but who have an increased risk of JE virus exposure due to their itineraries or activities. The highest rates of human disease have been reported from the Chiang Mai Valley. Several cases have recently been reported among travelers who visited resort or coastal areas of southern Thailand.

Rabies Vaccine

Despite government-sponsored mass vaccination campaigns for dogs and cats, rabies is still a risk in Thailand, particularly in Bangkok, where community dogs roam the streets. Preexposure vaccination is only recommended for travelers who have an occupation that puts them at risk for exposure (such as veterinarians), will be traveling for long periods of time, or are expatriates. Hospitals and clinics in Bangkok cater to the expatriate community and medical tourists, and rabies vaccine is readily available for preexposure and postexposure prophylaxis, although not all hospitals in Thailand carry human rabies immune globulin.

Malaria

Malaria is endemic in specific areas of Thailand, particularly the rural, forested areas that border Burma (Myanmar), Cambodia, and Laos, as well as the rural, forested areas of Phang Nga and Phuket. Prophylaxis is recommended for travelers visiting any of these areas (see Chapter 3, Malaria). Transmission in Thailand occurs year-round, and most cases are due to *Plasmodium falciparum*, with the rest due to *P. vivax* or mixed infection. Atovaquone-proguanil or doxycycline are the recommended antimalarial drugs for travelers in Thailand.

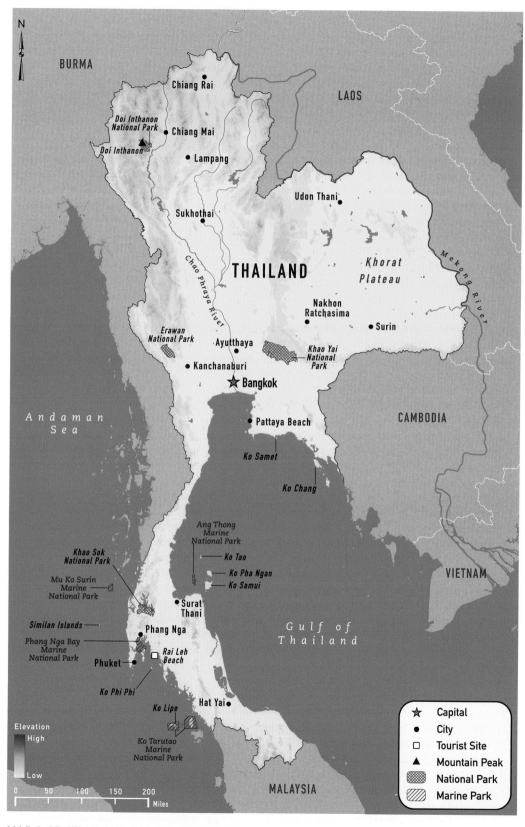

MAP 4-13. THAILAND DESTINATION MAP

Legend:
- ★ Capital
- ● City
- □ Tourist Site
- ▲ Mountain Peak
- National Park
- Marine Park

Elevation
High
Low

0 50 100 150 200 Miles

Dengue

Dengue is endemic throughout Thailand with large epidemics that occur every several years. Peak transmission occurs during the rainy season, although cases occur year-round even in non-epidemic years. Travelers to Thailand should take measures to protect themselves from daytime mosquito bites to prevent dengue (see Chapter 2, Protection against Mosquitoes, Ticks, & Other Insects & Arthropods).

Travelers' Diarrhea

Although the Thai Government and several nongovernmental organizations are leading projects to provide clean water across Thailand, and some hotels use their own filtration systems, water and food still contain harmful bacteria and other contaminants. Travelers should practice food and water precautions and bring an antibiotic for self-treatment. Because fluoroquinolone resistance is widespread in Thailand and other areas of Southeast Asia, azithromycin may be preferred (see Chapter 2, Travelers' Diarrhea).

Water and Soil Diseases

Melioidosis is highly endemic in northeast Thailand, and leptospirosis is reemerging primarily in the north and northeast regions of the country. For both diseases, most cases occur during the rainy season. Travelers who visit endemic areas should avoid contact with soil and water that could be contaminated and ensure that any open wounds are covered to prevent exposure. When contact cannot be avoided, travelers should wear protective clothing and footwear to reduce the risk of exposure. Skin lacerations, abrasions, or burns that have been contaminated with soil or surface water should be immediately and thoroughly cleaned.

Other Health and Safety Risks

Sexually Transmitted Diseases and HIV/AIDS

Thailand is a popular destination for sex tourism (see Chapter 3, *Perspectives*: Sex & Tourism), and although illegal, sex work is practiced openly across the country. A 100% condom program with sex workers helped slow the spread of HIV and other sexually transmitted diseases; however, approximately 530,000 people are living with HIV/AIDS in Thailand. Travelers should be aware of these risks and always use condoms during sex.

Safety and Security

Approximately 12,000 people are killed on the roads in Thailand each year, and a substantial proportion (82% in 2002) are killed while riding motorcycles. Motorcycles are a cheap, easy, and popular mode of transportation in Thailand, but they are also the most vulnerable vehicle on the road. If at all possible, travelers should avoid riding motorcycles and ride only if they wear a helmet.

In recent years, Thailand experienced a great deal of political unrest. With a new prime minister in office, the country remains divided but calm. Travelers should pay attention to the local news and monitor the US embassy websites and social media outlets to find out if and where protests and demonstrations will occur. Travelers should avoid these locations, since no one can predict whether protests will stay peaceful or turn violent.

BIBLIOGRAPHY

1. Bundhamcharoen K, Odton P, Phulkerd S, Tangcharoensathien V. Burden of disease in Thailand: changes in health gap between 1999 and 2004. BMC Public Health. 2011;11:53.
2. Chongsuvivatwong V, Chariyalertsak S, McNeil E, Aiyarak S, Hutamai S, Dupont HL, et al. Epidemiology of travelers' diarrhea in Thailand. J Travel Med. 2009 May–Jun;16(3):179–85.
3. Coker RJ, Hunter BM, Rudge JW, Liverani M, Hanvoravongchai P. Emerging infectious diseases in southeast Asia: regional challenges to control. Lancet. 2011 Feb 12;377(9765):599–609.
4. Howard RW. Western retirees in Thailand: motives, experiences, wellbeing, assimilation and future needs. Ageing Soc. 2008;28(2):145–63.

5. Kasempimolporn S, Sichanasai B, Saengseesom W, Puempumpanich S, Sitprija V. Stray dogs in Bangkok, Thailand: rabies virus infection and rabies antibody prevalence. Dev Biol. 2008;131:137–43.

6. Kositprapa C, Wimalratna O, Chomchey P, Chareonwai S, Benjavongkulchai M, Khawplod P, et al. Problems with rabies postexposure management: a survey of 499 public hospitals in Thailand. J Travel Med. 1998 Mar;5(1):30–2.

7. Tanaboriboon Y, Satiennam T. Traffic accidents in Thailand. IATSS Res. 2005;29(1):88–100.

8. US Agency for International Development. Thailand: HIV/AIDS health profile. Washington, DC: US Agency for International Development; 2010 [cited 2012 Sep 26]. Available from: http://transition.usaid.gov/our_work/global_health/aids/Countries/asia/thailand_profile.pdf.

9. Wichmann O, Yoon IK, Vong S, Limkittikul K, Gibbons RV, Mammen MP, et al. Dengue in Thailand and Cambodia: an assessment of the degree of underrecognized disease burden based on reported cases. PLoS Negl Trop Dis. 2011;5(3):e996.

10. Wiwanitkit V. Rate of malarial infection among foreigners in a tertiary hospital of Thailand: change of epidemiology and importance of travel medicine (1996–2005). J Vector Borne Dis. 2007 Sep;44(3):219–22.

11. Wuthiekanun V, Sirisukkarn N, Daengsupa P, Sakaraserane P, Sangkakam A, Chierakul W, et al. Clinical diagnosis and geographic distribution of leptospirosis, Thailand. Emerg Infect Dis. 2007 Jan;13(1):124–6.

VIETNAM

Nicole M. Smith, Michael F. Iademarco, Bryan K. Kapella

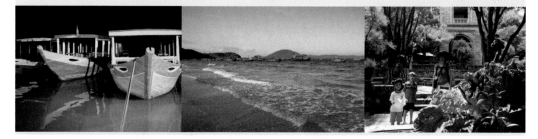

DESTINATION OVERVIEW

Vietnam has a population of approximately 90 million people, of whom about 70% live in rural areas. The total size of Vietnam is 127,243 mi² (331,114 km²), making it the 66th largest country in the world, comparable to Finland and Malaysia, or the combined size of Ohio, Kentucky, and Tennessee. It is located in Southeast Asia and borders China, Laos, and Cambodia. Vietnam is divided into 63 provinces. The terrain and climate vary, particularly between the north and the south and the mountainous and coastal areas.

Vietnam is an increasingly popular travel destination for business and tourism. Travelers often try to get a flavor for the entire country with at least a 10-day trip, or combine their Vietnam travels with other nearby Southeast Asia destinations such as Angkor Wat in Cambodia and Luang Prabang in Laos. There is no shortage of attractions in Vietnam, regardless of whether a traveler is interested in touring historical sites, shopping in ethnic markets or traditional trade villages, trekking or biking in hills or valleys, seeing native wildlife, cruising on the Mekong River, scuba diving in the sea, relaxing at a spa resort, visiting art galleries, or taking cooking lessons to understand the regional variations of Vietnam's cuisine.

A typical itinerary might start in the north and include visiting the capital, Hanoi; touring the UNESCO World Heritage site, Ha Long Bay, aboard a junk; and experiencing the rice fields and ethnic minorities in Sapa or Mai Chau. In the coastal region travelers often go to Hue, Hoi An, Danang, Dalat, and Nha Trang, each with their own charms and unique personalities. In the South travelers often choose to see Vietnam's largest, busiest, and most modern city, Ho Chi Minh City. From there, Phu Quoc Island, the Cu Chi tunnels, and floating markets of the Mekong Delta are easy trips.

HEALTH ISSUES

Immunizations

Travelers to Vietnam should be up-to-date on routine vaccines, such as measles-mumps-rubella, diphtheria-pertussis-tetanus, and influenza. Travelers should also protect themselves by getting vaccinated against typhoid and hepatitis A. Hepatitis B protection is advised, especially for long-term travelers and expatriates, given the high prevalence of chronic HBV infection in the population.

Japanese Encephalitis Vaccine

Because Japanese encephalitis (JE) is endemic throughout Vietnam, JE vaccination is recommended for all travelers who spend ≥1 month or more in the country during the transmission season and should be considered for short-term travelers who plan on spending time outside urban areas and may be involved in activities that expose them to the mosquitoes that transmit JE virus. Such activities may include camping, hiking, biking or other outdoor activities, or straying in accommodations without air conditioning, screens, or bed nets (see Chapter 3, Japanese Encephalitis). JE has seasonal peaks from May through October, especially in the northern part of the country, where the highest rates of JE disease occur in the northern provinces around Hanoi and the northwestern and northeastern provinces bordering China. Personalized advice during a thorough pre-travel consultation is important.

Rabies Vaccine

Travelers should receive preexposure immunizations against rabies if they will be spending a lot of time outdoors, have direct contact with wildlife, or will be in Vietnam for a prolonged period of time. Most dogs are not routinely vaccinated in Vietnam and are numerous even in urban areas. Special consideration should be given to vaccinating children. Care should also be taken to avoid contact with nonhuman primates, as several tourist destinations (for example, islands in Ha Long Bay and off Nha Trang) have macaques that are not afraid of humans and may be infected with herpes B virus as well as rabies. Human rabies immune globulin is usually available in larger cities, such as Hanoi and Ho Chi Minh City. Travelers should be encouraged to purchase travel health insurance that includes medical evacuation insurance in the event postexposure prophylaxis is unavailable.

Malaria

Most tourist itineraries do not include malarious areas of Vietnam. Malaria is primarily a concern in rural areas and is mostly caused by *Plasmodium falciparum*. There are rare cases in the Mekong Delta and none in the Red River Delta, the coast north of Nha Trang, or in larger cities such as Da Nang, Haiphong, Hanoi, Ho Chi Minh City, Nha Tran, and Qui Nhon. Travelers to the Mekong Delta should avoid exposure to mosquitos but do not need to take antimalarial drugs. Travelers to other parts of Vietnam where malaria is known to be circulating should take chemoprophylaxis appropriate to the specific places they will be visiting. Mefloquine resistance has been reported in some areas, so travel health clinicians may feel more comfortable recommending atovaquone-proguanil or doxycycline to travelers (see Chapter 3, Malaria).

Dengue

Dengue is endemic in Vietnam and although peak transmission occurs during the summer rainy season, dengue virus transmission occurs year-round. Travelers to Vietnam should take

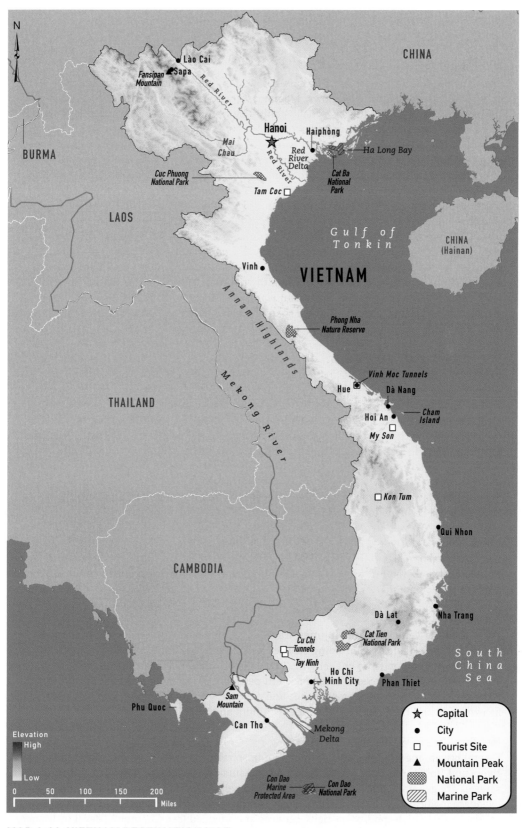

MAP 4-14. VIETNAM DESTINATION MAP

measures to protect themselves from daytime mosquito bites to prevent dengue
(see Chapter 2, Protection against Mosquitoes, Ticks, & Other Insects & Arthropods).

Avian Influenza

Vietnam continues to report sporadic cases of human infection with avian influenza A (H5N1) or "bird flu," as it is commonly known. Most people who have become infected had direct contact or close exposure to sick or dead poultry by visiting live bird or poultry markets or preparing or eating uncooked or undercooked bird products (such as meat, eggs, or blood). In extremely rare situations, a few people were infected as a result of close, prolonged contact with another person who was sick with avian influenza.

To avoid infection, travelers to an area affected by avian influenza should avoid direct contact with birds, including poultry (such as chickens and ducks) and wild birds; avoid touching surfaces that have bird droppings (feces) or other bird fluids on them; and avoid places where live birds are raised or kept.

In general, travelers should eat only bird meat or products that have been thoroughly cooked. Any dishes that contain uncooked (raw) or undercooked bird meat or products such as eggs and poultry blood should be avoided. For example, egg yolks should not be runny or liquid. Travelers should also practice healthy habits to help stop the spread of germs by washing hands often with soap and clean water or using an alcohol-based hand sanitizer (containing at least 60% alcohol) when soap and clean water are not available and hands are not visibly dirty.

Other Health and Safety Risks

Foodborne Illnesses

Drinking tap water should be avoided, as should beverages with ice. Travelers should avoid eating food or drinking beverages from street vendors and should avoid eating raw or undercooked meat, seafood, uncooked vegetables, and raw fruits that cannot be peeled by the traveler.

Travelers with seafood allergies should be particularly cautious in Vietnam, given the common use of fish and other seafood sauces in many dishes.

Skin Diseases

Skin rashes may result from the combination of heat and humidity or fungal infections. Efforts should be made to keep clothes, shoes, and linens clean and dry.

Noise and Air Pollution

Construction sounds and frequent honking of motorbike and car horns can be an annoyance. Travelers with allergies or asthma may find their conditions are exacerbated because of high levels of particulate matter and indoor air pollution.

Road Safety

To avoid motor vehicle–related injuries, travelers should fasten seat belts when riding in cars and wear a helmet when riding bicycles and motorbikes. Pedestrians may find road conditions in Vietnam to be challenging. Travelers are advised to walk facing traffic and, when crossing the street, to proceed at a consistent pace (not stopping or suddenly turning back). Pedestrians will observe that motorbikes and cars will go around them much like a school of fish will part and then regroup when it encounters an object.

Medical Care in Vietnam

Several private medical practices, clinics, and hospitals that serve foreigners are available in Hanoi and Ho Chi Minh City. However, blood transfusion services, inpatient care, and specialty services are generally not of high quality. Thus travelers should ensure that they have adequate medical evacuation insurance in case they need to be evacuated to Singapore or Bangkok where high-quality specialty services are provided (see Chapter 2, Travel Insurance, Travel Health Insurance, & Medical Evacuation Insurance). To ensure the quality of any needed medications, travelers may want to consider purchasing them through an expatriate or international travel clinic, even if the price is higher.

BIBLIOGRAPHY

1. Caramello P, Canta F, Balbiano R, Lipani F, Ariaudo S, De Agostini M, et al. A case of imported JE acquired during short travel in Vietnam. Are current recommendations about vaccination broader? J Travel Med. 2007 Sep–Oct;14(5):346–8.
2. Cuong HQ, Hien NT, Duong TN, Phong TV, Cam NN, Farrar J, et al. Quantifying the emergence of dengue in Hanoi, Vietnam: 1998–2009. PLoS Negl Trop Dis. 2011 Sep;5(9):e1322.
3. Emerson JW, Hsu A, Levy MA, de Sherbinin A, Mara V, Esty DC, et al. 2012 Environmental performance index and pilot trend environmental performance index: country profiles. New Haven: Yale Center for Environmental Law and Policy; 2012 [cited 2012 Sep 26]. Available from: http://epi.yale.edu/epi2012/countryprofiles.
4. Hanoi International Women's Club. Hanoi Guide. Hanoi: Hanoi Publishing House; 2008.
5. Phan HYT, Yano T. Road traffic noise policy in Vietnam. J Temporal Des Arch Environ. 2009;9(1):150–3.
6. Sniadack DH, Mendoza-Aldana J, Huyen DT, Van TT, Cuong NV, Olive JM, et al. Epidemiology of a measles epidemic in Vietnam 2008–2010. J Infect Dis. 2011 Jul;204 Suppl 1:S476–82.
7. Statistics Documentation Centre. General Statistics Office of Vietnam. Hanoi: General Statistics Office of Vietnam; 2012 [cited 2012 Sep 26]. Available from: http://www.gso.gov.vn/default_en.aspx?tabid=491.
8. Trung Dung D, Van De N, Waikagul J, Dalsgaard A, Chai JY, Sohn WM, et al. Fishborne zoonotic intestinal trematodes, Vietnam. Emerg Infect Dis. 2007 Dec;13(12):1828–33.
9. World Bank. Vietnam overview. Washington, DC: The World Bank Group; 2012 [cited 2012 Sep 26]. Available from: http://www.worldbank.org/en/country/vietnam/overview.
10. World Health Organization Representative Office in Viet Nam. Vietnam homepage. Hanoi: World Health Organization; 2012 [cited 2012 Sep 26]. Available from: http://www2.wpro.who.int/vietnam/home.htm.

The Middle East & North Africa

SAUDI ARABIA: HAJJ PILGRIMAGE
Qanta Ahmed, Victor Balaban

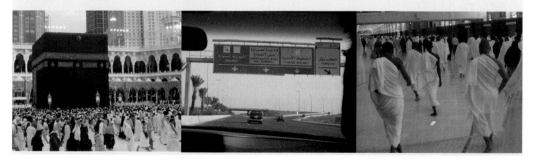

DESTINATION OVERVIEW

They will come to thee on foot and (mounted) on every kind of camel, lean on account of journeys through deep and distant mountain highways…(Quran 22:27)

The Hajj is the annual pilgrimage to Mecca, Saudi Arabia, and the largest mass gathering in the world. Every able-bodied adult Muslim who can afford to do so is required to make Hajj at least once in his or her lifetime. Hajj takes place from the 8th through the 12th of Dhu al-Hijja, the last month of the Islamic year. Because the Islamic calendar is lunar, the timing of Hajj varies with respect to the Gregorian calendar (for example, it was November 4–7 in 2011 and October 24–27 in 2012 and will be October 13–16 in 2013, and October 3–6 in 2014).

More than 2 million Muslims from >183 countries make Hajj each year (2.5 million in 2009), >11,000 of whom travel from the United States. Most international pilgrims fly into Jeddah and take a bus to Mecca. After arriving in Mecca, pilgrims go immediately to the Grand Mosque, which contains the Ka'aba, the most sacred site in Islam, and perform a *tawaf*, circling the Ka'aba 7 times counterclockwise. Because of the vast number of people (each floor of the 3-level mosque has a capacity of 750,000), a single *tawaf* can take hours. In addition to *tawaf*, pilgrims perform *sa'i*, walking or running 7 times between the hills of Safa and Marwah. Once in open air, this route is now enclosed by the Grand Mosque and can be traversed via air-conditioned tunnels, with separate sections for walkers, runners, and disabled pilgrims.

Hajj culminates on the Plain of Arafat, a few miles east of Mecca, where the Prophet Muhammad delivered his final sermon. Pilgrims spend the day in supplication, praying and reading the Quran; it is the pinnacle of most pilgrims' spiritual lives. The following day's ritual, the Stoning of the Devil at Jamaraat, is the site of some of the densest crowds during Hajj. During this ritual, pilgrims throw 7 tiny pebbles (specifically, no larger than a chickpea) at each of 3 white pillars. Because of the sheer number of people crowding around the pillars, panic can easily trigger crowd turbulence and stampede. In 2004, after 251 pilgrims were killed and another 244 injured, the Saudi government replaced the round pillars with wide, elliptical columns to reduce crowd densities. After a stampede in 2006 that killed 380 pilgrims and injured 289, the Jamaraat pedestrian bridge was demolished and replaced with a wider, multilevel bridge.

After Jamaraat, pilgrims traditionally sacrificed an animal to symbolize the ram that Abraham sacrificed instead of his son. In modern times, pilgrims must purchase a "sacrifice voucher" in Mecca and perform this sacrifice by proxy. Centralized, licensed abattoirs then perform the sacrifice on behalf of the pilgrim, and meat is immediately donated to charity, often reaching international locations. Each year, >600,000 animals are sacrificed. After a final *tawaf*, pilgrims leave Mecca, ending Hajj. Although it is not required as part of Hajj, many pilgrims extend their trips to travel to Medina to visit the Mosque of the Prophet, which contains the tomb of Mohammed and is the second holiest site in Islam.

HEALTH ISSUES

Immunizations

All pilgrims should be up-to-date with routine immunizations. In addition, hepatitis A and B and typhoid vaccines are recommended. Although a requirement for polio vaccine does not include pilgrims from the United States, it is best to ensure full vaccination against polio before travel. Current vaccination requirements are available from the website of the Saudi Arabian Ministry of Health (www.moh.gov.sa/en/Pages/Default.aspx).

Meningococcal Vaccine

Because of the intensely crowded conditions of the Hajj and high carrier rates of *Neisseria meningitidis* among pilgrims, outbreaks of meningococcal disease have historically been a problem during Hajj. In the aftermath of outbreaks in 2000 and 2001 that affected 1,300 and 1,109 people, respectively, the Saudi Ministry of Health began requiring all pilgrims and local at-risk populations to receive the meningococcal vaccine—Hajj visas cannot be issued without proof of vaccination. All adults and children aged >2 years must have received a single dose of quadrivalent A/C/Y/W-135 vaccine and must show proof of vaccination on a valid International Certificate of Vaccination or Prophylaxis. Hajj pilgrims must have had the meningococcal vaccine ≤3 years and ≥10 days before arriving in Saudi Arabia.

Respiratory Infections   *pneumonia*

Respiratory tract infections are common during Hajj; the most common cause of hospital admission is pneumonia. These risks underscore the need to follow the Advisory Committee on Immunization Practices recommendations for pneumococcal polysaccharide vaccine for pilgrims aged ≥65 years and for younger pilgrims with comorbidities. Seasonal influenza vaccine is recommended for all pilgrims. Behavioral interventions such as hand hygiene, wearing a face mask, cough etiquette, social distancing, and contact avoidance can be effective at mitigating respiratory illness among Hajj pilgrims.

Other Health and Safety Risks   *T/D, skin*
Communicable Diseases

Diarrheal disease is common during Hajj, and travelers should be educated on usual prevention measures and self-treatment. Environmental conditions during the summer months can be extremely hot, with air temperatures exceeding 122°F (50°C), further increasing risks for dehydration. Adequate fluid intake must be a priority for every pilgrim. Fortunately, millions of containers of water are distributed to pilgrims from refrigerated trucks located along the pilgrim route. In addition, Saudi authorities have erected thousands of sprinklers on top of 30-foot poles that spray a fine mist of water to cool pilgrims.

Long rituals of standing and walking, heat, sweating, and obesity contribute to the risk for chafing, leading to skin infections. Travelers should be advised to keep skin dry, use talcum powder, and be aware of any pain or soreness caused by garments. Any sores or blisters that

Tx Skin
Talcum
powder

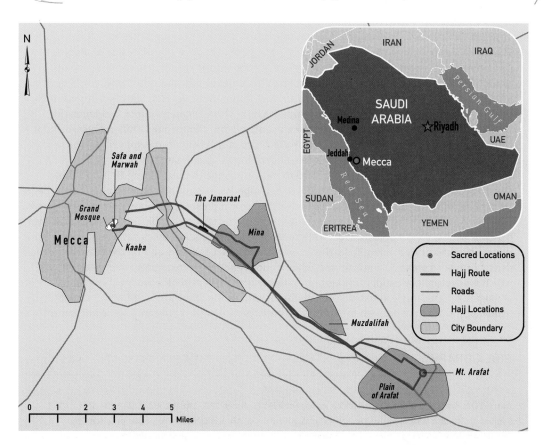

MAP 4-15. HAJJ DESTINATION MAP

develop should be disinfected and kept covered. Special attention should be paid to the feet, which are bare when inside the Grand Mosque.

At the end of Hajj, Muslim men must shave their heads, and unclean blades can transmit bloodborne pathogens, such as hepatitis B, hepatitis C, and HIV. Licensed barbers are tested for these bloodborne pathogens and are required to use disposable, single-use blades. Unfortunately, unlicensed barbers continue to operate by the roadside, where they use nonsterile blades on multiple men. Male travelers should be advised to be shaved only at officially designated centers, which are clearly marked.

Noncommunicable Diseases and Other Hazards

Cardiovascular disease is the primary cause of death during Hajj. Hajj is arduous even for young, healthy pilgrims, and many Muslims wait until they are older before making Hajj. Pilgrims who are caught up in the spiritual experience of Hajj may forget to take their usual medications. Consequently, travelers with preexisting cardiovascular disease should be advised of this risk and specifically consult with their doctors before leaving, ensure that they have an adequate supply of medication, adhere to their usual regimen, and immediately report to the nearest health center if they notice symptoms of cardiac decompensation.

Heat exhaustion and heatstroke are also leading causes of death, particularly when Hajj occurs during the summer. Pilgrims should stay hydrated, wear sunscreen, and seek shade when possible. Some rituals may also be performed at night to avoid daytime heat. Pilgrims can be reassured that night rituals have been advocated as legitimate by religious clerics.

Fire is a potential risk at Hajj. In 1997, open stoves set tents on fire, and the resulting blaze killed 343 pilgrims and injured more than 1,500. As a result, makeshift tents were replaced with permanent fiberglass structures; no pilgrim is allowed to set up his own tent or prepare his own food. Cooking in the tents is also prohibited.

Trauma

Trauma is a major cause of injury and death during Hajj. Pilgrims may walk long distances through or near dense traffic, and motor vehicle accidents are inevitable. The most feared trauma hazard, however, is stampede. In such dense crowds, little can be done to avoid or escape a stampede once it has begun, but the physical environment of the Hajj has been engineered specifically to minimize this risk. Past stampedes have often begun as minor incidents; the 2006 Hajj stampede, for example, began when some pilgrims tripped over fallen luggage, but it resulted in hundreds of injuries and deaths. Death usually results from asphyxiation or head trauma, and providing prompt treatment is next to impossible in large crowds.

The Saudi government is committed to mitigating health risks during Hajj, and it has spent >$25 billion to date, in efforts to prevent stampedes. The round columns at Jamaraat have been replaced with wider elliptical ones to dissipate crowd pressure and ease crowd density, and a new Jamaraat bridge has been built. The new bridge has a capacity to hold 5 million pilgrims over a 6-hour period. Bottlenecks have been engineered out, and large canopies have been added to protect pilgrims from the sun. To further protect themselves, travelers should try to avoid the most densely crowded areas during Hajj and, when options exist, perform rituals at nonpeak hours, which is advocated by Saudi religious authorities and underlines their concern about the safety of all pilgrims. For example, most pilgrims prefer to perform the Stoning of the Devil at midday, but Saudi authorities have decreed that it may be performed anytime between sunrise and sunset.

BIBLIOGRAPHY

1. Ahmed QA, Arabi YM, Memish ZA. Health risks at the Hajj. Lancet. 2006 Mar 25;367(9515):1008–15.
2. Balaban V, Stauffer WM, Hammad A, Afgarshe M, Abd-Alla M, Ahmed Q, et al. Protective practices and respiratory illness among US travelers to the 2009 Hajj. J Travel Med. 2012 May–Jun;19(3):163–8.
3. Gatrad AR, Sheikh A. Hajj: journey of a lifetime. BMJ. 2005 Jan 15;330(7483):133–7.

4. Memish ZA, Ahmed QA. Mecca bound: the challenges ahead. J Travel Med. 2002 Jul–Aug;9(4):202–10.

5. Shafi S, Memish ZA, Gatrad AR, Sheikh A. Hajj 2006: communicable disease and other health risks and current official guidance for pilgrims. Euro Surveill. 2005;10(12):E051215.2.

6. World Health Organization. Health conditions for travellers to Saudi Arabia pilgrimage to Mecca (Hajj). Wkly Epidemiol Rec. 2005 Dec 9;80(49–50):431–2.

EGYPT & NILE RIVER CRUISES
Ann M. Buff

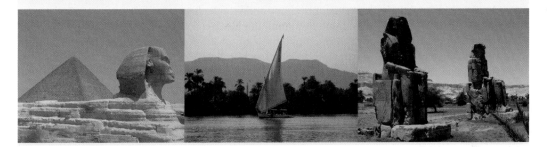

DESTINATION OVERVIEW

The Arab Republic of Egypt covers a land area >1,000,000 km², approximately the same size as Texas and New Mexico combined, and >95% of the country is desert. With an estimated 80 million people, Egypt accounts for one-fourth of the Arab world's population. Egypt has long been considered the cradle of civilization and may be the oldest tourist destination on earth. Throughout the world, Egypt is synonymous with the legends of the Pharaohs, the Great Pyramids, treasure-laden tombs, and hieroglyphs. Millions of travelers visit Egypt each year to see the ancient monuments and timeless river vistas along the Nile Valley.

A typical visit to Egypt includes arrival in the capital city of Cairo, the largest city in Africa and the Middle East, with a population of over 16 million. Considered the "Mother of the World" by Arabs, Cairo today is a modern, cosmopolitan mix of Arab, African, and European influences. Travelers generally spend at least a few days in Cairo seeing the Egyptian Antiquities Museum, the Pyramids at Giza, the Citadel and Mosque of Al-Azhar, and Khan al-Khalili bazaar.

Most travelers include an Upper Nile River cruise as part of their itineraries. Nile River cruises are usually 3–7 days, with embarkation in either Luxor or Aswan. Riverboats do not sail through Middle Egypt because of security concerns; therefore, most travelers take short domestic flights or trains from Cairo to Luxor or Aswan. Approximately 200 riverboats cruise the Nile, and the average boat accommodates 120 passengers. The largest boats accommodate upwards of 300 passengers; chartered yachts might have just a few cabins. Riverboats have a range of accommodations from basic to 5-star luxury, and nights aboard are generally spent cruising from one port to the next.

Virtually all Nile cruises sail between Luxor and Aswan. There are 3 usual Nile cruise durations and itineraries: a 3-night cruise from Aswan to Luxor (or the reverse), a 4-night cruise from Luxor to Aswan (or the reverse), and a 7-night cruise roundtrip from Luxor or Aswan. A standard itinerary is as follows:

> Day 1: Fly from Cairo to Aswan or Luxor. Stay in a hotel for the first night or board the boat directly and spend the afternoon and early the next morning visiting the sites (High Dam

and Philae Temple in Aswan or Karnak Temple, Luxor Temple, Valley of the Kings, and Hapshepsut Temple in Luxor).

> Days 2–6: Visit temples of Edfu, Esna, and Kom Ombo and enjoy the passing riverside scenes of ancient villages, minarets, farmers in *galabiyas*, and traditional *feluccas*. Most travelers have an early breakfast aboard and then depart the boat for sightseeing early in the day to avoid the crowds and heat. Most travelers will be back aboard by mid- to late afternoon. Dinner and entertainment follow in the evening.

> Final day: Disembark and return to Cairo or travel to a Red Sea resort.

Egypt is also a beach destination, with thousands of miles of Mediterranean and Red Sea coastlines. Alexandria, Egypt's second largest city, with >5 million people, is located on the Mediterranean Sea and has a string of beaches and wonderful seafood restaurants. The World War II battlefield of El-Alamein lies along the Mediterranean coast, and divers will find an array of sunken cities and wartime wrecks to explore offshore. Edged by coral reefs and teeming with tropical fish, the Sinai Peninsula has excellent diving, snorkeling, and beaches; Sharm el Sheikh is the most developed and visited area of the Sinai. Visits to Mount Sinai (7,497 ft [2,285 m] above sea level) and Saint Catherine's Monastery in the mountainous interior are also popular destinations. Egypt's Red Sea coast has more reefs offshore, with diving and snorkeling traditionally centered in Hurghada.

Popular among adventure travelers are desert jeep safaris and camel treks to remote oases and spectacular *wadis*. Many travelers start in Cairo or Assyut and follow the "Great Desert Circuit" through 4 oases and the White Desert.

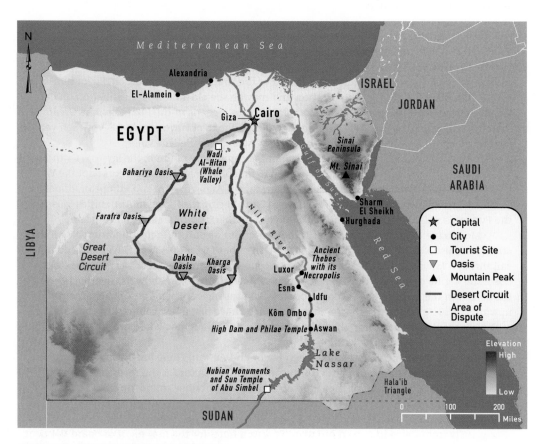

MAP 4-16. EGYPT DESTINATION MAP

In addition to being up-to-date on routine vaccines, hepatitis A and B and typhoid vaccines are recommended for travelers to Egypt. There is no risk of malaria. The estimated prevalences of hepatitis B and C virus infections (2%–7% and >10%, respectively) are among the highest in the world. Travelers should be cautioned to protect themselves from all bloodborne pathogens by avoiding unprotected sex, invasive medical and dental procedures, injection drug use, and tattooing. Modern hospitals and clinics cater to the large expatriate communities in Cairo and Alexandria and to tourists in the Red Sea resort areas.

Travelers' Diarrhea
In most large international tourist hotels, the tap water is heavily chlorinated and generally safe to drink but unpalatable. Tap water is not safe to drink in other locations. Eating thoroughly cooked meat and vegetables in tourist hotels, on Nile River cruise ships, and in tourist restaurants is generally safe. Eating raw or undercooked ground meat or shellfish should be avoided. As in many developing countries, the safety of uncooked vegetables and salads may be in question. The risk of diarrhea in Egypt is high. Travelers to Egypt should be provided with an antibiotic for empiric self-treatment of diarrhea.

Schistosomiasis
Schistosoma mansoni and *S. haematobium* are endemic in Egypt. Travelers to Egypt should avoid wading, swimming, or other contact with freshwater, including the Nile River and irrigation canals. Swimming in saline pools of desert oases, chlorinated swimming pools, the Mediterranean Sea, or Red Sea does not pose a risk for acquiring schistosomiasis.

Rabies
As in most other developing countries, rabies is endemic throughout Egypt. For most travelers on a package tour, the risk will be minimal. However, travelers should be aware that there are large numbers of stray dogs and cats in urban and tourist areas and should be advised to avoid contact with domestic or wild mammals. Rabies vaccine is readily available for preexposure and postexposure prophylaxis, and human rabies immune globulin (HRIG) is also available. Both rabies vaccine and HRIG are produced locally, but it is also possible to find imported rabies vaccine and HRIG (manufactured in the United States or Europe).

Environmental Concerns
Temperature and weather conditions vary widely in Egypt. The desert is extremely hot in the summer (>100°F; >38°C) and can be cold in the winter (<32°F; <0°C). Thirst is a late indicator of mild dehydration, and travelers should drink fluids regularly in the heat. Because sweat evaporates immediately, people can become dehydrated without realizing it. Travelers who are elderly or take diuretic, anticholinergic, or neuroleptic medications are at increased risk of heat-associated illnesses. To stay cool and protect themselves from sun exposure, travelers should wear a hat and lightweight, loose-fitting clothing and use sunscreen.

Sandstorms occur sporadically in the desert. Desert sand, dust, and smog can cause eye irritation and exacerbate asthma or other lung disorders. Travelers who wear contact lenses should make sure that they are carrying glasses and all their contact lens care supplies.

Motion Sickness
Generally, the Nile is a slow, smooth river. However, a variety of boats are employed for Nile cruises, and traffic on the Nile can be heavy. The combination of diesel fuel, heat, and motion can cause distress for travelers. Most travelers do not consider the possibility of motion sickness on a river, so they are unprepared. Onboard medical services vary greatly. Travelers who know that they are sensitive to motion should carry anti–motion sickness medication.

Insects

Even without the risk of malaria, mosquitoes and other biting insects can be problematic for travelers to Egypt, particularly in the summer months. Avoiding insect bites can minimize the risk of West Nile virus infection and dengue.

ACKNOWLEDGMENT

The author thanks Dr. Mohammad Abdel Sabour Diab, Professor of Pulmonary Medicine, Ain Shams University and Regional Staff Physician, Eastern Mediterranean Regional Office, World Health Organization, Cairo, Egypt, for his valuable contributions and insightful review.

BIBLIOGRAPHY

1. Gautret P, Adehossi E, Soula G, Soavi MJ, Delmont J, Rotivel Y, et al. Rabies exposure in international travelers: do we miss the target? Int J Infect Dis. 2010 Mar;14(3):e243–6.
2. Gautret P, Schwartz E, Shaw M, Soula G, Gazin P, Delmont J, et al. Animal-associated injuries and related diseases among returned travellers: a review of the GeoSentinel Surveillance Network. Vaccine. 2007 Mar 30;25(14):2656–63.
3. Lehman EM, Wilson ML. Epidemiology of hepatitis viruses among hepatocellular carcinoma cases and healthy people in Egypt: a systematic review and meta-analysis. Int J Cancer. 2009 Feb 1;124(3):690–7.
4. Nicolls DJ, Weld LH, Schwartz E, Reed C, von Sonnenburg F, Freedman DO, et al. Characteristics of schistosomiasis in travelers reported to the GeoSentinel Surveillance Network 1997-2008. Am J Trop Med Hyg. 2008 Nov;79(5):729–34.
5. Sievert W, Altraif I, Razavi HA, Abdo A, Ahmed EA, Alomair A, et al. A systematic review of hepatitis C virus epidemiology in Asia, Australia and Egypt. Liver Int. 2011 Jul;31 Suppl 2:61–80.

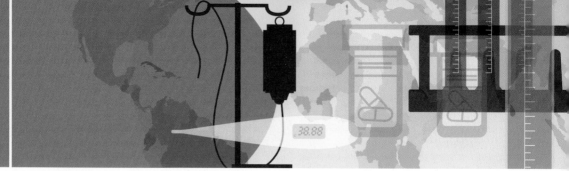

Post-Travel Evaluation

GENERAL APPROACH TO THE RETURNED TRAVELER

Jessica K. Fairley

THE POST-TRAVEL EVALUATION

Travel-related health problems have been reported in as many as 22%–64% of travelers to developing countries. Although most of these illnesses are mild, up to 8% of travelers are ill enough to seek care from a medical provider. Most post-travel infections become apparent soon after travel, but incubation periods vary, and some syndromes can present months to years after initial infection. When evaluating a patient with a probable travel-related illness, the clinician should consider the items summarized in Box 5-1.

The Severity of Illness

The first item to assess in ill returned travelers is the severity of illness. Is this a potentially life-threatening infection, such as malaria? A severe respiratory syndrome or signs of hemorrhagic fever are examples of cases that may also necessitate prompt involvement of public health authorities. See "Management" below for more details.

Travel Itinerary

The itinerary is crucial to formulating a differential diagnosis, because potential exposures differ depending on the region of travel. A febrile illness with nonspecific symptoms could be malaria, dengue, typhoid fever, or rickettsial disease, among others. Being able to exclude certain infections will avoid unnecessary testing. A study from the GeoSentinel Surveillance Network found that systemic febrile illness was more often associated with travel to sub-Saharan Africa or Southeast Asia, while acute diarrhea was more common from south-central Asia. The duration of travel is also important, since the risk of a travel-related illness increases with the length of the trip. A tropical medicine specialist can assist with the differential diagnosis and may be aware of outbreaks or the current prevalence of an infectious disease in an area.

Timing of Illness in Relation to Travel

Most ill travelers will seek medical attention within 1 month of return from their destination, because most common travel-related infections have short incubation periods. Occasionally, however, infections such as schistosomiasis, leishmaniasis, or Chagas disease can manifest months or even years later. Therefore, in unusual cases, a detailed history that extends beyond a few months before presentation can be helpful. The most common travel-related infections with short incubation periods are listed in Table 5-1.

Underlying Medical Illness

Comorbidities can affect the susceptibility to infection, as well as the clinical manifestations and severity of illness. An increasing number of immunosuppressed people (due to organ transplants, immune-modulating medications, HIV infection, or other primary or acquired immunodeficiencies) are international travelers (see Chapter 8, Immunocompromised Travelers).

Vaccines Received and Prophylaxis Used

The history of vaccinations and malaria chemoprophylaxis should be reviewed when evaluating an ill returned traveler. Less than half of US travelers to developing countries seek pre-travel medical advice and may not have received vaccines or taken antimalarial drugs. Although adherence to malaria chemoprophylaxis does not rule out the possibility of malaria, it reduces the risk and increases the chance of an alternative diagnosis. Fever and a rash in a traveler without an up-to-date measles vaccination would raise concern about measles. The most common vaccine-preventable diseases found in a large 2010 GeoSentinel study of returned travelers included enteric fever (typhoid and paratyphoid), viral hepatitis, and influenza. More than half of these patients with vaccine-preventable diseases were hospitalized.

Individual Exposure History

Knowledge of the patient's exposures during travel, including insect bites, contaminated food or water, or freshwater swimming, can also assist with the differential diagnosis. In addition to malarial parasites, mosquitoes can transmit viruses (such as dengue virus, yellow fever virus, and chikungunya virus) and filarial parasites (such as *Wuchereria bancrofti*). Depending on the clinical syndrome, a history of a tick bite could suggest a diagnosis of tickborne encephalitis, African tick-bite fever, or other rickettsial infections. Tsetse flies are large, and their bites are painful and often recalled by the patient. They can carry *Trypanosoma brucei*, the protozoan that causes African sleeping sickness. Freshwater swimming or other water contact can put the patient at risk for schistosomiasis, leptospirosis, and other diseases.

The purpose of the patient's trip and the type of accommodations can also influence the risk for acquiring certain diseases. Travelers who visit friends and relatives are at higher risk of malaria, typhoid fever, and certain other diseases, probably because, compared with tourists, they stay longer, travel to more remote destinations, have more contact with local water sources, and do not seek pre-travel advice (see Chapter 8, Immigrants Returning Home to Visit Friends & Relatives

Table 5-1. Illnesses associated with fever presenting in the first 2 weeks after travel

SYNDROME	POSSIBLE CAUSE
Systemic febrile illness with initial nonspecific symptoms	Malaria Dengue Typhoid fever Rickettsial diseases (such as scrub typhus, relapsing fever) East African trypanosomiasis Acute HIV infection Leptospirosis
Fever with central nervous system involvement	Meningococcal meningitis Malaria Arboviral encephalitis (such as Japanese encephalitis virus, West Nile virus) East African trypanosomiasis Angiostrongyliasis Rabies
Fever with respiratory complaints	Influenza Bacterial pneumonia Acute histoplasmosis or coccidioidomycosis, *Legionella* pneumonia Q fever Malaria Tularemia Pneumonic plague
Fever and skin rash	Dengue Measles Varicella Spotted-fever or typhus group rickettsiosis Typhoid fever Parvovirus B19 Mononucleosis Acute HIV infection

[VFRs]). Someone backpacking and camping in rural areas will also have a higher risk of certain diseases than those staying in luxury, air-conditioned hotels.

COMMON SYNDROMES

The most common clinical presentations after travel to developing countries include systemic febrile illness, acute diarrhea, and dermatologic conditions. These are described in more detail in the following sections of this chapter (Fever in Returned Travelers, Persistent Travelers' Diarrhea, and Skin & Soft Tissue Infections in Returned Travelers). Fever in a traveler returning from a malaria-endemic country needs to be evaluated immediately.

Respiratory Complaints

Respiratory complaints are frequent among returned travelers and are typically associated with common respiratory viruses (see Chapter 2, Respiratory Infections). Influenza is one of the most common vaccine-preventable diseases associated with international travel. Severe respiratory symptoms—especially associated with fever—in a returned traveler should alert the physician to common infectious diseases such as seasonal influenza, bacterial pneumonia, and malaria but could also suggest more unusual entities, such as Legionnaires' disease. In these suspected cases, local public health authorities and CDC should be alerted immediately.

Delayed onset and chronic cough after travel could be tuberculosis, especially in a long-term traveler or health care worker. Other uncommon infections causing respiratory illness after travel to specific regions are histoplasmosis, coccidioidomycosis, Q fever, plague, tularemia, and melioidosis. Helminth infections that produce pulmonary disease include strongyloidiasis, paragonimiasis, and schistosomiasis.

Eosinophilia

Eosinophilia in a returning traveler suggests a possible helminth infection. Allergic diseases, hematologic disorders, and a few other viral, fungal, and protozoan infections can also cause eosinophilia. Fever and eosinophilia can be present during pulmonary migration of parasites, such as hookworm, *Ascaris*, and *Strongyloides*. Acute schistosomiasis, or Katayama syndrome, is also a cause of fever and eosinophilia and can be associated with pulmonary infiltrates. Other parasitic infections associated with eosinophilia include chronic strongyloidiasis, visceral larval migrans, lymphatic filariasis, and acute trichinellosis. Findings in a recent outbreak of sarcocystosis in travelers returning from Tioman Island, Malaysia, included myalgia and eosinophilia. The affected travelers had eosinophilic myositis on muscle biopsy.

MANAGEMENT

Most post-travel illnesses can be managed on an outpatient basis, but some patients, especially those with systemic febrile illnesses, may need to be hospitalized. In a 2007 analysis of GeoSentinel data, 46% of returned travelers with systemic febrile illness were hospitalized. Severe presentations, such as acute respiratory distress, mental status change, and hemodynamic instability, require inpatient care. Clinicians should have a low threshold for admitting febrile patients if malaria is suspected. Confirmation of diagnosis can be delayed, and complications can occur rapidly. Management in an inpatient setting is especially important if the patient may not reliably follow up or when no one is at home to assist if symptoms worsen quickly. Consultation with an infectious diseases physician is recommended in severe travel-related infections, when management is complicated, or when the diagnosis remains unclear. A tropical medicine or infectious disease specialist should be involved in cases that require specialized treatment, such as neurocysticercosis, severe malaria, and leishmaniasis, among others. CDC provides on-call assistance with the diagnosis and management of parasitic infections at 404-718-4745 for parasitic infections other than malaria or 770-488-7788 (toll-free at 855-856-4713) for malaria, during business hours. After business hours, call the CDC Emergency Operations Center at 770-488-7100.

BIBLIOGRAPHY

1. Boggild AK, Castelli F, Gautret P, Torresi J, von Sonnenburg F, Barnett ED, et al. Vaccine preventable diseases in returned international travelers: results from the GeoSentinel Surveillance Network. Vaccine. 2010 Oct 28;28(46):7389–95.

2. CDC. Notes from the field: acute muscular sarcocystosis among returning travelers—Tioman Island, Malaysia, 2011. MMWR Morb Mortal Wkly Rep. 2012 Jan 20;61(2):37–8.

3. Chen LH, Wilson ME, Davis X, Loutan L, Schwartz E, Keystone J, et al. Illness in long-term travelers visiting GeoSentinel clinics. Emerg Infect Dis. 2009 Nov;15(11):1773–82.

4. Franco-Paredes C, Jacob JT, Hidron A, Rodriguez-Morales AJ, Kuhar D, Caliendo AM. Transplantation and tropical infectious diseases. Int J Infect Dis. 2010 Mar;14(3):e189–96.

5. Freedman DO, Weld LH, Kozarsky PE, Fisk T, Robins R, von Sonnenburg F, et al. Spectrum of disease and relation to place of exposure among ill returned travelers. N Engl J Med. 2006 Jan 12;354(2):119–30.

6. Hamer DH, Connor BA. Travel health knowledge, attitudes and practices among United States travelers. J Travel Med. 2004 Jan–Feb;11(1):23–6.

7. Hendel-Paterson B, Swanson SJ. Pediatric travelers visiting friends and relatives (VFR) abroad: illnesses,

barriers and pre-travel recommendations. Travel Med Infect Dis. 2011 Jul;9(4):192–203.

8. Hill DR. Health problems in a large cohort of Americans traveling to developing countries. J Travel Med. 2000 Sep–Oct;7(5):259–66.

9. Ryan ET, Wilson ME, Kain KC. Illness after international travel. N Engl J Med. 2002 Aug 15;347(7):505–16.

10. Schulte C, Krebs B, Jelinek T, Nothdurft HD, von Sonnenburg F, Loscher T. Diagnostic significance of blood eosinophilia in returning travelers. Clin Infect Dis. 2002 Feb 1;34(3):407–11.

11. Wilson ME, Weld LH, Boggild A, Keystone JS, Kain KC, von Sonnenburg F, et al. Fever in returned travelers: results from the GeoSentinel Surveillance Network. Clin Infect Dis. 2007 Jun 15;44(12):1560–8.

FEVER IN RETURNED TRAVELERS
Mary Elizabeth Wilson

INITIAL FOCUS

Fever commonly accompanies serious illness in returned travelers. Because it can signal a rapidly progressive infection such as malaria, the clinician must initiate early evaluation, especially in people who have visited areas with malaria in recent months (see Chapter 3, Malaria). The initial focus in evaluating a febrile returned traveler should be on identifying infections that are rapidly progressive, treatable, or transmissible. In some instances, public health officials must be alerted if the traveler may have been contagious en route or infected with a pathogen of public health importance (such as yellow fever) at the origin or destination.

USE OF HISTORY, LOCATION OF EXPOSURE, AND INCUBATION TO LIMIT DIFFERENTIAL DIAGNOSIS

Often the list of potential diagnoses is long, but multiple recent studies help to identify more common diagnoses. A large proportion of illnesses in returned travelers is caused by common, cosmopolitan infections (such as bacterial pneumonia or pyelonephritis), so these must be considered along with unusual infections. Because the geographic area of travel determines the relative likelihood of major causes of fever, it is essential to identify where the febrile patient has traveled and lived (Table 5-2). Details about activities (such as freshwater exposure in schistosomiasis-endemic areas, animal bites, sexual activities, or local medical care with injections) and accommodations in areas with malaria (bed nets, window screens, air conditioning) during travel may provide useful clues. Preparation before travel (such as hepatitis A vaccine or yellow fever vaccine) will markedly reduce the likelihood of some infections, so this is a relevant part of the history.

Because each infection has a characteristic incubation period (although the range is extremely wide with some infections), the time of exposures needs to be defined in different geographic areas (Table 5-3). This knowledge will allow the clinician to exclude some infections from the differential diagnosis. Most serious febrile infections manifest within the first month after return from tropical travel, yet infections related to travel exposures can occasionally occur months or even >1 year after return. In the United States, >90% of reported cases of *Plasmodium falciparum* malaria manifest within 30 days of return, but almost half of cases of *P. vivax* malaria manifest >30 days after return. A history of travel and residence should be an integral part of every medical history.

FINDINGS REQUIRING URGENT ATTENTION

Presence of associated signs, symptoms, or laboratory findings can focus attention on specific infections (Table 5-4). Findings that should prompt urgent attention include hemorrhage, neurologic impairment, and acute respiratory distress. Even if an initial physical examination is unremarkable, it is worth repeating the examination, as new findings may appear that will help in the diagnostic process (such as skin lesions or tender liver). Although most febrile illnesses in returned travelers are related to

Table 5-2. Common causes of fever, by geographic area

GEOGRAPHIC AREA	COMMON TROPICAL DISEASE CAUSING FEVER	OTHER INFECTIONS CAUSING OUTBREAKS OR CLUSTERS IN TRAVELERS
Caribbean	Dengue, malaria (Haiti)	Acute histoplasmosis, leptospirosis
Central America	Dengue, malaria (primarily *Plasmodium vivax*)	Leptospirosis, histoplasmosis, coccidioidomycosis
South America	Dengue, malaria (primarily *P. vivax*)	Bartonellosis, leptospirosis, histoplasmosis
South-central Asia	Dengue, enteric fever, malaria (primarily non-falciparum)	Chikungunya virus infection
Southeast Asia	Dengue, malaria (primarily non-falciparum)	Chikungunya virus infection, leptospirosis
Sub-Saharan Africa	Malaria (primarily *P. falciparum*), tickborne rickettsiae, acute schistosomiasis, filariasis	African trypanosomiasis

Table 5-3. Common infections, by incubation period

DISEASE	USUAL INCUBATION PERIOD (RANGE)	DISTRIBUTION
Incubation <14 Days		
Chikungunya	2–4 days (1–14 days)	Tropics, subtropics (Eastern Hemisphere)
Dengue	4–8 days (3–14 days)	Tropics, subtropics
Encephalitis, arboviral (Japanese encephalitis, tickborne encephalitis, West Nile virus, other)	3–14 days (1–20 days)	Specific agents vary by region
Enteric fever	7–18 days (3–60 days)	Especially in Indian subcontinent

continued

TABLE 5-3. COMMON INFECTIONS, BY INCUBATION PERIOD (continued)

Acute HIV	10–28 days (10 days to 6 weeks)	Worldwide
Influenza	1–3 days	Worldwide, can also be acquired en route
Legionellosis	5–6 days (2–10 days)	Widespread
Leptospirosis	7–12 days (2–26 days)	Widespread, most common in tropical areas
Malaria, *Plasmodium falciparum*	6–30 days (almost always within 3 months of travel; occasionally longer)	Tropics, subtropics
Malaria, *P. vivax*	8 days to 12 months (occasionally longer)	Widespread in tropics and subtropics
Spotted-fever rickettsiae	Few days to 2–3 weeks	Causative species vary by region
Incubation 14 Days to 6 Weeks		
Encephalitis, arboviral; enteric fever; acute HIV; leptospirosis; malaria	See above incubation periods for relevant diseases	See above distribution for relevant diseases
Amebic liver abscess	Weeks to months	Most common in developing countries
Hepatitis A	28–30 days (15–50 days)	Most common in developing countries
Hepatitis E	26–42 days (2–9 weeks)	Widespread
Acute schistosomiasis (Katayama syndrome)	4–8 weeks	Most common in sub-Saharan Africa
Incubation >6 Weeks		
Amebic liver abscess, hepatitis E, malaria, acute schistosomiasis	See above incubation periods for relevant diseases	See above distribution for relevant diseases
Hepatitis B	90 days (60–150 days)	Widespread
Leishmaniasis, visceral	2–10 months (10 days to years)	Asia, Africa, Latin America, southern Europe, and the Middle East
Tuberculosis	Primary, weeks; reactivation, years	Global distribution, rates and levels of resistance vary widely

Table 5-4. Common clinical findings and associated infections

COMMON CLINICAL FINDINGS	INFECTIONS TO CONSIDER AFTER TROPICAL TRAVEL
Fever and rash	Dengue, chikungunya, rickettsial infections, enteric fever (skin lesions may be sparse or absent), acute HIV infection, measles
Fever and abdominal pain	Enteric fever, amebic liver abscess
Undifferentiated fever and normal or low white blood cell count	Dengue, malaria, rickettsial infection, enteric fever, chikungunya
Fever and hemorrhage	Viral hemorrhagic fevers (dengue and others), meningococcemia, leptospirosis, rickettsial infections
Fever and eosinophilia	Acute schistosomiasis, drug hypersensitivity reaction, fascioliasis and other parasitic infections (rare)
Fever and pulmonary infiltrates	Common bacterial and viral pathogens, legionellosis, acute schistosomiasis, Q fever, leptospirosis
Fever and altered mental status	Cerebral malaria, viral or bacterial meningoencephalitis, African trypanosomiasis, scrub typhus
Mononucleosis syndrome	Epstein-Barr virus, cytomegalovirus, toxoplasmosis, acute HIV
Fever persisting >2 weeks	Malaria, enteric fever, Epstein-Barr virus, cytomegalovirus, toxoplasmosis, acute HIV, acute schistosomiasis, brucellosis, tuberculosis, Q fever, visceral leishmaniasis (rare)
Fever with onset >6 weeks after travel	*Plasmodium vivax* or *ovale* malaria, acute hepatitis (B, C, or E), tuberculosis, amebic liver abscess

5

infections, the clinician should bear in mind that other problems, including pulmonary emboli and drug hypersensitivity reactions, can be associated with fever.

CDC's Division of Global Migration and Quarantine is responsible for preventing the transmission of illnesses across US borders and, in particular, for preventing transmission of such illnesses into the United States. Fever accompanied by any of the following syndromes deserves further scrutiny, because it may indicate a disease of public health importance:

- Skin rash
- Difficulty breathing
- Shortness of breath
- Persistent cough
- Decreased consciousness
- Bruising or unusual bleeding (without previous injury)
- Persistent diarrhea
- Persistent vomiting (other than air or motion sickness)
- Jaundice
- Paralysis of recent onset

People who travel to visit friends and relatives (VFRs) often do not seek pre-travel medical advice. A review of GeoSentinel Surveillance Network data showed that a larger proportion of immigrant VFRs than tourist travelers presented with serious (requiring hospitalization), potentially preventable travel-related illnesses.

CHANGE OVER TIME

Clinicians have access to resources on the Internet that provide information about geographic-specific risks, disease activity, and other useful information, such as drug-susceptibility patterns for pathogens. Infectious diseases are dynamic, as is demonstrated by a review of adult returned travelers with fever and rash seen in 2006 and 2007 at a Paris hospital. The most common diagnosis was chikungunya fever, followed by dengue and African tick-bite fever. In contrast, because of the wide use of vaccine, hepatitis A infection is becoming less common in travelers.

Common infections in returned travelers may be seen at unexpected times of the year. Because influenza transmission can occur throughout the year in tropical areas, and the peak season in the Southern Hemisphere is May to August, clinicians in the Northern Hemisphere must be alert to the possibility of influenza outside the usual influenza season.

Travelers may acquire infections caused by common bacteria that are unusually resistant. Bacteria that produce the enzyme NDM-1 (New Delhi metallo-β-lactamase-1), which confers resistance to virtually all available antibiotics, have been found in infections acquired during travel, most often related to medical care (both elective and emergency). These bacteria have been most commonly reported after exposures in the Indian subcontinent. Enteric fever, the term used to describe either typhoid or paratyphoid fever, has also become increasingly resistant to fluoroquinolones (see Chapter 3, Typhoid & Paratyphoid Fever).

The tables in this section identify some common infections by presenting findings or other characteristics, by area of travel and by incubation periods. These highlight only the most common infections. The listed references and websites should be consulted for more detailed information. In most studies, a specific cause for fever is not identified in about 25% of returned travelers.

KEEP IN MIND

- Initial symptoms of life-threatening and self-limited infections can be identical.
- Fever in returned travelers is often caused by common, cosmopolitan infections, such as pneumonia and pyelonephritis, which should not be overlooked in the search for more exotic diagnoses.
- Patients with malaria may be afebrile at the time of evaluation but typically give a history of chills.
- Malaria is the most common cause of acute undifferentiated fever after travel to sub-Saharan Africa and to some other tropical areas.
- Malaria, especially *P. falciparum*, can progress rapidly. Diagnostic studies should be done promptly and treatment instituted immediately if malaria is diagnosed (see Chapter 3, Malaria).
- A history of taking malaria chemoprophylaxis does not exclude the possibility of malaria.
- Patients with malaria can have prominent respiratory (including acute respiratory distress syndrome), gastrointestinal, or central nervous system findings.
- Dengue is the most common cause of febrile illness among people who seek medical care after travel to Latin America or Asia.
- Viral hemorrhagic fevers are important to identify but are rare in travelers; bacterial infections, such as leptospirosis, meningococcemia, and rickettsial infections, can also cause fever and hemorrhage and should be always be considered because of the need to institute prompt, specific treatment.
- Sexually transmitted diseases, including acute HIV, can cause acute febrile infections.
- Consider infection control, public health implications, and requirements for reportable diseases.

5

BIBLIOGRAPHY

1. Bottieau E, Clerinx J, Schrooten W, Van den Enden E, Wouters R, Van Esbroeck M, et al. Etiology and outcome of fever after a stay in the tropics. Arch Intern Med. 2006 Aug 14–28;166(15):1642–8.

2. Bottieau E, Clerinx J, Van den Enden E, Van Esbroeck M, Colebunders R, Van Gompel A, et al. Infectious mononucleosis-like syndromes in febrile travelers returning from the tropics. J Travel Med. 2006 Jul–Aug;13(4):191–7.

3. Freedman DO, Weld LH, Kozarsky PE, Fisk T, Robins R, von Sonnenburg F, et al. Spectrum of disease and relation to place of exposure among ill returned travelers. N Engl J Med. 2006 Jan 12;354(2):119–30.

4. Hochedez P, Canestri A, Guihot A, Brichler S, Bricaire F, Caumes E. Management of travelers with fever and exanthema, notably dengue and chikungunya infections. Am J Trop Med Hyg. 2008 May;78(5):710–3.

5. Jensenius M, Davis X, von Sonnenburg F, Schwartz E, Keystone JS, Leder K, et al. Multicenter GeoSentinel analysis of rickettsial diseases in international travelers, 1996–2008. Emerg Infect Dis. 2009 Nov;15(11):1791–8.

6. Jensenius M, Fournier PE, Raoult D. Rickettsioses and the international traveler. Clin Infect Dis. 2004 Nov 15;39(10):1493–9.

7. Kumarasamy KK, Toleman MA, Walsh TR, Bagaria J, Butt F, Balakrishnan R, et al. Emergence of a new antibiotic resistance mechanism in India, Pakistan, and the UK: a molecular, biological, and epidemiological study. Lancet Infect Dis. 2010 Sep;10(9):597–602.

8. Leder K, Tong S, Weld L, Kain KC, Wilder-Smith A, von Sonnenburg F, et al. Illness in travelers visiting friends and relatives: a review of the GeoSentinel Surveillance Network. Clin Infect Dis. 2006 Nov 1;43(9):1185–93.

9. O'Brien D, Tobin S, Brown GV, Torresi J. Fever in returned travelers: review of hospital admissions for a 3-year period. Clin Infect Dis. 2001 Sep 1;33(5):603–9.

10. Ryan ET, Wilson ME, Kain KC. Illness after international travel. N Engl J Med. 2002 Aug 15;347(7):505–16.

11. Wilson ME, Freedman DO. Etiology of travel- related fever. Curr Opin Infect Dis. 2007 Oct;20(5):449–53.

12. Wilson ME, Weld LH, Boggild A, Keystone JS, Kain KC, von Sonnenburg F, et al. Fever in returned travelers: results from the GeoSentinel Surveillance Network. Clin Infect Dis. 2007 Jun 15;44(12):1560–8.

PERSISTENT TRAVELERS' DIARRHEA

Bradley A. Connor

Although most cases of travelers' diarrhea are acute and self-limited, a certain percentage of travelers will develop persistent (>14 days) gastrointestinal symptoms (see Chapter 2, Travelers' Diarrhea). The pathogenesis of persistent travelers' diarrhea generally falls into 1 of the following broad categories: 1) persistent infection or coinfection with a second organism not targeted by initial therapy, 2) previously undiagnosed gastrointestinal disease unmasked by the enteric infection, or 3) a postinfectious phenomenon.

PERSISTENT INFECTION

Most cases of travelers' diarrhea are the result of bacterial infection and are short-lived and self-limited. Travelers may experience prolonged diarrheal symptoms if they are immunosuppressed, are infected sequentially with diarrheal pathogens, or are infected with protozoan parasites. Parasites as a group are the pathogens most likely to be isolated from patients with persistent diarrhea, and their probability relative to bacterial infections increases with increasing duration of symptoms. Parasites may also be the cause of persistent diarrhea in patients already treated for a bacterial pathogen.

Giardia is by far the most likely persistent pathogen to be encountered. Suspicion for giardiasis should be particularly high when upper gastrointestinal symptoms predominate. Untreated, symptoms may last for months, even in immunocompetent hosts. The diagnosis can often be made through stool microscopy, antigen detection, or immunofluorescence. However, as *Giardia* infects the proximal small bowel, even multiple stool specimens may fail to detect it, and a duodenal aspirate may be necessary for definitive diagnosis. Given the high prevalence of *Giardia* in persistent travelers' diarrhea, empiric therapy is a reasonable option in the clinical setting after negative stool microscopy and in lieu of duodenal sampling. Other intestinal parasites that may cause persistent symptoms include *Cryptosporidium* species, *Entamoeba histolytica*, *Isospora belli*, *Microsporidia*, *Dientamoeba fragilis*, and *Cyclospora cayetanensis*.

Individual bacterial infections rarely cause persistence of symptoms, although persistent diarrhea has been reported in children infected with enteroaggregative or enteropathogenic *Escherichia coli* and among people with diarrhea due to *Clostridium difficile*. *C. difficile*–associated diarrhea may follow treatment of a bacterial pathogen with a fluoroquinolone or other antibiotic, or may even follow malaria chemoprophylaxis. This is especially important to consider in the patient with persistent travelers' diarrhea that seems refractory to multiple courses of empiric antibiotic therapy. The initial workup of persistent travelers' diarrhea should always include a *C. difficile* stool toxin assay. Treatment of *C. difficile* is with metronidazole, oral vancomycin, or fidaxomicin, although increasing reports of resistance to the first 2 drugs have been noted.

Persistent travelers' diarrhea has also been associated with tropical sprue and Brainerd diarrhea. These syndromes are suspected to result from infectious diseases, but specific pathogens have not been identified. Tropical sprue is associated with deficiencies of vitamins absorbed in the proximal and distal small bowel and most commonly affects long-term travelers to tropical areas. Investigation of an outbreak of Brainerd diarrhea among passengers on a cruise ship to the Galápagos Islands of Ecuador revealed that diarrhea persisted from 7 to more than 42 months and did not respond to antimicrobial therapy.

UNDERLYING GASTROINTESTINAL DISEASE

In some cases, persistence of gastrointestinal symptoms relates to chronic underlying gastrointestinal disease or susceptibility unmasked by the enteric infection. Most prominent among these is celiac disease, a systemic disease manifesting primarily with small bowel changes. In genetically susceptible people, villous atrophy and crypt hyperplasia are seen in response to exposure to antigens found in wheat, leading to malabsorption. The diagnosis is made by obtaining serologic tests, including tissue transglutaminase antibodies. A biopsy of the small bowel showing villous atrophy confirms the diagnosis. Treatment is with a wheat (gluten)-free diet.

Idiopathic inflammatory bowel disease, both Crohn disease and ulcerative colitis, may be seen after acute bouts of travelers' diarrhea. One prevailing hypothesis is that an initiating endogenous pathogen triggers inflammatory bowel disease in genetically susceptible people.

Depending on the clinical setting and age group, it may be necessary to do a more comprehensive search for other underlying causes of chronic diarrhea. Colorectal cancer should be considered, particularly in patients passing occult or gross blood rectally or with the onset of a new iron-deficiency anemia.

POSTINFECTIOUS PHENOMENA

In a certain percentage of patients who present with persistent gastrointestinal symptoms, no specific source will be found. Patients may experience temporary enteropathy following an acute diarrheal infection, with villous atrophy, decreased absorptive surface area, and disaccharidase deficiencies. This can lead to osmotic diarrhea, particularly when large amounts of lactose, sucrose, sorbitol, or fructose are consumed. Use of antimicrobial medications during the initial days of diarrhea may also lead to alterations in intestinal flora and diarrhea symptoms.

Occasionally, the onset of symptoms of irritable bowel syndrome (IBS) can be traced to an acute bout of gastroenteritis. IBS that develops after acute enteritis has been termed postinfectious (PI)-IBS. In the context of travelers' diarrhea, PI-IBS has been newly defined by the Rome III criteria as recurrent abdominal pain or discomfort associated with ≥2 of the following features:

- Improvement with defecation
- Onset associated with a change in the frequency of stool
- Onset associated with a change in form (appearance) of stool

To be labeled PI-IBS, these symptoms should follow an episode of gastroenteritis or travelers' diarrhea if the work-up for microbial pathogens and underlying gastrointestinal disease is negative. The role of small intestinal bacterial overgrowth in the pathogenesis of PI-IBS, especially when gas and bloating predominate, is being investigated.

EVALUATION

Three or more stool examinations should be performed for ova and parasites, including acid-fast stains for *Cryptosporidium*, *Cyclospora*, and *Isospora*; *Giardia* antigen testing; *C. difficile* toxin assay; and a D-xylose absorption test to determine if nutrients are being properly absorbed. Patients may also be given empiric treatment for *Giardia* infection. If underlying gastrointestinal disease is suspected, an initial evaluation should include serologic tests for celiac and inflammatory bowel disease. Subsequently, other studies to visualize both the upper and lower gastrointestinal tracts, with biopsies, may be indicated.

MANAGEMENT

Although US travelers are unlikely to become dehydrated or malnourished due to persistent diarrhea, hydration and nutritional support are of foremost importance. Dietary modifications may help those with malabsorption. If stools are bloody or when disease is caused by *C. difficile*, antidiarrheal medications such as loperamide or diphenoxylate should not be used in children and should be used cautiously, if at all, in adults. Probiotic medications have been shown to reduce the duration of persistent diarrhea among children in some settings. Antimicrobial medications may be useful in treating persistent diarrhea caused by parasites. Additional management strategies will depend on the specific cause of persistent diarrhea.

BIBLIOGRAPHY

1. Connor BA. Sequelae of traveler's diarrhea: focus on postinfectious irritable bowel syndrome. Clin Infect Dis. 2005 Dec 1;41 Suppl 8:S577–86.

2. Ford AC, Spiegel BM, Talley NJ, Moayyedi P. Small intestinal bacterial overgrowth in irritable bowel syndrome: systematic review and meta-analysis. Clin Gastroenterol Hepatol. 2009 Dec;7(12):1279–86.

3. Green PH, Jabri B. Coeliac disease. Lancet. 2003 Aug 2;362(9381):383–91.

4. Guerrant RL, Van Gilder T, Steiner TS, Thielman NM, Slutsker L, Tauxe RV, et al. Practice guidelines for the management of infectious diarrhea. Clin Infect Dis. 2001;32:331–50.

5. Jung IS, Kim HS, Park H, Lee SI. The clinical course of postinfectious irritable bowel syndrome: a five-year follow-up study. J Clin Gastroenterol. 2009 Jul;43(6):534–40.

6. Mintz ED, Weber JT, Guris D, Puhr N, Wells JG, Yashuk JC, et al. An outbreak of Brainerd diarrhea among travelers to the Galapagos Islands. J Infect Dis. 1998 Apr;177(4):1041–5.

7. Norman FF, Perez-Molina J, Perez de Ayala A, Jimenez BC, Navarro M, Lopez-Velez R. *Clostridium difficile*-associated diarrhea after antibiotic treatment for traveler's diarrhea. Clin Infect Dis. 2008 Apr 1;46(7):1060–3.

8. Osterholm MT, MacDonald KL, White KE, Wells JG, Spika JS, Potter ME, et al. An outbreak of a newly recognized chronic diarrhea syndrome associated with raw milk consumption. JAMA. 1986 Jul 25;256(4):484–90.

9. Porter CK, Tribble DR, Aliaga PA, Halvorson HA, Riddle MS. Infectious gastroenteritis and risk of developing inflammatory bowel disease. Gastroenterology. 2008 Sep;135(3):781–6.

10. Spiller R, Garsed K. Postinfectious irritable bowel syndrome. Gastroenterology. 2009 May;136(6):1979–88.

11. Spiller RC, Jenkins D, Thornley JP, Hebden JM, Wright T, Skinner M, et al. Increased rectal mucosal enteroendocrine cells, T lymphocytes, and increased gut permeability following acute *Campylobacter* enteritis and in post-dysenteric irritable bowel syndrome. Gut. 2000 Dec;47(6):804–11.

12. Taylor DN, Connor BA, Shlim DR. Chronic diarrhea in the returned traveler. Med Clin North Am. 1999 Jul;83(4):1033–52, vii.

SKIN & SOFT TISSUE INFECTIONS IN RETURNED TRAVELERS

Jay S. Keystone

DESCRIPTION

Skin problems are one of the most frequent medical problems in returned travelers. The largest case series of dermatologic problems in returned travelers from the GeoSentinel Surveillance Network showed that cutaneous larva migrans, insect bites, and bacterial infections were the most frequent skin problems in ill travelers who sought medical care, making up 30% of the 4,742 diagnoses (Table 5-5). In another review of 165 travelers who returned to France with skin problems, cellulitis, scabies, and pyoderma led the list of skin conditions. These data are biased in that they do not include skin problems that were diagnosed and, in many cases, easily managed during travel or that were self-limited.

Skin problems generally fall into 1 of the following categories: 1) those associated with fever, usually a rash or secondary bacterial infection (cellulitis, lymphangitis, bacteremia, toxin-mediated) and 2) those not associated with fever. Most skin problems are minor and are not accompanied by fever. Diagnosis of skin problems in returned travelers is based on the following:

- Pattern recognition of the lesions: papular, macular, nodular, linear, or ulcerative
- Location of the lesions: exposed versus unexposed skin surfaces
- Exposure history: freshwater, ocean, insects, animals, or human contact
- Associated symptoms: fever, pain, pruritus

It is important to recognize that skin conditions in returned travelers may not have a travel-related cause.

PAPULAR LESIONS

Insect bites, the most common cause of papular lesions, may be associated with secondary infection or hypersensitivity reactions. Bed bug and flea bites may produce grouped papules (see Box 2-4 for more information about bed bugs). Scabies infestation usually manifests as a generalized or regional pruritic, papular rash. Scabies burrows may present as papules or pustules in a short linear pattern on the skin.

Onchocerciasis may occur in long-stay travelers living in rural sub-Saharan Africa and, rarely, Latin America. It manifests as a generalized pruritic, papular dermatitis.

NODULAR OR SUBCUTANEOUS LESIONS, INCLUDING BACTERIAL SKIN INFECTIONS

Bacterial skin infections may occur more frequently after bites and other wounds in the tropics, particularly when good hygiene cannot be maintained. Organisms responsible are commonly *Staphylococcus aureus* or *Streptococcus pyogenes*. The presentations can include abscess formation, cellulitis, lymphangitis, or ulceration. Furunculosis, or recurrent pyoderma, may be the result of colonization of the skin and nasal mucosa with *S. aureus*. Boils may continue to occur weeks or months after a traveler returns and, if associated with *S. aureus*, definitive treatment usually involves decolonization with nasal mupirocin, a skin wash with an antimicrobial skin cleanser, and often an oral antibiotic combination including rifampin.

In addition to pyodermas, cellulitis or erysipelas may complicate excoriated insect bites or any trauma to the skin. Cellulitis and erysipelas manifest as areas of skin erythema, edema, and warmth in the absence of an underlying suppurative focus. Unlike cellulitis, erysipelas lesions are raised, there is a clear line of demarcation at the edge of the lesion, and the lesions are more likely to be associated with fever. Cellulitis, on the other hand, is more likely to be associated with lymphangitis. Cellulitis and erysipelas are usually caused by β-hemolytic streptococci; *S. aureus* (including methicillin-resistant strains) and gram-negative aerobic bacteria may also cause cellulitis. A recent study

Table 5-5. Skin lesions in returned travelers, by cause[1]

SKIN LESION	PERCENTAGE OF ALL DERMATOLOGIC DIAGNOSES (N = 4,742)
Cutaneous larva migrans	9.8
Insect bite	8.2
Skin abscess	7.7
Superinfected insect bite	6.8
Allergic rash	5.5
Rash, unknown origin	5.5
Dog bite	4.3
Superficial fungal infection	4.0
Dengue	3.4
Leishmaniasis	3.3
Myiasis	2.7
Spotted-fever group rickettsiae	1.5
Scabies	1.5
Cellulitis	1.5

[1] Modified from Lederman ER, Weld LH, Elyazar IR, et al. Dermatologic conditions of the ill returned traveler: an analysis from the GeoSentinel Surveillance Network. Int J Infect Dis. 2008;12(6):593–602.

from France of 60 returned travelers with skin and soft tissue infections found 35% had impetigo and 23% had cutaneous abscesses. Methicillin-susceptible S. aureus was detected in 43%, group A Streptococcus in 34%, and both in 23%.

Emerging antibiotic resistance among staphylococci and streptococci is problematic. Another common bacterial skin infection, especially in children in the tropics, is impetigo, due to S. aureus or S. pyogenes. Impetigo is a highly contagious superficial skin infection that generally appears on the arms, legs, or face as "honey-colored" or golden crustings formed from dried serum. Local care and a topical antibiotic such as mupirocin may be used, although a systemic antibiotic may be required. Emerging antibiotic resistance among staphylococci and streptococci complicates antimicrobial options.

Myiasis presents as a painful, boil-like lesion. It is caused by infestation with the larval stage of the African tumbu fly (Cordylobia anthropophaga) or the Latin American bot fly

(*Dermatobia hominis*). At the center of the lesion is a small punctum that allows the larva to breathe. Extraction of the fly larva can be difficult, especially of the bot fly; extraction may be facilitated by first asphyxiating the larvae, usually with an occlusive dressing or covering (such as a bottle cap filled with petroleum jelly) and then squeezing it out.

Tungiasis is caused by a sand flea (*Tunga penetrans*). The female burrows into the skin, usually the foot, and produces a nodular, pale, subcutaneous lesion with a central dark spot. The lesion expands as the female produces eggs in her uterus. Treatment involves extraction.

Loa loa filariasis can rarely occur in long-term travelers living in rural sub-Saharan Africa. The traveler may present with transient, migratory, subcutaneous, painful, or pruritic swellings produced by the adult nematode migration (Calabar swelling). Rarely, the worm can be visualized crossing the conjunctiva of the eye or eyelid. Eosinophilia is common. Loaiasis can be diagnosed by finding microfilariae in blood collected during daytime.

Gnathostomiasis is a nematode infection found primarily in Southeast Asia and less commonly in Africa and Latin America. Infection results from eating undercooked or raw freshwater fish. Infected travelers may experience transient, migratory, subcutaneous, pruritic, or painful swellings that may occur weeks or even years after exposure. The symptoms are due to migration of the worm through the body, and the central nervous system may be involved. Eosinophilia is common, and the diagnosis can be made by serology.

MACULAR LESIONS

Macular lesions are common and often non-specific and may be due to drug reactions or viral exanthems. Superficial mycoses, such as tinea versicolor and tinea corporis, may also present as macular lesions.

Tinea versicolor, due to *Malassezia furfur* (previously *Pityrosporum ovale*), is characterized by asymptomatic hypopigmented or hyperpigmented oval, slightly scaly patches measuring 1–3 cm, found on the upper chest, neck, and back. Diagnosis may be made by examination with a Wood's lamp or by placing a drop of methylene blue on a slide onto which clear cellulose acetate tape is placed sticky side down, after it has been touched

briefly to the skin lesions to pick up superficial scales. Detection of hyphae ("spaghetti") and spores ("meatballs") suggest the diagnosis. Treatment with topical or systemic azoles (ketoconazole, fluconazole) or terbinafine is recommended.

Tinea corporis (ringworm) may be caused by a number of different superficial fungi. The lesion is often a single lesion with an expanding red, raised ring, with a central area of clearing in the middle. Treatment is usually several weeks' application of a topical antifungal agent.

Lyme disease, a tickborne infection with *Borrelia burgdorferi*, is common in North America, Europe, and Russia (see Chapter 3, Lyme Disease). An infected traveler may present with ≥1 large erythematous patches, with or without central clearing, often surrounding a prior tick bite. The patient may not have noticed the tick bite.

LINEAR LESIONS

Cutaneous larva migrans, a skin infection with the larval stage of dog or cat hookworm (*Ancylostoma braziliense*), manifests as an extremely pruritic, serpiginous, linear lesion that advances within the skin relatively slowly (see Chapter 3, Cutaneous Larva Migrans). A similar lesion that may be more urticarial and that rapidly progresses may be due to **larva currens** (running larva) due to cutaneous migration of filariform larvae of *Strongyloides stercoralis*.

Phytophotodermatitis results from interaction of natural psoralens, most commonly from spilled lime juice, and ultraviolet radiation from the sun. The result is an exaggerated sunburn that gives rise to a linear, asymptomatic lesion that later develops hyperpigmentation. The hyperpigmentation may take weeks or months to resolve.

Lymphocutaneous spread of infection occurs when organisms spread along superficial cutaneous lymphatics, producing raised, linear, cordlike lesions; nodules or ulcers may also be found. Examples include sporotrichosis, *Mycobacterium marinum* infection (associated with exposure to water), leishmaniasis, bartonellosis (cat-scratch disease), *Nocardia* infection, tularemia, and blastomycosis.

SKIN ULCERS

Ulcerated skin lesions may result from *Staphylococcus* infections or may be the direct result of an unseen spider bite. The necrotic ulcer of anthrax is often surrounded by edema and usually results from handling animal hides or products. Rarely, a painless destructive ulcer with undermining edges may result from infection with Mycobacterium ulcerans (Buruli ulcer). Of particular concern is the ulcer (or less commonly, nodule) caused by **cutaneous leishmaniasis**. The main areas of risk are Latin America, the Mediterranean, the Middle East, Asia, and parts of Africa. The lesion is a chronic, usually painless ulcer, unless superinfected, with heaped-up margins on exposed skin surfaces. Special diagnostic techniques are necessary to confirm the diagnosis. Both topical and systemic treatments are effective; the species of the infection often determines the treatment modality. If cutaneous leishmaniasis is suspected, clinicians can contact CDC for further advice about diagnosis and treatment at 404-718-4745 or parasites@cdc.gov (see Chapter 3, Leishmaniasis, Cutaneous).

MISCELLANEOUS SKIN INFECTIONS
Skin Infections Associated with Water
Soft tissue infections can occur after both freshwater and saltwater exposure, particularly if there is associated trauma. Puncture wounds due to fishhooks and fish spines, lacerations due to inanimate objects during wading and swimming, and bites from fish or other sea creatures may be the source of the trauma leading to waterborne infections. Soft tissue infections associated with exposure to water or water-related animals include M. marinum, Aeromonas spp., Edwardsiella tarda, Erysipelothrix rhusiopathiae, and Vibrio vulnificus. A variety of skin and soft tissue manifestations may occur in association with these infections, including cellulitis, abscess formation, ecthyma gangrenosum, and necrotizing fasciitis. V. vulnificus infection may be especially severe in those with underlying liver disease and may manifest as a dramatic cellulitis with hemorrhagic bullae and sepsis. In general, infections caused by these organisms may be more severe in those who are immunosuppressed. M. marinum lesions are usually indolent and usually appear as solitary nodules or papules on an extremity, especially on the dorsum of feet and hands, which subsequently progress to shallow ulceration and scar formation. Occasionally, "sporotrichoid"

spread may occur as the lesions spread proximally along superficial lymphatics.

"Hot tub folliculitis" due to Pseudomonas aeruginosa may result from the use of spa pools or whirlpools or exposure to inadequately chlorinated swimming pools and hot tubs. Folliculitis typically develops 8–48 hours after exposure in contaminated water and consists of tender, pruritic papules, papulopustules, or nodules. Most patients have malaise, and some have low-grade fever. The condition is self-limited in 2–12 days; typically no antibiotic therapy is required.

Skin Infections Associated with Bites
Wound infections after dog and cat bites are caused by a variety of microorganisms. S. aureus; α-, β-, and γ-hemolytic streptococci; several genera of gram-negative organisms; and a number of anaerobic microorganisms have all been isolated. The prevalence of Pasteurella multocida isolates from dog bite wounds is 20%–50%; P. multocida is a major pathogen in cat bite wound infections. Splenectomized patients are at particular risk of severe cellulitis and sepsis due to Capnocytophaga canimorsus after a dog bite. Management of dog and cat bites includes consideration of rabies postexposure prophylaxis, tetanus immunization, and antibiotic prophylaxis. Primary closure of puncture wounds and dog bites to the hand should be avoided. Antibiotic prophylaxis for dog bites is controversial, although most experts would prophylactically treat splenectomized patients with amoxicillin-clavulanate. Since P. multocida is a common accompaniment of cat bites, prophylaxis with amoxicillin-clavulanate or a fluoroquinolone for 3–5 days should be considered.

FEVER AND RASH
Fever and rash in returned travelers are most often due to a viral infection.

Dengue is caused by 1 of 4 strains of dengue viruses (see Chapter 3, Dengue). The disease is transmitted by a day-biting Aedes mosquito often found in urban areas, and its incidence continues to increase. The disease is characterized by the abrupt onset of high fever, frontal headache (often accompanied by retroorbital pain), myalgia, and a faint macular rash that becomes evident on the second to fourth day of illness. A petechial rash may be found in classical dengue, as well as severe dengue (such as dengue hemorrhagic fever). PCR and serologic tests are available to diagnose dengue; the detection of IgM antibodies in the appropriate clinical scenario would support the diagnosis.

Chikungunya, a virus transmitted by a day-biting *Aedes* mosquito, has recently caused major outbreaks of illness in southeast Africa and South Asia (see Chapter 3, Chikungunya). Chikungunya fever is similar to dengue clinically, including the rash, although hemorrhage, shock, and death are not typical of Chikungunya. A major distinguishing feature is that arthritis or arthralgia is common with chikungunya (and may persist for months), whereas in dengue, myalgia is the major clinical feature. Similar to dengue, serologic tests are available. Treatment of the arthritis is with nonsteroidal antiinflammatory drugs.

South African tick typhus, or African tick-bite fever (*Rickettsia africae*), is the most frequent cause of fever and rash in southern Africa. Transmitted by ticks, the disease is characterized by fever and a papular or vesicular rash associated with localized lymphadenopathy and the presence of an eschar (a mildly painful 1- to 2-cm black necrotic lesion with an erythematous margin). Satellite lesions may be present. Diagnosis is usually one of clinical recognition and is confirmed by serology. Treatment is with doxycycline.

Rocky Mountain spotted fever (RMSF), although uncommon in travelers, is an important cause of fever and rash because of its potential severity and the need for early treatment. This tickborne infection is found in the United States, Mexico, and parts of Central and South America. Most patients with RMSF develop a rash between the third and fifth days of illness. The typical rash of RMSF begins on the ankles and wrists and spreads both centrally and to the palms and soles. The rash commonly begins as a maculopapular eruption and then becomes petechial, although in some patients it begins as petechial. Doxycycline is the treatment of choice.

The category of fever with rash is large, and providers caring for ill travelers should also consider the following diagnoses: enteroviruses, such as echovirus and coxsackievirus; hepatitis B virus; measles; Epstein-Barr virus; cytomegalovirus; typhus; leptospirosis; and HIV.

BIBLIOGRAPHY

1. Ansart S, Perez L, Jaureguiberry S, Danis M, Bricaire F, Caumes E. Spectrum of dermatoses in 165 travelers returning from the tropics with skin diseases. Am J Trop Med Hyg. 2007 Jan;76(1):184–6.

2. Bernard P. Management of common bacterial infections of the skin. Curr Opin Infect Dis. 2008 Apr;21(2):122–8.

3. Bowers AG. Phytophotodermatitis. Am J Contact Dermat. 1999 Jun;10(2):89–93.

4. Chapman AS, Bakken JS, Folk SM, Paddock CD, Bloch KC, Krusell A, et al. Diagnosis and management of tickborne rickettsial diseases: Rocky Mountain spotted fever, ehrlichioses, and anaplasmosis—United States: a practical guide for physicians and other health-care and public health professionals. MMWR Recomm Rep. 2006 Mar 31;55(RR-4):1–27.

5. Diaz JH. The epidemiology, diagnosis, management, and prevention of ectoparasitic diseases in travelers. J Travel Med. 2006 Mar–Apr;13(2):100–11.

6. Freedman DO, Weld LH, Kozarsky PE, Fisk T, Robins R, von Sonnenburg F, et al. Spectrum of disease and relation to place of exposure among ill returned travelers. N Engl J Med. 2006 Jan 12;354(2):119–30.

7. Heukelbach J, Feldmeier H. Epidemiological and clinical characteristics of hookworm-related cutaneous larva migrans. Lancet Infect Dis. 2008 May;8(5):302–9.

8. Hochedez P, Canestri A, Guihot A, Brichler S, Bricaire F, Caumes E. Management of travelers with fever and exanthema, notably dengue and chikungunya infections. Am J Trop Med Hyg. 2008 May;78(5):710–3.

9. Hochedez P, Canestri A, Lecso M, Valin N, Bricaire F, Caumes E. Skin and soft tissue infections in returning travelers. Am J Trop Med Hyg. 2009 Mar;80(3):431–4.

10. Huang DB, Ostrosky-Zeichner L, Wu JJ, Pang KR, Tyring SK. Therapy of common superficial fungal infections. Dermatol Ther. 2004;17(6):517–22.

11. Jensenius M, Davis X, von Sonnenburg F, Schwartz E, Keystone JS, Leder K, et al. Multicenter GeoSentinel analysis of rickettsial diseases in international travelers, 1996–2008. Emerg Infect Dis. 2009 Nov;15(11):1791–8.

12. Klion AD. Filarial infections in travelers and immigrants. Curr Infect Dis Rep. 2008 Mar;10(1):50–7.

13. Lederman ER, Gleeson TD, Driscoll T, Wallace MR. Doxycycline sensitivity of S. *pneumoniae* isolates. Clin Infect Dis. 2003 Apr 15;36(8):1091.

14. Lederman ER, Weld LH, Elyazar IR, von Sonnenburg F, Loutan L, Schwartz E, et al. Dermatologic conditions of the ill returned traveler: an analysis from the GeoSentinel Surveillance Network. Int J Infect Dis. 2008 Nov;12(6):593–602.

15. Magill AJ. Cutaneous leishmaniasis in the returning traveler. Infect Dis Clin North Am. 2005 Mar;19(1):241–66, x–xi.

16. Medical Letter Inc. Drugs for Parasitic Infections. 2nd ed. New Rochelle, NY: The Medical Letter, Inc; 2010.

17. Menard A, Dos Santos G, Dekumyoy P, Ranque S, Delmont J, Danis M, et al. Imported cutaneous gnathostomiasis: report of five cases. Trans R Soc Trop Med Hyg. 2003 Mar–Apr;97(2):200–2.

18. Nordlund JJ. Cutaneous ectoparasites. Dermatol Ther. 2009 Nov–Dec;22(6):503–17.

19. Nutman TB, Miller KD, Mulligan M, Reinhardt GN, Currie BJ, Steel C, et al. Diethylcarbamazine prophylaxis for human loiasis. Results of a double-blind study. N Engl J Med. 1988 Sep 22;319(12):752–6.

20. Oostvogel PM, van Doornum GJ, Ferreira R, Vink J, Fenollar F, Raoult D. African tickbite fever in travelers, Swaziland. Emerg Infect Dis. 2007 Feb;13(2):353–5.

21. Solomon M, Benenson S, Baum S, Schwartz E. Tropical skin infections among Israeli travelers. Am J Trop Med Hyg. 2011 Nov;85(5):868–72.

22. Tristan A, Bes M, Meugnier H, Lina G, Bozdogan B, Courvalin P, et al. Global distribution of Panton-Valentine leukocidin–positive methicillin-resistant *Staphylococcus aureus*, 2006. Emerg Infect Dis. 2007 Apr;13(4):594–600.

23. Walsh DS, Portaels F, Meyers WM. Buruli ulcer: advances in understanding *Mycobacterium ulcerans* infection. Dermatol Clin. 2011 Jan;29(1):1–8.

24. Wilson ME, Chen LH. Dermatologic infectious diseases in international travelers. Curr Infect Dis Rep. 2004 Feb;6(1):54–62.

SCREENING ASYMPTOMATIC RETURNED TRAVELERS

Michael Libman

CDC has no official guidelines or recommendations for screening those returning from international travel who are asymptomatic (see Chapter 9 for recommendations regarding the screening of newly arrived immigrants and refugees). Nevertheless, screening high-risk travelers, such as those who have spent an extended time in developing countries, can reveal occult infections, some of which can cause serious sequelae or have public health implications.

PARASITIC INFECTION

Asymptomatic travelers should not be screened for malaria. All travelers, especially those who did not take recommended malaria chemoprophylaxis during and after the trip, should be reminded to seek evaluation for unexplained fever and notify practitioners of recent travel.

Travelers are often concerned about "worms," but high-burden infections with common nematodes such as *Ascaris, Trichuris,* or hookworm are uncommon in returning travelers. Rarely, complications have been reported among initially asymptomatic travelers, such as migration of *Ascaris* into the biliary system, but the lifespan of most helminths—months to a few years—generally ensures eventual spontaneous cure and precludes ongoing transmission in industrialized countries. The exception is *Strongyloides*, which can cause serious complications. The duration of carriage is unlimited, and the original burden of infection is irrelevant. Unfortunately, diagnosis by stool examination is insensitive, and serologic methods are often required.

Testing for pathogenic protozoa in asymptomatic patients is not recommended. No evidence suggests that carriers are likely to develop symptoms at a later time, although minor, unreported symptoms could be alleviated, and transmission (which is rare in asymptomatic people) could be prevented. Stool microscopy for protozoa is expensive, relatively insensitive, poorly reproducible, and strongly influenced by the expertise of laboratory personnel. *Entamoeba histolytica* (pathogenic) cannot be distinguished from *E. dispar* (nonpathogenic) by microscopy, and several studies suggest that most travelers with *Entamoeba* identified on microscopy are carrying *E. dispar*.

Some extraintestinal helminths, particularly *Strongyloides* and *Schistosoma*, are capable of eventually causing subsequent serious illness in travelers who are asymptomatic upon return. Low-burden schistosomal infections, such as those typically found in travelers, are not likely to lead to the "classic" chronic complications, such as liver fibrosis or malignancy. However, complications due to ectopic egg migration can occur even in light infections and without warning, although these complications are unusual. Traditional tests for these infections, including stool examination for *Strongyloides* and *Schistosoma* spp. and urine tests for *S. haematobium*, all lack sensitivity, particularly in low-burden infections. For this reason, serologic testing has been advocated as the best screening tool, although it is expensive, available only in some commercial laboratories, and poorly standardized. Treatments for strongyloidiasis and schistosomiasis are inexpensive, easy, and effective. Serologic testing can be considered for travelers who had a prolonged or high-risk exposure (people with environmental exposures in an area of known high endemicity, for example), and all those found to be positive should be treated.

Reports of travelers with late complications from asymptomatic filarial infections are also very rare. Transmission of filarial infection typically requires longer-term exposure (generally >3 months in an endemic area) but should be considered in returning travelers with eosinophilia who have traveled to endemic countries, if no other pathogen commonly associated with eosinophilia can be identified. Filarial serology usually becomes positive only after adult forms have matured, which means waiting ≥3 months after exposure.

Eosinophil counts are commonly used to screen returning travelers when parasitic infection is a concern. This test can suggest the presence of invasive helminths but not protozoa. However, eosinophilia has poor sensitivity for detecting invasive helminths, and although specificity can be high, the low prevalence of infection in travelers means the positive predictive value is low (positive predictive value increases, however, with high-grade eosinophilia). Many cases of eosinophilia resolve spontaneously, and eosinophilia is also often due to noninfectious causes, such as allergy or drug reactions. Eosinophil counts can be repeated over several weeks or months before an extensive investigation is done. Counts may be highly variable over time, even within a single day, and eosinophilia can be suppressed by endogenous or exogenous steroids. Evaluation of absolute eosinophil counts, rather than by percentage of eosinophils among leukocytes, is more reproducible and predictive.

Asymptomatic trypanosomiasis among US residents who have traveled to endemic areas appears to be extremely rare. Screening asymptomatic travelers for trypanosomiasis is generally not recommended. For people traveling to areas of Latin America where Chagas disease is endemic, testing might be considered in cases of prolonged residence in primitive housing (such as with mud walls or thatched roofs) or when the large reduviid bugs have been seen in the residence. Asymptomatic Chagas disease among people who were born in Central or South America has been a concern in recent years, and these people would be candidates for Chagas disease screening, but the screening decision is not based on recent travel history. East African trypanosomiasis has occasionally affected travelers but is generally symptomatic. West African trypanosomiasis is very rarely reported in travelers.

NONPARASITIC ILLNESS

Casual sex with new partners, including with sex workers, is common among travelers, and the low rates of reported condom use are concerning. Returning travelers with acute HIV or hepatitis B virus infection pose public health risks, so screening for sexually transmitted infections should be considered.

The incidence of tuberculosis related to travel is difficult to assess. A history of work in high-prevalence settings such as health care institutions, prisons, or refugee camps should prompt screening. Doing pre- and post-travel skin tests is cumbersome, requiring as many

Table 5-6. Considerations for screening asymptomatic travelers

RISK OR EXPOSURE	SCREENING TEST
Stays <3–6 months	None
Stays >3–6 months, poor sanitation or hygiene	Eosinophil count, consider stool ova and parasites
Walking barefoot on soil potentially contaminated with human feces or sewage	*Strongyloides* serologic tests
Exposure to freshwater rivers, lakes, or irrigation canals	*Schistosoma* serologic tests
Sexual contact	Screen for sexually transmitted infections
Work in health care setting, close contact (>6 months) with population in a highly TB-endemic area	TB screening (TST or IGRA)

Abbreviations: TB, tuberculosis; TST, tuberculin skin testing; IGRA, interferon-γ release assay.

as 4 pre-travel visits for a 2-step test and 2 visits after potential exposure. An alternative is an interferon-γ release assay (IGRA), which is also less subject to false-positive results related to vaccination. IGRAs are expensive, but the cost may be offset by the reduced number of visits and medical costs. In most patients born and raised in nonendemic countries, the pre-travel test can be omitted.

For many long-term travelers, such as expatriate workers and some missionary and aid workers, a visit for asymptomatic screening may be their only interlude from a continuing assignment abroad and is an opportunity for a general health evaluation. The usual recommendations for the periodic health exam, which may include a routine blood count and chemistries, as well as screening for hypertension, diabetes, and malignancy, also apply.

CONCLUSIONS

Most recommendations for screening asymptomatic returning travelers are based on opinion and common sense, rather than convincing evidence. The following general recommendations apply (Table 5-6).

Short Stay (<3–6 Months)

The yield of screening is low and should be directed by specific risk factors revealed in the history. A history of prolonged (>2 weeks) digestive symptoms suggests protozoal infection. Exposure to freshwater in a region endemic for schistosomiasis, especially in Africa, merits consideration of microscopic stool and urine examination in the case of high-intensity exposure, with the addition of serologic testing to diagnose light infections, when egg shedding may not be consistent in travelers and in others who have not had schistosomiasis previously. Antibody tests do not distinguish between past and current infection. Serologic tests for *Strongyloides* should be considered in those who have a high risk of exposure, usually those who report that they frequently walked outdoors barefoot. A sexual history should be obtained. Work in a health care setting or other area at high risk for tuberculosis may merit screening.

Longer Stay

Stool examinations are of limited utility, but they can reassure the traveler. However, they may also identify a nonpathogenic protozoan, which could distress the traveler. Serologic tests for schistosomiasis and strongyloidiasis can be considered for those who report engaging in high-risk activities (exposure to fresh water or soil, respectively). An eosinophil count is usually done, although results should be interpreted cautiously, and repeat testing may be needed to assess trends in eosinophil count. Screening for sexually transmitted infections should be offered to all travelers. Tuberculin skin test or IGRA should be offered to those who have worked in a health care or similar setting or who have had intimate and prolonged contact with residents of an endemic area for ≥6 months. Possible exposure to blood-borne pathogens should be assessed. Any other screening should be guided by exceptional exposures or knowledge about local outbreaks.

BIBLIOGRAPHY

1. Baaten GG, Sonder GJ, van Gool T, Kint JA, van den Hoek A. Travel-related schistosomiasis, strongyloidiasis, filariasis, and toxocariasis: the risk of infection and the diagnostic relevance of blood eosinophilia. BMC Infect Dis. 2011;11:84.
2. MacLean JD, Libman M. Screening returning travelers. Infect Dis Clin North Am. 1998 Jun;12(2):431–43.
3. Whitty CJ, Carroll B, Armstrong M, Dow C, Snashall D, Marshall T, et al. Utility of history, examination and laboratory tests in screening those returning to Europe from the tropics for parasitic infection. Trop Med Int Health. 2000 Nov;5(11):818–23.

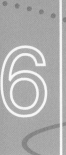
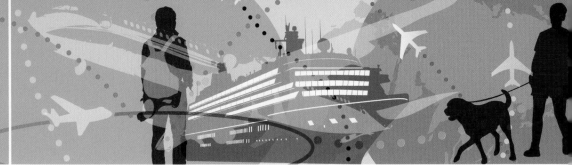

Conveyance & Transportation Issues

AIR TRAVEL

Karen J. Marienau, Petra A. Illig, Phyllis E. Kozarsky, Nancy M. Gallagher

Worldwide, >1 billion people travel by commercial aircraft every year, and this number is expected to double in the next 20 years. Travelers often have concerns about the health risks of flying in airplanes. Those with underlying illness need to be aware that the entire point-to-point travel experience, including buses, trains, taxis, and public waiting areas, can pose challenges. While illness may occur as a direct result of air travel, it is uncommon; the main concerns are:

- Exacerbations of chronic medical problems due to changes in air pressure, humidity, and oxygen concentration
- Relative immobility during flights (risk of thromboembolic disease, see Chapter 2, Deep Vein Thrombosis & Pulmonary Embolism)
- Close proximity to other passengers with certain communicable diseases
- Spraying of airplane cabins with insecticides (disinsection) before landing in certain destinations

EXACERBATION OF CHRONIC DISEASE

During flight, the aircraft cabin pressure is usually maintained at the equivalent of 6,000–8,000 ft (1,829–2,438 m) above sea level. Most healthy travelers will not notice any effects. However, for travelers with cardiopulmonary

diseases (especially those who normally require supplemental oxygen), cerebrovascular disease, anemia, or sickle cell disease, conditions in an aircraft can exacerbate underlying medical conditions. Aircraft cabin air is typically dry, usually 10%–20% humidity, which can cause dryness of the mucous membranes of the eyes and airways.

People with chronic illnesses, particularly those whose conditions may be unstable, should be evaluated by a physician to ensure they are fit for air travel. For those who require supplemental in-flight oxygen, the following must be taken into consideration:

- Federal regulations prohibit airlines from allowing passengers to bring their own oxygen aboard; passengers requiring in-flight supplemental oxygen should notify the airline ≥72 hours before departure.
- Information regarding the screening of respiratory equipment (such as oxygen canisters or portable oxygen concentrators) at airports in the United States and regulations regarding oxygen use on aircraft can be found at www.tsa.gov/travelers/airtravel.
- Airlines might not offer in-flight supplemental oxygen on all aircraft or flights; some airlines permit only portable oxygen concentrators.

- Travelers must arrange their own oxygen supplies while on the ground, at departure, during layovers, and on arrival. The National Home Oxygen Patients Association provides information to assist patients who require supplemental oxygen during travel (www.homeoxygen.org/airtrav.html).

BAROTRAUMA DURING FLIGHT

Barotrauma may occur when the pressure inside an air-filled, enclosed body space (such as the middle ear, sinuses, or abdomen) is not the same as air pressure inside the aircraft cabin. It most commonly occurs during rapid changes in environmental pressure, such as during ascent, when cabin pressure rapidly decreases, and during descent, when cabin pressure rapidly increases. Barotrauma most commonly affects the middle ear; it occurs when the eustachian tube is blocked and thus unable to equalize the air pressure in the middle ear with the outside cabin pressure. Middle ear barotrauma is usually not severe or dangerous and can usually be prevented or self-treated. It may rarely cause complications such as a perforated tympanic membrane, dizziness, permanent tinnitus, or hearing loss. The following suggestions may help avoid potential barotrauma:

- People with ear, nose, and sinus infections or severe congestion may wish to temporarily avoid flying to prevent pain or injury.
- Oral pseudoephedrine 30 minutes before flight departure, or a nonsteroidal anti-inflammatory agent, may alleviate symptoms.
- Travelers with allergies should continue their regular allergy medication.
- Travelers should stay hydrated to help avoid irritation of nasal passages and pharynx and to promote better function of the eustachian tubes.
- Travelers sensitive to abdominal bloating should avoid carbonated beverages and foods that can increase gas production.
- People who have had recent surgery, particularly intra-abdominal, neurologic, intrapulmonary, or intraocular procedures, should consult with their physicians before flying.

VENTILATION AND AIR QUALITY

All commercial jet aircraft built after the late 1980s and a few modified older aircraft recirculate 10%–50% of the air in the cabin mixed with outside air. The recirculated air passes through a series of filters 20–30 times per hour. In most newer-model airplanes, the recycled air passes through high-efficiency particulate air (HEPA) filters, which capture 99.9% of particles (bacteria, fungi, and larger viruses) 0.1–0.3 µm in diameter. Air flow occurs transversely across the plane in limited bands, and air is not forced up and down the length of the plane. As a result, the air cabin environment is not conducive to the spread of most infectious diseases.

IN-FLIGHT MEDICAL EMERGENCIES

Increasingly, large aircraft, combined with an aging flying population, makes the incidence of onboard medical emergencies likely to increase. Approximately 1 in 10,000 to 40,000 passengers has a medical incident during air transport. Of these, approximately 1 in 150,000 requires use of in-flight medical equipment or drugs. The most commonly encountered in-flight medical events, in order of frequency, are the following:

- Vasovagal syncope
- Gastrointestinal events
- Respiratory events
- Cardiac events
- Neurologic events

Deaths aboard commercial aircraft have been estimated at 0.3 per 1 million passengers; approximately two-thirds of these are caused by cardiac problems. Air carriers in the United States that fly with a maximum payload capacity of >7,500 pounds and with ≥1 flight attendant (typically those aircraft with a capacity of ≥30 passengers) are now required to carry ≥1 approved automatic external defibrillator and an emergency medical kit. The kit is required to have the items specified by the Federal Aviation Administration (for contents, see www.faa.gov/regulations_policies/advisory_circulars/index.cfm/go/document.information/documentID/22516).

Although flight attendants receive training in basic first aid procedures, they are generally not certified in emergency medical response. Many airlines use ground-based medical consultants via radio or phone communication to assist volunteer passenger responders and flight attendants in managing medical cases.

The goal of managing in-flight medical emergencies is to stabilize the passenger until ground-based medical care can safely be reached; it should not be considered a method of maintaining the original flight route in order to reach the scheduled destination. The captain must, therefore, weigh the needs of the ill passenger with other safety considerations such as weather, landing conditions, and terrain. Certain routes, such as transoceanic flights, may severely restrict diversion options, while others may present a number of safe landing choices. In the latter circumstance, consideration should be given to choosing an airport that has timely access to a medical facility.

IN-FLIGHT TRANSMISSION OF COMMUNICABLE DISEASES

Communicable diseases may be transmitted to other travelers during air travel; therefore, people who are acutely ill, or still within the infectious period for a specific disease, should delay their travel until they are no longer contagious. Travelers should be up-to-date on routine vaccinations and receive destination-specific vaccinations before travel. Travelers should be reminded to wash their hands frequently and thoroughly (or use an alcohol-based hand sanitizer containing ≥60% alcohol), especially after using the toilet and before preparing or eating food, and to cover their noses and mouths when coughing or sneezing.

If a passenger with a communicable disease is identified as having flown on a particular flight (or flights), passengers who may have been exposed may be contacted by public health authorities for possible screening or prophylaxis. When necessary, public health authorities will obtain contact information from the airline for potentially exposed travelers so they may be contacted and offered intervention. Notifying a passenger of potential exposure to a communicable disease during a flight is facilitated if he or she has provided the airline with accurate and up-to-date contact information.

Tuberculosis

Mycobacterium tuberculosis is transmitted from person to person via airborne respiratory droplet nuclei. Although the risk of transmission onboard aircraft is low, CDC recommends conducting passenger contact investigations for flights ≥8 hours if the person with tuberculosis (TB) is sputum smear positive for acid-fast bacilli and has cavitation on chest radiograph or has multidrug-resistant TB. People known to have active TB disease should not travel by commercial air (or any other commercial means) until they are determined to be noninfectious. State health department TB controllers are valuable resources for advice (www.tbcontrollers.org/community/statecityterritory).

Neisseria meningitidis

Meningococcal disease (caused by *Neisseria meningitidis*) is transmitted by direct contact with respiratory droplets and secretions and can be rapidly fatal. Therefore, close contacts need to be quickly identified and provided with prophylactic antimicrobial agents. Antimicrobial prophylaxis should be considered for any of the following:

- Household member traveling with the ill traveler
- Travel companion with very close contact
- Passenger seated directly next to the ill traveler on flights ≥8 hours

Measles

Measles (rubeola) is a viral illness transmitted by respiratory droplets or direct contact, but it can also be spread via airborne routes. Most measles cases diagnosed in the United States are imported from countries where measles is endemic. Travelers should ensure they are immune to measles before travel. Infants aged 6–11 months who will be traveling overseas should receive 1 dose of measles-mumps-rubella (MMR) vaccine before travel. However, this dose will not count as part of the recommended immunization schedule of 2 doses, which begins at age 12–15 months. An ill traveler is considered infectious during a flight of any duration if he or she traveled during the 4 days before rash onset through 4 days after rash onset. Flight-related contact investigations are initiated as quickly as possible so postexposure prophylaxis may be provided to susceptible travelers. MMR vaccine given within 72 hours of exposure or immune globulin given within 6 days of exposure may prevent measles or minimize its severity.

Influenza

Transmission of the influenza virus aboard aircraft has been documented, but data are limited. Transmission is thought to be primarily due to large droplets; therefore, passengers seated closest to the source case are believed to be most at risk for exposure. Influenza vaccine is routinely recommended each year for all people aged ≥6 months who do not have contraindications.

See the CDC Travelers' Health website (www.cdc.gov/travel and wwwnc.cdc.gov/travel/page/air-travel-cruise-ships.htm) for additional information. Travel advice specific for air crews may be found in Chapter 8.

DISINSECTION

To reduce the accidental spread of mosquitoes and other vectors via airline cabins and luggage compartments, a number of countries require disinsection of all inbound flights. The World Health Organization (WHO) and the International Civil Aviation Organization (ICAO) specify 2 approaches for aircraft disinsection:

- Spraying the aircraft cabin with an aerosolized insecticide (usually 2% phenothrin) while passengers are on board

- Treating the aircraft's interior surfaces with a residual insecticide while the aircraft is empty

Some countries use a third method, in which aircraft are sprayed with an aerosolized insecticide while passengers are not on board.

Disinsection is not routinely done on incoming flights to the United States. Although disinsection, when done appropriately, was declared safe by WHO in 1995, there is still much debate about the safety of the agents and methods used. Guidelines for disinsection have been updated for the revised International Health Regulations (www.who.int/ihr/en). Many countries, including the United States, reserve the right to increase the use of disinsection in case of increased threat of vector or disease spread. An updated list of countries that require disinsection and the types of methods used is available at the Department of Transportation website (http://ostpxweb.dot.gov/policy/safetyenergyenv/disinsection.htm).

BIBLIOGRAPHY

1. Aerospace Medical Association Task Force. Medical guidelines for airline travel, 2nd ed. Aviat Space Environ Med. 2003 May;74(5 Suppl):A1–19.
2. Bagshaw M, DeVoll JR, Jennings RT, McCrary BF, Northrup SE, Rayman RB, et al. Medical Guidelines for Airline Passengers. Alexandria, VA: Aerospace Medical Association; 2002 [cited 2012 Sep 26]. Available from: http://www.asma.org/asma/media/asma/Travel-Publications/paxguidelines.pdf.
3. Bagshaw M, Nicolls DN. The aircraft cabin environment. In: Keystone JS, Freedman DO, Kozarsky PE, Connor BA, Nothdurft HO, editors. Travel Medicine. 3rd ed. Philadelphia: Saunders Elsevier; 2013. p. 405–12.
4. CDC. Exposure to patients with meningococcal disease on aircrafts—United States, 1999–2001. MMWR Morb Mortal Wkly Rep. 2001 Jun 15;50(23):485–9.
5. CDC. Multistate measles outbreak associated with an international youth sporting event—Pennsylvania, Michigan, and Texas, August–September 2007. MMWR Morb Mortal Wkly Rep. 2008 Feb 22;57(7):169–73.
6. CDC. Public health interventions involving travelers with tuberculosis—US ports of entry, 2007–2012. MMWR Morb Mortal Wkly Rep. 2012 Aug 3;61:570–3.
7. Delaune EF 3rd, Lucas RH, Illig P. In-flight medical events and aircraft diversions: one airline's experience. Aviat Space Environ Med. 2003 Jan;74(1):62–8.

8. Han K, Zhu X, He F, Liu L, Zhang L, Ma H, et al. Lack of airborne transmission during outbreak of pandemic (H1N1) 2009 among tour group members, China, June 2009. Emerg Infect Dis. 2009 Oct;15(10):1578–81.
9. Illig P. Passenger health. In: Curdt-Christiansen C, Draeger J, Kriebel J, Antunano M, editors. Principles and Practice of Aviation Medicine. Hackensack, NJ: World Scientific; 2009. p. 667–708.
10. Kenyon TA, Valway SE, Ihle WW, Onorato IM, Castro KG. Transmission of multidrug-resistant *Mycobacterium tuberculosis* during a long airplane flight. N Engl J Med. 1996 Apr 11;334(15):933–8.
11. Marsden AG. Outbreak of influenza-like illness [corrected] related to air travel. Med J Aust. 2003 Aug 4;179(3):172–3.
12. Mayo Clinic. Airplane ear: definition. Rochester, MN: Mayo Clinic; 2010 [cited 2012 Sep 26]. Available from: http://www.mayoclinic.com/health/airplane-ear/DS00472.
13. Mirza S, Richardson H. Otic barotrauma from air travel. J Laryngol Otol. 2005 May;119(5):366–70.
14. Moser MR, Bender TR, Margolis HS, Noble GR, Kendal AP, Ritter DG. An outbreak of influenza aboard a commercial airliner. Am J Epidemiol. 1979 Jul;110(1):1–6.
15. Nelson K, Marienau K, Schembri C, Redd S. Measles transmission during air travel, United States, December 1, 2008–May 31, 2011. In: 2012 International

Conference on Emerging Infectious Diseases Program and Abstracts Book. Atlanta: CDC; 2012. p. 127.

16. Rosenkvist L, Klokker M, Katholm M. Upper respiratory infections and barotraumas in commercial pilots: a retrospective survey. Aviat Space Environ Med. 2008 Oct;79(10):960–3.

17. World Health Organization. Tuberculosis and Air Travel: Guidelines for Prevention and Control. 3rd ed. Geneva: World Health Organization; 2008 [cited 2012 Sep 26]. Available from: http://www.who.int/tb/publications/2008/WHO_HTM_TB_2008.399_eng.pdf.

CRUISE SHIP TRAVEL

Douglas D. Slaten, Kiren Mitruka

INTRODUCTION

Cruise travel continues to gain popularity. In 2010, the North American cruise industry, which makes up most of the global cruise market, comprised 205 ships that carried nearly 15 million passengers to destinations. Of these, almost 10 million passengers left from US ports, and Florida accounted for two-thirds of all US departures. The Caribbean is the top destination, followed by the Mediterranean, Europe, and Alaska. The average length of a cruise is 7 days, although voyages range from a few hours ("voyages to nowhere") to several months for around-the-world cruises. An average-sized cruise ship carries 2,200 passengers; however, cruise ship capacities continue to increase, and "mega ships" can exceed 5,000 passengers. The crew-to-passenger ratio is roughly 1:2. The median age of a cruise ship passenger is 48 years, and more than one-quarter are ≥60. To a certain extent, cruise lines target different population groups, and longer cruises often attract older passengers.

Although most passengers on North American cruise ships are from the United States or Canada, cruise ships bring together large numbers of people from a variety of communities and backgrounds. Communicable diseases can be introduced onboard by embarking passengers and crew members or acquired during visits to seaports. The crowded, semienclosed environment of the cruise ship facilitates transmission of communicable diseases either person to person or from contaminated food, water, or environmental surfaces. Crew members who remain onboard can sustain transmission of infectious diseases. The stress of travel can worsen chronic conditions in specific groups, such as pregnant women and the elderly, who may also be more seriously affected by infectious diseases.

HEALTH AND SAFETY REGULATIONS

The World Health Organization's International Health Regulations (IHR), which were revised in 2005 and implemented in 2007, provide international standards for ship and port sanitation, disease surveillance, and response to infectious diseases. The intent of the IHR (2005), binding in 194 countries, is to help the international community prevent and respond to acute public health risks worldwide, while avoiding unnecessary interference with international traffic and trade (www.who.int/ihr/en).

The US Coast Guard enforces safety, security, and environmental regulations in US waters and on the high seas. CDC ensures health and sanitation aboard ships with international itineraries arriving at US ports. US federal quarantine regulations require such ships to immediately report all shipboard deaths and certain illnesses suggestive of communicable diseases. CDC's 20 quarantine stations respond to these reports, providing recommendations to prevent the spread of illness (www.cdc.gov/quarantine/index.html). Since 1975, CDC's Vessel Sanitation Program (VSP) has also helped the cruise ship industry prevent and control gastrointestinal illnesses by inspecting cruise ships, monitoring gastrointestinal illnesses, and responding to outbreaks, updates of which are posted on its website (www.cdc.gov/nceh/vsp).

Guidelines of Health Canada's Cruise Ship Inspection Program (www.hc-sc.gc.ca/hl-vs/travel-voyage/general/ship-navire-eng.php) are harmonized with those of VSP.

CRUISE SHIP MEDICAL CAPABILITIES

Medical facilities on cruise ships can vary widely depending on a number of factors, such as ship size, itinerary, length of cruise, and passenger demographics. Generally, shipboard medical clinics are comparable to ambulatory care centers. Although no official agency regulates medical practice aboard cruise ships, consensus-based guidelines have been published, which cruise lines are encouraged to adopt. The Cruise Lines International Association (CLIA), representing 26 major cruise lines that account for >97% of the North American cruise market (www.cruising.org), developed industrywide guidelines in 1995 to promote the following standard of care among cruise ship medical facilities:

- Provide emergency medical care for passengers and crew
- Stabilize patients and initiate reasonable diagnostic and therapeutic interventions
- Facilitate the evacuation of seriously ill or injured patients

The American College of Emergency Physicians, Section of Cruise Ship and Maritime Medicine, provides more detailed Health Care Guidelines for Cruise Ship Medical Facilities (www.acep.org/practres.aspx?LinkIdentifier=id&id=29980&fid=2184&Mo=No). Recognizing that the needs of individual ships can vary, these guidelines describe desired physician qualifications (3 years' postgraduate training in general and emergency medicine or board certification in emergency medicine, family practice, or internal medicine) and nurse competencies. They also outline recommended shipboard medical care capabilities, including medications, supplies, equipment (such as laboratory and x-ray) and preparedness planning.

ILLNESSES AND INJURY ABOARD CRUISE SHIPS

Cruise ship medical clinics deal with a wide variety of illnesses and injuries. Most health-related events are treated or managed onboard. However, evacuation and shoreside consultation for medical, surgical, and dental problems are not infrequent; 3%–11% of all conditions reported on a cruise ship are urgent or an emergency.

Published reviews of cruise ship medical logs have shown that most (69%–88%) passenger dispensary visits on cruise ships were due to medical conditions; respiratory (19%–29%) and gastrointestinal (9%) illnesses were the most frequently reported diagnoses. Injuries, typically from slips, trips, or falls, accounted for 12%–18% of medical visits.

Deaths on cruise ships are most often due to cardiovascular events. The most frequently documented cruise ship outbreaks involve respiratory infections (influenza and legionellosis), gastrointestinal infections (norovirus), and vaccine-preventable diseases other than influenza, such as rubella and varicella (chickenpox). To reduce the risk of onboard introduction of communicable diseases by embarking passengers, most ships conduct preembarkation medical screening followed by specific management of contagious passengers according to cruise line protocols and the medical judgment of onboard physicians. CDC guidance to cruise ships for commonly reported conditions (varicella, influenzalike illness) is available on the CDC Travelers' Health website (wwwnc.cdc.gov/travel/page/travel-industry-cruise.htm). Passengers acutely ill with communicable diseases should delay travel until they are no longer contagious. Ill passengers are encouraged to use onboard medical facilities for optimal care and to maximize reporting of potential public health events.

SPECIFIC HEALTH RISKS
Gastrointestinal Illness

VSP conducts twice-yearly, unannounced inspections of ships carrying ≥13 passengers with international itineraries that call on US seaports. Cruise ships report to VSP the total number of cases of gastrointestinal illness evaluated by the medical staff before arrival at a US port. In recent years, outbreaks of gastroenteritis on cruise ships (defined as ≥3% of passengers or crew with reported symptoms of acute gastrointestinal illness during a voyage) have continued, despite good cruise ship environmental health standards and high VSP inspection scores. Most cruise ship gastrointestinal outbreaks are due to norovirus, which is also the leading cause of sporadic cases and outbreaks of gastroenteritis in the United States. Characteristics of norovirus that facilitate outbreaks are a low infective dose, easy person-to-person transmissibility, prolonged viral shedding, no long-term immunity, and the organism's ability to survive routine cleaning procedures. Vigilance in hand hygiene is key to reducing spread of norovirus (see Chapter 3, Norovirus).

Gastrointestinal outbreaks on cruise ships from food and water sources have been associated with Salmonella, enterotoxigenic Escherichia coli, Shigella, Vibrio, Staphylococcus aureus, Clostridium perfringens, Cyclospora, hepatitis E virus, and Trichinella.

Respiratory Illness
Influenza

Influenza seasons in the Northern and Southern Hemispheres typically occur at opposite times of the year. Since passengers and crew originate from all regions of the world, shipboard outbreaks of influenza A and B can occur year-round. Outbreaks usually result from the importation of influenza by embarking passengers and crew, followed by person-to-person spread.

During the 2009 influenza A (H1N1) pandemic, cruise line medical personnel made case-by-case decisions regarding the boarding of passengers with influenzalike illness. Travelers, particularly those at high risk for influenza-related complications, should receive the current seasonal influenza vaccine, if available, ≥2 weeks before travel. Cruise ships have the capacity to manage cases of influenzalike illness according to CDC recommendations (wwwnc.cdc.gov/travel/page/guidance-cruise-ships-flu.htm). Onboard control measures travelers can expect include isolation of ill people, encouragement of respiratory hygiene and cough etiquette, antiviral treatment of ill people, and prophylaxis of high-risk contacts.

Legionellosis (Legionnaires' Disease)

Legionnaires' disease is a severe pneumonia caused by inhalation or possibly aspiration of warm, aerosolized water containing Legionella organisms. The organism is not transmitted from person to person. Symptom onset is typically 2–10 days after exposure, and older (≥65 years) travelers and those with underlying medical conditions are at increased risk for infection.

Contaminated ships' whirlpool spas and potable water supply systems are the most commonly implicated sources of shipboard Legionella outbreaks, although improvements in ship design and standardization of spa and water supply disinfection have reduced the risk of Legionella growth and colonization. Most cruise ships can perform Legionella urine antigen testing. In evaluating returned travelers for Legionnaires' disease, clinicians should collect respiratory secretions for culture, which is essential to identifying the source of infection, in addition to collecting urine for antigen testing. People with suspected Legionnaire's disease require prompt antibiotic treatment.

About 20%–25% of all Legionnaires' disease reported to CDC is travel-associated. CDC should be informed of any travel-associated Legionnaires' disease cases by sending an e-mail to travellegionella@cdc.gov.

Vaccine-Preventable Diseases

Although each cruise ship voyage typically introduces a new cohort of passengers, crew members remain onboard for extended periods. And although most cruise ship passengers are from countries (mainly the United States and Canada) with routine vaccination programs, crew members tend to originate from developing countries, some with low immunization rates. In past cruise ship investigations involving vaccine-preventable diseases, 11% of crew members were found to be acutely infected with or susceptible to rubella, and 13% of crew, mostly from tropical countries, were susceptible to or acutely infected with varicella.

Crew members should have documented proof of immunity to vaccine-preventable diseases. Passengers should be up-to-date with routine vaccinations before travel, as well as any required or recommended vaccinations at their destinations. Women of childbearing age should be immune to rubella before cruise ship travel.

Vectorborne Diseases

Cruise ship port visits may include countries where vectorborne diseases, such as malaria, dengue, and yellow fever, are endemic. Yellow fever vaccination certificates may be required by some countries for entry. Although cruise lines may schedule arrival and departure times to avoid peak mosquito-biting periods, personal protection is still necessary. Preventive measures include the following:

- Using an effective insect repellent (see Chapter 2, Protection against Mosquitoes, Ticks, & Other Insects & Arthropods)
- Taking antimalarial chemoprophylaxis based on a destination- and activity-specific risk assessment (see Chapter 3, Malaria)
- Remaining in well-screened or air-conditioned areas
- Minimizing areas of exposed skin by wearing long-sleeved shirts, long pants, boots, and hats

Other Health Concerns

Stresses of cruise ship travel include varying temperature and weather conditions, as well as unaccustomed changes in diet and physical activity. Foreign travel increases the likelihood of risk-taking behaviors such as alcohol misuse, drug use, and unsafe sex. In spite of modern stabilizer systems, seasickness is a common complaint and likely unrelated to location of passenger cabins (see Chapter 2, Motion Sickness).

PREVENTIVE MEASURES FOR CRUISE SHIP TRAVELERS
Before and During Travel

Cruise ship travelers often have complex itineraries due to multiple, short port visits. Although most of these port visits do not include overnight stays off the cruise ship, many exotic trips have options for travelers to venture off the ship for ≥1 nights. Therefore, cruise ship travelers may be uncertain about potential exposures and which antimicrobial prophylaxis, immunizations, and preventive measures should be considered. Box 6-1 summarizes recommendations for cruise travelers and clinicians advising cruise travelers in pre-travel preparation and healthy behaviors during travel.

After Travel

Travelers who become ill after returning home should inform their health care providers of where they have traveled. Clinicians should report suspected communicable diseases in recently returned cruise ship travelers to public health authorities. Gastrointestinal illnesses related to cruise ship travel should be reported to the CDC VSP (by calling 800-CDC-INFO [800-232-4636] or by visiting www.cdc.gov and clicking on "Contact CDC-INFO"). Clinicians should inform CDC of any travel-associated Legionnaires' disease cases by sending an e-mail to travellegionella@cdc.gov. Other suspected communicable illnesses should be reported to the CDC Quarantine Station with jurisdiction over the cruise ship's port of arrival (www.cdc.gov/quarantine).

BOX 6-1. CRUISE TRAVEL HEALTH PRECAUTIONS

Advice for Clinicians Giving Pre-Travel Cruise Consultations
Risk Assessment and Risk Communication
- Discuss itinerary, including season, duration of travel, and activities at port stops.
- Review the traveler's medical and immunization history, allergies, and special health needs.
- Discuss relevant travel-specific health hazards and risk reduction.
- Provide the traveler with documentation of his or her medical history, immunizations, and medications.

Immunization and Risk Management
- Provide immunizations that are routinely recommended (age-specific), required (yellow fever), and recommended based on risk.
- Discuss food and water precautions and insect bite prevention.
- Older travelers, especially those with a history of heart disease, should carry a baseline EKG to facilitate onboard or overseas medical care.

Medications Based on Risk and Need
- Consider malaria chemoprophylaxis if itinerary includes port stops in malaria-endemic areas.
- Consider motion sickness medications for self-treatment (see Chapter 2, Motion Sickness).

(continued)

BOX 6-1. CRUISE TRAVEL HEALTH PRECAUTIONS (continued)

Precautions for Cruise Ship Travelers

Pre-Travel

- Evaluate the type and length of the planned cruise in the context of personal health requirements.
- Consult medical and dental care providers before cruise travel.
- Consider additional insurance for overseas health care and medical evacuation.
- Carry prescription medications in their original containers, with a copy of the prescription and accompanying physician's letter.
- Defer travel while acutely ill.

During Travel

- Wash hands frequently with soap and water or use an alcohol-based sanitizer containing ≥60% alcohol.
- Follow safe food and water precautions when eating off the ship at ports of call.
- Use measures to prevent insect bites during port visits, especially in malaria- or dengue-endemic areas.
- Use sun protection.
- Maintain good fluid intake, but avoid excessive alcohol consumption.
- Avoid contact with ill people.
- If sexually active, practice safe sex.

BIBLIOGRAPHY

1. Carling PC, Bruno-Murtha LA, Griffiths JK. Cruise ship environmental hygiene and the risk of norovirus infection outbreaks: an objective assessment of 56 vessels over 3 years. Clin Infect Dis. 2009 Nov 1;49(9):1312–7.

2. CDC. Cruise-ship–associated Legionnaires' disease, November 2003–May 2004. MMWR Morb Mortal Wkly Rep. 2005 Nov 18;54(45):1153–5.

3. CDC. Rubella among crew members of commercial cruise ships—Florida, 1997. MMWR Morb Mortal Wkly Rep. 1998 Jan 9;46(52–53):1247–50.

4. Cramer EH, Blanton CJ, Blanton LH, Vaughan GH, Jr., Bopp CA, Forney DL. Epidemiology of gastroenteritis on cruise ships, 2001–2004. Am J Prev Med. 2006 Mar;30(3):252–7.

5. Cramer EH, Slaten DD, Guerreiro A, Robbins D, Ganzon A. Management and control of varicella on cruise ships: a collaborative approach to promoting public health. J Travel Med. 2012 Jul;19(4):226–32.

6. Dahl E. Medical practice during a world cruise: a descriptive epidemiological study of injury and illness among passengers and crew. Int Marit Health. 2005;56(1–4):115–28.

7. Dahl E. Passenger accidents and injuries reported during 3 years on a cruise ship. Int Marit Health. 2010;61(1):1–8.

8. Gahlinger PM. Cabin location and the likelihood of motion sickness in cruise ship passengers. J Travel Med. 2000 May–Jun;7(3):120–4.

9. Guyard C, Low DE. *Legionella* infections and travel associated legionellosis. Travel Med Infect Dis. 2011 Jul;9(4):176–86.

10. Hill CD. Cruise ship travel. In: Keystone JS, Freedman DO, Kozarsky PE, Connor BA, Nothdurft HO, editors. Travel Medicine. 3rd ed. Philadelphia: Saunders Elsevier; 2013. p. 349–55.

11. Kornylo K, Henry R, Slaten D. Respiratory disease on cruise ships. Clin Infect Dis. 2012 Mar 1;54(5):v–vi.

12. Lawson CJ, Dykewicz CA, Molinari NA, Lipman H, Alvarado-Ramy F. Deaths in international travelers arriving in the United States, July 1, 2005 to June 30, 2008. J Travel Med. 2012 Mar–Apr;19(2):96–103.

13. Mouchtouri VA, Nichols G, Rachiotis G, Kremastinou J, Arvanitoyannis IS, Riemer T, et al. State of the art: public health and passenger ships. Int Marit Health. 2010;61(2):49–98.

14. Novaro GM, Bush HS, Fromkin KR, Shen MY, Helguera M, Pinski SL, et al. Cardiovascular emergencies in cruise ship passengers. Am J Cardiol. 2010 Jan 15;105(2):153–7.

15. Uyeki TM, Zane SB, Bodnar UR, Fielding KL, Buxton JA, Miller JM, et al. Large summertime influenza A outbreak among tourists in Alaska and the Yukon Territory. Clin Infect Dis. 2003 May 1;36(9):1095–102.

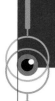

Perspectives

WHAT TO EXPECT WHEN TRAVELING DURING AN INTERNATIONAL OUTBREAK

Todd W. Wilson, Nicole J. Cohen

OVERVIEW

Outbreaks of communicable diseases have occurred throughout history, dramatically shaping the human experience. One of the most recognizable examples of an outbreak with terrible consequences for both human health and culture was the fourteenth-century plague epidemic, or "Black Death," thought to have been caused by *Yersinia pestis*, which killed up to 60% of Europe's population and also spread to Asia and Africa, possibly reducing the global population by 17%.

In recent times, diseases such as severe acute respiratory syndrome (SARS) have appeared, seemingly from nowhere, and resulted in high numbers of deaths and illness among those infected. And throughout history—most recently in 2009—new strains of influenza have emerged, circled the globe, and caused social disruption and economic upheaval. These diseases and others like them, which emerge, spread rapidly via travel across international borders, and have serious or initially unknown health effects, have led countries to take public health measures at borders that affect travelers.

Severe Acute Respiratory Syndrome

The 2003 outbreak of SARS has been well chronicled. This newly discovered pathogen was quickly spread by an infected traveler who left Guangdong Province, China, and arrived in Hong Kong, where he infected 10 other people staying in a hotel, leading directly or indirectly to cases in 8 countries. The combined influence of World Health Organization (WHO) travel advisories and media attention to SARS affected traveler behavior to the extent that tourist arrivals in East Asian airports dropped 41% from April 1 to April 21, 2003.

2009 Influenza A (H1N1)

In March 2009, a new strain of influenza A (H1N1) began spreading in Mexico. Within 30 days, cases occurred in US states bordering Mexico. Within 90 days, WHO declared that a pandemic, or global outbreak of H1N1 influenza, was occurring. Analysis of preliminary passenger volume data for the largest airline carriers between Mexico and the United States indicated that during April 27 through May 17, 2009, northbound volume dropped 42%, and southbound volume dropped 57%, compared with the previous year.

TRAVELER HEALTH SCREENING IS ALWAYS IN PLACE

Modern travel and trade rely on global circumnavigation in <24 hours. Therefore, each new outbreak of disease has the potential to affect travelers and the travel industry. When disease threats emerge, countries may take border measures that range from minimal to invasive, regardless of available evidence of the efficacy of those measures. These interventions vary between and within countries, because public health interventions are usually locally driven.

To understand what to expect during an emergency, it is important to know that health screening of travelers is always in place at international ports of entry into most countries. Usually, the form of screening is minimal and routine, since the risk for major threats to health is low most of the time. When increased health screening occurs, it is usually consistent with the threat of an identified contagious disease with the potential for spread through travel. Below is a list of public health measures used internationally, ranked in order from the least to the most invasive, that may be used to detect or control infection in international travelers, depending on the situation:

- Visual screening—observation of travelers conducted by customs or public health officers at ports of entry, typically without direct interaction with travelers, usually in place at all times
- Health education for travelers—health communications intended to educate international travelers about a particular disease and border screening measures in place, including travel health alert notices or other printed material handed to travelers upon arrival, announcements or posters in transit areas, public service or social media announcements, and website information
- Travel warning—a notice published by government health authorities advising people to avoid travel to an area where a disease outbreak has been identified
- Passenger locator form—a form used by health officials to gather contact information for travelers believed to have been potentially exposed to an infectious disease during travel, for the purpose of locating or providing information to the travelers
- Traveler's health declaration form—a form often considered a legal, signed document, similar to a customs declaration form, that is used by customs or health officials at ports of entry to gather information related to a traveler's health, prior itinerary, and exposure to infection
- Direct questioning—interview of travelers by customs or health officials to evaluate symptoms and exposure history, to assess the risk of disease exposure or infection
- Temperature check—measurement of a traveler's temperature to identify a fever; can be done remotely by using a thermal imaging camera or through the use of a thermometer
- Detention—holding in custody a traveler suspected of being infected with a communicable disease of concern, to allow further medical screening and examination by public health officials
- Isolation—separating and restricting the movement of an ill person who has a communicable disease of concern from those who are healthy, to minimize disease spread by preventing further transmission
- Quarantine—separating and restricting the movement of people who are well but may have been exposed to a communicable disease, to monitor their health and prevent possible transmission to others, until it is determined that they are not infected

Ultimately, for a given outbreak, the decision on which health measures to use, and how extensively each measure is implemented, will depend on the transmissibility and severity of the disease in question.

WHAT TO EXPECT DURING AN INTERNATIONAL DISEASE OUTBREAK

Whether it is a person's first international trip or that person is a seasoned international traveler, chances are he or she has planned the itinerary carefully to make the trip an enjoyable travel experience. Factoring in some amount of risk and being aware of as many chance variables as possible can help mitigate some of the negative repercussions, should an outbreak of illness occur that impacts travel. The following situations have been observed in nearly all international outbreaks of disease during the modern travel era since the 1960s:

- Travel delays—Travel into, out of, or within certain regions may be affected by border health measures or behavior of travelers.
- Inconsistent information—Early in an outbreak, information may change rapidly, be conflicting, or later be determined to be incorrect, while governments, health officials, and the travel industry work to define the situation and provide reliable information.
- Canceled flights, ship voyages, trains, buses, or routes—Travel cancelations can occur suddenly, especially for air travel, which can be particularly sensitive to shifts in passenger demand and is often unpredictable during outbreaks.
- Voluntary cessation of travel—Travelers may choose to postpone their travel because of official travel warnings, travel advisories, or concerns about their health, border measures, or the possibility of being stranded in a foreign country. Large decreases in travel volume can decrease travel options, and travel schedules may be disrupted, especially to and from the countries most affected by the outbreak.

- Increase in travel—People traveling in affected countries in the early stages of an emerging outbreak may seek unplanned return journeys, as people try to avoid infection or seek health care in their home countries.
- Grounding of flights—In extreme circumstances, flights may be unavailable in a region for a period of time, as occurred in the United States after September 11, 2001, and in the spring of 2010, when clouds of ash resulting from eruptions from Iceland's Eyjafjallajökull volcano stalled air traffic over Europe. Although these instances were emergency disasters and not illness outbreaks, they demonstrate the sensitivity of air travel to health and safety threats.
- Entry or exit screening—The set of border health measures described earlier in this section may be applied, in whole or in part, at international borders, either to prevent the introduction of infection into the country (entry screening) or to prevent infected people from leaving and spreading infection to other countries (exit screening).

Guidelines and practices for what governments ask of travelers on arrival or exit may differ from country to country. Some countries maintain national control over all ports of entry and exit, while in other countries such control is delegated to state, provincial, or local authorities. In either case, requirements and procedures may differ widely and change over time. Flexibility, honesty, and compliance are essential to a successful interaction with public health and other government officials during international travel.

Below is a list of actions travelers might experience upon arrival to or exit from a country during an infectious disease outbreak. This list is not comprehensive or exhaustive. Travelers may be asked or forced to comply with ≥1 of the following:

- Have their temperatures taken either by thermal imaging camera or oral or ear thermometer

- Provide personal contact information and details about their travel itineraries
- Respond to questions regarding symptoms of illness or exposure to ill people
- Undergo a medical evaluation for infection, including diagnostic testing, such as nasal or throat swabs or blood tests
- Be isolated from other people until they are determined to be noninfectious
- Be hospitalized and given medical treatment if they test positive for or are otherwise diagnosed with an infectious disease of public health concern
- Be quarantined for a specified period of time if they were exposed to someone who is suspected or confirmed to be infected
- Monitor their health during and after travel and report any symptoms they develop to health officials
- Forego communications with family, friends, or traveling companions for a certain period
- Be denied boarding on an airplane, ship, bus, or train, if it is determined they are infectious or may have been exposed to a communicable disease of public health concern

TRAVELERS' RIGHTS AND RESPONSIBILITIES

The United States, acting through the Department of State, takes action to protect US citizens who are abroad via a number of diplomatic channels. However, in the event of an outbreak or epidemic, any country has the right to enact measures to protect its citizens from ill travelers entering its borders or to protect global health from ill travelers exiting the country. These border measures may infringe on the individual rights of any traveler who appears to be infected with or exposed to a disease of public health concern. The ability of the Department of State to intervene in such situations is limited. In effect, if a person chooses to travel abroad, he or she should be aware of the potential for the complete disruption of his or her journey by an outbreak or epidemic of public health significance. Travelers should be up-to-date on routine vaccinations and receive any vaccinations or prophylaxis recommended or required for their destinations. CDC recommends that if a person is planning to travel internationally and feels ill or has symptoms such as fever, rash, or cough, he or she should consult with a medical provider and postpone travel until the illness or symptoms have resolved. Similarly, if a traveler becomes ill during or after international travel, he or she should seek medical attention and postpone further travel until the illness or symptoms have resolved. If an infectious disease is suspected, the traveler should call ahead before arriving at the medical facility, to avoid infecting other patients and staff.

Travelers can consult the embassies of the countries in their travel itineraries for information about health interventions and procedures that may affect their travel, although in some instances, inquiries or embassy websites do not provide correct or up-to-date information. The Department of State website may be helpful (http://travel.state.gov/travel/tips/brochures/brochures_1215.html). Up-to-date information regarding infectious disease risks related to travel may be found at the CDC website (www.cdc.gov/travel). Finally, because of the potential for delays and unexpected costs arising from an outbreak of communicable disease, CDC strongly recommends that travelers consider purchasing travel insurance to cover possible trip cancellations, requirements for health care abroad, or possible emergency medical evacuations (see Chapter 2, Travel Insurance, Travel Health Insurance, & Medical Evacuation Insurance).

BIBLIOGRAPHY

1. Barry JM. Observations on past influenza pandemics. Disaster Med Public Health Prep. 2009 Dec;3 Suppl 2:S95–9.

2. Berro A, Gallagher N, Yanni E, Lipman H, Whatley A, Bossak B. World Health Organization (WHO) travel recommendations during the 2003 SARS outbreak: lessons learned for mitigating influenza pandemic and globally emerging infectious diseases. Board 109. International Conference on Emerging Infectious Diseases; 2009 Mar 16–19; Atlanta, Georgia.

3. CDC. Update: outbreak of severe acute respiratory syndrome—worldwide, 2003. MMWR Morb Mortal Wkly Rep. 2003 Mar 28;52(12):241–6, 248.

4. Chan M. World now at the start of 2009 influenza pandemic. Geneva: World Health Organization; 2009 [cited 2012 Sep 26]. Available from: http://www.who.int/mediacentre/news/statements/2009/

h1n1_pandemic_phase6_20090611/en/index.html.

5. Christian MD, Poutanen SM, Loutfy MR, Muller MP, Low DE. Severe acute respiratory syndrome. Clin Infect Dis. 2004 May 15;38(10):1420–7.

6. Hays JN. Epidemics and Pandemics: Their Impacts on Human History. Santa Barbara, CA: ABC-CLIO; 2005.

7. Snowden FM. Emerging and reemerging diseases: a historical perspective. Immunol Rev. 2008 Oct;225:9–26.

8. World Health Organization. International Health Regulations (2005). Geneva: World Health Organization; 2005 [cited 2012 Sep 26]. Available from: http://www.who.int/ihr/en/.

9. World Health Organization. Public health measures taken at international borders during early stages of pandemic influenza A (H1N1) 2009: preliminary results. Wkly Epidemiol Rec. 2010 May 21;85(21):186–95.

DEATH DURING TRAVEL

Clare A. Dykewicz, Nicole J. Cohen

OBTAINING US DEPARTMENT OF STATE ASSISTANCE

When a US citizen dies outside the United States, the deceased person's family members, domestic partner, or legal representative should notify US consular officials at the Department of State. Consular personnel are available 24 hours a day, 7 days a week, to provide assistance to US citizens for overseas emergencies.

- If a family member, domestic partner, or legal representative is in the foreign country with the deceased US citizen, he or she should contact the nearest US embassy or consulate for assistance. Contact information for US embassies, consulates, and consular agencies overseas may be found at the Department of State website (www.usembassy.gov).

- If a family member, domestic partner, or legal representative is located in the United States or Canada, he or she should call the Department of State's Office of Overseas Citizens Services in Washington, DC, from 8 AM to 8 PM Eastern Time, Monday through Friday, at 888-407-4747 (toll-free) or 202-501-4444. For emergency assistance after working hours or on weekends and holidays, call the Department of State switchboard at 202-647-4000 and ask to speak with the Overseas Citizens Services Duty Officer. In addition, the US embassy closest to or in the country where the US citizen died can provide assistance (www.usembassy.gov).

Emergency services provided by US consular officials can include advising the family, domestic partner, or legal representative about options and costs for disposing of the remains and personal effects of the deceased. Preparing and returning human remains to the United States can be an expensive and lengthy process. The Department of State does not pay for these expenses; they are the responsibility of the deceased person's family, domestic partner, or legal representative. Consular officials may also serve as provisional conservators of the deceased person's estate, if no other legal representative is present in the foreign country where the death occurred.

IMPORTATION OF HUMAN REMAINS FOR INTERMENT OR CREMATION
General Guidance

Except for cremated remains, human remains intended for interment (placement in a grave or tomb) or cremation after entry into the United States must be accompanied by a death certificate stating the cause of death. A death certificate is an official document signed by a coroner, physician, or other official authorized to make a declaration of cause of death. Death certificates written in a language other than English must be accompanied by an English translation.

Remains of a Person Known or Suspected to Have Died from a Quarantinable Communicable Disease

Federal quarantine regulations (42 CFR Part 71.55) state that the remains of a person who is known or suspected to have died from a quarantinable communicable disease may not be brought into the United States unless the remains are cremated, properly embalmed and placed in a hermetically sealed casket, or accompanied by a CDC permit to allow importation of human remains, issued by the CDC director.

Quarantinable communicable diseases include cholera, diphtheria, infectious tuberculosis, plague, smallpox, yellow fever, viral hemorrhagic fevers (Lassa, Marburg, Ebola, Crimean-Congo, or others not yet isolated or named), severe acute respiratory syndrome (SARS), and influenza caused by novel or reemergent influenza viruses that are causing or have the potential to cause a pandemic. A hermetically sealed casket is one that is airtight and secured against the escape of microorganisms. It should be accompanied by valid documentation certifying that it is hermetically sealed.

If a CDC permit is obtained to allow importation of human remains, CDC may impose additional conditions for importation. Permits for the importation of human remains of a person known or suspected to have died from a quarantinable communicable disease may be obtained from CDC's Division of Global Migration and Quarantine by calling 866-694-4867 (toll-free) or the CDC Emergency Operations Center at 770-488-7100. A copy of the CDC permit must accompany the human remains at all times during shipment.

Remains of a Person Who Died of Any Cause Other than a Quarantinable Communicable Disease

When the cause of death is anything other than a quarantinable communicable disease, the remains may be cleared, released, and authorized for entry into the United States if 1 of the following conditions is met:

1. The remains meet the standards for importation found in 42 CFR 71.55: the remains are cremated or properly embalmed and placed in a hermetically sealed casket or are accompanied by a permit issued by the CDC director.
2. The remains are shipped in a leakproof container. A leakproof container is one that is puncture resistant and sealed so that there is no leakage of fluids outside the container during handling, storage, transport, or shipping.

CDC may also require additional measures, including detention, disinfection, disinfestation, fumigation, or other related measures, if there is evidence that the human remains are or may be infected or contaminated with a communicable disease and that such measures are necessary to prevent the introduction, transmission, or spread of communicable diseases into the United States.

EXPORTATION OF HUMAN REMAINS

CDC places no restrictions on the exportation of human remains outside the United States, although other federal, state, and local regulations may apply. Exporters of human remains and travelers taking human remains out of the United States should be aware that the importation requirements

of the destination country must be met. Information regarding these requirements may be obtained from the appropriate foreign embassy or consulate.

BIBLIOGRAPHY

1. CDC. Guidance for importation of human remains into the United States for interment or subsequent cremation. Atlanta: CDC; 2012 [cited 2012 Sep 26]. Available from: http://www.cdc.gov/quarantine/human-remains.html.

2. CDC. Quarantine stations: quarantine station contact lists and jurisdictions. Atlanta: CDC; 2012 [cited 2012 Sep 26]. Available from: http://www.cdc.gov/quarantine/QuarantineStations.html.

3. Federal Register. Executive order 13295 of April 4, 2003—revised list of quarantinable communicable diseases. Washington, DC: Federal Register; 2003. p. 17255.

4. US Customs and Border Protection. Requirements for importing bodies in coffins/ashes in urns. Washington, DC: US Department of Homeland Security; 2012 [cited 2012 Sep 26]. Available from: https://help.cbp.gov/app/answers/detail/a_id/237/~/requirements-for-importing-bodies-in-coffins-ashes-in-urns.

5. US Department of Health and Human Services. Title 42. Public Health. Chapter 1. Public Health Service, Department of Health and Human Services. Part 71. Foreign Quarantine. US Government Printing Office; 2001.

6. US Department of State. Country specific information. Washington, DC: US Department of State; 2012 [cited 2012 Sep 26]. Available from: http://travel.state.gov/travel/cis_pa_tw/cis/cis_4965.html.

7. US Department of State. Death or injury of an American citizen abroad Washington, DC: US Department of State; 2012 [cited 2012 Sep 26]. Available from: http://travel.state.gov/travel/tips/emergencies/death/death_3878.html

8. US Department of State. Emergencies and crises. Washington, DC: US Department of State; 2012 [cited 2012 Sep 26]. Available from: http://travel.state.gov/travel/tips/emergencies/emergencies_1212.html.

9. US Department of State. Return of remains of deceased US citizens. Washington, DC: US Department of State; 2012 [cited 2012 Sep 26]. Available from: http://travel.state.gov/travel/tips/emergencies/death/death_1191.html.

TAKING ANIMALS & ANIMAL PRODUCTS ACROSS INTERNATIONAL BORDERS

G. Gale Galland, Robert J. Mullan, Heather Bair-Brake

CDC restricts the importation of animals, vectors, and products, such as trophies, that may pose an infectious disease threat to humans. These restrictions apply to some pets, such as dogs and cats, as well as turtles, nonhuman primates, African rodents, civets, and bats, as well as products made from these animals (see www.cdc.gov/animalimportation/index.html). Animals taken out of the United States are subject, upon return, to the same regulations as those entering for the first time.

In addition to CDC, the US Department of Agriculture (USDA) and the Fish and Wildlife Service (FWS) have jurisdiction over the importation of some animals into the United States. States may also have additional restrictions on the importation of animals.

ANIMAL HEALTH CERTIFICATES
CDC regulations do not require general health certificates for animals (including dogs or cats) entering the United States. However, health certificates may be required for entry of animals into some states and may be required by airlines in order to transport animals. Before departure, travelers should check with the

public health veterinarian in their destination state and with the airline for any certificate requirements.

DOGS

Dogs are subject to inspection and may be denied entry into the United States if they have evidence of an infectious disease that can be transmitted to humans or if they have not been vaccinated against rabies. If a dog appears to be ill, further examination by a licensed veterinarian, at the owner's expense, may be required before it is released for official entry into the United States.

Rabies vaccination is required for all dogs entering the United States from a country where rabies is present. Unless a dog is being imported from a country considered "rabies-free" by the World Health Organization (Table 3–14), it must be accompanied by a current, valid rabies vaccination certificate that includes the following information:

- The breed, sex, age, color, markings, and other identifying information for the dog
- Date of rabies vaccination
- Signature of a licensed veterinarian
- Date of expiration of vaccination (Rabies certificates have expiration dates that range from 1 to 3 years from the date of vaccination, depending on the type of vaccine given.)

Dogs must be ≥3 months old before getting a rabies vaccine for the first time. Since it takes 30 days for the vaccine to take effect, dogs must have had their first rabies vaccination ≥30 days prior to arrival.

- If dogs arrive in the United States unvaccinated, CDC requires that they receive a rabies vaccine within 4 days of arrival at their final US destination and within 10 days of entry into the United States. They must be confined for the 30-day period until the vaccination takes effect.
- If dogs arrive that have received their first rabies vaccine <30 days before arrival, CDC requires that the dogs be confined for the remainder of the 30-day period.
- Older dogs that have had prior rabies vaccination may be given a rabies vaccine up to the day of travel. Dogs that arrive in the United States with an expired rabies

vaccination must be confined until they are revaccinated.

Dogs that do not meet CDC's rabies vaccination requirement may enter the United States only if the importer or owner completes a legal document called a *confinement agreement*. A copy of the confinement agreement (CDC Form 75.37) can be found on the CDC website at www.cdc.gov/animalimportation/dogs.html. By signing a confinement agreement, the importer or owner promises to confine the animal until it is fully vaccinated against rabies. Confinement agreements must be completed for:

- Dogs not accompanied by a current, valid rabies certificate
- Dogs <4 months of age
- Dogs that received their first rabies vaccination <30 days prior to arrival in the United States

Confinement is defined as isolation away from people and other animals, except for contact necessary for the dog's care. Conditions of the confinement agreement are as follows:

- The dog must be kept confined at a place of the owner's choosing, including the owner's home, until a rabies vaccination has been obtained, until 30 days have passed since vaccination, or both (depending on whether it is the dog's first rabies vaccine).
- If the dog is allowed out of its enclosure, the owner must muzzle the dog and use a leash.
- The dog may not be sold or transferred from the responsibility of the importer during the confinement period.

Routine rabies vaccination of dogs is recommended in the United States and required by most state and local health authorities. Check with state authorities at the final destination to determine any state requirements for rabies vaccination. State-specific information is found at www.aphis.usda.gov/import_export/animals/animal_import/animal_imports_states.shtml. All pet dogs arriving in the state of Hawaii and the territory of Guam, even from the US mainland, are subject to locally imposed quarantine requirements. For more information about animal importation in Hawaii, consult http://hawaii.gov/hdoa/ai/aqs/info or call 808-483-7151. For more information about animal importation in Guam, see www.guamcourts.org/CompilerofLaws/GAR/09GAR/09GAR001-1.pdf or call 671-475-1426.

CATS

Cats are subject to inspection at US ports of entry and must appear healthy on arrival. If a cat appears to be ill, further examination by a licensed veterinarian, at the owner's expense, may be required before entry is permitted. Cats are not required to have proof of rabies vaccination for importation into the United States. States may require rabies vaccination for cats, however, so check with state and local health authorities at the final destination to determine any state requirements for rabies vaccination. All pet cats arriving in the state of Hawaii and the territory of Guam, even from the US mainland, are subject to locally imposed quarantine requirements. For more information about animal importation in Hawaii, consult http://hawaii.gov/hdoa/ai/aqs/info or call 808-483-7151. For more information about animal importation in Guam, see www.guamcourts.org/CompilerofLaws/GAR/09GAR/09GAR001-1.pdf or call 671-475-1426.

OTHER ANIMALS, ANIMAL PRODUCTS, AND VECTORS

Nonhuman Primates (Monkeys, Apes)

Nonhuman primates can transmit a variety of serious diseases to humans, including Ebola hemorrhagic fever and tuberculosis. Nonhuman primate entry into the United States is restricted (see www.cdc.gov/animalimportation/monkeys.html). Nonhuman primates may only be imported into the United States by a CDC-registered importer and only for scientific, educational, or exhibition purposes. Nonhuman primates may not be imported as pets. All nonhuman primates are considered endangered or threatened and require additional FWS permits for importation. Nonhuman primates that leave the United States may only return through a registered importer, and only if they are imported for science, education, or exhibition.

Turtles

Turtles can transmit *Salmonella* to humans, and because turtles are often kept as pets,

restrictions apply to their importation. More information is available at www.cdc.gov/animalimportation/turtles.html. A person may import ≤6 viable turtle eggs or live turtles with a carapace (shell) length of <4 in (10 cm) for noncommercial purposes. More turtles may be imported with CDC permission but only for science, education, or exhibition. CDC has no restrictions on the importation of live turtles with a carapace length ≥4 in. Check with USDA or FWS regarding additional requirements to import turtles.

African Rodents and Civets

To reduce the risk of introducing monkeypox and the severe acute respiratory syndrome (SARS) coronavirus, live African rodents and civets, as well as potentially infectious products made from these animals, may not be imported into the United States (see www.cdc.gov/animalimportation/africanrodents.html or www.cdc.gov/animalimportation/civets.html). Exceptions may be made for animals imported for science, education, or exhibition purposes, with permission from CDC.

Bats

Bats are reservoirs of many viruses that can infect humans, including rabies virus, Nipah virus, and SARS coronavirus. To reduce the risk of introducing these viruses, the importation of all live bats requires a CDC permit. Because they may be endangered species, bats also require additional permits issued by FWS. The application for a CDC import permit for bats can be found at www.cdc.gov/animalimportation/bats.html.

Other Animals, Trophies, Animal Products, and Vectors

Certain live animals, hosts, or vectors of human disease, including insects, biological materials, tissues, and other unprocessed animal products, may pose an infectious disease risk to humans and be restricted from entry. For example, goatskin souvenirs (such as goatskin drums) from Haiti have been associated with human anthrax cases, and CDC restricts their entry into the United States. Potentially infectious nonhuman primate trophies may be imported if they have been treated to render them noninfectious or if accompanied by a permit issued by CDC. In some circumstances, restricted items may be admitted with a permit from CDC for science, education, or exhibition (see www.cdc.gov/od/eaipp). FWS and USDA may also have requirements for animal products and trophies.

Travelers planning to import horses, ruminants, swine, poultry or other birds, or dogs used for handling livestock should contact the National Center for Import and Export (a part of USDA's Animal Plant Health Inspection Service) at 301-851-3300 or visit www.aphis.usda.gov to learn about additional requirements.

Travelers planning to import fish, reptiles, spiders, wild birds, rabbits, bears, wild members of the cat family, or other wild or endangered animals should contact FWS at 800-344-9453 (toll-free general number), 703-358-1949 (FWS Office of Law Enforcement), or visit www.fws.gov/le/travelers.html.

For additional CDC information regarding animal and animal product importations, travelers should visit www.cdc.gov/animalimportation/index.html or contact CDC INFO by calling toll-free at 800-CDC-INFO (800-232-4636) or by visiting www.cdc.gov and clicking on "Contact CDC-INFO."

RESCUING ANIMALS FROM OVERSEAS

Each year, travelers rescue dogs and cats from other countries and bring them back into the United States. Although done with the best of intentions, rescuing and importing stray animals from foreign countries create potential human health risks. The potential for bites and scratches among fearful and stressed animals puts the traveler at a higher risk for injury and infectious disease. Animals that are infected with zoonotic diseases may not show any outward signs of being ill. Therefore, all rescued animals should be examined by a licensed veterinarian both before departure and after arrival in the United States. If the intent of travel is to rescue animals, participants should discuss rabies preexposure prophylaxis with their physician.

TRAVELING ABROAD WITH A PET

Travelers planning to take a companion animal to a foreign country should be advised to meet the entry requirements of the destination country and transportation guidelines of the airline. To obtain this information, travelers should contact the country's embassy in Washington, DC, or the nearest consulate (see www.state.gov/s/cpr/rls/fco). Travelers also need to be aware that such travel is not inconsequential for the pet, and there is often substantial morbidity and mortality in pets associated with such travel.

BIBLIOGRAPHY

1. CDC. Human rabies prevention—United States, 1999. Recommendations of the Advisory Committee on Immunization Practices (ACIP). MMWR Recomm Rep. 1999 Jan 8;48(RR-1):1–21.
2. CDC. Multistate outbreak of monkeypox—Illinois, Indiana, and Wisconsin, 2003. MMWR Morb Mortal Wkly Rep. 2003 Jun 13;52(23):537–40.
3. CDC. Rabies in a dog imported from Iraq—New Jersey, June 2008. MMWR Morb Mortal Wkly Rep. 2008 Oct 3;57(39):1076–8.
4. DeMarcus TA, Tipple MA, Ostrowski SR. US policy for disease control among imported nonhuman primates. J Infect Dis. 1999 Feb;179 Suppl 1:S281–2.
5. Dobson AP. What links bats to emerging infectious diseases? Science. 2005 Oct 28;310(5748):628–9.
6. Editorial: bongo-drum disease. Lancet. 1974 Jun 8;1(7867):1152.
7. McQuiston JH, Wilson T, Harris S, Bacon RM, Shapiro S, Trevino I, et al. Importation of dogs into the United States: risks from rabies and other zoonotic diseases. Zoonoses Public Health. 2008 Oct;55(8–10):421–6.
8. National Association of State Public Health Veterinarians, Inc. Compendium of animal rabies prevention and control, 2009. MMWR Recomm Rep. 2009;58(RR-1):1–15.
9. Stam F, Romkens TE, Hekker TA, Smulders YM. Turtle-associated human salmonellosis. Clin Infect Dis. 2003 Dec 1;37(11):e167–9.
10. Wu D, Tu C, Xin C, Xuan H, Meng Q, Liu Y, et al. Civets are equally susceptible to experimental infection by two different severe acute respiratory syndrome coronavirus isolates. J Virol. 2005 Feb;79(4):2620–5.

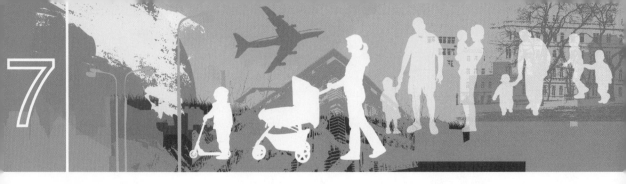

7

International Travel with Infants & Children

TRAVELING SAFELY WITH INFANTS & CHILDREN

Nicholas Weinberg, Michelle Weinberg, Susan A. Maloney

OVERVIEW

The number of children who travel or live outside their home countries has increased dramatically. In 2010, an estimated 2.2 million US resident children aged ≤18 years traveled internationally. Although data about the incidence of pediatric illnesses associated with international travel are limited, the risks that children face while traveling are likely similar to those their parents face. Children are less likely to receive pre-travel advice. In a review of children with post-travel illnesses seen at clinics in the GeoSentinel Surveillance Network, only 51% of all children and 32% of the children visiting friends and relatives (VFRs) had received pre-travel medical advice, compared with 59% of adults. The most commonly reported health problems among children are:

- Diarrheal illnesses
- Dermatologic conditions, including animal bites
- Systemic febrile illnesses, especially malaria
- Respiratory disorders

Motor vehicle and water-related injuries are also major health problems for child travelers. In assessing a child who is planning international travel, clinicians should:

- Review routine childhood and travel-related vaccinations. The pre-travel visit is an opportunity to ensure that children are up-to-date on routine vaccinations.
- Assess all anticipated travel-related activities.
- Provide preventive counseling and interventions tailored to specific risks, including special travel preparations and treatment that may be required for infants and children with underlying conditions, chronic diseases, or immunocompromising conditions. Older adolescents traveling in a student group or program may require counseling about disease prevention and the risks of sexually transmitted infections, empiric treatment and management of common travel-related illnesses, sexual assault, and drug and alcohol use during international travel (see Chapter 8, Study Abroad & Other International Student Travel).
- Give special consideration to the risks of children who are VFR travelers in developing countries. Conditions may include increased risk of malaria, intestinal parasites, and tuberculosis.
- Consider counseling adults and older children to take a course in basic first aid before travel.

DIARRHEA

Diarrhea and associated gastrointestinal illness are among the most common travel-related problems affecting children. Infants and children with diarrhea can become dehydrated more quickly than adults. The etiology of travelers' diarrhea (TD) in children is similar to that in adults (see Chapter 2, Travelers' Diarrhea).

Prevention

For infants, breastfeeding is the best way to reduce the risk of foodborne and waterborne illness. Infant formulas available abroad may not be the same as in the United States; parents feeding their child formula should consider whether they need to bring formula from home.

Water served to young children, including water used to prepare infant formula, should be disinfected (see Chapter 2, Water Disinfection for Travelers). In some parts of the world, bottled water may also be contaminated and should be disinfected before consumption.

Similarly, food precautions should be followed diligently. Foods served to children should be thoroughly cooked and eaten while still hot; fruits eaten raw should be peeled by the caregiver immediately before consumption. Additionally, caution should be used with fresh dairy products, which may not be pasteurized and may be diluted with untreated water. For short trips, parents may want to bring a supply of safe snacks from home for times when the children are hungry and the available food may not be appealing or safe. See Chapter 2, Food & Water Precautions for more information.

Scrupulous attention should be paid to handwashing and cleaning bottles, pacifiers, teething rings, and toys that fall to the floor or are handled by others; water used to clean these items should be potable. Parents should be particularly careful to wash hands well after diaper changes, especially for infants with diarrhea, to avoid spreading infection to themselves and other family members. When proper handwashing facilities are not available, an alcohol-based hand sanitizer (containing ≥60% alcohol) can be used as a disinfecting agent. However, because alcohol-based hand sanitizers are not effective against certain types of germs, hands should be washed with soap and water as soon as possible. Additionally, alcohol does not remove organic material; visibly soiled hands should be washed with soap and water.

Chemoprophylaxis with antibiotics is not generally used in children.

Treatment

Antiemetics and Antimotility Drugs

Because of potential side effects, antiemetics are generally not recommended for self- or family-administered treatment of children with vomiting and TD. Because of the association between salicylates and Reye syndrome, bismuth subsalicylate (BSS), the active ingredient in both Pepto-Bismol and Kaopectate, is not generally recommended to treat diarrhea in children aged <12 years. However, some clinicians use it off-label with caution in certain circumstances. Caution should be taken in administering BSS to children with viral infections, such as varicella or influenza, because of the risk for Reye syndrome. BSS is not recommended for children aged <3 years. A recent Cochrane Collaboration Review of the use of antiemetics for reducing vomiting related to acute gastroenteritis in children and adolescents showed some benefits with ondansetron, metoclopramide, or dimenhydrinate. However, the routine use of these medications for emesis associated with TD has not yet been determined and is not generally recommended.

Antimotility drugs, such as loperamide and diphenoxylate, are rarely given to small children. Loperamide is not recommended for children aged <6 years. Diphenoxylate and atropine combination tablets are not recommended for children aged <2 years. These drugs should be used with caution in children because of potential side effects (See Chapter 2, Travelers' Diarrhea).

Antibiotics

Few data are available regarding empiric treatment of TD in children. The antimicrobial options for empiric treatment of TD in children are limited. In practice, when an antibiotic is indicated for moderate to severe diarrhea, some clinicians prescribe azithromycin as a single daily dose (10 mg/kg) for 3 days. Physicians can prescribe unreconstituted azithromycin powder before travel, with instructions from the pharmacist for mixing it into an oral suspension if it becomes necessary to use it. Although resistance breakpoints have not yet been determined, elevated minimum inhibitory concentrations for azithromycin have been reported for some gastrointestinal pathogens. Therefore, patients should be counseled to seek medical attention if they do not improve after empiric treatment. Clinicians should review possible contraindications, such as QT prolongation and cardiac arrhythmias with azithromycin, before prescribing medications for empiric treatment of TD.

Although fluoroquinolones are frequently used for the empiric treatment of TD in adults, they are not approved by the Food and Drug Administration for this purpose among children aged <18 years because of cartilage damage seen in animal studies. The American Academy of Pediatrics suggests that fluoroquinolones be considered for the treatment of children with severe infections caused by multidrug-resistant strains of *Shigella* species, *Salmonella* species, *Vibrio cholerae*, or *Campylobacter jejuni*. Clinicians should be aware that fluoroquinolone resistance in gastrointestinal organisms has been reported from some countries, particularly in Southeast Asia. Routine use of fluoroquinolones for chemoprophylaxis or empiric treatment for TD among children is not recommended.

Management

The biggest threat to the infant with diarrhea and vomiting is dehydration. Fever or increased ambient temperature increases fluid loss and speeds dehydration. Adults traveling with children should be counseled about the signs and symptoms of dehydration and the proper use of oral rehydration salts (ORS). Medical attention may be required for an infant or young child with diarrhea who has:

- Signs of moderate to severe dehydration
- Bloody diarrhea
- Temperature >101.5°F (38.6°C)
- Persistent vomiting (unable to maintain oral hydration)

The mainstay of management of TD is adequate hydration.

ORS Use and Availability

Parents should be advised that dehydration is best prevented and treated by use of ORS, in addition to the infant's usual food. ORS should be provided to the infant by bottle, cup, oral syringe (often available in pharmacies), or spoon while medical attention is obtained. Low-osmolarity ORS is the most effective in preventing dehydration, although other formulations are available and may be used if they are more acceptable to young children. Homemade sugar-salt solutions are not recommended. Adults traveling with children should be counseled that sports drinks, which are designed to replace water and electrolytes lost through sweat, do not contain the same proportions of electrolytes as the solution recommended by the World Health Organization for rehydration during diarrheal illness. However, if ORS is not readily available, children should be offered whatever safe, palatable liquid they will take until ORS is obtained.

ORS packets are available at stores or pharmacies in almost all developing countries. ORS is prepared by adding 1 packet to boiled or treated water. Travelers should be advised to check packet instructions carefully to ensure that the salts are added to the correct volume of water. ORS solution should be consumed or discarded within 12 hours if held at room temperature or 24 hours if kept refrigerated.

A dehydrated child will usually drink ORS avidly; travelers should be advised to give it to the child as long as the dehydration persists. As dehydration lessens, the child may refuse the salty-tasting ORS solution, and another safe liquid can be offered. An infant or child who has been vomiting will usually keep ORS down if it is offered by spoon or oral syringe in small sips; these small amounts must be offered frequently, however, so the child can receive an adequate volume of ORS. Older children will often drink well by sipping through a straw. Severely dehydrated children, however, often will be unable to drink adequately. Severe dehydration is a medical emergency that usually requires administration of fluids by intravenous or intraosseous routes.

In general, children weighing <22 lb (10 kg) who have mild to moderate dehydration should be administered 2–4 oz (60–120 mL) ORS for each diarrheal stool or vomiting episode. Children who weigh ≥22 lb (10 kg) should receive 4–8 oz (120–240 mL) of ORS for each diarrheal stool or vomiting episode. The American Academy of Pediatrics

7

provides detailed guidance on rehydration for vomiting and diarrhea; see "Care Advice" at www.healthychildren.org/English/tips-tools/Symptom-Checker/Pages/Vomiting-With-Diarrhea.aspx.

ORS packets are available in the United States from Jianas Brothers Packaging Company (816-421-2880; http://rehydrate.org/resources/jianas.htm). ORS packets may also be available at stores that sell outdoor recreation and camping supplies. In addition, Cera Products (843-842-2600 or 888-237-2598; www.ceraproductsinc.com) markets a rice-based, rather than glucose-based, product.

Dietary Modification

Breastfed infants should continue nursing on demand. Formula-fed infants should continue their usual formula during rehydration. They should receive a volume that is sufficient to satisfy energy and nutrient requirements. Lactose-free or lactose-reduced formulas are usually unnecessary. Diluting formula may slow resolution of diarrhea and is not recommended. Older infants and children receiving semisolid or solid foods should continue to receive their usual diet during the illness. Recommended foods include starches, cereals, pasteurized yogurt, fruits, and vegetables, following safe food selection guidelines. Foods that are high in simple sugars, such as soft drinks, undiluted apple juice, gelatins, and presweetened cereals, can exacerbate diarrhea by osmotic effects and should be avoided. In addition, foods high in fat may not be tolerated because of their tendency to delay gastric emptying.

The practice of withholding food for ≥24 hours is not recommended. Early feeding can decrease changes in intestinal permeability caused by infection, reduce illness duration, and improve nutritional outcome. Highly specific diets (such as the BRAT [bananas, rice, applesauce, and toast] diet) have been commonly recommended; however, similar to juice-based and clear fluid diets, such severely restrictive diets have no scientific basis and should be avoided.

MALARIA

Malaria is among the most serious and life-threatening diseases that can be acquired by pediatric international travelers. Pediatric VFR travelers are at particularly high risk for acquiring malaria if they do not receive chemoprophylaxis.

Children with malaria can rapidly develop high levels of parasitemia. They are at increased risk for severe complications of malaria, including shock, seizures, coma, and death. Initial symptoms of malaria in children may mimic many other common causes of pediatric febrile illness and therefore may result in delayed diagnosis and treatment. Clinicians should counsel adults traveling with children in malaria-endemic areas to use preventive measures, be aware of the signs and symptoms of malaria, and seek prompt medical attention if they develop.

Antimalarial Drugs

Pediatric doses for malaria chemoprophylaxis are provided in Table 3-9. Pediatric doses of medications used for treatment are included in Table 3-7. All dosing should be calculated on the basis of body weight. Medications used for infants and young children are the same as those recommended for adults, except under the following circumstances:

- Doxycycline should not be given to children aged <8 years because of the risk of teeth staining.
- Atovaquone-proguanil should not be used for prophylaxis in children weighing <5 kg (11 lb) because of lack of data on safety and efficacy.

Chloroquine, mefloquine, and atovaquone-proguanil have a bitter taste. Before departure, pharmacists can be asked to pulverize tablets and prepare gelatin capsules with calculated pediatric doses. Mixing the powder in a small amount of food or drink can facilitate the administration of antimalarial drugs to infants and children. Additionally, any compounding pharmacy can alter the flavoring of malaria medication tablets so that children are more willing to take them. Assistance with finding a compounding pharmacy is available on the International Academy of Compounding Pharmacists' website (www.iacprx.org). Because overdose of antimalarial drugs, particularly chloroquine, can be fatal, medication should be stored in childproof containers and kept out of the reach of infants and children.

Personal Protection Measures

Children should sleep in rooms with air conditioning or screened windows or sleep under bed nets, when available. Mosquito netting should be used over infant carriers. Children can reduce skin exposed to mosquitoes by wearing long pants and long sleeves while outdoors in areas where malaria is transmitted. Clothing and mosquito nets can be treated with insect repellents such as permethrin, a repellent and insecticide that repels and kills ticks, mosquitoes, and other arthropods. Permethrin remains effective through multiple washings. Clothing and bed nets should be retreated according to the product label. Permethrin should not be applied to the skin. Although permethrin provides longer duration protection, recommended repellents that can be applied to skin (DEET [N,N-diethyl-*m*-toluamide], picaridin, oil of lemon eucalyptus [OLE] or PMD, and IR3535) can also be used on clothing and mosquito nets. See Chapter 2, Protection against Mosquitoes, Ticks, & Other Insects & Arthropods for more details about these protective measures.

Repellent Use

CDC recommends the use of repellents containing 1 of the following active ingredients, which are registered with the US Environmental Protection Agency, according to the product labels: DEET, picaridin, OLE or PMD, and IR3535. Most repellents can be used on children aged >2 months, with the following considerations:

- Products containing OLE specify that they should not be used on children aged <3 years.
- Repellent products must state any age restriction. If none is stated, the Environmental Protection Agency has not required a restriction on the use of the product.
- Many repellents contain DEET as the active ingredient. The concentration of DEET varies considerably among products. The duration of protection varies with the DEET concentration: higher concentrations protect longer. Products with DEET concentration above 50% do not offer a marked increase in protection time. The American Academy of Pediatrics recommends:
  > ≤30% DEET should be used on children aged >2 months.
  > Repellents with DEET should not be used on infants aged <2 months.

Repellents can be applied to exposed skin and clothing; however, they should not be applied under clothing. Repellents should never be used over cuts, wounds, or irritated skin. Young children should not be allowed to handle the product. When using repellent on a child, an adult should apply it to his or her own hands and then rub them on the child, with the following considerations:

- Avoid the child's eyes and mouth, and apply sparingly around the ears.
- Do not apply repellent to children's hands, since children tend to put their hands in their mouths.
- Heavy application and saturation are generally unnecessary for effectiveness. If biting insects do not respond to a thin film of repellent, then apply a bit more.
- After returning indoors, wash treated skin with soap and water or bathe. This is particularly important when repellents are used repeatedly in a day or on consecutive days.

Products that contain both repellents and sunscreen are generally not recommended, because instructions for use are different and the need to reapply sunscreen is usually more frequent than with repellent alone. In general, apply sunscreen first, then apply repellent. Mosquito coils should be used with caution in the presence of children to avoid burns and inadvertent ingestion.

For more information about repellent use, see Chapter 2, Protection against Mosquitoes, Ticks, & Other Insects & Arthropods.

DENGUE

Pediatric VFR travelers who may have frequent and prolonged travel may have risk similar to children living in dengue-endemic areas. Among 8 children who were diagnosed with acute dengue infection after visiting friends and relatives in the Caribbean, 3 developed either dengue hemorrhagic fever or dengue shock syndrome. Children traveling to areas with dengue should use the same mosquito protection measures described for malaria. However, families should be counseled that, unlike the mosquitoes that transmit malaria, the *Aedes* mosquitoes that transmit dengue bite during

7

the daytime. Clinicians should consider dengue in children with fever if they have recently been in an endemic area. For more information about dengue, see Chapter 3, Dengue.

INFECTION AND INFESTATION FROM SOIL CONTACT

Children are more likely than adults to have contact with soil or sand, and therefore, they may be exposed to diseases caused by infectious stages of parasites present in soil, including ascariasis, hookworm infestation, cutaneous or visceral larva migrans, trichuriasis, and strongyloidiasis. Children and infants should wear protective footwear and play on a sheet or towel rather than directly on the ground. Clothing should not be dried on the ground. In countries with a tropical climate, clothing or diapers dried in the open air should be ironed before use to prevent infestation with fly larvae.

ANIMAL BITES AND RABIES

Worldwide, rabies is more common in children than adults. In addition to the potential for increased contact with animals, children are also more likely to be bitten on the head or neck, leading to more severe injuries. Children and their families should be counseled to avoid all stray or unfamiliar animals and to inform adults of any contact or bites. Bats throughout the world are considered to have the potential to transmit rabies virus. Mammal-associated injuries should be washed thoroughly with water and soap (and povidone iodine if available), and the child should be evaluated promptly to assess the need for rabies postexposure prophylaxis. Because rabies vaccine and rabies immune globulin may not be unavailable in certain destinations, families should seriously consider purchasing medical evacuation insurance.

AIR TRAVEL

Although air travel is safe for healthy newborns, infants, and children, a few issues should be considered in preparation for travel. Children with chronic heart or lung problems may be at risk for hypoxia during flight, and a physician should be consulted before travel. Making sure that children can be safely restrained during a flight is a safety consideration. Severe turbulence or crash can create enough momentum that a parent cannot hold onto a child:

- Children should be placed in a rear-facing Federal Aviation Authority–approved child-safety seat until they are aged ≥1 year and weigh ≥20 lb.
- Children aged ≥1 year and 20–40 lb should use a forward-facing Federal Aviation Authority–approved child-safety seat.
- Children who weigh >40 lb can be secured in the aircraft seat belt.

Ear pain can be troublesome for infants and children during descent. Pressure in the middle ear can be equalized by swallowing or chewing:

- Infants should nurse or suck on a bottle.
- Older children can try chewing gum.
- Antihistamines and decongestants have not been shown to be of benefit.

There is no evidence that air travel exacerbates the symptoms or complications associated with otitis media. Travel to different time zones, jet lag, and schedule disruptions can disturb sleep patterns in infants and children, as well as adults.

INJURIES
Vehicle-Related

MVA #1 death cause

Vehicle-related injuries are the leading cause of death in children who travel. While traveling in automobiles and other vehicles, children weighing ≤40 lb should be restrained in age-appropriate car seats or booster seats, as described above. These seats often must be carried from home, since availability of well-maintained and approved seats may be limited abroad. In general, children are safest traveling in the rear seat; no one should ever travel in the bed of a pickup truck. Families should be counseled that in many developing countries, cars may lack front or rear seatbelts. They should attempt to arrange transportation in vehicles or rent vehicles with seatbelts and other safety features.

Drowning and Water-Related Illness and Injuries _#2 death_

Drowning is the second leading cause of death in young travelers. Children may not be familiar with hazards in the ocean or in rivers. Swimming pools may not have protective fencing to keep toddlers from falling into the pool. Close supervision of children around water is essential. Water safety devices such as life vests may not be available abroad, and families should consider bringing these from home. Protective footwear is important to avoid injury in many marine environments. Schistosomiasis is a risk to children and adults in endemic areas. While in schistosomiasis-endemic areas (see Map 3-12), children should not swim in fresh, unchlorinated water such as lakes or ponds.

Accommodations

Conditions at hotels and other lodging may not be as safe as those in the United States, and accommodations should be carefully inspected for exposed wiring, pest poisons, paint chips, or inadequate stairway or balcony railings.

ALTITUDE

Children are as susceptible to altitude illness as adults. Young children who cannot talk can show nonspecific symptoms, such as loss of appetite and irritability. They may have unexplained fussiness and change in sleep and activity patterns. Older children may complain of headache or shortness of breath. If children demonstrate unexplained symptoms after an ascent, it may be necessary to descend to see if they improve. Acetazolamide is not approved for pediatric use for altitude illness, but it is generally safe in children when used for other indications.

SUN EXPOSURE

Sun exposure, and particularly sunburn before age 15 years, is strongly associated with melanoma and other forms of skin cancer (see Chapter 2, Sunburn). Exposure to UV light is highest near the equator, at high altitudes, during midday (10 AM–4 PM), and where light is reflected off water or snow. Sunscreens are generally recommended for use in children aged >6 months. Sunscreens (or sun blocks), either physical (such as titanium or zinc oxides) or chemical (SPF ≥15 and providing protection from both UVA and UVB), should be applied as directed and reapplied, as needed, after sweating and water exposure. Babies aged <6 months require extra protection from the sun

because of their thinner and more sensitive skin; severe sunburn for this age group is considered a medical emergency. Babies should be kept in the shade and wear clothing that covers the entire body. A minimal amount of sunscreen can be applied to small exposed areas, including the infant's face and hands.

Sun-blocking shirts are available that are made for swimming and preclude having to rub sunscreen over the entire trunk. Hats and sunglasses also reduce sun injury to skin and eyes. If both sunscreen and a DEET-containing insect repellent are applied, the sun protection factor (SPF) of the sunscreen may be diminished by one-third, and covering clothing should be worn or time in the sun decreased accordingly.

OTHER GENERAL CONSIDERATIONS
Travel Stress

Changes in schedule, activities, and environment can be stressful for children. Including children in planning for the trip and bringing along familiar toys or other objects can decrease these stresses. For children with chronic illnesses, decisions regarding timing and itinerary should be made in consultation with the child's health care providers.

Insurance

As for any traveler, insurance coverage for illnesses and injuries while abroad should be verified before departure. Consideration should be given to purchasing special medical evacuation insurance for airlifting or air ambulance to an area with adequate medical care (see Chapter 2, Travel Insurance, Travel Health Insurance, & Medical Evacuation Insurance).

Identification

In case family members become separated, each infant or child should carry identifying information and contact numbers in his or her own clothing or pockets. Because of concerns about illegal transport of children across international borders, if only 1 parent is traveling with the child, he or she may need to carry relevant custody papers or a notarized permission letter from the other parent.

BIBLIOGRAPHY

1. American Academy of Pediatrics. Insect repellents. Elk Grove Village, IL: American Academy of Pediatrics; 2012 [cited 2012 Sep 26]. Available from: http://www. healthychildren.org/English/safety-prevention/at-play/Pages/Insect-Repellents.aspx.

2. American Academy of Pediatrics. Sun safety. Elk Grove Village, IL: American Academy of Pediatrics; 2012 [cited 2012 Sep 26]. Available from: http://www. healthychildren.org/English/safety-prevention/at-play/Pages/Sun-Safety.aspx.

3. American Academy of Pediatrics. Vomiting with diarrhea. Elk Grove Village, IL: American Academy of Pediatrics; 2012 [cited 2012 Sep 26]. Available from: http://www.healthychildren.org/English/tips-tools/Symptom-Checker/Pages/Vomiting-With-Diarrhea.aspx.

4. Bradley JS, Jackson MA, Committee on Infectious Diseases. The use of systemic and topical fluoroquinolones. Pediatrics. 2011 Oct;128(4):e1034–45.

5. DuPont HL, Ericsson CD, Farthing MJ, Gorbach S, Pickering LK, Rombo L, et al. Expert review of the evidence base for prevention of travelers' diarrhea. J Travel Med. 2009 May–Jun;16(3):149–60.

6. Fedorowicz Z, Jagannath VA, Carter B. Antiemetics for reducing vomiting related to acute gastroenteritis in children and adolescents. Cochrane Database Syst Rev. 2011(9):1–71.

7. Hagmann S, Neugebauer R, Schwartz E, Perret C, Castelli F, Barnett ED, et al. Illness in children after international travel: analysis from the GeoSentinel Surveillance Network. Pediatrics. 2010 May;125(5):e1072–80.

8. Han P, Balaban V, Marano C. Travel characteristics and risk-taking attitudes in youths traveling to nonindustrialized countries. J Travel Med. 2010 Sep–Oct;17(5):316–21.

9. Herbinger KH, Drerup L, Alberer M, Nothdurft HD, Sonnenburg F, Loscher T. Spectrum of imported infectious diseases among children and adolescents returning from the tropics and subtropics. J Travel Med. 2012 May–Jun;19(3):150–7.

10. Hunziker T, Berger C, Staubli G, Tschopp A, Weber R, Nadal D, et al. Profile of travel-associated illness in children, Zurich, Switzerland. J Travel Med. 2012 May–Jun;19(3):158–62.

11. King CK, Glass R, Bresee JS, Duggan C. Managing acute gastroenteritis among children: oral rehydration, maintenance, and nutritional therapy. MMWR Recomm Rep. 2003 Nov 21;52(RR-16):1–16.

12. Krishnan N, Purswani M, Hagmann S. Severe dengue virus infection in pediatric travelers visiting friends and relatives after travel to the Caribbean. Am J Trop Med Hyg. 2012 Mar;86(3):474–6.

13. Murphy ME, Montemarano AD, Debboun M, Gupta R. The effect of sunscreen on the efficacy of insect repellent: a clinical trial. J Am Acad Dermatol. 2000 Aug;43(2 Pt 1):219–22.

14. US Department of Commerce, Office of Travel and Tourism Industries. Profile of US resident travelers visiting overseas destinations: 2010 outbound. 2011 [cited 2012 Sep 26]. Available from: http://tinet.ita.doc.gov/outreachpages/download_data_table/2010_Outbound_Profile.pdf.

15. van Rijn SF, Driessen G, Overbosch D, van Genderen PJ. Travel-related morbidity in children: a prospective observational study. J Travel Med. 2012 May–Jun;19(3):144–9.

VACCINE RECOMMENDATIONS FOR INFANTS & CHILDREN

Sheila M. Mackell

Vaccinating children for travel requires careful evaluation. Whenever possible, children should complete the routine immunizations of childhood on a normal schedule. However, travel at an earlier age may require accelerated schedules. **Not all travel-related vaccines are effective in infants, and some are specifically contraindicated.**

The recommended childhood and adolescent immunization schedule is depicted in Table 7-1. Table 7-2 depicts the catch-up schedule for children and adolescents who start their vaccination schedule late or who are >1 month behind. This table also describes the recommended minimum intervals between doses for children who need to be vaccinated

Table 7-1. Recommended immunization schedule for ages 0–18 years—United States, 2013

For those who fall behind or start late, provide catch-up vaccination at the earliest opportunity as indicated by the green bars below. To determine minimum intervals between doses, see the catch-up schedule, Table 7-2. School entry and adolescent vaccine age groups are in bold.

Vaccines	Birth	1 mo	2 mos	4 mos	6 mos	9 mos	12 mos	15 mos	18 mos	19-23 mos	2-3 yrs	4-6 yrs	7-10 yrs	11-12 yrs	13-15 yrs	16-18 yrs
Hepatitis B[1] (Hep B)	1st dose	2nd dose			3rd dose											
Rotavirus[2] (RV) RV-1 (2-dose series); RV-5 (3-dose series)			1st dose	2nd dose	See footnote 2											
Diphtheria, tetanus, & acellular pertussis[3] (DTap: <7 yrs)			1st dose	2nd dose	3rd dose		4th dose					5th dose				
Tetanus, diphtheria & acellular pertussis[3] (Tdap: ≥7 yrs) (Tdap)														(Tdap)		
Haemophilus influenzae type b5 (Hib)			1st dose	2nd dose	See footnote 5		3rd or 4th dose see footnote 5									
Pneumococcal conjugate[6a,c] (PCV13)			1st dose	2nd dose	3rd dose		4th dose									
Pneumococcal polysaccharide[6b,c] (PPSV23)																
Inactivated Poliovirus[7] (IPV) (<18 years)			1st dose	2nd dose	3rd dose							4th dose				
Influenza[8] (IIV; LAIV) 2 doses for some: see footnote 8					Annual vaccination (IIV only)						Annual vaccination (IIV or LAIV)					
Measles, mumps, rubella[9] (MMR)							1st dose					2nd dose				
Varicella[10] (VAR)							1st dose					2nd dose				
Hepatitis A[11] (HepA)							2 dose series, see footnote 11									
Human papillomavirus[12] (HPV2): females only; HPV4: males and females)														(3 dose series)		
Meningococcal[13] (HibMenCY ≥6wks; MCV4-D≥9 mos; MCV4-CRM ≥ 2 yrs.)			see footnote 13											1st dose		booster

- Range of recommended ages for all children
- Range of recommended ages for catch-up Immunization
- Range of recommended ages for certain high-risk groups
- Range of recommended ages during which catch up is encouraged and for certain high-risk groups
- Not routinely recommended

This schedule includes recommendations in effect as of January 2013. Any dose not administered at the recommended age should be administered at a subsequent visit, when indicated and feasible. The use of a combination vaccine generally is preferred over separate injections of its equivalent component vaccines. Vaccination providers should consult the relevant Advisory Committee on Immunization Practices (ACIP) statement for detailed recommendations, available online at www.cdc.gov/vaccines/pubs/acip-list.htm. Clinically significant adverse events that follow vaccination should be reported to the Vaccine Adverse Event Reporting System (VAERS) online (www.vaers.hhs.gov) or by telephone (800-822-7967). Suspected cases of vaccine-preventable diseases should be reported to the state or local health department. Additional information, including precautions and contraindications for vaccination, is available from CDC online (www.cdc.gov/vaccines) or by telephone (call CDC-INFO toll-free at 800-232-4636). This schedule is approved by the ACIP (www.cdc.gov/vaccines/acip/index.html), the American Academy of Pediatrics (www.aap.org), and the American Academy of Family Physicians (www.aafp.org).

1. **Hepatitis B (HepB) vaccine.** (Minimum age: birth)
   Routine vaccination:
   At birth:
   - Administer monovalent HepB vaccine to all newborns before hospital discharge.
   - For infants born to hepatitis B surface antigen (HBsAg)–positive mothers, administer HepB vaccine and 0.5 mL of hepatitis B immune globulin (HBIG) within 12 hours of birth. These infants should be tested for HBsAg and antibody to HBsAg (anti-HBs) 1–2 months after completion of the HepB series, at age 9–18 months (preferably at the next well-child visit).

- If the mother's HBsAg status is unknown, within 12 hours of birth, administer HepB vaccine to all infants regardless of birth weight. For infants weighing <2,000 g, administer HBIG in addition to HepB vaccine within 12 hours of birth. Determine the mother's HBsAg status as soon as possible and, if she is HBsAg-positive, also administer HBIG for infants weighing ≥2,000 g (no later than age 1 week).

Doses following the birth dose:
- The second dose should be administered at age 1–2 months. Monovalent HepB vaccine should be used for doses administered before age 6 weeks.
- Infants who did not receive a birth dose should receive 3 doses of a HepB-containing vaccine on a schedule of 0, 1–2 months, and 6 months starting as soon as feasible (see Table 7-2).
- The minimum interval between dose 1 and dose 2 is 4 weeks, and between dose 2 and 3 is 8 weeks. The final (third or fourth) dose in the HepB vaccine series should be administered no earlier than age 24 weeks and ≥16 weeks after the first dose.
- Administration of a total of 4 doses of HepB vaccine is recommended when a combination vaccine containing HepB is administered after the birth dose.

Catch-up vaccination:
- Unvaccinated people should complete a 3-dose series.
- A 2-dose series (doses separated by ≥4 months) of adult formulation Recombivax HB is licensed for use in children aged 11–15 years.
- For other catch-up issues, see Table 7-2.

2. **Rotavirus (RV) vaccines.** (Minimum age: 6 weeks for both RV-1 [Rotarix] and RV-5 [Rota Teq])

Routine vaccination:
- Administer a series of RV vaccine to all infants as follows:
- If RV-1 is used, administer a 2-dose series at ages 2 and 4 months.
- If RV-5 is used, administer a 3-dose series at ages 2, 4, and 6 months.
- If any dose in the series was RV-5 or vaccine product is unknown for any dose in the series, a total of 3 doses of RV vaccine should be administered.

Catch-up vaccination:
- The maximum age for the first dose in the series is 14 weeks, 6 days.
- Vaccination should not be initiated for infants aged ≥15 weeks, 0 days.
- The maximum age for the final dose in the series is 8 months, 0 days.
- If RV-1 (Rotarix) is administered for the first and second doses, a third dose is not indicated.
- For other catch-up issues, see Table 7-2.

3. **Diphtheria and tetanus toxoids and acellular pertussis (DTaP) vaccine.** (Minimum age: 6 weeks)

Routine vaccination:
- Administer a 5-dose series of DTaP vaccine at ages 2, 4, 6, 15–18 months, and 4–6 years. The fourth dose may be administered as early as age 12 months, provided ≥6 months have elapsed since the third dose.

Catch-up vaccination:
- The fifth (booster) dose of DTaP vaccine is not necessary if the fourth dose was administered at age ≥4 years.
- For other catch-up issues, see Table 7-2.

4. **Tetanus and diphtheria toxoids and acellular pertussis (Tdap) vaccine.** (Minimum age: 10 years for Boostrix, 11 years for Adacel.)

Routine vaccination:
- Administer 1 dose of Tdap vaccine to all adolescents aged 11–12 years.
- Tdap can be administered regardless of the interval since the last tetanus and diphtheria toxoid–containing vaccine.
- Administer 1 dose of Tdap vaccine to pregnant adolescents during each pregnancy (preferred during 27–36 weeks' gestation) regardless of the number of years from prior Td or Tdap vaccination.

Catch-up vaccination:
- People aged 7–10 years who are not fully immunized with the childhood DTaP vaccine series should receive Tdap vaccine as the first dose in the catch-up series; if additional doses are needed, use Td vaccine. For these children, an adolescent Tdap vaccine should not be given.
- People aged 11–18 years who have not received Tdap vaccine should receive a dose, followed by tetanus and diphtheria toxoids (Td) booster doses every 10 years thereafter.
- An inadvertent dose of DTaP vaccine administered to children ages 7–10 years can count as part of the catch-up series. This dose can count as the adolescent Tdap dose, or the child can later receive a Tdap booster dose at age 11–12 years.
- For other catch-up issues, see Table 7-2.

5. *Haemophilus influenzae* type b (Hib) conjugate vaccine. (Minimum age: 6 weeks)

Routine vaccination:
- Administer a Hib vaccine primary series and a booster dose to all infants. The primary series doses should be administered at ages 2, 4, and 6 months; however, if PRP-OMP (PedvaxHIB or Comvax) is administered at ages 2 and 4 months, a dose at age 6 months is not indicated. One booster dose should be administered at age 12–15 months.
- Hiberix (PRP-T) should only be used for the booster (final) dose in children aged 12 months through 4 years who have received ≥1 dose of Hib.

Catch-up vaccination:
- If dose 1 was administered at age 12–14 months, administer booster (as final dose) ≥8 weeks after dose 1.
- If the first 2 doses were PRP-OMP (PedvaxHIB or Comvax) and were administered at age <11 months, the third (and final) dose should be administered at age 12–15 months and ≥8 weeks after the second dose.
- If the first dose was administered at age 7–11 months, administer the second dose ≥4 weeks later and a final dose at age 12–15 months, regardless of Hib vaccine (PRP-T or PRP-OMP) used for first dose.
- For unvaccinated children age ≥15 months, administer only 1 dose.
- For other catch-up issues, see Table 7-2.

Vaccination of people with high-risk conditions:
- Hib vaccine is not routinely recommended for patients aged >5 years. However, 1 dose of Hib vaccine should be administered to unvaccinated or partially vaccinated people aged ≥5 years who have leukemia, malignant neoplasms, anatomic/functional asplenia (including sickle cell disease), HIV infection, or other immunocompromising conditions.

6a. **Pneumococcal conjugate vaccine (PCV).** (Minimum age: 6 weeks)

Routine vaccination:
- Administer a series of PCV13 vaccine at ages 2, 4, and 6 months with a booster at age 12–15 months.

continued

- For children aged 14–59 months who have received an age-appropriate series of 7-valent PCV (PCV7), administer a single supplemental dose of 13-valent PCV (PCV13).

Catch-up vaccination:

- Administer 1 dose of PCV13 to all healthy children aged 24–59 months who are not completely vaccinated for their age.
- For other catch-up issues, see Table 7-2.

Vaccination of people with high-risk conditions:

- For children aged 24–71 months with certain underlying medical conditions (see footnote 6c), administer 1 dose of PCV13 if 3 doses of PCV were received previously, or administer 2 doses of PCV13 ≥8 weeks apart if fewer than 3 doses of PCV were received previously.
- A single dose of PCV13 may be administered to previously unvaccinated children aged 6–18 years who have anatomic/functional asplenia (including sickle cell disease), HIV infection or an immunocompromising condition, cochlear implant, or cerebrospinal fluid leak. See *MMWR* 2010;59(No. RR-11), available at www.cdc.gov/mmwr/pdf/rr/rr5911.pdf.
- Administer PPSV23 ≥8 weeks after the last dose of PCV to children aged ≥2 years with certain underlying medical conditions (see footnotes 6b and 6c).

6b. **Pneumococcal polysaccharide vaccine (PPSV23).** (Minimum age: 2 years)

Vaccination of people with high-risk conditions:

- Administer PPSV23 ≥8 weeks after the last dose of PCV to children aged ≥2 years with certain underlying medical conditions (see footnote 6c). A single revaccination with PPSV should be administered after 5 years to children with anatomic/functional asplenia or an immunocompromising condition.

6c. **Medical conditions for which PPSV would be indicated in children aged ≥2 years and for which use of PCV13 is indicated in children aged 24–71 months:**

- Immunocompetent children with: chronic heart disease (particularly cyanotic congenital heart disease and cardiac failure), chronic lung disease (including asthma if treated with high-dose oral corticosteroid therapy), diabetes mellitus, cerebrospinal fluid leaks, or cochlear implant.
- Children with anatomic/functional asplenia (sickle cell disease and other hemoglobinopathies, congenital or acquired asplenia, or splenic dysfunction).
- Children with immunocompromising conditions: HIV infection; chronic renal failure and nephrotic syndrome; diseases associated with treatment with immunosuppressive drugs or radiation therapy, including malignant neoplasms, leukemias, lymphomas and Hodgkin disease, or solid organ transplantation; or congenital immunodeficiency.

7. **Inactivated poliovirus vaccine (IPV).** (Minimum age: 6 weeks)

Routine vaccination:

- Administer a series of IPV at ages 2, 4, and 6–18 months, with a booster at age 4–6 years. The final dose in the series should be administered on or after the fourth birthday and ≥6 months after the previous dose.

Catch-up vaccination:

- In the first 6 months of life, minimum age and minimum intervals are only recommended if the infant is at risk for imminent exposure to circulating poliovirus (i.e., travel to a polio-endemic region or during an outbreak).

- If ≥4 doses are administered before age 4 years, an additional dose should be administered at age 4–6 years.
- A fourth dose is not necessary if the third dose was administered at age ≥4 years and ≥6 months after the previous dose.
- If both OPV and IPV were administered as part of a series, a total of 4 doses should be administered, regardless of the child's current age.
- IPV is not routinely recommended for US residents aged ≥18 years.
- For other catch-up issues, see Table 7-2.

8. **Influenza vaccines.** (Minimum age: 6 months for inactivated influenza vaccine [IIV]; 2 years for live, attenuated influenza vaccine [LAIV])

Routine vaccination:

- Administer influenza vaccine annually to all children beginning at age 6 months. For most healthy nonpregnant people aged 2–49 years, either LAIV or IIV may be used. However, LAIV should NOT be administered to some people, including 1) those with asthma, 2) children 2–4 years who had wheezing in the past 12 months, or 3) those who have any other underlying medical conditions that predispose them to influenza complications. For all other contraindications to use of LAIV, see *MMWR* 2010;59(No. RR-8), available at www.cdc.gov/mmwr/pdf/rr/rr5908.pdf.
- Administer 1 dose to people aged ≥9 years.
- For children aged 6 months through 8 years:
  > For the 2012–13 season, administer 2 doses (separated by ≥4 weeks) to children who are receiving influenza vaccine for the first time. For additional guidance, follow dosing guidelines in the 2012 ACIP influenza vaccine recommendations, *MMWR* 2012;61:613–8(RR-32), available at www.cdc.gov/mmwr/pdf/wk/mm6132.pdf.
  > For the 2013–14 and 2014–15 seasons, follow future dosing guidelines in the published ACIP influenza vaccine recommendations.

9. **Measles, mumps, and rubella (MMR) vaccine.** (Minimum age: 12 months for routine vaccination)

Routine vaccination:

- Administer the first dose of MMR vaccine at age 12–15 months, and the second dose at age 4–6 years. The second dose may be administered before age 4 years, provided ≥4 weeks have elapsed since the first dose.
- Administer 1 dose of MMR vaccine to infants aged 6–11 months before departure from the United States for international travel. These children should be revaccinated with 2 doses of MMR vaccine, the first at age 12–15 months (12 months if the child remains in an area where disease risk is high) and the second ≥4 weeks later.
- Administer 2 doses of MMR vaccine to children aged ≥12 months, before departure from the United States for international travel. The first dose should be administered on or after age 12 months and the second dose ≥4 weeks later.

Catch-up vaccination:

- Ensure that all school-aged children and adolescents have had 2 doses of MMR vaccine; the minimum interval between the 2 doses is 4 weeks.

10. **Varicella (VAR) vaccine.** (Minimum age: 12 months)

Routine vaccination:

- Administer the first dose of VAR vaccine at age 12–15 months and the second dose at age 4–6 years. The second dose may be administered before age 4 years, provided ≥3 months have elapsed since

continued

the first dose. If the second dose was administered ≥4 weeks after the first dose, it can be accepted as valid.

Catch-up vaccination:

- Ensure that all people aged 7–18 years without evidence of immunity (see *MMWR* 2007;56 [No. RR-4], available at www.cdc.gov/mmwr/pdf/rr/rr5604.pdf) have 2 doses of varicella vaccine. For children aged 7–12 years, the recommended minimum interval between doses is 3 months (if the second dose was administered ≥4 weeks after the first dose, it can be accepted as valid); for people aged ≥13 years, the minimum interval between doses is 4 weeks.

11. **Hepatitis A (HepA) vaccine.** (Minimum age: 12 months)

    Routine vaccination:

    - Initiate the 2-dose HepA vaccine series for children between ages 12–23 months; separate the 2 doses by 6–18 months.
    - Children who have received 1 dose of HepA vaccine before age 24 months should receive a second dose 6–18 months after the first dose.
    - For anyone aged ≥2 years who has not already received the complete HepA vaccine series, completion of 2 doses of HepA vaccine separated by 6–18 months may be administered if immunity against hepatitis A virus infection is desired.

    Catch-up vaccination:

    - The minimum interval between the 2 doses is 6 months.

    Special populations:

    - Administer 2 doses of HepA vaccine ≥6 months apart to previously unvaccinated people who live in areas where vaccination programs target older children, or who are at increased risk for infection.

12. **Human papillomavirus (HPV) vaccines (HPV4 [Gardasil] and HPV2 [Cervarix]).** (Minimum age: 9 years)

    Routine vaccination:

    - Administer a 3-dose series of HPV vaccine on a schedule of 0, 1–2, and 6 months to all adolescents aged 11–12 years. Either HPV4 or HPV2 may be used for girls, and only HPV4 may be used for boys.
    - The vaccine series can be started beginning at age 9 years.
    - Administer the second dose 1–2 months after the first dose and the third dose 6 months after the first dose (≥24 weeks after the first dose).

    Catch-up vaccination:

    - Administer the vaccine series to girls (either HPV2 or HPV4) and boys (HPV4) at age 13–18 years if not previously vaccinated.
    - Use recommended routine dosing intervals (see above) for vaccine series catch-up.

13. **Meningococcal conjugate vaccines (MCV4).** (Minimum age: 6 weeks for HibMenCY, 9 months for Menactra [MCV4-D], 2 years for Menveo [MCV4-CRM])

    Routine vaccination:

    - Administer MCV4 vaccine at age 11–12 years, with a booster dose at age 16 years.
    - Adolescents aged 11–18 years with HIV infection should receive a 2-dose primary series of MCV4, ≥8 weeks apart (see *MMWR* 2011;60:1018–9[RR-30], available at www.cdc.gov/mmwr/pdf/wk/mm6030.pdf).
    - For children aged 9 months through 10 years with high-risk conditions, see below.

    Catch-up vaccination:

    - Administer MCV4 vaccine at age 13–18 years if not previously vaccinated.
    - If the first dose is administered at age 13–15 years, a booster dose should be administered at age

16–18 years with a minimum interval of ≥8 weeks from the preceding dose.

- If the first dose is administered at age ≥16 years, a booster dose is not needed.
- For other catch-up issues, see Table 7-2.

Vaccination of people with high-risk conditions:

- For children aged <19 months with anatomic/ functional asplenia (including sickle cell disease), administer an infant series of HibMenCY at 2, 4, 6, and 12–15 months.
- For children 2–18 months with persistent complement component deficiency, administer either an infant series of HibMenCY at 2, 4, 6, and 12–15 months or a 2-dose primary series of MCV4-D starting at 9 months, ≥8 weeks apart.
- For children 19–23 months with persistent complement component deficiency who have not received a complete series of Hib-MenCY or MCV4-C, administer 2 primary doses of MCV4-D ≥8 weeks apart.
- For children ≥24 months with persistent complement component deficiency or anatomic/functional asplenia (including sickle cell disease), who have not received a complete series of HibMenCY or MCV4-D, administer 2 primary doses of either MCV4-D or MCV4-CRM. If MCV4-D (Menactra) is administered to a child with asplenia (including sickle cell disease), do not administer MCV4-D until 2 years of age and ≥4 weeks after the completion of all PCV13 doses (see *MMWR* 2011;60:1391–2[RR-40], available at www.cdc.gov/ mmwr/pdf/wk/mm6040.pdf).
- For children ≥9 months old who are residents of or travelers to countries in the African meningitis belt or the Hajj, administer an age-appropriate formulation and series of MCV4 for protection against serogroups A and W-135. Prior receipt of HibMenCY is not sufficient for children traveling to the meningitis belt or the Hajj (see *MMWR* 2011;60:1391–2[RR-40], available at www. cdc.gov/mmwr/pdf/wk/mm6040.pdf).
- For children who are present during outbreaks caused by a vaccine serogroup, administer or complete an age- and formulation-appropriate series of HibMenCY or MCV4.
- For booster doses among people with high-risk conditions, refer to www.cdc.gov/vaccines/pubs/ACIP-list.htm#mening.

Additional Information

- For contraindications and precautions for use of a vaccine and for additional information regarding that vaccine, vaccination providers should consult the relevant ACIP statement available online at www.cdc. gov/vaccines/pubs/acip-list.htm.
- For the purposes of calculating intervals between doses, 4 weeks=28 days. Intervals of ≥4 months are determined by calendar months.
- Information on travel vaccine requirements and recommendations is available at wwwnc.cdc.gov/ travel/page/vaccinations.htm.
- For vaccination of people with primary and secondary immunodeficiencies, see Table 13. Vaccination of persons with primary and secondary immunodeficiencies, General Recommendations on Immunization (ACIP), available at http://www.cdc.gov/mmwr/preview/ mmwrhtml/rr6002a1.htm?s_cid=rr6002a1_e#Tab13; and American Academy of Pediatrics. Passive immunization. In: Pickering LK, Baker CJ, Kimberlin DW, Long SS eds. Red Book: 2012 Report of the Committee on Infectious Diseases. 29th ed. Elk Grove Village, IL: American Academy of Pediatrics.

Table 7-2. Catch-up immunization schedule for children 4 months through 18 years who start late or who are more than 1 month behind—United States, 2013

The table below provides catch-up schedules and minimum intervals between doses for children whose vaccinations have been delayed. A vaccine series does not need to be restarted, regardless of the time that has elapsed between doses. Use the section appropriate for the child's age. Always use this table in conjunction with the accompanying recommended immunization schedule for ages 0–18 years (Table 7-1) and its respective footnotes.

VACCINE	MINIMUM AGE FOR DOSE 1	MINIMUM INTERVAL BETWEEN DOSES			
		DOSE 1 TO DOSE 2	DOSE 2 TO DOSE 3	DOSE 3 TO DOSE 4	DOSE 4 TO DOSE 5
People Aged 4 Months through 6 Years					
Hepatitis B[1]	Birth	**4 weeks**	**8 weeks** (and ≥16 weeks after first dose; minimum age for the final dose is 24 weeks)		
Rotavirus[2]	6 weeks	**4 weeks**	**4 weeks**[2]		
Diphtheria-Tetanus-Pertussis[3,4]	6 weeks	**4 weeks**	**4 weeks**	**6 months**	**6 months**[3]
Haemophilus influenzae type b[5]	6 weeks	**4 weeks** if first dose administered at age <12 months **8 weeks (as final dose)** if first dose administered at age 12–14 months **No further doses needed** if first dose administered at age ≥15 months	**4 weeks**[5] if current age is <12 months **8 weeks (as final dose)**[5] if current age is ≥12 months and first dose administered at age <12 months and second dose administered at age <15 months **No further doses needed** if previous dose administered at age ≥15 months	**8 weeks (as final dose)** This dose only necessary for children aged 12–59 months who received 3 doses before age 12 months	

Vaccine	Minimum Age for Dose 1	Minimum Interval Between Dose 1 to Dose 2	Minimum Interval Between Dose 2 to Dose 3	Minimum Interval Between Dose 3 to Dose 4
Pneumococcal[6]	6 weeks	**4 weeks** if first dose administered at age <12 months **8 weeks (as final dose for healthy children)** if first dose administered at age ≥12 months or current age 24–59 months **No further doses needed** for healthy children if first dose administered at age ≥24 months	**4 weeks** if current age is <12 months **8 weeks (as final dose for healthy children)** if current age is ≥12 months **No further doses needed** for healthy children if previous dose administered at age ≥24 months	**8 weeks (as final dose)** This dose only necessary for children aged 12–59 months who received 3 doses before age 12 months or for children at high risk who received 3 doses at any age
Inactivated Poliovirus[7]	6 weeks	**4 weeks**	**4 weeks**	**6 months**[7] (minimum age 4 years for final dose)
Meningococcal[13]	6 weeks	**8 weeks**[13]	see footnote 13	see footnote 13
Measles-Mumps-Rubella[9]	12 months	**4 weeks**		
Varicella[10]	12 months	**3 months**		
Hepatitis A[11]	12 months	**6 months**		
People Aged 7 through 18 Years				
Tetanus-Diphtheria or Tetanus-Diphtheria-Pertussis[3,4]	7 years[3,4]	**4 weeks**	**4 weeks** if first dose administered at age <12 months **6 months** if first dose administered at age ≥12 months	**6 months** if first dose administered at age <12 months

continued

TABLE 7-2. CATCH-UP IMMUNIZATION SCHEDULE FOR CHILDREN 4 MONTHS THROUGH 18 YEARS WHO START LATE OR WHO ARE MORE THAN 1 MONTH BEHIND—UNITED STATES, 2013 (continued)

VACCINE	MINIMUM AGE FOR DOSE 1	MINIMUM INTERVAL BETWEEN DOSES			
		DOSE 1 TO DOSE 2	DOSE 2 TO DOSE 3	DOSE 3 TO DOSE 4	DOSE 4 TO DOSE 5
Human Papillomavirus[12]	9 years	Routine dosing intervals are recommended[12]			
Hepatitis A[11]	12 months	**6 months**			
Hepatitis B[1]	Birth	**4 weeks**	**8 weeks** [and ≥16 weeks after first dose]		
Inactivated Poliovirus[7]	6 weeks	**4 weeks**	**4 weeks**[7]	**6 months**[7]	
Meningococcal[13]	6 weeks	**8 weeks**[13]			
Measles–Mumps–Rubella[9]	12 months	**4 weeks**			
Varicella[10]	12 months	**3 months** if current age is <13 years **4 weeks** if current age is ≥13 years			

Use the footnotes from Table 7-1 as footnotes for this table.

on an accelerated schedule, which may be necessary before international travel. Proof of yellow fever vaccination is required for entry into certain countries.

MODIFYING THE IMMUNIZATION SCHEDULE FOR INADEQUATELY IMMUNIZED INFANTS AND YOUNGER CHILDREN BEFORE INTERNATIONAL TRAVEL

Several factors influence recommendations for the age at which a vaccine is administered, including age-specific risks of the disease and its complications, the ability of people of a given age to develop an adequate immune response to the vaccine, and potential interference with the immune response by passively transferred maternal antibody.

The routine immunization schedules for infants and children in the United States do not provide specific guidelines for those traveling internationally before the age when specific vaccines and toxoids are routinely recommended. Recommended age limitations are based on potential adverse events (yellow fever vaccine), lack of efficacy data or inadequate immune response (polysaccharide vaccines and influenza vaccine), maternal antibody interference (measles-mumps-rubella vaccine), or lack of safety data. In deciding when to travel with a young infant or child, parents should be advised that the earliest opportunity to receive routinely recommended immunizations in the United States (except for the dose of hepatitis B vaccine at birth) is at age 6 weeks.

Routine Infant and Childhood Vaccinations
Hepatitis B Vaccine
Hepatitis B virus (HBV) is a cause of acute and chronic hepatitis, cirrhosis, and hepatocellular carcinoma. There are >350 million chronically infected people worldwide. The risk of chronic infection is highest when infection occurs in infancy or childhood and declines with age. Infants and children who have not previously been vaccinated and who are traveling to areas where HBV is intermediately or highly endemic are at risk if they are directly exposed to blood (or body fluids containing blood) from the local population. HBV transmission could occur in children if they receive blood transfusions not

screened for HBV surface antigen (HBsAg), are exposed to unsterilized medical or dental equipment, or have continuous close contact with local residents who have open skin lesions (impetigo, scabies, or scratched insect bites).

Hepatitis B vaccine is recommended for all infants in the United States, with the first dose administered soon after birth and before hospital discharge. Infants who did not receive a birth dose of hepatitis B vaccine are recommended to be vaccinated on a 0, 1-month, and 6-months schedule. Infants, children, and adolescents who will travel should receive 3 doses of hepatitis B vaccine before traveling:

- The interval between doses 1 and 2 should be ≥4 weeks.
- The interval between doses 2 and 3 should be ≥8 weeks.
- The interval between doses 1 and 3 should be ≥16 weeks.
- The third dose should not be given before the infant is age 24 weeks.
- An accelerated schedule of 0, 1, 2, and 12 months is an option; the last dose may be given on return from travel.
- A 2-dose series is licensed for adolescents aged 11–15 years, and doses can be separated by 4–6 months.

Diphtheria and Tetanus Toxoid and Pertussis Vaccine
Diphtheria, tetanus, and pertussis each occur worldwide and are endemic in countries with low immunization levels. Infants and children leaving the United States should be immunized before traveling. Optimum protection against diphtheria, tetanus, and pertussis is achieved with ≥3 but preferably 4 doses of diphtheria and tetanus toxoids and acellular pertussis vaccine (DTaP). Two doses of DTaP received at intervals ≥4 weeks apart can provide some protection; however, a single dose offers little protective benefit. Parents should be informed that infants and children who have not received ≥3 doses of DTaP might not be fully protected against pertussis.

The usual series includes 5 doses given at ages 2, 4, 6, 15–18 months, and 4–6 years. The fifth dose is not necessary if the fourth dose in the primary series was given after the child's fourth birthday.

The schedule can be accelerated as soon as the infant is age 6 weeks, with the second and third doses given 4 weeks after each preceding dose. The fourth dose should not be given before the infant is age 12 months and should be separated from the third dose by ≥6 months. The fifth (booster) dose should not be given before the child is age 4 years.

Haemophilus influenzae Type b Conjugate Vaccine

Haemophilus influenzae type b (Hib) is an endemic disease worldwide that can cause fatal meningitis, epiglottitis, and other invasive diseases. Infants and children should have optimal protection before traveling. Routine Hib vaccination beginning at age 2 months is recommended for all US children. The first dose may be given when an infant is as young as 6 weeks. Children aged <6 weeks should not be given Hib vaccine, because it may induce immune tolerance to subsequent vaccines.

A primary series consists of 2 or 3 doses (depending on the brand of vaccine used) with a minimum interval of 4 weeks between doses. A booster dose is recommended when the infant is age ≥12 months and ≥8 weeks have passed since the previous dose. If Hib vaccination is started when the infant or child is age ≥7 months, fewer doses are required.

Considerations for travel by age include the following:

- If previously unvaccinated, infants aged <15 months should receive ≥2 vaccine doses before travel. An interval as short as 4 weeks between these 2–3 doses is acceptable.
- Unvaccinated infants and children aged 15–59 months should receive a single dose of Hib vaccine.
- Children aged >59 months, adolescents, and adults do not need to be vaccinated unless a specific condition exists, such as functional or anatomic asplenia, immunodeficiency, immunosuppression, or HIV infection.

If different brands of vaccine are administered, a total of 3 doses of Hib conjugate vaccine completes the primary series. After completion of the primary infant vaccination series, any of the licensed Hib conjugate vaccines may be used for the booster dose when the infant is age 12–15 months.

Polio Vaccine

Although polio has been eliminated in the United States, poliovirus continues to circulate in other parts of the world. In the United States, all infants and children should receive 4 doses of inactivated poliovirus vaccine (IPV) at ages 2, 4, 6–18 months, and 4–6 years. If accelerated protection is needed, the minimum age for the first dose is 6 weeks and the minimum interval between the first and second doses and between the second and third doses is 4 weeks. The minimum interval between the third and fourth doses is 6 months. The final dose in the IPV series should be administered at age ≥4 years, regardless of the number of previous doses. If a child has received 4 doses of poliovirus vaccine before the fourth birthday, a fifth dose is recommended; the minimum interval between the fourth and fifth doses should be ≥6 months.

Rotavirus Vaccine

Rotavirus is the most common cause of severe gastroenteritis in infants and young children worldwide. In developing countries, rotavirus gastroenteritis is responsible for approximately 500,000 deaths per year among children aged <5 years. Routine rotavirus vaccination beginning at age 2 months is recommended for all US infants.

Two rotavirus vaccines, RotaTeq (RV5) and Rotarix (RV1), are licensed for use in US infants. RV5 is administered orally in a 3-dose series at ages 2, 4, and 6 months. RV1 is administered orally in a 2-dose series at ages 2 and 4 months (see Table 7-3). The minimum age for the first dose of rotavirus vaccine is 6 weeks; the maximum age for the first dose is 14 weeks, 6 days. Vaccination should not be initiated for infants aged ≥15 weeks, 0 days because of insufficient data on the safety of the first dose of rotavirus vaccine in older infants. The minimum interval between doses of rotavirus vaccine is 4 weeks. All doses should be administered before age 8 months, 0 days.

Measles, Mumps, and Rubella Vaccine

Measles is an endemic, highly communicable disease in many countries; outbreaks may occur in countries throughout the world where vaccination rates are suboptimal, including Europe. International travelers are

Table 7-3. Schedule for administration of rotavirus vaccine

	RV5 (ROTATEQ; MERCK)	RV1 (ROTARIX; GLAXOSMITHKLINE)
Number of doses in series	3	2
Recommended ages for doses	2, 4, and 6 months	2 and 4 months
Minimum age for first dose	6 weeks	
Maximum age for first dose	14 weeks, 6 days	
Minimum interval between doses	4 weeks	
Maximum age for last dose	8 months, 0 days	

at increased risk for measles exposure. Infants and children should be protected against measles, and the 2-dose immunization series should be completed before traveling, if possible. While the risk for serious disease from either mumps or rubella is low, these diseases circulate in many parts of the world, and vaccination is recommended.

Monovalent measles, mumps, and rubella vaccines are not currently available in the United States. The Advisory Committee for Immunization Practices (ACIP) recommends that measles-mumps-rubella (MMR) or measles-mumps-rubella-varicella (MMRV) vaccines be administered when any of the individual components is indicated as part of the routine immunization schedule. MMRV vaccine is licensed for children aged 12 months to 12 years. However, the risk of seizures after vaccination is increased if MMRV is used for the first dose in the series between the ages of 12 and 47 months. So for this dose, MMR and varicella administered separately are preferred over MMRV. The combination product MMRV is generally recommended for the second dose of the series, or for the first dose if it is given to a child aged 47 months through 12 years.

Two doses of MMR are routinely recommended for all children, usually at age 12 months and again at age 4–6 years. The second dose of MMR can be given as soon as 28 days after the first dose.

Children traveling abroad should be vaccinated at an earlier age than children remaining in the United States if their travel schedule requires departure prior to the usual dosing of vaccines. Children aged 6–11 months should receive 1 dose of MMR vaccine. Infants vaccinated before age 12 months should be vaccinated with 2 additional doses of MMR or MMRV vaccine on or after the first birthday, according to the routinely recommended schedule. Children aged ≥12 months traveling internationally should receive 2 doses of MMR vaccine, separated by ≥28 days.

Varicella Vaccine

Varicella (chickenpox) is an endemic disease throughout the world. Two doses of varicella vaccine are routinely recommended for all children and adolescents without evidence of varicella immunity. The first dose is recommended at age 12–15 months. The second dose is recommended at age 4–6 years but can be given earlier, provided that ≥3 months have passed since the first dose.

Efforts should be made to ensure varicella immunity before age 13 years, because varicella disease can be more severe among older children and adults. Children aged ≥13 should receive 2 doses of varicella vaccine 4–8 weeks apart.

Vaccination is not necessary for children with a history of documented chickenpox. When a history of chickenpox is uncertain, the vaccine should be given.

Meningococcal Vaccine

Meningococcal disease, caused by the bacterium *Neisseria meningitidis*, is associated with high morbidity and mortality. Epidemics occur in sub-Saharan Africa during the dry season, December through June (see Map 3-11), and CDC recommends that travelers be vaccinated before traveling to this region. Meningococcal vaccination is a requirement to enter Saudi Arabia when traveling to Mecca during the annual Hajj. Health requirements and recommendations for US travelers planning to travel to Saudi Arabia for Hajj are available each year on the CDC Travelers' Health website after these recommendations are determined (www.cdc.gov/travel).

Three vaccines are available in the United States that protect against the 4 serogroups of *N. meningitidis* (A, C, Y, and W-135): 2 meningococcal conjugate vaccines (MenACWY) and 1 meningococcal polysaccharide vaccine (MPSV4). The 2 conjugate vaccines are differentiated by their protein conjugate. A 1-dose primary series of MenACWY-D (Menactra) is licensed for people aged 2–55 years; a 2-dose primary series of MenACWY-D is licensed for children aged 9–23 months. MenACWY-Crm (Menveo) is licensed for people aged 2–55 years.

Routine MenACWY booster vaccination is recommended in adolescents 5 years after the first dose. CDC recommends routine vaccination of people with MenACWY at age 11 or 12 years, with a booster dose at age 16 years. For adolescents who receive the first dose at age 13-15 years, a one-time booster dose should be administered, preferably at age 16–18 years. People who receive their first dose of MenACWY at or after age 16 years do not need a booster dose, unless they remain at continued risk for meningococcal disease.

Meningococcal vaccine is also recommended for children aged 9 months through 10 years who travel to or reside in areas where *N. meningitidis* is hyperendemic or epidemic. A conjugate product is preferred where licensed for a person's age group, and providers should take care to use a meningococcal vaccine that is licensed for a particular age. MPSV4 (licensed for people aged ≥2 years) can be used when neither MenACWY vaccine is available.

Age considerations:

- The serogroup A polysaccharide in MPSV4 induces an antibody response in some children as young as 3 months. Thus, vaccinating infants traveling to high-risk areas can provide some degree of protection.
- For children vaccinated with either MPSV4 or MenACWY at age <7 years, revaccination with MenACWY in 3 years is recommended, if the children remain at high risk for infection and every 5 years thereafter, if they remain at continued risk.
- For children vaccinated with either MPSV4 or MenACWY at age ≥7 years, revaccination with MenACWY is recommended in 5 years if they remain at high risk and every 5 years thereafter if they remain at continued risk.

Pneumococcal Vaccines

Streptococcus pneumoniae is a leading cause of illness and death worldwide. In the United States, 2 vaccines are available to prevent pneumococcal disease: the 13-valent pneumococcal conjugate vaccine (PCV13) is recommended for routine use in children aged ≤5 years, and the pneumococcal polysaccharide vaccine (PPSV23) is recommended for children and adults aged ≥2 years who have certain underlying medical conditions and for all adults aged ≥65 years. Before March 2010, the 7-valent conjugate vaccine (PCV7) was used. Licensure of PCV13 with its improved serotype protection has replaced PCV7 on the same schedule.

All infants should be vaccinated with PCV13. Infant vaccination provides the earliest protection, and children aged <2 years have high rates of pneumococcal disease. The primary series for PCV13 includes 3 doses given at ages 2, 4, and 6 months, with a fourth (booster) dose at age 12–15 months. Children who have been completely vaccinated with PCV7 should receive a single dose of PCV13 between the ages of 14 and 59 months. For children at risk of invasive *S. pneumoniae* disease, this supplemental dose is recommended through age 71 months.

Children aged ≥2 years who are at high risk for pneumococcal disease (such as those

7

with sickle cell disease, asplenia, HIV, chronic illness, or immunocompromising conditions) should receive a dose of PPSV23 ≥2 months after their last dose of PCV13. A second dose of PPSV23 is recommended 5 years after the first dose of PPSV23 for people aged ≥2 years who are immunocompromised, have sickle cell disease, or have functional or anatomic asplenia.

All healthy children aged 24–59 months who have not completed any recommended schedule for PCV7 should receive 1 dose of PCV13. All children up to age 71 months who have underlying medical conditions and have received 3 doses of PCV7 should receive 1 dose of PCV13. This includes those who have previously received PPSV23. All children aged 24–59 months who have underlying medical conditions and have received <3 doses and have not received any doses after age 12 months should receive 2 doses of PCV13 ≥8 weeks apart. A single dose of PCV13 vaccine is recommended for children 6–18 years with immunocompromising conditions, cerebrospinal fluid leak, or cochlear implants.

Influenza Vaccine

Influenza viruses circulate predominantly in the winter months in temperate regions (typically November–April in the Northern Hemisphere and April–September in the Southern Hemisphere) but can occur year-round in tropical climates. ACIP recommends annual influenza vaccination of all people aged ≥6 months as the most effective measure for preventing influenza and its associated complications. Prevention of influenza is particularly important for people who are (or who live with those who are) at increased risk for influenza-related complications, such as children aged <5 years (particularly infants aged <6 months, who are not eligible for influenza vaccination), people with medical conditions (such as immunosuppression, diabetes, asthma, pregnancy, and neurologic disorders) and children and adolescents who are receiving long-term aspirin therapy.

Two types of influenza vaccines are available for use in the United States for children: trivalent inactivated vaccine (TIV), administered by intramuscular injection; and live, attenuated influenza vaccine (LAIV), administered by nasal spray. LAIV is approved for use only in healthy people aged 2–49 years who are not pregnant. LAIV may result in an increase in asthma or reactive airway disease in children aged <5 years; therefore, LAIV should not be administered to children aged <2 years or to children aged 2–4 years who have a history of wheezing in the past year or who have been diagnosed with asthma.

Children receiving TIV should be administered an age-appropriate dose (0.25 mL for those aged 6–35 months and 0.5 mL for those aged ≥36 months). One dose of influenza vaccine per season is recommended for most people. Children aged <9 years who have not received ≥2 doses of seasonal influenza vaccine since July 1, 2010 should receive 2 doses separated by a 4-week interval. Only 1 dose per year is needed in previously unvaccinated children aged ≥9 years. More specific information about these influenza vaccine recommendations can be found on the CDC website (www.cdc.gov/flu).

Hepatitis A Vaccine or Immune Globulin for Hepatitis A

Hepatitis A virus (HAV) is endemic in most parts of the world, and children traveling to these areas are at increased risk for acquiring HAV infection. Although HAV is often not severe in infants and children aged <5 years, infected children may transmit the infection to older children and adults, who are at risk for severe disease.

Hepatitis A vaccine

Hepatitis A vaccine is a routine immunization of childhood in the United States. It is recommended for all children at age 1 year (12–23 months), although vaccination coverage is currently ≤50%. Vaccination should be ensured for all children traveling to areas where there is an intermediate or high risk of HAV infection. Because of the potential interference by maternal antibody, the hepatitis A vaccine is not approved for children aged <1 year. The HAV vaccine series consists of 2 doses ≥6 months apart. One dose of monovalent hepatitis A vaccine administered at any time before departure can provide adequate protection for most healthy children. The second dose is necessary for long-term protection.

Immune globulin

Children aged <1 year who are traveling to high-risk areas can receive immune globulin (IG). For optimal protection, children aged

≥1 year who are immunocompromised or have chronic medical conditions and who are planning to depart to a high-risk area in <2 weeks should receive the initial dose of vaccine, along with IG (0.02 mL/kg intramuscularly) at a separate anatomic injection site.

IG does not interfere with the response to yellow fever vaccine but can interfere with the response to other live injected vaccines (such as MMR and varicella vaccines). Administration of MMR vaccine should be delayed for ≥5 months (immunocompetent children) or ≥6 months (immunocompromised children) and varicella vaccine for >5 months after administration of IG. IG should not be administered for 2 weeks after measles-, mumps-, rubella-, and varicella-containing vaccines unless the benefits exceed those of vaccination. If IG is given during this time, the child should be revaccinated with the live MMR and varicella vaccines ≥3 months after administration of IG. When travel plans do not allow adequate time to administer live vaccines and IG before travel, the severity of the diseases and their epidemiology at the destination will help determine the most appropriate course of preparation.

Human Papillomavirus Vaccine

Human papillomavirus (HPV) infection can be prevented with 2 licensed vaccines. One vaccine, HPV4, protects against HPV types 6, 11, 16, and 18; the other, HPV2, protects against types 16 and 18. Both protect against cervical cancer, and HPV4 also protects against genital warts. HPV vaccination is recommended for girls aged 11–12 years with catch-up vaccination recommended through 26 years. HPV vaccination is recommended for boys aged 11–12 years with catch-up vaccination recommended through age 21 years. HPV2 is licensed for girls/women aged 10–25 years and HPV4 is licensed for girls/women and boys/men aged 9–26 years. The schedule for both vaccines is 3 doses at 0, 1–2, and 6 months. The minimum interval between dose 1 and dose 2 is 4 weeks. Dose 3 should be given ≥12 weeks after dose 2.

Other Vaccines
Yellow Fever Vaccine

Yellow fever, a disease transmitted by mosquitoes, is endemic in certain areas of Africa and South America (see Maps 3-16 and 3-17).

Proof of yellow fever vaccination is required for entry into some countries (see Chapter 3, Travel Vaccines & Malaria Information, by Country). Infants and children aged ≥9 months can be vaccinated if they travel to countries within the yellow fever-endemic zone.

Infants aged <9 months are at higher risk for developing encephalitis from yellow fever vaccine, a live virus vaccine. Vaccination of infants should be considered on an individual basis. Although the incidence of these adverse events has not been clearly defined, 14 of 18 reported cases of postvaccination encephalitis were in infants aged <4 months. One fatal case confirmed by viral isolation was in a 3-year-old child.

Travelers with infants aged <9 months should be advised against traveling to areas within the yellow fever-endemic zone. ACIP recommends that yellow fever vaccine *never* be given to infants aged <6 months. Infants ages 6–8 months should be vaccinated only if they must travel to areas of ongoing epidemic yellow fever and if a high level of protection against mosquito bites is not possible (see Chapter 3, Yellow Fever). Physicians considering vaccinating infants aged 6–8 months may contact their respective state health departments or CDC toll-free at 800-CDC-INFO (800-232-4636).

Typhoid Vaccine

Typhoid fever is caused by the bacterium *Salmonella enterica* serotype Typhi. Vaccination is recommended for travelers to areas where there is a recognized risk of exposure to S. Typhi.

Two typhoid vaccines are available: Vi capsular polysaccharide vaccine (ViCPS) administered intramuscularly and oral live attenuated vaccine (Ty21a). Both vaccines induce a protective response in 50%–80% of recipients. The ViCPS vaccine can be administered to children who are aged ≥2 years, with a booster dose 2 years later, if continued protection is needed. The Ty21a vaccine, which consists of a series of 4 capsules (1 taken every other day) can be administered to children aged ≥6 years. A booster series for Ty21a should be taken every 5 years, if indicated. The capsule cannot be opened for administration but must be swallowed whole. All 4 doses should be taken ≥1 week before potential exposure.

Japanese Encephalitis Vaccine

Japanese encephalitis (JE) virus is transmitted by mosquitoes and is endemic throughout Asia. The risk can be seasonal in temperate climates and year-round in more tropical climates. The risk to short-term travelers and those who confine their travel to urban centers is low. Travelers who plan to travel for ≥1 month or take up residence in an endemic area should be vaccinated against JE. The decision to vaccinate a child should follow the more detailed recommendations in Chapter 3, Japanese Encephalitis.

JE-Vax, an inactivated mouse brain–derived vaccine, was licensed in the United States in 1992 for use in travelers aged ≥1 year. However, JE-Vax is no longer manufactured, and all remaining doses expired in 2011. A new, inactivated Vero cell culture–derived JE vaccine (trade name Ixiaro [Intercell Biomedical]) was licensed by the Food and Drug Administration in 2009 for use in the United States for travelers aged ≥17 years. Ixiaro is not approved for use in children aged <17 years. Pediatric clinical trials are being conducted to enable licensure of Ixiaro for use in children.

Three options exist for children who require JE protection: 1) enrollment in a clinical trial through the manufacturer, 2) off-label use of Ixiaro, and 3) obtaining vaccine at a travel clinic in the destination country. All options require discussion with the traveling family. Details can be obtained at www.cdc.gov/ncidod/dvbid/jencephalitis/children.htm and through the manufacturer.

Rabies Vaccine

Rabies virus causes an acute viral encephalitis that is virtually 100% fatal. Traveling children may be at increased risk of rabies exposure, mainly from dogs who roam the streets in developing countries. Bat bites carry a potential risk of rabies throughout the world. There are 2 strategies to prevent rabies in humans:

- Avoiding animal bites or scratches.
- A 3-shot preexposure immunization series, on days 0, 7, and 21 or 28. In the event of a subsequent possible rabies virus exposure, the child will require 2 more doses of rabies vaccine on days 0 and 3. The decision whether to obtain preexposure immunization for children should follow the recommendations in Chapter 3, Rabies.

For children who have not received preexposure immunization and may have been exposed to rabies, a weight-based dose of human rabies immune globulin and a series of 4 rabies vaccine injections are required on days 0, 3, 7, and 14.

BIBLIOGRAPHY

1. Broder KR, Cortese MM, Iskander JK, Kretsinger K, Slade BA, Brown KH, et al. Preventing tetanus, diphtheria, and pertussis among adolescents: use of tetanus toxoid, reduced diphtheria toxoid and acellular pertussis vaccines—recommendations of the Advisory Committee on Immunization Practices (ACIP). MMWR Recomm Rep. 2006 Mar 24;55(RR-3):1–34.
2. CDC. Epidemiology and Prevention of Vaccine-Preventable Diseases. 12th ed. Atkinson W, Wolfe S, Hamborsky J, editors. Washington, DC: Public Health Foundation; 2012 [cited 2012 Sep 26]. Available from: http://www.cdc.gov/vaccines/pubs/pinkbook/index.html.
3. CDC. Licensure of a 13-valent pneumococcal conjugate vaccine (PCV13) and recommendations for use among children—Advisory Committee on Immunization Practices (ACIP), 2010. MMWR Morb Mortal Wkly Rep. 2010 Mar 12;59(9):258–61.
4. CDC. Notice to readers: recommendation from the Advisory Committee on Immunization Practices (ACIP) for use of quadrivalent meningococcal conjugate vaccine (MCV4) in children aged 2–10 years at increased risk for invasive meningococcal disease. MMWR Morb Mortal Wkly Rep. 2007;56(48):1265–6.
5. CDC. Recommendation of the Advisory Committee on Immunization Practices (ACIP) for use of quadrivalent meningococcal conjugate vaccine (MenACWY-D) among children aged 9 through 23 months at increased risk for invasive meningococcal disease. MMWR Morb Mortal Wkly Rep. 2011 Oct 14;60(40):1391–2.
6. CDC. Recommendations for use of a booster dose of inactivated Vero cell culture–derived Japanese encephalitis vaccine: Advisory Committee on Immunization Practices, 2011. MMWR Morb Mortal Wkly Rep. 2011 May 27;60(20):661–3.
7. CDC. Revised recommendations of the Advisory Committee on Immunization Practices to vaccinate all persons aged 11–18 years with meningococcal conjugate vaccine. MMWR Morb Mortal Wkly Rep. 2007 Aug 10;56(31):794–5.

7

8. CDC. Update on Japanese encephalitis vaccine for children: United States, May 2011. MMWR Morb Mortal Wkly Rep. 2011 May 27;60(20):664–5.

9. CDC. Updated recommendations for use of meningococcal conjugate vaccines—Advisory Committee on Immunization Practices (ACIP), 2010. MMWR Morb Mortal Wkly Rep. 2011 Jan 28;60(3):72–6.

10. CDC. Updated recommendations of the Advisory Committee on Immunization Practices (ACIP) regarding routine poliovirus vaccination. MMWR Morb Mortal Wkly Rep. 2009 Aug 7;58(30):829–30.

11. Cortese MM, Parashar UD. Prevention of rotavirus gastroenteritis among infants and children: recommendations of the Advisory Committee on Immunization Practices (ACIP). MMWR Recomm Rep. 2009 Feb 6;58(RR-2):1–25.

12. Fiore AE, Shay DK, Broder K, Iskander JK, Uyeki TM, Mootrey G, et al. Prevention and control of seasonal influenza with vaccines: recommendations of the Advisory Committee on Immunization Practices (ACIP), 2009. MMWR Recomm Rep. 2009 Jul 31;58(RR-8):1–52. Erratum in: MMWR Recomm Rep. 2009 Aug 21;58(32):896–7.

13. Fiore AE, Wasley A, Bell BP. Prevention of hepatitis A through active or passive immunization: recommendations of the Advisory Committee on Immunization Practices (ACIP). MMWR Recomm Rep. 2006 May 19;55(RR-7):1–23.

14. Fischer M, Lindsey N, Staples JE, Hills S. Japanese encephalitis vaccines: recommendations of the Advisory Committee on Immunization Practices (ACIP). MMWR Recomm Rep. 2010 Mar 12;59(RR-1):1–27.

15. Marin M, Broder KR, Temte JL, Snider DE, Seward JF. Use of combination measles, mumps, rubella, and varicella vaccine: recommendations of the Advisory Committee on Immunization Practices (ACIP). MMWR Recomm Rep. 2010 May 7;59(RR-3):1–12.

16. Mast EE, Margolis HS, Fiore AE, Brink EW, Goldstein ST, Wang SA, et al. A comprehensive immunization strategy to eliminate transmission of hepatitis B virus infection in the United States: recommendations of the Advisory Committee on Immunization Practices (ACIP) part 1: immunization of infants, children, and adolescents. MMWR Recomm Rep. 2005 Dec 23;54(RR-16):1–31.

17. Rupprecht CE, Briggs D, Brown CM, Franka R, Katz SL, Kerr HD, et al. Use of a reduced (4-dose) vaccine schedule for postexposure prophylaxis to prevent human rabies: recommendations of the Advisory Committee on Immunization Practices. MMWR Recomm Rep. 2010 Mar 19;59(RR-2):1–9.

18. Staples JE, Gershman M, Fischer M. Yellow fever vaccine: recommendations of the Advisory Committee on Immunization Practices (ACIP). MMWR Recomm Rep. 2010 Jul 30;59(RR-7):1–27.

TRAVEL & BREASTFEEDING
Katherine Shealy, Jessica Allen

The medical preparation of a traveler who is breastfeeding differs only slightly from that of other travelers and depends in part on whether the mother and child will be separated or together during travel. Most mothers should be advised to continue breastfeeding their infants throughout travel. Before departure, mothers may wish to carry with them a list of local breastfeeding resources at their destination. Clinicians may be able to help breastfeeding mothers find out about available breastfeeding support experts at their destination through sources that include:

- International Board-Certified Lactation Consultants (IBCLCs)—health professionals in approximately 50 countries who specialize in the clinical management of breastfeeding (www.iblce.org).
- La Leche League Leaders (LLLLs)—trained and accredited volunteer mothers in approximately 60 countries who provide mother-to-mother breastfeeding support and help (www.llli.org).

Mothers who plan to use a breast pump while traveling may need an electrical current adapter and converter and should have a backup option available, including written instructions for hand expression (for more detailed instructions about hand expression, see www.workandpump.com/handexpression.htm).

IMMUNIZATIONS AND MEDICATIONS

In almost all situations, clinicians can and should select immunizations and medications that are compatible with breastfeeding. In most circumstances, it is inappropriate to counsel mothers to wean in order to be vaccinated or to withhold vaccination due to breastfeeding status.

Breastfeeding and lactation do not affect maternal or infant dosage guidelines for any immunization or medication; children always require their own immunization or medication, regardless of maternal dose. In the absence of documented risk to the breastfeeding child of a particular maternal medication, the known risks of stopping breastfeeding generally outweigh a theoretical risk of exposure via breastfeeding.

Immunizations

Breastfeeding mothers and children should be vaccinated according to routine, recommended schedules; only preventive vaccinia (smallpox) vaccine is contraindicated for use in breastfeeding mothers. Administration of most live and inactivated vaccines does not affect breastfeeding, breast milk, or the process of lactation.

Special Consideration: Yellow Fever Vaccination

Whether this vaccine is excreted in human milk is unknown. However, at least 3 cases of yellow fever vaccine–associated neurologic disease have been documented in infants, presumably associated with breastfeeding transmission of yellow fever vaccine virus. No testing has been done to detect the yellow fever vaccine virus in breast milk, so it can only be said that the vaccine virus was transmitted during breastfeeding, but it has not been definitively determined that transmission occurred via the breast milk. Therefore, breastfeeding is a precaution to yellow fever vaccination, and women should be cautioned to avoid this vaccination while breastfeeding. Since risk exists and there are many gaps in knowledge, breastfeeding mothers should be discouraged from traveling to yellow fever–endemic areas. However, if travel to a yellow fever–endemic area cannot be avoided or postponed, then the mother should be vaccinated.

Medications

The American Academy of Pediatrics (AAP) 2001 Policy Statement: The Transfer of Drugs and Other Chemicals into Human Milk provides an overview of the compatibility or effects on breastfeeding of approximately 250 drugs. The pharmaceutical reference guide, Medications and Mothers' Milk, is updated every 2 years and provides a comprehensive review of the compatibility or effects on breastfeeding of approximately 1,000 drugs, including generic and trade names, AAP recommendations, risk categories, pharmacologic properties, interactions with other drugs, suitable alternatives, theoretic and relative child dose, pediatric half-life, and many other concerns.

Special Consideration: Antimalarial Medications

Since chloroquine and mefloquine may be safely prescribed to infants, both are considered safe to prescribe to mothers who are breastfeeding. Most experts consider short-term use of doxycycline compatible with breastfeeding. Primaquine may be used for breastfeeding mothers and children with normal glucose-6-phosphate dehydrogenase (G6PD) levels. Breastfeeding mothers should not use atovaquone-proguanil when the breastfeeding infant weighs <5 kg (about 11 lb).

AIR TRAVEL

X-rays used in airport screenings have no effect on breastfeeding, breast milk, or the process of lactation. Airlines typically consider breast pumps as personal items to be carried onboard, similar to laptop computers, handbags, and diaper bags.

Before departure, mothers who will be traveling by air and expect to have expressed milk with them during travel need to carefully plan how they will transport their milk. Airport security regulations for passengers carrying expressed milk vary internationally and are subject to change. In the United States, the Transportation Security Administration (TSA) recognizes expressed milk in the category of liquid medications that may be carried on, regardless of whether the breastfeeding child is traveling, as long as it is declared before screening. TSA recommends that travelers carrying expressed milk have with them a printed copy of the TSA website page www.tsa.gov/travelers/airtravel/children/formula.shtm to help prevent problems at security checkpoints.

Travelers carrying expressed milk in checked luggage should refer to cooler pack storage guidelines in "Proper Handling and Storage of Human Milk" on CDC's website (www.cdc.gov/breastfeeding/recommendations/handling_breastmilk.htm) to protect milk during travel. Expressed milk is not considered a biohazard. International Air Transport Authority regulations for shipping category B biological substances (UN 3373) do not apply to expressed milk; it is considered a food for individual use. Travelers shipping frozen milk should follow guidelines for shipping other frozen foods and liquids. Expressed milk does not need to be declared at US Customs upon return to the United States.

TRAVELING WITH A BREASTFEEDING CHILD

Breastfeeding provides unique benefits to mothers and children traveling together. Health clinicians should explain clearly to breastfeeding mothers the value of continuing breastfeeding during travel. Exclusive breast milk feeding (only breast milk, no other food or drink) protects infants from exposure to contamination and pathogens via foods or liquids. Additionally, feeding only at the breast protects infants from exposure to contamination from containers (bottles, cups, utensils).

Breastfeeding infants require no water supplementation, even in extreme heat environments. Breastfeeding protects children from eustachian tube pain and collapse during air travel, especially during ascent and descent, by allowing them to stabilize and gradually equalize internal and external air pressure, which cannot be replicated by sucking on a bottle or pacifier.

Clinicians should offer information to breastfeeding mothers so that they are better able to continue breastfeeding during travel. Frequent, unrestricted breastfeeding opportunities ensure the mother's milk supply remains ample and the child's nutrition and hydration are ideal. Safe use of a fabric infant carrier helps maintain breastfeeding by increasing breastfeeding opportunities and skin-to-skin contact with the child, while also protecting the child from environmental hazards and easing the burden of carrying a heavy child. Mothers who are concerned about breastfeeding away from home may breastfeed modestly with the child in a fabric carrier. In many countries around the world, breastfeeding in public places is more widely practiced than in the United States. US federal legislation protects mothers' and children's right to breastfeed on federal property, which includes US Customs areas, embassies, and consulates overseas.

Special Consideration: Travelers' Diarrhea

Exclusive breastfeeding protects infants against travelers' diarrhea. Breastfeeding is ideal rehydration therapy. Children who are suspected of having travelers' diarrhea should breastfeed more frequently. Children in this situation should not be offered other fluids or foods that replace breastfeeding. Breastfeeding mothers with travelers' diarrhea should continue breastfeeding and increase their own fluid intake. The organisms that cause travelers' diarrhea do not pass through breast milk. Breastfeeding mothers should not use bismuth subsalicylate compounds, because they may transfer salicylate to the child. Use of oral rehydration salts is fully compatible with breastfeeding.

TRAVELING WITHOUT A BREASTFEEDING CHILD

A breastfeeding mother traveling without her breastfeeding infant or child may wish to express and store a supply of milk to be fed to the infant or child during her absence. Building a supply to be fed in her absence takes time and patience and is most successful when begun gradually, many weeks in advance of the mother's departure. Infants who have never drunk milk from a bottle or cup need opportunities to practice this skill with another caregiver before the mother's departure.

A mother's milk supply can diminish if she does not express milk while away from her nursing child, but this does not need to be a reason to stop breastfeeding. Clinicians should help mothers determine the best course for breastfeeding based on a variety of factors, including the amount of time she has to prepare for her trip, her flexibility of time while traveling, her options for express-ing and storing milk while traveling, the duration of her travel, and her destination. A mother who returns to her nursing infant or child can continue breastfeeding and, if necessary, supplement as needed until her milk supply returns to its prior level. Often,

after a mother returns from travel, her nurs-ing infant or child will help bring her milk supply to its prior level. However, nurs-ing infants or children who are separated from their mother for an extended time may have difficulty transitioning back to breastfeeding.

BIBLIOGRAPHY

1. The Academy of Breastfeeding Medicine Protocol Committee. ABM clinical protocol #8: human milk storage information for home use for full-term infants. Breastfeeding Medicine [Internet]. 2010 [cited 2012 Sep 26]. Available from: http://www.bfmed.org/Resources/Protocols.aspx.
2. American Academy of Pediatrics Committee on Drugs. Transfer of drugs and other chemicals into human milk. Pediatrics. 2001 Sep;108(3):776–89.
3. CDC. Transmission of yellow fever vaccine virus through breast-feeding—Brazil, 2009. MMWR Morb Mortal Wkly Rep. 2010 Feb 12;59(5):130–2.
4. CDC. Update: universal precautions for prevention of transmission of human immunodeficiency virus, hepatitis B virus, and other bloodborne pathogens in health-care settings. MMWR Morb Mortal Wkly Rep. 1988 Jun 24;37(24):377–82, 87–8.
5. Hale TW. Medications and mothers' milk 2008. 13th ed. Amarillo, TX: Pharmasoft Medical Publishing; 2008.
6. Kroger AT, Sumaya CV, Pickering L, Atkinson WL. General recommendations on immunization—recommendations of the Advisory Committee on Immunization Practices (ACIP). MMWR Recomm Rep. 2011 Jan 28;60(2):1–64.
7. Sachdev HP, Krishna J, Puri RK, Satyanarayana L, Kumar S. Water supplementation in exclusively breastfed infants during summer in the tropics. Lancet. 1991 Apr 20;337(8747):929–33.
8. Section on Breastfeeding. Breastfeeding and the use of human milk. Pediatrics. 2012 Mar;129(3):e827–41.
9. Staples JE, Gershman M, Fischer M. Yellow fever vaccine: recommendations of the Advisory Committee on Immunization Practices (ACIP). MMWR Recomm Rep. 2010 Jul 30;59(RR-7):1–27.

INTERNATIONAL ADOPTION

Cynthia R. Howard, Chandy C. John

OVERVIEW

In 2011, 9,504 internationally adopted chil-dren arrived in the United States, compared with an average of 21,400 each year from 2003 through 2007 and 13,700 each year from 2008 through 2010. The number of internationally adopted children and their countries of birth are in constant flux. Consequently, the epide-miology of diseases in these children shifts. In 2011, the 12 most common countries of ori-gin for internationally adopted children were, in descending order, China, Ethiopia, Russia, South Korea, Ukraine, India, Philippines, Colombia, Taiwan, Uganda, Haiti, and Nigeria (Map 7-1). In 2011, 15% of internationally adopted children were aged <1 year, 55% were aged 1–4 years, and 30% were aged ≥5 years; 56% were girls.

Families traveling to unite with their adoptive child, siblings who wait at home for the child's arrival, extended family mem-bers, and child care providers all are at risk for acquiring infectious diseases secondary to travel or contact with the newly arrived child. International adoptees are usually underimmunized and are at increased risk for infections such as measles, hepatitis A, and hepatitis B because of crowded living conditions, malnutrition, lack of clean water, lack of immunizations, and exposure to endemic diseases that are not common in the United States. Challenges in providing care to

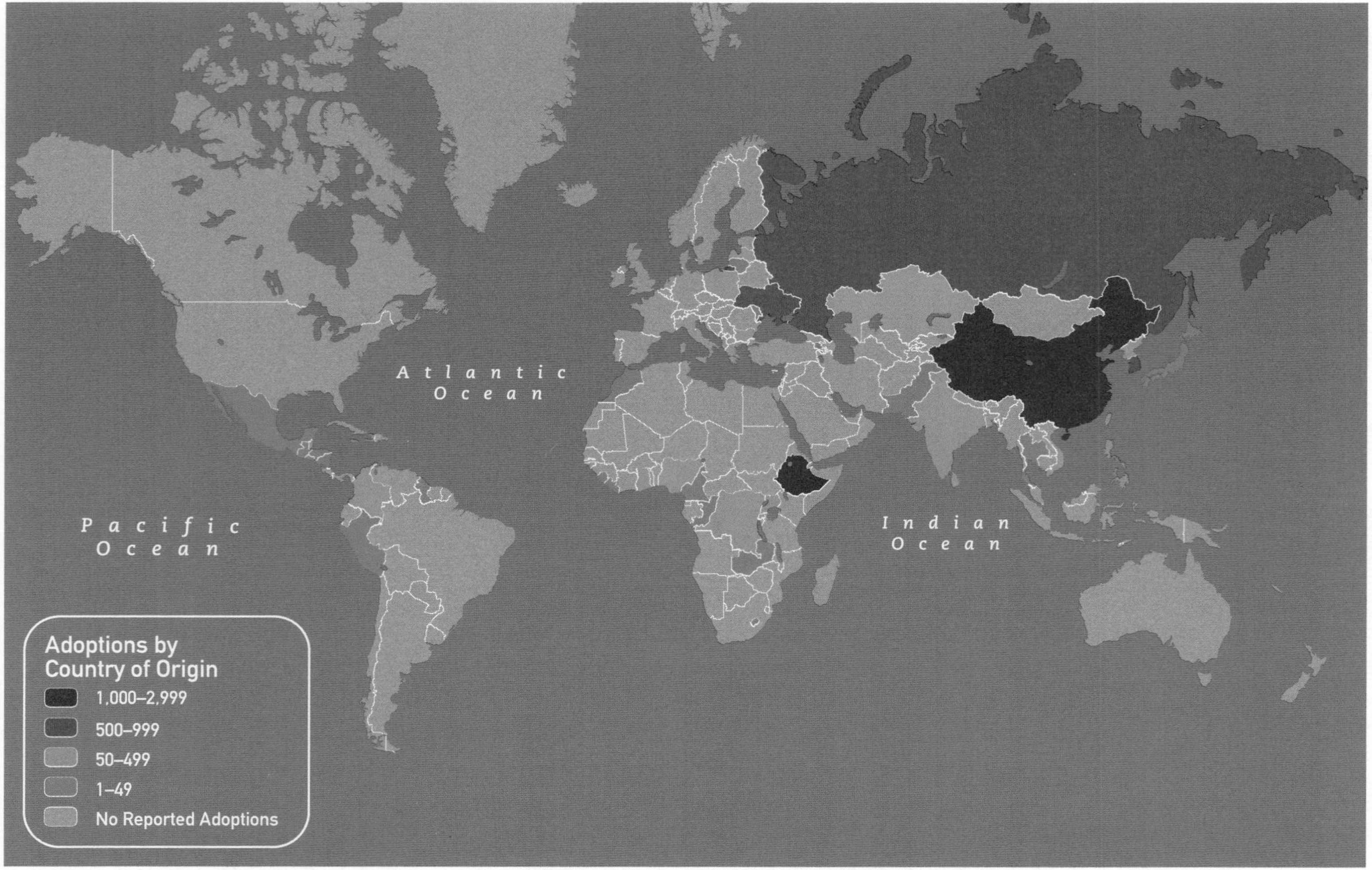

MAP 7-1. COUNTRIES OF ORIGIN OF ADOPTED CHILDREN IMMIGRATING TO THE UNITED STATES, 2011[1]

Adoptions by Country of Origin
- 1,000–2,999
- 500–999
- 50–499
- 1–49
- No Reported Adoptions

[1] Data from US Department of Homeland Security. Yearbook of Immigration Statistics: 2011. Washington, DC: US Department of Homeland Security, Office of Immigration Statistics; 2012.

INTERNATIONAL TRAVEL WITH INFANTS & CHILDREN

internationally adopted children include the absence of medical history, lack of availability of biological family history, questionable reliability of immunization records, variation in preadoption living standards, varying disease epidemiology in the countries of origin, the presence of previously unidentified medical problems, and the increased risk for developmental delays in these children.

TRAVEL PREPARATION FOR ADOPTIVE PARENTS AND THEIR FAMILIES

A pre-travel visit is strongly recommended for prospective adoptive parents. In preparation, the travel health provider must know the disease risks in the adoptive child's country of origin and the medical and social histories of the adoptee (if available), as well as which family members will be traveling, their immunization and medical histories, the season of travel, and length of stay in the country.

Family members who remain at home, including extended family, should be current on their routine immunizations, as recommended by the Advisory Committee on Immunization Practices (ACIP). Protection against measles, hepatitis A, and hepatitis B must be ensured for everyone who will be in the household or providing care for the adopted child. Measles immunity or 2 doses of MMR vaccine separated by ≥28 days should be documented for all people born in or after 1957. ACIP recommends that unprotected family members and close contacts of the adopted child be immunized against hepatitis A virus (HAV) before the child's arrival. Most adult family members will also require immunization with hepatitis B vaccine. Adults who have not received the tetanus-diphtheria-acellular pertussis (Tdap) vaccine, including adults >65 years old, should receive a single dose of Tdap to protect against *Bordetella pertussis* in addition to tetanus and diphtheria. Family members should ensure they have completed the recommended age-appropriate polio vaccine series; a one-time inactivated polio booster is also recommended for adults who have completed the primary series in the past.

Prospective adoptive parents and any children traveling with them should receive advice on travel safety, food safety, immunization, malaria chemoprophylaxis, diarrhea prevention and treatment, and other travel-related health issues, as outlined elsewhere in this book. Instructions on car seats, injury prevention, food safety, and air travel apply equally to the adoptive child, so the travel health provider should also be familiar with and provide information on these child-specific issues.

OVERSEAS MEDICAL EXAMINATION OF THE ADOPTED CHILD

All immigrants, including infants and children adopted internationally by US citizens, must undergo a medical examination in their country of origin, performed by a physician designated by the Department of State. The medical examination is used primarily to detect certain serious contagious diseases that may make the immigrant ineligible for a visa. Prospective adoptive parents should not rely on this medical examination to detect all possible disabilities and illnesses. Laboratory results from the country of origin may be unreliable.

The medical examination consists of a brief physical examination and a medical history. A chest radiograph examination for tuberculosis (TB) and a blood test for syphilis are required for immigrants aged ≥15 years. Immigration applicants aged <15 years are tested only if there is reason to suspect any of these diseases. However, children aged 2–14 years who are coming from countries with an estimated TB incidence of ≥20 cases per 100,000 population per year must have a tuberculin skin test or interferon-γ release assay (IGRA) before arrival in the United States. TB incidence exceeds this rate in all the top 12 countries from which children were adopted internationally in 2011.

Additional information about the medical examination and the vaccination exemption form for internationally adopted children is available on the Department of State website at http://adoption.state.gov/adoption_process/how_to_adopt/health.php and http://travel.state.gov/pdf/DS-1981.pdf, respectively.

FOLLOW-UP MEDICAL EXAMINATION AFTER ARRIVAL IN THE UNITED STATES

The adopted child should have a medical examination within 2 weeks of arrival in the United States, or earlier if the child has fever, anorexia, diarrhea, or vomiting. Items to consider during medical examination of an adopted child include the following:

- Temperature (fever requires further investigation)
- General appearance: alert, interactive
- Anthropometric measurements: height/age, weight/age, weight/height, head circumference/age
- Facial features: length of palpebral fissures, philtrum, upper lip (fetal alcohol syndrome: short palpebral fissures, thin upper lip, indistinct philtrum)
- Hair: texture, color
- Eyes: jaundice, pallor, strabismus, visual acuity screen
- Ears: hearing screen
- Mouth: palate, teeth
- Neck: thyroid (enlargement secondary to hypothyroidism, iodine deficiency)
- Heart: murmurs
- Chest: symmetry, Tanner stage breasts
- Abdomen: liver or spleen enlargement
- Skin: Mongolian spots, scars, Bacillus Calmette-Guérin (BCG) scar
- Lymph nodes: enlargement suggestive of TB
- Back: scoliosis and neurocutaneous findings
- Genitalia: Tanner stage, presence of both testicles

In addition, all children should receive a complete neurodevelopmental examination by a clinician with experience in child development. Further evaluation will depend on the country of origin, the age of the child, previous living conditions, nutritional status, developmental status, and the adoptive family's specific questions. Concerns raised during the preadoption medical review may dictate further investigation.

SCREENING FOR INFECTIOUS DISEASES

The current panel of tests for infectious diseases recommended by the American Academy of Pediatrics (AAP) for screening internationally adopted children is as follows:

- Hepatitis B virus (HBV) serologic testing (repeat at 6 months if negative)
- Syphilis serologic testing
- HIV 1 and 2 serologic testing
- Complete blood cell count with differential and red blood cell indices

- Stool examination for ova and parasites (3 specimens)
- Stool examination for *Giardia intestinalis* and *Cryptosporidium* antigen (1 specimen)
- TST or IGRA (repeat at 6 months if negative)

Additional screening tests may be useful, depending on the child's country of origin or specific risk factors. These screens include HAV, hepatitis C virus (HCV), and Chagas disease serologic tests; malaria smears; and *Helicobacter pylori* antigen screening of stool if there is persistent abdominal pain or refractory anemia.

Gastrointestinal Parasites

Gastrointestinal parasites have been found in up to 74% of internationally adopted children. *G. intestinalis* is the most common parasite identified. The highest rates of infection have been reported from Ukraine and Ethiopia. Three stool samples collected in the early morning, 2–3 days apart, and placed in a container with preservative are recommended for ova and parasite analysis. Only 1 of these samples needs to be analyzed for *Giardia* antigen and *Cryptosporidium* antigen. Although theoretically possible, transmission of intestinal parasites from internationally adopted children to family and school contacts has not been reported. Stool samples should be cultured for enteric bacterial pathogens for any child with diarrhea.

Hepatitis A

HAV serology is useful in identifying the infant or child from a HAV-endemic area who may be asymptomatic but is acutely infected and shedding virus. In 2007 and early 2008, multiple cases of hepatitis A secondary to exposure to a newly arrived internationally adopted child were reported in the United States. Some of these cases involved extended family members who were not living in the household. Identification of acutely infected toddlers new to the United States is necessary to prevent further transmission. In addition, identifying children who have natural immunity and do not need the HAV vaccine is cost-effective.

Hepatitis B

HBV surface antigen (HBsAg) has been reported in 1%–5% of newly arrived adoptees.

Because of widespread use of the HBV vaccine, the prevalence of HBV infection has decreased. Children found to be positive for HBsAg should be retested for confirmation. Results of a positive HBsAg test should be reported to the state health department. HBV is highly transmissible within the household. All members of households adopting children with chronic HBV infection must be immunized and should have follow-up antibody titers to determine whether levels consistent with immunity have been achieved. Children with chronic HBV infection should receive additional tests for HBV e antigen, hepatitis D virus antibody, and liver function; they should also have a consultation with a pediatric gastroenterologist. Repeat screening at 6 months after arrival should be done on all children who initially test negative for HBV surface antibody.

Hepatitis C

Routine screening for HCV is not recommended. However, AAP suggests that clinicians consider HCV serologic screening for children from Russia, Eastern Europe, Egypt, and China. HCV screening for children from other areas may be indicated depending on presence of symptoms consistent with hepatitis and on histories of prevalence in the country of origin, receipt of blood products, and maternal drug use.

Syphilis

Screening for *Treponema pallidum* is recommended for all internationally adopted children. Initial screening may be done with either a nontreponemal or treponemal test, but any positive result must be confirmed by using the opposite test. Care must be taken in interpreting either test method. Treponemal tests remain positive for life in most cases even after successful treatment and are specific for treponemal diseases, which include syphilis and other diseases (such as yaws, pinta, and bejel) that are seen in tropical countries. If syphilis cannot be satisfactorily excluded, a full evaluation for disease must be undertaken and antitreponemal treatment given.

HIV

Clinical symptoms of malnutrition, long-term institutionalization, and acquired immunodeficiency may overlap, but positive HIV antibodies in children aged <18 months may reflect maternal antibody and not infection. Assaying for HIV DNA with PCR will confirm the diagnosis of HIV in the infant or child. Standard screening for HIV is with ELISA antibody testing, but some experts recommend PCR for any infant aged <6 months on arrival. If PCR testing is done, 2 negative results from assays administered 1 month apart, ≥1 of which is done after the age of 4 months, are necessary to exclude infection. Some experts recommend repeating the screen for HIV antibodies 6 months after arrival.

Chagas Disease

Chagas disease is endemic throughout much of Mexico, Central America, and South America. Risk of Chagas disease varies by region within endemic countries. Although the risk of Chagas disease is likely low in adopted children from endemic countries, treatment of infected children is very effective. If a child comes from a country with endemic Chagas disease, testing for Chagas disease should be considered. Serologic testing when the child is aged >1 year will avoid possible false-positive results due to maternal antibody.

Malaria

Thick and thin malaria smears should be obtained immediately for any febrile child newly arrived from a malaria-endemic area. A child with fever should have 3 sets of malaria smears ≥12 hours apart to exclude the diagnosis.

Tuberculosis

Internationally adopted children are at 4–6 times the risk for TB than their US-born peers. The TST of purified protein derivative is indicated for all children, regardless of their BCG status. TST results must be interpreted carefully for internationally adopted children; guidelines may be found in the bibliography. For children aged ≥5 years, IGRAs (such as QuantiFERON-TB Gold) are an acceptable screening alternative to the TST. IGRAs have the advantage of not requiring a follow-up visit for testing or requiring individual interpretation of results (although results may be termed "indeterminate" by the laboratory). In addition, they appear to be more specific than the TST for M. *tuberculosis* infection in children who have had BCG vaccination. However, the TST remains the most widely used screening test for TB in children. A chest radiograph and complete physical examination to assess for pulmonary and extrapulmonary TB are indicated for all children with positive TST results. Hilar lymphadenopathy is a more sensitive finding for TB in young children than are pulmonary infiltrates or cavitation. A repeat TST 3–6 months after arrival is recommended for children who initially test negative. Children who have a positive TST result but have no evidence of active disease should be treated with isoniazid for 9 months. If active disease is found, every effort should be made to isolate the organism and determine sensitivities, particularly if the child is from a region of the world with a high rate of multidrug-resistant TB, such as Russia, Eastern Europe, South Africa, or Asia.

Eosinophilia

An eosinophil count >450 cells/mm³ in an internationally adopted child may warrant further evaluation. One option for children who appear well is to repeat a complete blood count with differential 4 weeks after the initial test. If eosinophilia persists, further investigations should be based on the child's country of origin and might include evaluation for *Strongyloides stercoralis, Toxocara canis, Schistosoma* species, *Ancylostoma* species, *Trichinella spiralis*, intestinal parasites that can migrate through tissues, and filarial worms.

SCREENING FOR NONINFECTIOUS DISEASES

Several screening tests for noninfectious diseases should be performed in all or select internationally adopted children. Serum levels of thyroid-stimulating hormone, iron, iron-binding capacity, transferrin, ferritin, C-reactive protein, total vitamin D 25-hydroxy, and lead should be measured in all internationally adopted children. Hemoglobin electrophoresis and testing glucose-6-phosphate dehydrogenase deficiency should be performed on all children from sub-Saharan Africa. In certain circumstances, neurologic and psychological testing may also be considered.

IMMUNIZATIONS

The US Immigration and Nationality Act requires that any person seeking an immigrant visa for permanent residency must show proof of having received the ACIP-recommended vaccines (Table 7-1) before immigration. This requirement applies to all immigrant infants and children entering the United States, but internationally adopted children aged <10 years are exempt from the overseas immunization requirements. Adoptive parents are required to sign a waiver indicating their intention to comply with the immunization requirements within 30 days of the infant's or child's arrival in the United States.

Most children throughout the developing world receive BCG, oral polio, measles, diphtheria, tetanus, and pertussis vaccines per the original immunization schedule of the United Nations Expanded Programme of Immunizations (begun in 1974). In many developing countries, HBV and *Haemophilus influenzae* type B vaccines have become more widely available. Upon arrival in the United States, >90% of newly arrived internationally adopted children need catch-up immunizations to meet ACIP guidelines. Varicella, pneumococcal conjugate, rubella, mumps, and *Haemophilus influenzae* type b vaccines are often not available in developing countries.

Reliability of vaccine records appears to differ by, and even within, country of origin. Providers can choose 1 of 2 approaches for vaccination of internationally adopted children. The first is to reimmunize regardless of immunization record. The second, applicable to children aged ≥6 months, is to test antibody titers to the vaccines reportedly administered and reimmunize only for those diseases to which the child has no protective titers. Immunity to *B. pertussis* is an exception; antibody titers do not correlate with immune status to *B. pertussis*. However, protective antibody levels to diphtheria and tetanus imply protective antibody levels to *B. pertussis*.

Most experts recommend serologic testing for infants and children aged ≥6 months. MMR is not given in most countries of origin. Measles vaccine is administered as a single antigen. Unless the child has had mumps and rubella, administration of the MMR vaccine is recommended over serologic testing. Varicella testing for children coming from tropical countries is not recommended before

7

age 12 years, unless there is a history of disease. In the tropics, varicella is a disease of adolescents and adults.

Immunizations should be given according to the current ACIP schedule for catch-up vaccination. If the infant is <6 months old and there is uncertainty regarding immunization status or validity of the immunization record, the child should be re-immunized according to the ACIP schedule.

BIBLIOGRAPHY

1. American Academy of Pediatrics. Medical evaluation of internationally adopted children for infectious diseases. In: Pickering LK, editor. Red Book: 2012 Report of the Committee on Infectious Diseases. 29th ed. Elk Grove Village, IL; 2012. p. 191–3.
2. CDC. CDC immigration requirements: technical instructions for tuberculosis screening and treatment: using cultures and directly observed therapy. 2009 [cited 2012 Sep 26]. Available from: http://www.cdc.gov/immigrantrefugeehealth/pdf/tuberculosis-ti-2009.pdf.
3. CDC. Recommended adult immunization schedule—United States. MMWR Morb Mortal Wkly Rep. 2010;59(1):1–4.
4. CDC. Recommended immunization schedules for persons aged 0 through 18 years—United States, 2010. MMWR Morb Mortal Wkly Rep. 2010;58(51, 52):1–4.
5. Chen LH, Barnett ED, Wilson ME. Preventing infectious diseases during and after international adoption. Ann Intern Med. 2003 Sep 2;139(5 Pt 1):371–8.
6. Lee PJ. Vaccines for travel and international adoption. Pediatr Infect Dis J. 2008 Apr;27(4):351–4.
7. Mandalakas AM, Detjen AK, Hesseling AC, Benedetti A, Menzies D. Interferon-gamma release assays and childhood tuberculosis: systematic review and meta-analysis. Int J Tuberc Lung Dis. 2011 Aug;15(8):1018–32.
8. Mandalakas AM, Kirchner HL, Iverson S, Chesney M, Spencer MJ, Sidler A, et al. Predictors of *Mycobacterium tuberculosis* infection in international adoptees. Pediatrics. 2007 Sep;120(3):e610–6.
9. Mazurek GH, Jereb J, Vernon A, LoBue P, Goldberg S, Castro K. Updated guidelines for using interferon gamma release assays to detect *Mycobacterium tuberculosis* infection—United States, 2010. MMWR Recomm Rep. 2010 Jun 25;59(RR-5):1–25.
10. Mazzulli T. Laboratory diagnosis of infection due to viruses, *Chlamydia*, *Chlamydophila*, and *Mycoplasma*. In: Long SS, Pickering LK, Prober CG, editors. Principles and Practice of Pediatric Infectious Diseases. 3rd ed. China: Churchill Livingstone; 2008.
11. Miller LC. International adoption: infectious diseases issues. Clin Infect Dis. 2005 Jan 15;40(2):286–93.
12. Schulte JM, Maloney S, Aronson J, San Gabriel P, Zhou J, Saiman L. Evaluating acceptability and completeness of overseas immunization records of internationally adopted children. Pediatrics. 2002 Feb;109(2):E22.
13. Staat MA, Rice M, Donauer S, Mukkada S, Holloway M, Cassedy A, et al. Intestinal parasite screening in internationally adopted children: importance of multiple stool specimens. Pediatrics. 2011 Sep;128(3):e613–22.
14. Stauffer WM, Kamat D, Walker PF. Screening of international immigrants, refugees, and adoptees. Prim Care. 2002 Dec;29(4):879–905.
15. US Department of Homeland Security, Office of Immigration Statistics. Yearbook of Immigration Statistics: 2011. Washington, DC: US Department of Homeland Security; 2012 [cited 2012 Sep 26]. Available at http://www.dhs.gov/yearbook-immigration-statistics.

7

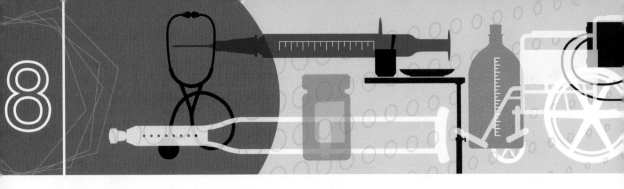

Advising Travelers with Specific Needs

IMMUNOCOMPROMISED TRAVELERS

Camille Nelson Kotton, David O. Freedman

APPROACH TO THE IMMUNOCOMPROMISED TRAVELER

The pre-travel preparation of travelers with immune suppression due to any medical condition, drug, or treatment must address several categories of concern:

- Is the traveler's underlying medical condition stable? The travel health provider may need to contact the traveler's primary and specialty care providers (with the patient's permission) to discuss the traveler's fitness to travel, give specific medical advice for the proposed itinerary, and verify the drugs and doses composing the usual maintenance regimen.
- Do the conditions, medications, and treatments of the traveler constitute contraindications to, decrease the effectiveness of, or increase the toxicity of any of the disease-prevention measures recommended for the proposed trip? Depending on the destination, these measures include, but are not limited to, immunizations and drugs used for malaria chemoprophylaxis and management of travelers' diarrhea.
- Could any of the disease-prevention measures recommended for the proposed trip destabilize the underlying medical condition, directly or through drug interactions?

- Are there specific health hazards at the destination that would exacerbate the underlying condition or be more severe in an immunocompromised traveler? If so, can specific interventions be recommended to mitigate these risks?

The traveler's immune status is particularly relevant to immunizations. Overall considerations for vaccine recommendations, such as destination and the likely risk of exposure to disease, are the same for immunocompromised travelers as for other travelers. The risk of a severe outcome from a vaccine-preventable disease must be weighed against potential adverse events from administering a live vaccine to an immunocompromised patient. In some complex cases when travelers cannot tolerate recommended immunizations or prophylaxis, the traveler should consider changing the itinerary, altering the activities planned during travel, or deferring the trip.

For purposes of clinical assessment and approach to immunizations, immunocompromised travelers fall into 1 of 4 groups, based on mechanism and level of immune suppression. Vaccine recommendations for different categories of immunocompromised adults are shown in Table 8-1.

Table 8-1. Immunization of immunocompromised adults

	HIV INFECTION, CD4 CELLS ≥200/mm³	SEVERE IMMUNOSUPPRESSION (HIV/AIDS), CD4 CELLS <200/mm³	SEVERE IMMUNOSUPPRESSION (NOT HIV-RELATED)	ASPLENIA	RENAL FAILURE	CHRONIC LIVER DISEASE, DIABETES
Live Vaccines						
Bacillus Calmette-Guérin (BCG)	X	X	X	U	U	U
Influenza, live attenuated (LAIV)	X	X	X	U	X	X
Measles-mumps-rubella (MMR)	R[1]	X[1]	X[1]	U	U	U
Typhoid, Ty21a	X	X	X	U	U	U
Varicella (adults)[2]	U	X	X	U	U	U
Yellow fever[3]	P[3]	X[3]	X	U	W	W
Zoster	C[4]	X[4]	X	U	U	U
Inactivated Vaccines						
Haemophilus influenzae type b (Hib)	C[5]	C[5]	R	R	U	U
Hepatitis A[6]	U	U	U	U	U	U
Hepatitis B[6]	U[7]	U[7]	U[7]	U[7]	R[8]	U[7]
Influenza (inactivated)	R	R	R	R	R	R

continued

TABLE 8-1. IMMUNIZATION OF IMMUNOCOMPROMISED ADULTS (continued)

	HIV INFECTION, CD4 CELLS ≥200/mm³	SEVERE IMMUNOSUPPRESSION (HIV/AIDS), CD4 CELLS <200/mm³	SEVERE IMMUNOSUPPRESSION (NOT HIV-RELATED)	ASPLENIA	RENAL FAILURE	CHRONIC LIVER DISEASE, DIABETES
Japanese encephalitis[9]	U	U	U	U	U	U
Meningococcal conjugate	C[10]	C[10]	U	R[10]	U	U
PCV13 followed by PPSV23[11]	R	R	R	R	R	C
Polio (IPV)	U	U	U	U	U	U
Rabies	U	U	U	U	U	U
Td or Tdap	R	R	R	R	R	R
Typhoid, Vi	U	U	U	U	U	U

Abbreviations: X, Contraindicated (per the Advisory Committee on Immunization Practices [ACIP]); U, Use as indicated for normal hosts; R, Recommended for all in this patient category; P, Precaution (per ACIP); W, Warning—medical conditions for which no data regarding YF vaccine exist but for which varying degrees of immune deficit might be present and could increase the risk of serious adverse events following vaccination; providers should carefully weigh vaccine risks and benefits before deciding to vaccinate such patients; C, Consider; PCV13, 13-valent pneumococcal conjugate vaccine; PPSV23, 23-valent pneumococcal polysaccharide vaccine.

[1] MMR vaccination should be considered for all symptomatic HIV-infected patients with CD4 counts ≥200/mm³ without evidence of measles immunity. Immune globulin may be administered for short-term protection of those facing high risk of measles and for whom MMR vaccine is contraindicated.

[2] Varicella vaccine should not be administered to people who have cellular immunodeficiencies, but people with impaired humoral immunity (including congenital or acquired hypoglobulinemia or dysglobulinemia) may be vaccinated. Immunocompromised hosts should receive 2 doses of vaccine spaced at 3-month intervals.

[3] See details in Chapter 3. Yellow Fever. YF vaccination is a precaution for asymptomatic HIV-infected people with CD4 cell counts of 200–499/mm³ YF vaccination is not a precaution for people with asymptomatic HIV infection and CD4 cell counts ≥500. YF vaccine is also considered contraindicated by ACIP for symptomatic HIV patients without AIDS and with CD4 counts ≥200/mm³.

[4] Also contraindicated by ACIP for symptomatic HIV patients without AIDS and with CD4 counts ≥200/mm³.

[5] Decision should be based on consideration of the individual patient's risk of Hib disease and the effectiveness of the vaccine for that person. In some settings, the incidence of Hib disease may be higher among HIV-infected adults than among HIV-uninfected adults, and the disease can be severe in these patients.

[6] Routinely indicated for all men who have sex with men, people with multiple sexual partners, hemophiliacs, patients with chronic hepatitis, and injection drug users.

[7] Test for antibodies to hepatitis B virus surface antigen serum titer after vaccination, and revaccinate if initial antibody response is absent or suboptimal (<10 mIU/mL). HIV-infected nonresponders may react to a subsequent vaccine course if CD4 cell counts rise to 500/mm³ after institution of highly active antiretroviral therapy. See text for discussion of other immunocompromised groups.

[8] Use special double-dose vaccine formulation. Test for antibodies to hepatitis B virus surface antigen after vaccination and revaccinate if initial antibody response is absent or suboptimal (<10 mIU/mL).

[9] As with most inactivated vaccines, no safety or efficacy data exist regarding the use of Ixiaro in immunocompromised people. Immunocompromised people may have a diminished immune response to Ixiaro.

[10] Two doses ≥2 months apart for asplenic and HIV-infected patients.

[11] Previously unimmunized asplenic, HIV-infected, or immunocompromised adults aged ≥19 years should receive 1 dose of 13-valent pneumococcal conjugate vaccine [PCV13] followed by 1 dose of pneumococcal polysaccharide vaccine (PPSV23) ≥8 weeks later. People with these conditions previously immunized with PPSV23 should follow catch-up guidelines per ACIP.

MEDICAL CONDITIONS WITHOUT SIGNIFICANT IMMUNOLOGIC COMPROMISE

With regard to travel immunizations, travelers whose health status places them in one of the following groups are not considered significantly immunocompromised and should be prepared as any other traveler, although the nature of the previous or underlying disease needs to be kept in mind.

1. Travelers receiving corticosteroid therapy under any of the following circumstances:
   > Short- or long-term daily or alternate-day therapy with <20 mg of prednisone or equivalent.
   > Long-term, alternate-day treatment with short-acting preparations.
   > Maintenance physiologic doses (replacement therapy).
   > Steroid inhalers.
   > Topical steroids (skin, ears, or eyes).
   > Intraarticular, bursal, or tendon injection of steroids.
   > If >1 month has passed since high-dose steroids (≥20 mg per day of prednisone or equivalent for >2 weeks) have been used. However, after short-term (<2 weeks) therapy with daily or alternate-day dosing of ≥20 mg of prednisone or equivalent, some experts will wait 2 weeks before administering measles vaccine.
2. HIV patients with >500/mm³ CD4 T lymphocytes.
3. Travelers with a history of cancer who received their last chemotherapy treatment ≥3 months previously and whose malignancy is in remission.
4. Bone marrow transplant recipients who are >2 years posttransplant, not on immunosuppressive drugs, and without graft-versus-host disease.
5. Travelers with autoimmune disease (such as systemic lupus erythematosus, inflammatory bowel disease, or rheumatoid arthritis) who are not being treated with immunosuppressive or immunomodulatory drugs, although definitive data are lacking.
6. Travelers with multiple sclerosis (MS) who are not on immunosuppressive or immunomodulatory agents and those who are not experiencing an exacerbation of disease. Although the risks of using live-virus vaccines for those with MS have been debated, the National MS Society

and CDC recommend following CDC guidelines for vaccination in those who lack prior immunity, who are not on immunosuppressive or immunomodulatory agents, and who are not experiencing an exacerbation of disease.

MEDICAL CONDITIONS AND TREATMENTS ASSOCIATED WITH LIMITED IMMUNE DEFICITS

Asymptomatic HIV Infection

Asymptomatic HIV-infected adults with CD4 cell counts of 200–500/mm³ are considered to have limited immune deficits. CD4 counts increased by antiretroviral drugs, rather than nadir counts, should be used to categorize HIV-infected people. The exact time at which reconstituted lymphocytes are fully functional is not well defined. To achieve a maximal vaccine response with minimal risk, many clinicians advise a delay of 3 months after reconstitution, if possible, before immunizations are administered. Although seroconversion rates and geometric mean titers of antibody in response to vaccines may be less than those measured in healthy controls, most vaccines can elicit seroprotective levels of antibody in most HIV-infected patients in this category.

Transient increases in HIV viral load, which return quickly to baseline, have been observed after administration of several different vaccines to HIV-infected people. The clinical significance of these increases is not known, but they do not preclude the use of any vaccine.

The combination measles, mumps, rubella, and varicella (MMRV) vaccine is contraindicated in anyone with HIV.

Multiple Sclerosis

Inactivated vaccines are generally considered safe for people with MS, although vaccination should be delayed during clinically significant relapses until patients have stabilized or begun to improve from the relapse, typically 4–6 weeks after it began. Administration of tetanus, hepatitis B, or influenza vaccines does not appear to increase the short-term risk of relapses in people with MS. However, published studies are lacking on the safety and efficacy of other vaccines (such as those against hepatitis A, human papilloma virus, meningitis, pertussis, pneumonia, polio, and typhoid). Inactivated vaccines are theoretically safe for people being treated with an

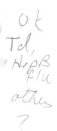

interferon medication, glatiramer acetate, mitoxantrone, fingolimod, or natalizumab, although efficacy data are lacking.

A few published studies suggest that measles, rubella, varicella, and zoster vaccines may be safe in people with stable MS if administered 1 month before starting or 1 month after discontinuing immunosuppressive therapy. Modern MS therapy includes aggressive and early immunomodulatory therapy for almost all MS patients, even those with stable disease. Live-virus vaccines should not be given to people with MS during therapy with immunosuppressants, such as mitoxantrone, azathioprine, methotrexate, or cyclophosphamide; during chronic corticosteroid therapy; or during therapy with the agents listed in Table 8-2. However, patients on glatiramer acetate and interferons have more limited immune deficits. Yellow fever vaccine and smallpox vaccine have not been well studied in people with MS and should only be given if there is a compelling reason to do so (such as unavoidable direct exposure and the risks of potential adverse events are carefully weighed against the likelihood of exposure to these potentially fatal illnesses); these decisions should be made in consultation with the patient's neurologist.

Other Chronic Conditions

Chronic medical conditions that may be associated with varying degrees of immune deficit include asplenia, chronic renal disease, chronic liver disease (including hepatitis C), diabetes mellitus, and complement deficiencies. Because no information is available regarding possible increased adverse events or decreased vaccine efficacy following administration of live, attenuated viral or bacterial antigen vaccines to patients with these diseases, caution should be used when considering the administration of live vaccines to such patients. Factors to consider in assessing the general level of immune competence of these patients include disease severity, duration, clinical stability, complications, and comorbidities (see the next section in this chapter, Travelers with Chronic Illnesses).

A blunted response to hepatitis B vaccine has been reported in patients with chronic liver disease; a decreased response to hepatitis B vaccine has also been observed in patients with diabetes. Additional doses of hepatitis B vaccine

beyond the primary 3-dose series may be necessary. Double-dose hepatitis B vaccine preparations are used to promote optimal immunization of people with chronic renal failure and other patients with absent or suboptimal response to standard hepatitis B vaccine doses. Adjuvanted hepatitis B candidate vaccines undergoing clinical trials appear to be more effective for immunization of liver transplant patients and patients with renal insufficiency.

Asplenic patients are susceptible to overwhelming sepsis with encapsulated bacterial pathogens. Although response to vaccines may be less than in people with a functioning spleen, many clinical guidelines recommend immunization against meningococcal, pneumococcal, and *Haemophilus influenzae* disease in these patients, regardless of travel plans.

- Limited data show that vaccine response in people who have had a splenectomy was more impaired if splenectomy was performed because of hematologic malignancy rather than for splenic trauma.
- The meningococcal A/C/Y/W-135 conjugate vaccine is indicated for both pediatric and adult populations at risk.
- The polysaccharide-protein conjugate vaccine against disease due to H. *influenzae* type b (Hib conjugate vaccine) appears to elicit an increased immune response and duration of protection in vaccine recipients, and many experienced clinicians recommend a single dose for splenectomized patients.
- *Streptococcus pneumoniae* vaccine is recommended for asplenic patients (Table 8-1).

People with terminal complement deficiencies appear to have increased susceptibility to meningococcal infections and should be immunized against meningococcal disease.

MEDICAL CONDITIONS AND TREATMENTS ASSOCIATED WITH SEVERE IMMUNE COMPROMISE

Severe Immune Compromise (Non-HIV)

Severely immunocompromised people include those who have active leukemia or lymphoma, generalized malignancy, aplastic anemia, graft-versus-host disease, or congenital immunodeficiency; others in this category include people who have received recent radiation therapy, people who have had solid-organ or bone marrow transplants (within 2 years of transplantation), or transplant recipients who are still taking immunosuppressive drugs.

People with chronic lymphocytic leukemia have poor humoral immunity, even early in the disease course, and rarely respond to vaccines. Complete revaccination with standard childhood vaccines should begin 12 months after bone marrow transplantation. However, measles, mumps, and rubella (MMR) vaccine should be administered 24 months after transplant if the recipient is presumed to be immunocompetent. Experience using varicella vaccine in transplant recipients is insufficient; however, if a decision is made to vaccinate with varicella vaccine, the vaccine should be administered a minimum of 24 months after transplantation if the recipient is presumed to be immunocompetent. Influenza vaccine should be administered 6 months after transplant and annually thereafter.

For solid-organ transplants, the risk of infection is highest in the first year after transplant, so travel to high-risk destinations should be postponed until after that time.

Vaccine doses received while concurrently receiving immunosuppressive therapy or during the 2 weeks before starting therapy are not considered valid. At least 3 months after therapy is discontinued, patients should be revaccinated with all vaccines that are still indicated. People taking any of the following categories of medications are considered severely immunocompromised:

- **High-dose corticosteroids**—Most clinicians consider a dose of either >2 mg/kg of body weight or ≥20 mg per day of prednisone or equivalent in people who weigh >10 kg, when administered for ≥2 weeks, as sufficiently immunosuppressive to raise concern about the safety of vaccination with live-virus vaccines. Furthermore, the immune response to vaccines may be impaired. Clinicians should wait ≥1 month after discontinuation of high-dose systemic corticosteroid therapy before administering a live-virus vaccine.
- **Alkylating agents** (such as cyclophosphamide)
- **Antimetabolites** (such as azathioprine, 6-mercaptopurine)
- **Transplant-related immunosuppressive drugs** (such as cyclosporine, tacrolimus,

sirolimus, mycophenolate mofetil, and mitoxantrone)
- **Cancer chemotherapeutic agents,** excluding tamoxifen but including low-dose methotrexate weekly regimens, are classified as severely immunosuppressive, as evidenced by increased rates of opportunistic infections and blunting of responses to certain vaccines among patient groups. Limited studies show that methotrexate monotherapy had no effect on the response to influenza vaccine, but it did impair the response to pneumococcal vaccine.
- **Tumor necrosis factor (TNF) blockers** such as etanercept, adalimumab, certolizumab pegol, golimumab, and infliximab blunt the immune response to certain vaccines and certain chronic infections. When used alone or in combination regimens with methotrexate to treat rheumatoid disease, TNF blockers were associated with an impaired response to influenza vaccine and to pneumococcal vaccine.
  > Despite measurable impairment of the immune response, postvaccination antibody titers were often sufficient to provide protection for most people; therefore, treatment with TNF blockers does not preclude immunization against influenza and pneumococcal disease.
  > The use of live vaccines is contraindicated according to the prescribing information for most of these therapies.
- Other biologic agents that are immunosuppressive or immunomodulatory, as outlined in Table 8-2.

Severe Immune Compromise Due to Symptomatic HIV/AIDS

Knowledge of the HIV-infected traveler's current CD4 T-lymphocyte count is necessary for pre-travel consultation. HIV-infected people with CD4 cell counts <200/mm^3, history of an AIDS-defining illness, or clinical manifestations of symptomatic HIV are considered to have severe immunosuppression (see Chapter 3, HIV Infection) and should not receive live attenuated viral or bacterial vaccines because of the risk that the vaccine could cause serious systemic disease. The response to inactivated vaccines also will be suboptimal; thus, vaccine doses received by HIV-infected people while CD4 cell counts are <200/mm^3 should

Table 8-2. Immunosuppressive biologic agents that preclude vaccination against yellow fever, measles-mumps-rubella, varicella, or zoster[1]

GENERIC NAME	TRADE NAME	MECHANISM/TARGET OF ACTION
Abatacept	Orencia	CTLA-4
Adalimumab	Humira	TNF blocker
Alefacept	Amevive	CD2
Alemtuzumab	Campath	Anti-CD52
Anakinra	Kineret	IL-1
Basiliximab	Simulect	IL-2R/CD25
Bevacizumab	Avastin	VEGF
Certolizumab pegol	Cimzia	TNF blocker
Cetuximab	Erbitux	EGFR
Daclizumab	Zenapax	IL-2R
Etanercept	Enbrel	TNF blocker
Glatiramer acetate	Copaxone	Immunomodulatory; target unknown
Golimumab	Simponi	TNF blocker
Ibritumomab tiuxetan	Zevalin	CD20 with radioisotope
Imatinib mesylate	Gleevec, STI 571	Signal transduction inhibitor/protein-tyrosine kinase inhibitor
Infliximab	Remicade	TNF blocker
Interferon alfa	Pegasys, PegIntron	Block hepatitis C viral replication
Interferon beta-1a	Avonex, Rebif	Immunomodulatory; target unknown
Interferon beta-1b	Betaseron	Immunomodulatory; target unknown

continued

Natalizumab	Tsabri	α4-integrin
Panitumumab	Vectibix	EGFR
Rilonacept	Arcalyst	IL-1
Rituximab	Rituxan	CD20
Sunitinib malate	Sutent	Multikinase inhibitor
Tocilizumab	Actemra	IL-6
Tositumomab	Bexxar	CD20 with radioisotope
Trastuzumab	Herceptin	Human EGFR 2 (HER2)
Ustekinumab	Stelara	IL-12, IL-23

Abbreviations: CTLA, cytotoxic T-lymphocyte antigen; TNF, tumor necrosis factor; CD, cluster of differentiation; IL, interleukin; VEGF, vascular endothelial growth factor; EGFR, epidermal growth factor receptor.

[1] This table is based primarily on conservative expert opinions, given the lack of clinical data. Numerous agents are often given in combination with other agents (especially chemotherapy) and are immunosuppressive when given together. The list provides examples but is not inclusive of all biologic agents that suppress or modulate the immune system. Not all therapeutic monoclonal antibodies or other biologic agents result in immunosuppression; details of individual agents not listed here must be reviewed before determining whether live viral vaccines can be given. Some of these agents are less immunosuppressive than others; specifically, interferon used for hepatitis C and interferon and glatiramer acetate given to multiple sclerosis patients are immunomodulators, but clinical data to support safety with live-virus vaccines are lacking. The period of time clinicians should wait after discontinuation of these before administering a live-virus vaccine is not specified by the Advisory Committee on Immunization Practices (ACIP) or other authoritative guidelines. Consultation with the prescribing physician (and possibly a hospital pharmacist) is recommended for management of individual patients and guidance in estimating a particular patient's degree of immunosuppression. No basis exists for interpreting laboratory studies of immune parameters with vaccine safety or efficacy. Some experts recommend waiting 1 month after discontinuing etanercept and 3 months after discontinuing the other TNF blockers. Lymphocyte-depleting agents such as alemtuzumab and rituximab may cause prolonged immunosuppression. Restarting immunosuppression after live-virus vaccination has not been studied, but some experts would recommend at least a 1-month period.

be ignored, and the person should be revaccinated ≥3 months after immune reconstitution with antiretroviral therapy.

In newly diagnosed, treatment-naïve patients with CD4 cell counts <200/mm³, travel should be delayed pending reconstitution of CD4 cell counts with antiretroviral therapy. This delay will minimize risk of infection and avoid immune reconstitution illness during the travel.

Household Contacts

Household contacts of severely immunocompromised patients may be given live-virus vaccines such as yellow fever, MMR, or varicella vaccines but should not be given the live attenuated influenza vaccine. Immunocompromised patients should be aware of the risk of transmission of oral polio vaccine virus by the fecal-oral route in parts of the world where that vaccine is still given. Smallpox vaccine (mostly in military personnel) is also transmissible to immunocompromised patients.

SPECIAL CONSIDERATIONS FOR IMMUNOCOMPROMISED TRAVELERS
Yellow Fever Vaccine

Travelers with severe immune compromise should be strongly discouraged from travel to destinations that present a true risk for yellow fever (YF). They should not undergo YF vaccination, as there is a risk of developing a serious adverse event, such as life-threatening yellow fever vaccine-associated viscerotropic disease. If travel to an area where YF vaccine is recommended (see Maps 3-16 and 3-17) is unavoidable and the vaccine is not given, these travelers should be informed of the risk of YF, carefully instructed in methods to avoid mosquito bites, and be provided with a vaccination medical waiver (see Chapter 3, Yellow Fever).

Patients with conditions that the Advisory Committee on Immunization Practices considers precautions to administration of YF vaccine, such as asymptomatic HIV (see "Precautions" in Chapter 3, Yellow Fever), may be offered YF vaccine if travel to YF-endemic areas is unavoidable; recipients should be monitored closely for possible adverse effects. As vaccine response may be suboptimal, such vaccinees are candidates for serologic testing 1 month after vaccination. For information about serologic testing, contact your state health department or CDC's Division of Vector-Borne Diseases at 970–221-6400. Data from clinical and epidemiologic studies are insufficient at this time to evaluate the actual risk of severe adverse effects associated with YF vaccine among recipients with limited immune deficits.

If international travel requirements, and not true exposure risk, are the only reasons to vaccinate a traveler with asymptomatic HIV-infection or a limited immune deficit, the physician should provide a waiver letter. Travelers should be warned that vaccination waiver documents may not be accepted by some countries; if the waiver is rejected, the option of deportation might be preferable to receipt of YF vaccine at the destination.

Response to Vaccination

Response to vaccination may be muted in immunocompromised hosts, and potential travelers should be informed about this. The decrease in response to vaccination is not particularly predictable based on the immunosuppressive regimen. In general, serologic testing for response to most travel-related vaccines is neither clinically recommended nor readily available to practicing clinicians.

Malaria Chemoprophylaxis

Immunocompromised travelers to malaria-endemic areas should be prescribed appropriate drugs for malaria chemoprophylaxis and receive counseling about mosquito bite avoidance—the same as for immunocompetent travelers (see Chapter 3, Malaria). However, special concerns for immunocompromised travelers include any of the following possibilities:

- Drugs used for malaria chemoprophylaxis may interact with drugs in the traveler's maintenance regimen.
- The underlying medical condition will predispose the immunocompromised traveler to more serious disease from malaria infection.
- A malaria infection and the drugs used to treat the malaria infection may exacerbate the underlying disease.

The severity of malaria is increased in HIV-infected people: malaria infection increases HIV viral load and thus may exacerbate disease progression. There is a lack of published data on the safety and efficacy of CDC-recommended antimalarial regimens in the HIV-infected traveler taking highly active antiretroviral therapy (HAART) while traveling to malaria-endemic areas. Table 8-3 gives some examples of potential interactions between drugs used for malaria chemoprophylaxis and those used in HAART regimens:

- Tetracyclines have no clinically significant interactions expected with the protease inhibitors and nonnucleoside reverse transcriptase inhibitors, so doxycycline might be a reasonable recommendation for malaria chemoprophylaxis in a traveler on HAART going to a malaria-endemic area.
- Atovaquone-proguanil might be a reasonable malaria chemoprophylaxis choice for a traveler whose HAART regimen includes nelfinavir (protease inhibitor) and nevirapine (nonnucleoside reverse transcriptase inhibitor). Atovaquone is not expected to have any significant interaction with common nucleoside reverse transcriptase inhibitors, although no data are available for proguanil.

Table 8-3. Potential interactions between malaria drugs and HIV[1,2] or transplant-related[3] drugs

DRUG	PROTEASE INHIBITORS	NRTIs	NNRTIs	CALCINEURIN INHIBITORS (TACROLIMUS, CYCLOSPORINE A)
Mefloquine	Potential interaction with all protease inhibitors	No available data	Decreased levels of mefloquine with efavirenz or nevirapine	Could cause prolonged QT interval or elevated calcineurin inhibitor levels
Atovaquone-proguanil	Atovaquone: potential interactions with indinavir, ritonavir, lopinavir, atazanavir, darunavir, tipranavir Proguanil: potential interactions with ritonavir and lopinavir	Atovaquone: no clinically significant interaction expected Proguanil: no available data	Atovaquone: potential interaction with efavirenz Proguanil: potential interaction with efavirenz	No available data
Doxycycline	No clinically significant interactions expected	No available data	No clinically significant interactions expected	Could cause elevated calcineurin inhibitor levels
Chloroquine	Potential interaction with ritonavir only	No available data	No clinically significant interactions expected	Could cause prolonged QT interval or elevated calcineurin inhibitor levels
Primaquine	No clear data	No available data	No available data	Could cause elevated calcineurin inhibitor levels

Abbreviations: NRTI, nucleoside reverse transcriptase inhibitor; NNRTI, nonnucleoside reverse transcriptase inhibitor.

[1] Adapted from Table 2 in Bhadelia N, Klotman M, Caplivski D. The HIV-positive traveler. Am J Med. 2007 Jul;120(7):574–80, and information available at www.hiv-druginteractions.org.

[2] All potential interactions within an HIV drug class are noted in the table. There are no drug combinations with absolute contraindications to coadministration.

[3] Adapted from Table 3 in Kotton CN, Hibberd PL. Travel medicine and the solid organ transplant recipient. Am J Transplant. 2009 Dec;9 Suppl 4:S273–81.

- New classes of antiretroviral drugs include entry inhibitors and integrase inhibitors, and little data are available. Since new drugs and drug combinations for HIV treatment are under continuous development, clinicians are encouraged to review the most current information regarding possible drug interactions. An interactive web-based resource for checking on drug interactions involving HAART drugs is found at the University of Liverpool website (www.hiv-druginteractions.org).

Artemisinin combination therapy, consisting of 6 oral doses of artemether-lumefantrine taken over 3 days, is one of the recommended treatments for uncomplicated malaria due to *Plasmodium falciparum*. For severe malaria infections, intravenous artesunate is available in the United States through an investigational new drug protocol by CDC (see Chapter 3, Malaria). Limited data have raised concerns that parasite clearance of *P. falciparum* after therapy with artemisinins may be delayed in malaria patients coinfected with HIV compared with those who are HIV seronegative, raising the possibility that the host's immunity affects the efficacy of antimalarial drug treatment. The use of quinidine (and by implication quinine) in patients taking nelfinavir or ritonavir is contraindicated because of potential cumulative cardiotoxicity. However, if a patient has severe and complicated malaria, there may be no choice. In these circumstances, as in others, quinidine should be used only with close monitoring. In addition, careful monitoring should accompany quinidine therapy in patients taking amprenavir, delavirdine, or the lopinavir-ritonavir combination. Although the clinical significance, if any, is not known, several protease inhibitors have been shown in laboratory testing to inhibit the growth of malaria parasites.

Similarly, organ transplant recipients may have drug interactions between their chronic immunosuppression and agents used for malaria prophylaxis and treatment. Mefloquine, doxycycline, chloroquine, and primaquine may increase calcineurin inhibitor levels (tacrolimus and cyclosporine A), and sulfadoxine-pyrimethamine may decrease their levels. Some travel-related prophylactic medications need to be dose-adjusted according to altered hepatic or renal function.

Some clinical case reports suggest that asplenic people may be at higher risk of acquisition and complications of malaria, so asplenic travelers to malaria areas should be counseled to adhere conscientiously to the malaria chemoprophylaxis regimen prescribed for them.

Enteric Infections

Many foodborne and waterborne infections, such as those caused by *Salmonella*, *Campylobacter*, *Giardia*, and *Cryptosporidium*, can be severe or become chronic in immunocompromised people. Enteroaggregative *Escherichia coli* is an emerging enteric pathogen causing persistent diarrhea among children, adults, and HIV-infected people.

Safe food and beverage precautions should be followed by all travelers, but travelers' diarrhea can occur despite strict adherence.

Selection of antimicrobials to be used for self-treatment of travelers' diarrhea may require special consideration of potential drug interactions among patients already taking medications for chronic medical conditions. Fluoroquinolones and rifaximin are active against several enteric pathogens and are not known to have significant interactions with HAART drugs. However, macrolide antibiotics may have significant interactions with HAART drugs (Table 8-4) and with organ transplant–related immunosuppression. Emerging therapies for diarrhea in HIV/AIDS patients may involve probiotics such as *Lactobacillus rhamnosus* GR-1, *L. reuteri* RC-14, and others.

Waterborne infections might result from swallowing water during recreational activities. To reduce the risk for cryptosporidiosis and giardiasis, patients should avoid swallowing water during swimming and should not swim in water that might be contaminated (with sewage or animal waste, for example).

Attention to hand hygiene, including frequent and thorough handwashing, is the best prevention against gastroenteritis. Hands should be washed after contact with public surfaces and also after any contact with animals or their living areas.

Reducing Risk for Other Diseases

Geographically focal infections that pose an increased risk of severe outcome for immunocompromised people include visceral leishmaniasis and several fungal infections acquired by inhalation (such as *Penicillium marneffei* infection in Southeast Asia and coccidioidomycosis in the Americas). Many developing areas have high rates of tuberculosis (TB), and establishing the TB status of immunocompromised travelers going to such destinations may be helpful in the evaluation of any subsequent travel-associated illness. Depending on the traveler's degree of immune suppression, the baseline TB status may be assessed by obtaining a tuberculin skin test, chest radiograph, or *Mycobacterium tuberculosis* antigen-specific interferon-γ assay.

Patients with advanced HIV and transplant recipients frequently take either primary or secondary prophylaxis for one or more opportunistic infections (such as *Pneumocystis*, *Mycobacterium*, and *Toxoplasma* spp.). Complete adherence to all indicated regimens should be confirmed before travel (see Chapter 3, HIV Infection).

8

Table 8-4. Potential interactions between antibiotics for travelers' diarrhea and HIV[1] or transplant-related[2] drugs

DRUG	PROTEASE INHIBITORS	NRTIs	NNRTIs	CALCINEURIN INHIBITORS (TACROLIMUS, CYCLOSPORINE A)
Fluoroquinolones	No clinically significant interactions	No clinically significant interactions	No clinically significant interactions	Could cause prolonged QT interval or elevated fluoroquinolone levels; dose per renal function
Macrolides	Possible increased levels of clarithromycin with ritonavir, atazanavir, and lopinavir	Decreased levels of zidovudine with clarithromycin; no data available for azithromycin	Possible interactions with clarithromycin, efavirenz, and nevirapine	Possible increased levels of calcineurin inhibitors
Rifaximin	No available data	No available data	No available data	No available data; could decrease levels of calcineurin inhibitors

Abbreviations: NRTI, nucleoside reverse transcriptase inhibitor; NNRTI, nonnucleoside reverse transcriptase inhibitor.

[1] Adapted from Table 2 in Bhadelia N, Klotman M, Caplivski D. The HIV-positive traveler. Am J Med. 2007 Jul;120(7):574–80.
[2] Adapted from Table 3 in Kotton CN, Hibberd PL. Travel medicine and the solid organ transplant recipient. Am J Transplant. 2009 Dec;9 Suppl 4:S273–81.

BIBLIOGRAPHY

1. Agarwal N, Ollington K, Kaneshiro M, Frenck R, Melmed GY. Are immunosuppressive medications associated with decreased responses to routine immunizations? A systematic review. Vaccine. 2012 Feb 14;30(8):1413–24.

2. Anukam KC, Osazuwa EO, Osadolor HB, Bruce AW, Reid G. Yogurt containing probiotic *Lactobacillus rhamnosus* GR-1 and *L. reuteri* RC-14 helps resolve moderate diarrhea and increases CD4 count in HIV/AIDS patients. J Clin Gastroenterol. 2008 Mar;42(3):239–43.

3. Beran J. Safety and immunogenicity of a new hepatitis B vaccine for the protection of patients with renal insufficiency including pre-haemodialysis and haemodialysis patients. Expert Opin Biol Ther. 2008 Feb;8(2):235–47.

4. Bhadelia N, Klotman M, Caplivski D. The HIV-positive traveler. Am J Med. 2007 Jul;120(7):574–80.

5. Boerbooms AM, Kerstens PJ, van Loenhout JW, Mulder J, van de Putte LB. Infections during low-dose methotrexate treatment in rheumatoid arthritis. Semin Arthritis Rheum. 1995 Jun;24(6):411–21.

6. Brinkman DM, Jol-van der Zijde CM, ten Dam MM, teBoekhorst PA, ten Cate R, Wulffraat NM, et al. Resetting the adaptive immune system after autologous stem cell transplantation: lessons from responses to vaccines. J Clin Immunol. 2007 Nov;27(6):647–58.

7. CDC. Vaccination of persons with primary and secondary immune deficiencies. In: Atkinson W, Wolfe S, Hamborsky J, editors. Epidemiology and Prevention of Vaccine-Preventable Diseases. 12th ed. Washington, DC: Public Health Foundation; 2012. p. A-23 [cited 2012 Sep 30]. Available from: http://www.cdc.gov/vaccines/pubs/pinkbook/downloads/appendices/A/immuno-table.pdf.

8. Cohen C, Karstaedt A, Frean J, Thomas J, Govender N, Prentice E, et al. Increased prevalence of severe malaria in HIV-infected adults in South Africa. Clin Infect Dis. 2005 Dec 1;41(11):1631–7.

9. Eigenberger K, Sillaber C, Greitbauer M, Herkner H, Wolf H, Graninger W, et al. Antibody responses to pneumococcal and hemophilus vaccinations in splenectomized patients with hematological malignancies or trauma. Wien Klin Wochenschr. 2007;119(7–8):228–34.

10. Farez MF, Correale J. Yellow fever vaccination and increased relapse rate in travelers with multiple sclerosis. Arch Neurol. 2011 Oct;68(10):1267–71.

11. Geretti AM, Doyle T. Immunization for HIV-positive individuals. Curr Opin Infect Dis. 2010 Feb;23(1):32–8.

12. Kamya MR, Gasasira AF, Yeka A, Bakyaita N, Nsobya SL, Francis D, et al. Effect of HIV-1 infection on antimalarial treatment outcomes in Uganda: a population-based study. J Infect Dis. 2006 Jan 1;193(1):9–15.

13. Kaplan JE, Benson C, Holmes KH, Brooks JT, Pau A, Masur H, et al. Guidelines for prevention and treatment of opportunistic infections in HIV-infected adults and adolescents: recommendations from CDC, the National Institutes of Health, and the HIV Medicine Association of the Infectious Diseases Society of America. MMWR Recomm Rep. 2009 Apr 10;58(RR-4):1–207.

14. Kotton CN, Hibberd PL, AST Infectious Diseases Community of Practice. Travel medicine and the solid organ transplant recipient. Am J Transplant. 2009 Dec 9;(Suppl 4):S273–81.

15. Laurence JC. Hepatitis A and B immunizations of individuals infected with human immunodeficiency virus. Am J Med. 2005 Oct;118 Suppl 10A:75S–83S.

16. Loebermann M, Winkelmann A, Hartung HP, Hengel H, Reisinger EC, Zettl UK. Vaccination against infection in patients with multiple sclerosis. Nat Rev Neurol. 2011;8(3):143–51.

17. Matulis G, Juni P, Villiger PM, Gadola SD. Detection of latent tuberculosis in immunosuppressed patients with autoimmune diseases: performance of a *Mycobacterium tuberculosis* antigen-specific interferon gamma assay. Ann Rheum Dis. 2008 Jan;67(1):84–90.

18. Mishra LC, Bhattacharya A, Sharma M, Bhasin VK. HIV protease inhibitors, indinavir or nelfinavir, augment antimalarial action of artemisinin in vitro. Am J Trop Med Hyg. 2010 Jan;82(1):148–50.

19. Nevens F, Zuckerman JN, Burroughs AK, Jung MC, Bayas JM, Kallinowski B, et al. Immunogenicity and safety of an experimental adjuvanted hepatitis B candidate vaccine in liver transplant patients. Liver Transpl. 2006 Oct;12(10):1489–95.

20. Skinner-Adams TS, McCarthy JS, Gardiner DL, Andrews KT. HIV and malaria co-infection: interactions and consequences of chemotherapy. Trends Parasitol. 2008 Jun;24(6):264–71.

21. Visser LG. TNF-α antagonists and immunization. Curr Infect Dis Rep. 2011 Jun;13(3):243–7.

TRAVELERS WITH CHRONIC ILLNESSES

Deborah Nicolls Barbeau

GENERAL TRAVEL PREPARATION: PRACTICAL CONSIDERATIONS

Although traveling abroad can be relaxing and rewarding, the physical demands of travel can be stressful, particularly for travelers with underlying chronic illnesses. With adequate preparation, however, those with chronic illnesses can have safe and enjoyable trips. The following is a list of general recommendations for patients with chronic illnesses:

- Ensure that any chronic illnesses are well controlled. Patients with an underlying illness should see their physicians to ensure that the management of their illness is optimized.

- Recommend seeking pre-travel consultation early, ≥4–6 weeks before departure, to ensure adequate time to respond to immunizations and, in some circumstances, to try medications before travel (see the Immunocompromised Travelers section earlier in this chapter).

- Ask about previous health-related issues encountered during travel, such as complications during air travel.

- Provide a physician's letter. The letter should be on office letterhead stationery, outlining existing medical conditions, medications prescribed (including generic names), and any equipment required to manage the condition. Travelers with underlying medical conditions should consider choosing a medical assistance company that allows them to store their medical history predeparture so it can be accessed worldwide if needed (see Chapter 2, Obtaining Health Care Abroad for the Ill Traveler).

- Advise travelers to pack medications in their original containers in carry-on luggage and to carry a copy of their prescriptions. Ensure the traveler has sufficient quantities of medications for the entire trip, plus extra in case of unexpected delays. Since medications should be taken based on elapsed time and not time of day, travelers may need guidance on scheduling when to take medications during and after crossing time zones.
- Educate regarding drug interactions (see Chapter 2, Interactions among Travel Vaccines & Drugs). Medications (such as warfarin) used to treat chronic medical illnesses may interact with medications prescribed for self-treatment of travelers' diarrhea or malaria chemoprophylaxis. Discuss all medications used, either daily or on an as-needed basis.
- Suggest supplemental insurance. Three types of insurance policies can be considered: 1) trip cancellation in the event of illness; 2) supplemental insurance so that money paid for health care abroad may be reimbursed, since most medical insurance policies do not cover health care in other countries; and 3) medical evacuation insurance (see Chapter 2, Travel Insurance, Travel Health Insurance, & Medical Evacuation Insurance).
- Help devise a health plan. This plan should give instructions for managing minor problems or exacerbations of underlying illnesses and should include information about medical facilities available in the destination country (see Chapter 2, Obtaining Health Care Abroad for the Ill Traveler).
- Recommend that the traveler wear a medical alert bracelet or carry medical information on his or her person (various brands of jewelry or tags, even electronic, are available).
- Advise travelers to keep well-hydrated, wear loose-fitting clothing, and walk and stretch at regular intervals during long-distance travel (see Chapter 2, Deep Vein Thrombosis & Pulmonary Embolism).

- Always advise the traveler about packing a health kit (see Chapter 2, Travel Health Kits).

SPECIFIC CHRONIC ILLNESSES

Issues related to specific chronic medical illnesses are addressed in Table 8-5. These recommendations should be used in conjunction with the other recommendations given throughout this book. Below is a noninclusive list of additional resources for information:

- American Association of Kidney Patients (www.aakp.org)
- American Diabetes Association (www.diabetes.org)
- American Heart Association (www.heart.org)
- American Lung Association (www.lungusa.org)
- American Thoracic Society (www.thoracic.org)
- Anticoagulation Forum (www.acforum.org)
- British Thoracic Society (www.brit-thoracic.org.uk)
- Crohn's and Colitis Foundation of America (www.ccfa.org)
- Global Dialysis (www.globaldialysis.com)
- International Self-Monitoring Association of Oral Anticoagulated Patients (www.ismaap.org)
- National Multiple Sclerosis Society (www.nationalmssociety.org)
- US Transportation Security Administration (www.tsa.gov)
- US Department of State (www.state.gov)

Also, many health care facilities outside the United States are accredited by the Joint Commission International, an affiliate of the Joint Commission, which is the largest accreditor of US-based health care organizations. A list of accredited international facilities is available at their website (www.jointcommissioninternational.org).

If travelers or their health care providers have concerns about fitness for air travel or the need to obtain a medical certificate before travel, the medical unit affiliated with the specific airline is a valuable source for information. Remember to notify the airline in advance if oxygen or other equipment is needed on the plane. The TSA Cares Help Line (toll-free at 855-787-2227) can also provide information on how to prepare for the airport security screening process with respect to a particular disability or medical condition.

Table 8-5. Special considerations for travelers with chronic medical illnesses

CONDITION	ABSOLUTE AND RELATIVE CONTRAINDICATIONS TO AIRLINE TRAVEL	PRE-TRAVEL CONSIDERATIONS	IMMUNIZATION CONSIDERATIONS	MISCELLANEOUS
Cardiovascular diseases	Following acute coronary syndrome: • those at very low risk—within 3 days after event • medium risk—within 10 days • high risk or awaiting further intervention or treatment—defer air travel until disease is stable Unstable angina CHF, severe, decompensated Uncontrolled hypertension CABG within 14 days CVA within 2 weeks Elective percutaneous coronary intervention within 2 days Uncontrolled arrhythmia Eisenmenger syndrome Severe symptomatic valvular heart disease	Supplemental oxygen Plan for self-management of dehydration and volume overload; may include adjusting medications Bring copy of recent EKG Bring pacemaker or AICD card DVT precautions	Influenza Pneumococcal Hepatitis B	Have sublingual nitroglycerine available in carry-on bag Mefloquine not recommended for people with cardiac conduction abnormalities, particularly for those with ventricular arrhythmias Self-monitoring and management of INR should be tailored to the individual patient by the anticoagulant primary provider

Condition				
Pulmonary diseases	Severe, labile asthma Recent hospitalization for acute respiratory illness Bullous lung disease Active lower respiratory infection Pneumothorax within 2–3 weeks Pleural effusion within 14 days High supplemental oxygen requirements at baseline Major chest surgery within 10–14 days	Supplemental oxygen Discuss with airline need for other equipment on plane (such as nebulizer) Plan for self-management of exacerbations (including COPD, asthma) DVT precautions	Influenza Pneumococcal Hepatitis B	Consider carrying a short course of antibiotics and steroids, as appropriate, for exacerbations Consider advising an inhaler be available in carry-on bag, even if not routinely used
Gastrointestinal diseases	Surgery, including laparoscopic, within 10–14 days Gastrointestinal bleed within 24 hours Colonoscopy within 24 hours Partial bowel obstruction Liver failure (especially cirrhosis or heavy alcohol use)	Emphasize food and water precautions Consider prescribing prophylactic antibiotic for TD Recommend avoiding undercooked seafood, if cirrhosis or heavy alcohol use (*Vibrio vulnificus*)	Influenza Pneumococcal Hepatitis A Hepatitis B	May experience increased colostomy output during air travel H₂ blockers and PPIs increase susceptibility to TD Use mefloquine with caution in any chronic liver disease For YF vaccine, see the Immunocompromised Travelers section earlier in this chapter
Renal failure and chronic renal insufficiency	None	Emphasize food and water precautions Plan for self-management of dehydration, which can worsen renal function Arrange dialysis abroad, if needed Adjust medications for CrCl	Influenza Pneumococcal Hepatitis B	Know HIV, hepatitis C, and hepatitis B status Atovaquone-proguanil contraindicated when CrCl <30 mL/min AAKP and Global Dialysis websites can help with finding dialysis centers; check for JCI accreditation For YF vaccine, see the Immunocompromised Travelers section earlier in this chapter

continued

TABLE 8-5. SPECIAL CONSIDERATIONS FOR TRAVELERS WITH CHRONIC MEDICAL ILLNESSES (continued)

CONDITION	ABSOLUTE AND RELATIVE CONTRAINDICATIONS TO AIRLINE TRAVEL	PRE-TRAVEL CONSIDERATIONS	IMMUNIZATION CONSIDERATIONS	MISCELLANEOUS
Diabetes mellitus	None	Plan for self-management of dehydration, diabetic foot, and pressure sores Insulin adjustments Should check FSBG at 4- to 6-hour intervals during air travel Discuss changes in insulin regimen or oral agent with diabetes specialist Provide physician's letter stating need for all equipment, including syringes, glucose meter, and supplies	Influenza Pneumococcal Hepatitis B	Keep insulin and all glucose meter supplies in carry-on bag Bring food and supplies needed to manage hypoglycemia during travel Check feet daily for pressure sores For YF vaccine, see the Immunocompromised Travelers section earlier in this chapter
Severe allergic reactions	None	Plan for managing allergic reactions while traveling and consider bringing a short course of steroids for possible allergic reactions Should carry injectable epinephrine and antihistamines (H_1 and H_2 blockers)—always have on person		Many airlines already have policies in place for dealing with peanut allergies Make sure to carry injectable epinephrine in case of a severe reaction while in flight
Autoimmune and rheumatologic diseases	None	Should have a baseline TST or IGRA before starting TNF blockers.	Immunosuppressive medications and TNF blockers may alter response to immunizations Live attenuated vaccines may be contraindicated	Particular emphasis should be placed on food and water precautions and hand hygiene

Abbreviations: CHF, congestive heart failure; CABG, coronary artery bypass graft; CVA, cerebrovascular accident; EKG, electrocardiogram; AICD, automatic implantable cardioverter defibrillators; DVT, deep vein thrombosis; INR, international normalized ratio; COPD, chronic obstructive pulmonary disease; TD, travelers' diarrhea; PPIs, proton-pump inhibitors; YF, yellow fever; CrCl, creatinine clearance; AAKP, American Association of Kidney Patients; JCI, Joint Commission International; FSBG, fingerstick blood glucose; TST, tuberculin skin test; IGRA, interferon-γ release assay; TNF, tumor necrosis factor.

BIBLIOGRAPHY

1. Aerospace Medical Association. Medical Guidelines for Airline Travel. 2nd ed. Alexandria, VA: Aerospace Medical Association; 2003 [cited 2012 Sep 23]. Available from: http://www.asma.org/asma/media/asma/Travel-Publications/medguid.pdf.

2. Aerospace Medical Association. Useful tips for airline travel. Alexandria, VA: Aerospace Medical Association; 2005 [cited 2012 Sep 23]. Available from: http://www.asma.org/asma/media/asma/Travel-Publications/tips_for_travelers.pdf.

3. Ahmedzai S, Balfour-Lynn IM, Bewick T, Buchdahl R, Coker RK, Cummin AR, et al. Managing passengers with stable respiratory disease planning air travel: British Thoracic Society recommendations. Thorax. 2011 Sep;66 Suppl 1:i1–30.

4. Chandran M, Edelman SV. Have insulin, will fly: diabetes management during air travel and time zone adjustment strategies. Clin Diabetes. 2003;21(2):82–5.

5. McCarthy AE, Burchard GD. The travelers with pre-existing disease. In: Keystone JS, Freedman DO, Kozarsky PE, Connor BA, Nothdurft HD, editors. Travel Medicine. 3rd ed. Philadelphia: Saunders Elsevier; 2013. p. 258–63.

6. Ringwald J, Strobel J, Eckstein R. Travel and oral anticoagulation. J Travel Med. 2009 Jul–Aug;16(4):276–83.

7. Schwartz M. Travel and oral anticoagulants. J Travel Med. 2009 Sep–Oct;16(5):369–70.

8. Simons FE. Anaphylaxis. J Allergy Clin Immunol. 2008 Feb;121(2 Suppl):S402–7.

9. Smith D, Toff W, Joy M, Dowdall N, Johnston R, Clark L, et al. Fitness to fly for passengers with cardiovascular disease. Heart. 2010 Aug;96 Suppl 2:ii1–16.

PREGNANT TRAVELERS
I. Dale Carroll

INTRODUCTION

Pregnancy is an altered state of health that requires special considerations. With careful preparation, however, most pregnant women are able to travel safely.

PRE-TRAVEL EVALUATION

The pre-travel evaluation of a pregnant traveler (Box 8-1) should begin with a careful medical and obstetric history, with particular attention to gestational age and evaluation for high-risk conditions. A visit with an obstetrician should be a part of the pre-travel assessment, which should include an ultrasound—to establish the gestational age of the pregnancy and identify any potential problems—and evaluation of the mother's blood type and Rh status. The traveler should be provided with a copy of her prenatal records and physician's contact information. Checking for immunity to various infectious diseases may obviate the need for some vaccines.

A review of the patient's travel itinerary, including destinations, types of accommodation, and planned activities, should guide pre-travel health advice. Preparation includes educating the patient regarding avoidance of travel-associated risks, the management of minor pregnancy discomforts, and recognition of more serious complications. Bleeding, premature labor, and premature rupture of the fetal membranes are conditions that require urgent medical attention.

Pregnant travelers should pack a travel health kit that includes a blood pressure monitor, hemorrhoid cream, antiemetic drugs, prenatal vitamins, medication for vaginitis or yeast infection, talcum powder, and support hose, in addition to the items recommended for all travelers (see Chapter 2, Travel Health Kits).

CONTRAINDICATIONS FOR TRAVEL DURING PREGNANCY

Although travel is rarely contraindicated during a normal pregnancy, complicated pregnancies require extra consideration and may warrant a recommendation that travel be delayed (Box 8-2). Pregnant travelers should be advised that the risk of obstetric complications is highest in the first and third trimesters.

BOX 8-1. PRE-TRAVEL CONSULTATION CHECKLIST FOR PREGNANT TRAVELERS

- Ultrasound to establish a reliable due date and to confirm normal pregnancy
- Check for immunity to infectious diseases, for example, hepatitis A and B, rubella, varicella, measles, pertussis
- Update routine immunizations: tetanus-diphtheria-pertussis, influenza (inactivated), polio, including hepatitis A and B
- Destination risk considerations
  > Infectious disease
    > Malaria
    > Outbreak of disease requiring a live virus vaccine
    > Outbreak of a disease for which no vaccine is available but which has a high risk of maternal or fetal illness or death
    > Sexually transmitted diseases
    > Food and water precautions
    > Insect exposure
  > Environmental: altitude, heat, humidity, pollution
  > Medical services available during transit and at destination
- Travel risk assessment
  > Mode of travel, destination, length of travel, and style
  > Planned activities such as climbing, water sports, snorkeling
- Supplemental travel insurance, travel health insurance, and medical evacuation insurance (research specific coverage information and limitations for pregnancy-related health issues)
- Signs and symptoms for which care should be sought immediately
  > Pelvic or abdominal pain
  > Bleeding
  > Rupture of membranes
  > Contractions
  > Symptoms of preeclampsia (unusual swelling, severe headaches, nausea and vomiting, vision changes)
  > Vomiting, diarrhea, dehydration
  > Symptoms of potential deep vein thrombosis or pulmonary embolism (unusual swelling of leg with pain in calf or thigh, unusual shortness of breath)
- Recommendations
  > Immunizations that reflect actual risk of disease and probable benefit
  > Malaria chemoprophylaxis, if indicated
  > Preventive measures to decrease the above risks
- Paperwork
  > Check airline and cruise line policies
  > Letter confirming due date and fitness to travel
  > Copy of medical records
  > Letter for customs regarding medications
  > Exemption letter or waiver for required vaccines
- Preparing for obstetric care
  > Check coverage by medical insurance
  > Arrange travel insurance, travel health insurance, and medical evacuation insurance
  > Arrange medical assistance
  > Arrange for obstetric care at destination
- Comfort arrangements
  > Loose clothing and comfortable shoes
  > Pillows, support hose
  > Bottled water
  > Upgrade flight seating if possible
  > Lighten itinerary if not accustomed to planned activities
- Postpone travel if risks outweigh benefits

- **Absolute Contraindications**
  - > Abruptio placentae
  - > Active labor
  - > Incompetent cervix
  - > Premature labor
  - > Premature rupture of membranes
  - > Suspected ectopic pregnancy
  - > Threatened abortion, vaginal bleeding
  - > Toxemia, past or present

- **Relative Contraindications**
  - > Abnormal presentation
  - > Fetal growth restriction
  - > History of infertility
  - > History of miscarriage or ectopic pregnancy
  - > Maternal age <15 or >35 years
  - > Multiple gestation
  - > Placenta previa or other placental abnormality

PLANNING FOR EMERGENCY CARE

Obstetric emergencies are often sudden and life-threatening. Travel to remote locations or areas in some developing countries where obstetric care may be less than the standard at home is inadvisable. For a woman in the third trimester of pregnancy, it is advisable to identify a medical facility in her destination that could manage complications of pregnancy, her delivery, a caesarean section, and neonatal problems. Some complications may be managed so that the mother could travel to a facility where she could receive advanced obstetric care, but some conditions are contraindications for any travel (Box 8-2). In such cases, it may be preferable to transport help to the patient rather than transport the patient.

Many general health insurance policies do not cover complications of pregnancy overseas. Supplemental travel health insurance should be strongly considered to cover both pregnancy-related problems and care of the neonate, as needed. Evacuation insurance with a policy that includes coverage of pregnancy-related complications is highly encouraged as well.

TRANSPORTATION CONSIDERATIONS

Pregnant women should be advised to wear seatbelts, when available, on all forms of transport, including airplanes, cars, and buses. A diagonal shoulder strap with a lap belt provides the best protection, with the straps carefully placed above and below the abdominal bulge. When only a lap belt is available, it should be worn low, between the abdomen and the pelvis.

Air Travel

Most commercial airlines allow pregnant travelers to fly until 36 weeks' gestation. Some limit international travel earlier in pregnancy, and some require documentation of gestational age. Travelers should check with the airline to find out their specific requirements or guidance for pregnant women. Air cabins of most commercial jetliners are pressurized to 6,000–8,000 ft (1,829–2,438 m) above sea level; the lower oxygen tension should not cause fetal problems in a normal pregnancy, but women with preexisting cardiovascular problems, sickle cell disease, or severe anemia (hemoglobin <80 g/L) may experience the effects of low arterial oxygen saturation. Risks of air travel include potential exposure to communicable diseases, immobility, and the common discomforts of flying. Abdominal distention and pedal edema frequently occur. The pregnant traveler may benefit from an upgrade in airline seating and should seek convenient and practical accommodations (such as close proximity to the toilet). Loose clothing and comfortable shoes should be recommended.

Some experts report that the risk of deep vein thrombosis in pregnancy is 5–10 times higher than for nonpregnant women, estimated to be 1 in 1,000. Preventive measures include frequent stretching, walking and isometric leg exercises, and wearing graduated compression stockings.

Cosmic radiation during air travel poses little threat, but may be a consideration for pregnant travelers who are frequent fliers (such as air crew). Older airport security machines are magnetometers and are not harmful to the fetus. Newer security machines use backscatter x-ray scanners, which emit low levels of radiation; most experts agree that the risk of radiation exposure from these scanners is extremely low.

Cruise Ship Travel

Most cruise lines restrict travel beyond 28 weeks of pregnancy, and some as early as 24 weeks. Pregnant travelers may be required to carry a physician's note stating that they are fit to travel and including the estimated date of delivery. Pregnant women should check with the cruise line to find out their specific requirements or guidance. The pregnant patient planning a cruise should be advised regarding motion sickness, gastrointestinal and respiratory infections, and the risk of falls on a moving vessel.

ENVIRONMENTAL CONSIDERATIONS

Air pollution may cause more health problems during pregnancy, as ciliary clearance of the bronchial tree is slowed and mucus more abundant. Body temperature regulation is not as efficient during pregnancy, and temperature extremes cause more stress on the gravid woman. In addition, an increase in core temperature, such as with heat prostration or heat stroke, may harm the fetus. The vasodilatory effect of a hot environment might also cause fainting. For these reasons, accommodation should be sought in air-conditioned quarters and activities restricted in hot environments.

Pregnant women should avoid activities at high altitude unless trained for and accustomed to such activities. Women unaccustomed to high altitudes may experience exaggerated breathlessness and palpitations. The common symptoms of acute mountain sickness (insomnia, headache, and nausea) are frequently also associated with pregnancy, and it may be difficult to distinguish the cause of the symptoms. No studies or case reports show harm to a fetus if the mother travels briefly to high altitudes during pregnancy. However, it may be prudent to recommend that pregnant women not stay at sleeping altitudes >12,000 ft (3,658 m), if possible. Although compelling reasons to use acetazolamide may exist, most experts recommend simply a slower ascent with adequate time for acclimatization. Probably the largest concern regarding high-altitude travel in pregnancy is that many high-altitude destinations are inaccessible and far from medical care.

ACTIVITIES

Pregnant travelers should be discouraged from undertaking unaccustomed vigorous physical activity. Swimming and snorkeling during pregnancy are generally safe, but waterskiing has resulted in falls that inject water into the birth canal. Most experts advise against scuba diving for pregnant women because of the risk of fetal gas embolism during decompression. Riding bicycles, motorcycles, or animals presents risk of trauma to the abdomen.

INFECTIOUS DISEASES

Pregnant women who develop travelers' diarrhea or other gastrointestinal infection may be more vulnerable to dehydration than are nonpregnant travelers. Strict hand hygiene and food and water precautions should be stressed (see Chapter 2, Food & Water Precautions). Bottled or boiled water is preferable to chemically treated or filtered water. Iodine-containing compounds should not be used to purify water for pregnant women because of potential effects on the fetal thyroid (see Chapter 2, Water Disinfection for Travelers). The treatment of choice for travelers' diarrhea is prompt and vigorous oral hydration; however, azithromycin may be given to pregnant women if clinically indicated. Use of bismuth subsalicylate is contraindicated.

Hepatitis A and E are both spread by the fecal-oral route. Hepatitis A has been reported to increase the risk of placental abruption and premature delivery. Hepatitis E is more likely to cause severe disease during pregnancy and may result in a case-fatality ratio of 15%–30%; when acquired during the third trimester, it is also associated with fetal complications and fetal death. Some foodborne illnesses of particular concern during pregnancy include toxoplasmosis and listeriosis. The risk during pregnancy is that the infection will cross the placenta and cause spontaneous abortion, stillbirth, or congenital infection. Risk of fetal infection increases with the length of gestation, but severity of infection is decreased. The patient should be warned, therefore, to avoid unpasteurized cheeses and undercooked meat products. Parasitic diseases are less common but may cause concern, particularly in women who are visiting friends and relatives in developing areas. In general, intestinal helminths rarely cause enough illness to warrant treatment during pregnancy. Most intestinal helminths, in fact, can safely be addressed with symptomatic treatment until the pregnancy is over. On the other hand, protozoan intestinal infections, such as *Giardia*, *Entamoeba histolytica*, and *Cryptosporidium*, often do require treatment. These parasites may cause acute gastroenteritis, chronic malabsorption resulting in fetal growth restriction, and in the case of *E. histolytica*, invasive disease, including amebic liver abscess and colitis. Pregnant women are advised to avoid swimming or wading in freshwater lakes, streams, and rivers that may harbor schistosomes.

Pregnant women should avoid mosquito bites when traveling in areas endemic for arboviruses or malaria. Preventive measures include the use of bed nets and insect repellents and wearing protective clothing (see Chapter 2, Protection against Mosquitoes, Ticks, & Other Insects & Arthropods).

Respiratory and urinary infections and vaginitis are also more likely to occur and to be more severe in pregnancy.

MEDICATIONS

Various systems are used to classify drugs in regard to their safety in pregnancy. In most cases, it is preferable to refer to specific data regarding the effects of a given drug during pregnancy rather than simply to depend on a classification.

Analgesics that can be used during pregnancy include acetaminophen and some narcotics. Aspirin may increase the incidence of abruption, and other antiinflammatory agents could cause premature closure of the ductus arteriosus. Constipation may require a mild bulk laxative. Several simple remedies are often effective in relieving the symptoms of morning sickness, and these may prevent motion sickness. Nonprescription remedies include ginger, which as a powder can be mixed with food or drinks such as tea. It is also available in candy, such as lollipops. Similarly, pyridoxine (vitamin B6) is effective in reducing symptoms of morning sickness and is available in tablet form, as well as

lozenges and lollipops. Antihistamines, such as meclizine and dimenhydrinate, are often used in pregnancy and appear to have a good safety record.

VACCINES

In the best possible scenario, a woman should be up-to-date on routine vaccinations before she becomes pregnant. The most effective way of protecting the infant against many diseases is to immunize the mother. Tetanus, diphtheria, and pertussis (Tdap) vaccine, if not previously received, is recommended during pregnancy for women to protect the woman from getting pertussis and to pass protective antibiotics to her newborn. To optimize the concentration of maternal antibodies transferred to the fetus, Tdap should be given preferably during the third or late second trimester (after 20 weeks' gestation). Annual influenza vaccine (inactivated) is recommended during any trimester if pregnancy coincides with influenza season. Certain vaccines, including meningococcal polysaccharide (MPSV4), inactivated polio vaccine (IPV), and hepatitis A and B vaccines, that are considered safe during pregnancy may be indicated based on risk. Rabies postexposure prophylaxis with rabies immune globulin and vaccine should be administered after any moderate- or high-risk exposure to rabies; preexposure vaccine may be considered for travelers when the risk of exposure is substantial.

Most live-virus vaccines, including measles-mumps-rubella (MMR) vaccine, varicella vaccine, and live attenuated influenza vaccine (LAIV), are contraindicated during pregnancy; the exception is yellow fever vaccine, for which pregnancy is considered a precaution by Advisory Committee on Immunization Practices (ACIP). If travel is unavoidable, and the risks for yellow fever virus exposure are felt to outweigh the risks of vaccination, a pregnant woman should be vaccinated. If the risks for vaccination are felt to outweigh the risks for yellow fever virus exposure, pregnant women should be issued a medical waiver to fulfill health regulations. Because pregnancy might affect immunologic function, serologic testing to document an immune response to yellow fever vaccine should be considered. Postexposure management of a nonimmune pregnant woman exposed to measles or varicella may be managed by administering immune globulin (IG) within 6 days for measles or varicella-zoster IG within 10 days for varicella. Women planning to become pregnant should be advised to wait 4 weeks after receipt of a live-virus vaccine before conceiving. For certain travel-related vaccines, including Japanese encephalitis vaccine and typhoid vaccine, data are insufficient for a specific recommendation for use in pregnant women. A summary of current ACIP guidelines for vaccinating pregnant women is available at www.cdc.gov/vaccines/pubs/preg-guide.htm.

MALARIA CHEMOPROPHYLAXIS

Malaria may be much more serious in pregnant than in nonpregnant women. Malaria in pregnancy may be characterized by heavy parasitemia, severe anemia, and sometimes profound hypoglycemia, and may be complicated by cerebral malaria and acute respiratory distress syndrome. Placental sequestration of parasites may result in fetal loss due to abruption, premature labor, or miscarriage. An infant born to an infected mother is apt to be of low birth weight, and, although rare, congenital malaria is a concern.

Because no prophylactic regimen provides complete protection, pregnant women should avoid or delay travel to malaria-endemic areas. However, if travel is unavoidable, pregnant women should take precautions to avoid mosquito bites, and use of an effective prophylactic regimen is essential.

Chloroquine and mefloquine are the drugs of choice for pregnant women for destinations with chloroquine-sensitive and chloroquine-resistant malaria, respectively. Doxycycline is contraindicated because of teratogenic effects on the fetus after the fourth month of pregnancy. Primaquine is contraindicated in pregnancy because the infant cannot be tested for G6PD deficiency, putting the infant at risk for hemolytic anemia. Atovaquone-proguanil is not recommended because of lack of available safety data. A list of the available antimalarial drugs and their uses and contraindications during pregnancy can be found in Table 3-10 and in Chapter 3, Malaria.

BIBLIOGRAPHY

1. ACOG Committee on Obstetric Practice. ACOG Committee Opinion No. 443: Air travel during pregnancy. Obstet Gynecol. 2009 Oct;114(4):954–5.
2. Brenner B. Prophylaxis of travel-related thrombosis in women. Thromb Res. 2009;123 Suppl 3:S26–9.
3. Carroll ID, Williams DC. Pre-travel vaccination and medical prophylaxis in the pregnant traveler. Travel Med Infect Dis. 2008 Sep;6(5):259–75.
4. CDC. General recommendations on immunization—recommendations of the Advisory Committee on Immunization Practices (ACIP). MMWR Recomm Rep. 2011 Jan 28;60(2):1–64.
5. CDC. Guidelines for vaccinating pregnant women. Atlanta: CDC; 2012 [cited 2012 Sep 23]. Available from: http://www.cdc.gov/vaccines/pubs/preg-guide.htm.
6. Dotters-Katz S, Kuller J, Heine RP. Parasitic infections in pregnancy. Obstet Gynecol Surv. 2011 Aug;66(8):515–25.
7. Hezelgrave NL, Whitty CJ, Shennan AH, Chappell LC. Advising on travel during pregnancy. BMJ. 2011;342:d2506.
8. Irvine MH, Einarson A, Bozzo P. Prophylactic use of antimalarials during pregnancy. Can Fam Physician. 2011 Nov;57(11):1279–81.
9. Mehta P, Smith-Bindman R. Airport full-body screening: what is the risk? Arch Intern Med. 2011 Jun 27;171(12):1112–5.
10. Niermeyer S. The pregnant altitude visitor. Adv Exp Med Biol. 1999;474:65–77.
11. Phillips-Howard PA, Wood D. The safety of antimalarial drugs in pregnancy. Drug Saf. 1996 Mar;14(3):131–45.
12. Rietveld AE. Malaria prevention for special groups: pregnant women, infants and young children. In: Schlagenhauf P, editor. Travelers' Malaria. Hamilton, ON: BC Decker; 2001. p. 303–23.

TRAVELERS WITH DISABILITIES
Megan Crawley O'Sullivan

OVERVIEW

Travelers with disabilities are defined as travelers whose mobility is reduced because of a physical incapacity (sensory or locomotor), an intellectual deficiency, age, illness, or another cause, and who may require special attention and adaptation of the transportation services that are available to all passengers. The medical preparation of a traveler with a stable, ongoing disability does not essentially differ from that of any other traveler. The following recommendations may assist in ensuring safe, accessible travel:

- Assess each international itinerary on an individual basis, in consultation with specialized travel agencies or tour operators.
- Consult travel health providers for additional recommendations.
- Use print and internet resources.

AIR TRAVEL
Regulations and Codes

In 1986, Congress passed the Air Carrier Access Act to ensure that people with disabilities are treated without discrimination in a way consistent with the safe carriage of all passengers. The regulations established by the Department of Transportation (DOT) apply to all flights of US airlines, as well as flights to or from the United States by foreign carriers.

Because of the act, carriers may not refuse transportation on the basis of a disability. However, there are a few exceptions; for example, the carrier may refuse transportation if the person with a disability would endanger the health or safety of other passengers or if transporting the person would be a violation of Federal Aviation Administration safety rules. (Travelers and their physicians can learn more about these exceptions and other aspects of the act at http://airconsumer.ost.dot.gov/publications/horizons.htm). Air carriers are also obliged to accept a declaration by a passenger that he or she is self-reliant. A medical certificate, which is a written statement from the passenger's physician saying that the passenger is capable of completing the flight safely without requiring extraordinary medical care, can be required only in specific situations (for example, if a person intends to travel with a possible communicable disease, will require a stretcher or oxygen, or if the person's medical condition can be reasonably expected to affect the operation of the flight).

International Air Transport Association (IATA) member airlines voluntarily adhere to codes of practice that are similar to US legislation based on guidance from the International Civil Aviation Organization. However, smaller airlines overseas may not be IATA members. If a traveler's plans include flying between foreign countries while abroad, one must check with the overseas airlines to ensure that the carriers adhere to accessibility standards for disabled passengers.

The Transportation Security Administration (TSA) has established a program for screening travelers with disabilities and their equipment, mobility aids, and devices. TSA permits prescriptions, liquid medications, and other liquids needed by people with disabilities and medical conditions.

Assistance and Accommodations

When a traveler with a disability requests assistance, the airline is obliged to meet certain accessibility requirements. For example, carriers must provide access to the aircraft door (preferably by a level entry bridge), an aisle seat, and a seat with removable armrests. However, aircraft with <30 seats are generally exempt from these requirements. Any aircraft with >60 seats must have an onboard wheelchair, and personnel must help move the wheelchair from a seat to the lavatory area. However, airline personnel are not required to transfer passengers from wheelchair to wheelchair, wheelchair to aircraft seat, or wheelchair to lavatory seat. In addition, airline personnel are not obliged to assist with feeding, visiting the lavatory, or dispensing medication to travelers. Only wide-body aircraft with ≥2 aisles are required to have fully accessible lavatories. Travelers with disabilities who require assistance should travel with a companion or attendant. However, carriers may not, without reason, require a person with a disability to travel with an attendant.

Airlines may not require advance notice of a passenger with a disability; however, they may require up to 48 hours' advance notice and 1-hour advance check-in for certain accommodations that require preparation time, such as the following services (if they are available on the flight):

- Medical oxygen for use on board the aircraft
- Carriage of an incubator
- Hook-up for a respirator to the aircraft electrical power supply
- Accommodation for a passenger who must travel in a stretcher
- Transportation of an electric wheelchair on a flight scheduled on an aircraft with <60 seats
- Provision by the airline of hazardous material packaging for a battery used in a wheelchair or other assistive devices
- Accommodation for a group of ≥10 people with disabilities who travel as a group
- Provision of an onboard wheelchair to be used on an aircraft that does not have an accessible lavatory

DOT maintains a toll-free hotline (800-778-4838, available 9 AM–5 PM, Eastern Time, Monday through Friday, except federal holidays) to provide general information to consumers about the rights of air travelers with disabilities and to assist air travelers with time-sensitive disability-related issues.

Assessment and Preparation
With the high incidence of cardiopulmonary disease and millions of people traveling by air, many people are at risk for hypoxia and respiratory symptoms while flying. Generally, patients with an oxygen saturation >95% by pulse oximetry do not require supplemental oxygen, and those with a saturation <92% will require it during air travel. The hypoxia altitude simulation test can identify those patients (with an oxygen saturation 92%–95% by pulse oximetry) who may benefit from oxygen supplementation during air travel, decreasing their risk for cardiopulmonary effects of induced hypoxia at higher altitudes.

Internationally standardized codes for classifying disabled passengers and their needs are available in all computerized reservations systems. Passengers with disabilities should use travel agents experienced in the use of the disability coding; it is critical that codes and interairline messages are sequentially entered for all flights. The delivering carrier is always responsible for a traveler with a disability until a subsequent carrier physically accepts responsibility for that passenger.

SERVICE ANIMALS
Service animals are not exempt from compliance with quarantine regulations and so may not be allowed to travel to all international destinations. They are also subject to US animal import regulations on return (see Chapter 6, Taking Animals & Animal Products across International Borders). However, carriers must permit guide dogs or other service animals with identification to accompany a person with a disability on a flight. Carriers must permit a service animal to accompany a traveler with a disability to any assigned seat, unless the animal obstructs an aisle or other area that must remain clear to facilitate an emergency evacuation, in which case the passenger will be assigned another seat.

CRUISE SHIPS
US companies or entities conducting programs or tours on cruise ships have obligations regarding access for travelers with disabilities, even if the ship itself is of foreign registry. However, all travelers with disabilities should check with individual cruise lines regarding availability of requested or needed items before booking. Cruises are available that cater to travelers with special needs, such as dialysis patients.

USEFUL LINKS
- Department of Transportation, Aviation Consumer Protection Division
  - > New Horizons Information for the Air Traveler with a Disability (http://airconsumer.ost.dot.gov/publications/horizons.htm#NewEnvironment)
  - > Aviation Consumer Protection and Enforcement Rules (see links under Part 382, Passengers with Disabilities) (http://airconsumer.ost.dot.gov/rules/rules.htm)
  - > Passengers with Disabilities (site provides a summary of the main

- points of the DOT rule, Title 14 CFR Part 382) (http://airconsumer.ost.dot.gov/publications/disabled.htm)
- Transportation Security Administration—travelers with disabilities and medical conditions (www.tsa.gov/travelers/airtravel/specialneeds)
- MossRehab ResourceNet (www.mossresourcenet.org/travel.htm)
- American Council of the Blind—lists cruises, books, useful telephone numbers, and links to products for purchase (www.acb.org)

- Society for Accessible Travel and Hospitality (www.sath.org)
- Aerospace Medical Association—medical publications for airline travel (http://www.asma.org/publications/medical-publications-for-airline-travel)
- Mobility International USA (www.miusa.org)
  > Preparing for Departure (www.miusa.org/ncde/goingabroad/survivalsteps/preparingtodepart)
  > Equipment and Tools that Make Traveling with a Disability Easy (www.miusa.org/ncde/tipsheets/tools)

BIBLIOGRAPHY

1. Bucks C. A World of Options: a Guide to International Exchange, Community Service and Travel for Persons with Disabilities. 3rd ed. Eugene, OR: ILR Press; 1997.

2. Dine CJ, Kreider ME. Hypoxia altitude simulation test. Chest. 2008 Apr;133(4):1002–5.

IMMIGRANTS RETURNING HOME TO VISIT FRIENDS & RELATIVES (VFRs)
Jay S. Keystone

DEFINITION OF VFR

A traveler categorized as a VFR is an immigrant, ethnically and racially distinct from the majority population of the country of residence (a higher-income country), who returns to his or her home country (lower-income country) to visit friends or relatives. Included in the VFR category are family members, such as the spouse or children, who were born in the country of residence. Some experts have recently recommended that the term VFR refer to all those visiting friends and relatives regardless of the traveler's country of origin; however, this more recently proposed definition may be too broad and not take into consideration cultural, economic, and attitudinal issues. Thus in this review, the more classic definition is used.

DISPROPORTIONATE INFECTIOUS DISEASE RISKS IN VFRs

Altered migration patterns to North America in the past 30 years have resulted in many immigrants originating from Asia, Southeast Asia, and Latin America instead of Europe. Although 12% of the US population is foreign born, in 2010 a total of 35% of those from the United States traveling overseas listed VFR as a reason for travel. VFRs experience a higher incidence of travel-related infectious diseases, such as malaria, typhoid fever, tuberculosis, hepatitis A, and sexually transmitted diseases, than do other groups of international travelers, for a number of reasons:

- Lack of awareness of risk
- ≤30% have a pre-travel health care encounter
- Financial barriers to pre-travel health care
- Clinics are not geographically convenient
- Cultural and language barriers with health care providers
- Lack of trust in the medical system
- Last-minute travel plans and longer trips
- Travel to higher-risk destinations, such as staying in homes and living the local lifestyle that often includes lack of safe food and water and bed net use

- Belief that they are immune (VFR health beliefs likely contribute to lower rates of vaccination against hepatitis A and typhoid and infrequent use of malaria chemoprophylaxis, compared with other international travelers.)

Malaria

In 2010, 54% of imported malaria cases in US civilians occurred among VFRs. Data from GeoSentinel Surveillance Network show that among ill travelers who present for medical care, VFRs are 8 times more likely to be diagnosed with malaria than are tourist travelers. Reports from the United Kingdom show similar results for VFR versus tourist travelers to West Africa. Many VFRs assume they are immune; however, in most VFRs, especially those who left their countries of origin years previously, immunity has waned and is no longer protective. In recent years, a number of VFRs have died of malaria on their return to North America; in 2010, 53% of those with severe malaria for whom the purpose of travel was known were VFRs, mostly returned from West Africa.

Other Infections

In the United States, 66% of typhoid cases occur in VFRs, mostly from South Asia and Latin America; 90% of paratyphoid A cases are imported from South Asia as well. Most typhoid isolates showed lower sensitivity to fluoroquinolones. A recent Canadian study showed that 94% of typhoid cases in Quebec were in VFRs, mostly from the Indian subcontinent.

VFR children aged <15 years are at highest risk for hepatitis A, and many are asymptomatic. The Quebec study cited above showed that 65% of hepatitis A cases were in VFRs aged <20 years. In a British study, most cases were acquired in South Asia. Other diseases, such as tuberculosis, hepatitis A and B, cholera, and measles, occur more commonly in VFRs after travel.

PRE-TRAVEL HEALTH COUNSELING FOR VFRs

Table 8-6 summarizes VFR health risks and prevention recommendations. It is important to increase awareness among travelers regarding their unique risks for travel-related infections and the barriers to travel health services. If possible, clinics should incorporate culturally sensitive educational materials, provide language translators, and provide handouts in multiple languages (see www.tropical.umn.edu/TTM/VFR/index.htm).

Vaccinations

Travel immunization recommendations and requirements for VFRs are the same as those for US-born travelers. It is crucial, however, to first try to establish whether the immigrant traveler has had routine immunizations (such as measles and tetanus) or has a history of the diseases. Adult travelers, in the absence of documentation of immunizations, may be considered to be nonimmune, and age-appropriate vaccinations (or serologic studies to check for antibody status) should be provided, with 2 caveats:

- Immunity to hepatitis A should not be assumed; many young adults and adolescents from developing countries are still susceptible. Pre-travel serologic testing for both hepatitis A and B may be worthwhile.
- Consider varicella immunization for immigrants from South and Southeast Asia and Latin America. These travelers may be more susceptible, because infection occurs at an older age in tropical than in temperate regions. Also, rates of death and complications from varicella disease are higher in adults than in children.

Malaria Prevention

VFR travelers to endemic areas should not only be encouraged to take prophylactic medications, but also be reminded of the benefits of barrier methods of prevention, such as bed nets and insect repellents, particularly for children (see Chapter 2, Protection against Mosquitoes, Ticks, & Other Insects & Arthropods). VFRs should be advised that drugs such as chloroquine and pyrimethamine, as well as proguanil monotherapy, are no longer effective in most areas, especially in sub-Saharan Africa. These medications are often readily available and inexpensive in their home countries but are not efficacious.

VFRs should also be encouraged to purchase their medications before traveling to ensure good drug quality. Studies in Africa and Southeast Asia show that one-third to half of antimalarial drugs purchased locally were counterfeit or substandard; a recently published study from Laos showed that 88% of oral artesunate sold in pharmacies was of poor quality.

8

Table 8-6. Diseases for which VFR travelers are at increased risk, proposed reasons for risk variance, and recommendations to reduce risks specific to travelers visiting friends and relatives[1]

SPECIFIC DISEASES	REASON FOR RISK VARIANCE[2]	RECOMMENDATIONS TO STRESS WITH VFR TRAVELERS
Foodborne and waterborne illness	Social and cultural pressure (eat the meal served by hosts)	Frequent handwashing Avoid high-risk foods (dairy products, undercooked foods) Simplify treatment regimens (single dose, such as azithromycin, 1,000 mg, or ciprofloxacin, 500 mg) Discuss food preparation
Fish-related toxins and infections	Eating high-risk foods Less pre-travel advice	Avoidance counseling about specific foods (such as raw freshwater fish)
Malaria	Longer stays Higher-risk destinations Less pre-travel advice leading to less use of chemoprophylaxis and fewer personal protection measures Belief that already immune	Education on malaria, mosquito avoidance, and the need for chemoprophylaxis Consider cost of chemoprophylaxis Use of insecticide-treated bed nets
Tuberculosis (particularly multidrug-resistant)	Increased close contact with local population Increased contact with HIV-coinfected people	Check PPD 2–3 months after return if history of negative tuberculin skin test and long stay (>3 months) Educate about tuberculosis signs, symptoms, and avoidance
Bloodborne and sexually transmitted diseases	More likely to seek substandard local care Cultural practices (tattoos, female genital mutilation) Longer stays and increased chance of blood transfusion Higher likelihood of sexual encounters with local population	Discuss high-risk behaviors, including tattoos, piercings, dental work, sexual encounters Encourage purchase of condoms before travel Consider providing syringes, needles, and intravenous catheters for long-term travel
Schistosomiasis and geohelminths	Limited access to piped-in water in rural areas for bathing and washing clothes	Avoid freshwater exposure Use liposomal DEET preparation with freshwater exposures[3] Discourage children from playing in dirt Use ground cover Use protective footwear

continued

TABLE 8-6. DISEASES FOR WHICH VFR TRAVELERS ARE AT INCREASED RISK, PROPOSED REASONS FOR RISK VARIANCE, AND RECOMMENDATIONS TO REDUCE RISKS SPECIFIC TO TRAVELERS VISITING FRIENDS AND RELATIVES[1] (continued)

SPECIFIC DISEASES	REASON FOR RISK VARIANCE[2]	RECOMMENDATIONS TO STRESS WITH VFR TRAVELERS
Respiratory problems	Increased close exposure to fires, smoking, or pollution	Prepare for asthma exacerbations by considering stand-by bronchodilators and steroids
Zoonotic diseases (such as rickettsial infections, leptospirosis, viral fevers, leishmaniasis, anthrax)	Rural destinations Staying with family where animals are kept Increased exposure to insects Increased exposure to mice and rats Sleeping on floors	Avoid animals Wash hands Wear protective clothing Check for ticks daily Avoid thatched roofs and mud walls in Latin America Avoid sleeping at floor level
Envenomations (snakes, spiders, scorpions)	Sleeping on floors	Avoid sleeping at floor level Wear shoes outdoors at night
Toxin ingestion (medication adverse events, heavy metal ingestion)	Purchase of local medications Use of traditional therapies Use of contaminated products (such as pottery with lead glaze) Eating contaminated freshwater fish	Anticipate need and purchase medications before travel Counsel avoidance of known traditional medications (such as Hmong bark tea with aspirin) and high-risk items (such as large reef fish)
Yellow fever and Japanese encephalitis (risk is decreased in adults)	Unclear, partial immunity from previous exposure or vaccination	Avoid mosquitoes by taking protective measures and receiving vaccination when appropriate
Dengue (especially risk of severe dengue)	Severe dengue occurs on repeat exposure to a different serotype of dengue; VFRs more likely to have had previous exposure	Avoid mosquitoes by taking protective measures

Abbreviations: VFR, visiting friends and relatives; PPD, tuberculin purified protein derivative; DEET, *N,N*-diethyl-*m*-toluamide.

[1] Adapted from: Bacaner N, Stauffer W, Boulware DR, Walker PF, Keystone JS. Travel medicine considerations for North American immigrants visiting friends and relatives. JAMA. 2004;291(23):2856–64.
[2] Hypothesis unless referenced to support assertions.
[3] In animal models, DEET (liposomal preparations) prevents *Schistosoma* cercariae from penetrating the skin.

BIBLIOGRAPHY

1. Angell SY, Cetron MS. Health disparities among travelers visiting friends and relatives abroad. Ann Intern Med. 2005 Jan 4;142(1):67–72.
2. Arguin PM. A definition that includes first and second generation immigrants returning to their countries of origin to visit friends and relatives still makes sense to me. J Travel Med. 2010 May–Jun;17(3):147–9.
3. Bacaner N, Stauffer B, Boulware DR, Walker PF, Keystone JS. Travel medicine considerations for North American immigrants visiting friends and relatives. JAMA. 2004 Jun 16;291(23):2856–64.
4. Barnett ED, Christiansen D, Figueira M. Seroprevalence of measles, rubella, and varicella in refugees. Clin Infect Dis. 2002 Aug 15;35(4):403–8.

5. Barnett ED, MacPherson DW, Stauffer WM, Loutan L, Hatz CF, Matteeli A, et al. The visiting friends or relatives traveler in the 21st century: time for a new definition. J Travel Med. 2010 May–Jun;17(3):163–70.

6. Bate R, Coticelli P, Tren R, Attaran A. Antimalarial drug quality in the most severely malarious parts of Africa—a six country study. PLoS One. 2008;3(5):e2132.

7. Bui YG, Trepanier S, Milord F, Blackburn M, Provost S, Gagnon S. Cases of malaria, hepatitis A, and typhoid fever among VFRs, Quebec (Canada). J Travel Med. 2011 Nov–Dec;18(6):373–8.

8. Greenaway C, Dongier P, Boivin JF, Tapiero B, Miller M, Schwartzman K. Susceptibility to measles, mumps, and rubella in newly arrived adult immigrants and refugees. Ann Intern Med. 2007 Jan 2;146(1):20–4.

9. Gupta SK, Medalla F, Omondi MW, Whichard JM, Fields PI, Gerner-Smidt P, et al. Laboratory-based surveillance of paratyphoid fever in the United States: travel and antimicrobial resistance. Clin Infect Dis. 2008 Jun 1;46(11):1656–63.

10. Hendel-Paterson B, Swanson SJ. Pediatric travelers visiting friends and relatives (VFR) abroad: illnesses, barriers and pre-travel recommendations. Travel Med Infect Dis. 2011 Jul;9(4):192–203.

11. Jacobsen KH, Koopman JS. Declining hepatitis A seroprevalence: a global review and analysis. Epidemiol Infect. 2004 Dec;132(6):1005–22.

12. Leder K, Tong S, Weld L, Kain KC, Wilder-Smith A, von Sonnenburg F, et al. Illness in travelers visiting friends and relatives: a review of the GeoSentinel Surveillance Network. Clin Infect Dis. 2006 Nov 1;43(9):1185–93.

13. Lynch MF, Blanton EM, Bulens S, Polyak C, Vojdani J, Stevenson J, et al. Typhoid fever in the United States, 1999–2006. JAMA. 2009 Aug 26;302(8):859–65.

14. Pavli A, Maltezou HC. Malaria and travellers visiting friends and relatives. Travel Med Infect Dis. 2010 May;8(3):161–8.

15. Schilthuis HJ, Goossens I, Ligthelm RJ, de Vlas SJ, Varkevisser C, Richardus JH. Factors determining use of pre-travel preventive health services by West African immigrants in The Netherlands. Trop Med Int Health. 2007 Aug;12(8):990–8.

16. US Department of Commerce, Office of Travel and Tourism Industries. Profile of US resident travelers visiting overseas destinations: 2010 outbound. Washington, DC: US Department of Commerce; 2010 [cited 2012 Sep 23]. Available from: http://tinet.ita.doc.gov/outreachpages/download_data_table/2010_Outbound_Analysis.pdf.

17. US Department of Commerce, US Census Bureau. Foreign Born. Washington, DC: US Department of Commerce; 2010 [cited 2012 Sep 23]. Available from: http://www.census.gov/population/foreign/data/cps2010.html.

18. US Department of Commerce, US Census Bureau. US Census Bureau announces 2010 Census population counts—apportionment counts delivered to president. Washington, DC: US Department of Commerce; 2010 [cited 2012 Sep 23]. Available from: http://2010.census.gov/news/releases/operations/cb10-cn93.html.

ADVICE FOR AIR CREWS

Phyllis E. Kozarsky

OVERVIEW

As airlines expand their reach and air crews are asked to travel to more exotic destinations, these travelers need to prepare ahead of time for the exposures they may encounter. To some degree, air crews are similar to all travelers to such destinations, but the differences require some modifications of travel health guidance for several reasons:

- Layovers are short, often 24–48 hours.
- Travel is frequent.
- Travel to new destinations may be on short notice.
- Despite short travel times, air crews may be more adventuresome and thus have more risk than typical package tourists.
- Air crews interact with each other frequently, and misinformation spreads quickly.
- Air crews may perceive themselves to be low risk because of their generally healthy status and because their exposure time in-country is short.

Given these factors, it is worth noting some guidelines for this special group. In general, air carriers traveling to destinations in the developing world try to inform their crews about health issues they may face. However, airlines do not necessarily have available on their staff occupational health or other providers who are experts in travel medicine, and the airlines may not be aware of special risks at their destinations. Air crews and clinicians seeing such travelers should, therefore, encourage airlines to avail themselves of professionals who are knowledgeable in the field and who can help determine recommendations for the various destinations served.

Pilots often know some of the medications and classes of medications that are not permitted while flying, so clinicians should always discuss medication options. Medications with central nervous system adverse events should not be prescribed, and pilots should take a trial between trips of any medication that could have side effects that may interfere with flying. Pilots and flight attendants should also be aware that certain foods and beverages contain trace amounts of products that could cause a drug screen to turn positive. They should also consider the effects on health and drug tests of drinking too much water (possibly causing hyponatremia). If questions arise, an aeromedical examiner should be consulted who will know the Federal Aviation Administration rules for what medications can and cannot be taken by pilots. These physicians are responsible for certifying that pilots are fit to fly, and they examine pilots regularly.

Although any travel health provider can see and advise flight crews, it is important to ask the crew member what the airline may require, in addition to what is required or recommended to maintain the person's health while traveling. If in doubt, the travel health provider should contact the airline medical director or occupational health department for guidance. For example, some air crews primarily fly domestic routes or routes to Western Europe or Japan, so would not fly to a region of yellow fever risk in their normal daily work. However, an airline may require that crew members without contraindications be vaccinated against yellow fever, so that the airline has flexibility to shift crews and be able to address any urgent need.

GENERAL HEALTH MEASURES
Although pilots are required to have periodic physician visits to ensure they are fit to fly, these may not address some issues that may affect them when they travel internationally, particularly to destinations in the developing world. Flight attendants and others should also consider asking their health care providers about these recommendations:

- Administering a periodic tuberculin skin test, if traveling frequently to destinations where the prevalence of tuberculosis is much higher than in the United States, where the incidence of antimicrobial resistance is higher, and where the crew member will be in close contact with crowds (www.who.int/tb/challenges/mdr/en).
- Checking at each visit to make sure that routine immunizations are up-to-date (see below).
- Immunizing against seasonal influenza every year when the vaccine becomes available.

In addition, all medications for chronic conditions should be carried in extra quantities, as they may not be available at some locations, and even if available and less costly, may be counterfeit or be of poor quality (see Chapter 2, *Perspectives*: Pharmaceutical Quality & Counterfeit Drugs). The business of manufacturing counterfeit medications in developing countries is huge and growing; it is impossible to tell from the packaging or pills if they are counterfeit. Some counterfeit drugs contain little or no active ingredient, and others contain toxic contaminants.

Vaccinations
Because of the frequency of travel to international destinations, air crews may be exposed to various diseases that are not common in the United States. For example, measles can be a life-threatening illness for adults; it is more common in most of the world, including Europe, because of lack of mandatory childhood immunization against the disease in many countries. International flight crews should consider a travel health visit to ensure as complete protection as possible. Some may have short notice before traveling to new destinations; thus, air crew members should be asked about this possibility during their visit, so that vaccinations for an upcoming trip—that may not be imminent—may be given, or a series may be started early. Providers should educate travelers about health risks in the

various destinations; whether certain vaccinations are administered will depend on the traveler's tolerance for risk.

Routine Vaccinations

All travelers should make sure they are up-to-date with routine vaccinations (see the separate sections on these diseases in Chapter 3):

- **Measles**—A person born in the United States before 1957 is assumed to be immune to measles. People born after 1957 should have documentation of having had the disease or having had 2 vaccine doses against measles. Measles vaccine is typically given as MMR (measles-mumps-rubella).
- **Varicella**—Strongly recommended for travelers with no history of chickenpox.
- **Polio**—A single booster is recommended as an adult. Although transmission of the polio virus is not a problem in the Western Hemisphere, it remains a risk in some countries in sub-Saharan Africa and in Asia.
- **Diphtheria-tetanus-pertussis**—Administered at 10-year intervals (a single booster of the triple combination, and thereafter Td) for complete protection.
- **Hepatitis B**—Administered to all children and adolescents in the United States, it is advisable for frequent travelers because of the unpredictability of exposure.
- **Hepatitis A**—Administered to all children in the United States, it is advisable for all travelers.
- **Influenza**—Recommended annually for all people.
- **Others**—Any age-related (such as varicella-zoster) or health maintenance-related (such as pneumococcal) vaccinations should be considered.

Special Vaccinations for Travel

Although there are no established guidelines or recommendations for the use of travel vaccinations in pilots and other air crews, it may be reasonable to offer meningococcal, Japanese encephalitis, yellow fever, and typhoid vaccine to this special population because of their frequent, short-stay, and at times unpredictable travel and destinations. As well, they are generally a group who travel frequently beyond work, so they should always be asked during a consultation whether they plan other travel itineraries that can be addressed at the same time.

Malaria Chemoprophylaxis

Crew members are typically informed by their airline as to which destinations harbor malaria. Some European and Asian air carriers have longer experience flying to destinations where malaria is endemic, and these airlines have various policies with respect to its prevention. Although there may be malaria transmission in some areas of destination countries, sometimes there is none in the capitals or the larger urban areas to which the major American carriers fly (such as in China or the Philippines). This is generally not the case in sub-Saharan Africa, where there can be substantial exposure during a short 24-hour layover (however, in Kenya, there is no malaria risk in Nairobi). Although there may be little risk at the hotels in the destination, risk may be increased at the international airports and during unpredictable delays in transit. Even during short single stops (for example, in West Africa en route to South Africa), there is some risk when the aircraft doors are open. Little published data are available on the risk of malaria for flight crews with short layovers, but some information suggests that it is less than that for tourists.

Unfortunately, experience in American air crews to malaria-endemic destinations has shown that air crews continue to acquire malaria, as well as develop severe and complicated disease. Some illness may result from lack of awareness of airline recommendations, failure to take precautions against mosquito bites, lack of compliance with antimalarial prophylaxis, and inaccurate information regarding toxicity of medication.

Flight crew members should have easy access to educational materials and chemoprophylaxis and, if desired, should be able to have an individual risk assessment for preventive measures. For destinations where the prevalence of malaria is high (countries in West Africa, for example), crew members should take prophylaxis for layovers. For other destinations where crews are thought to be at low risk based on local intensity of transmission, accommodations, and personal behaviors, they may be advised to use insect repellents and take no chemoprophylaxis. Flight crews should always:

- Educate themselves as much as possible about malaria.

- Understand the importance of personal protective measures such as repellents, and use them properly.
- Take chemoprophylaxis if recommended.
- Know that if fever or chills occur after exposure, it is a medical emergency.
- Know how they can get medical assistance at their destinations or at home in the event of symptoms or signs of malaria.

There are several options for malaria chemoprophylaxis, depending on the destination city. The combination of country-specific recommendations that can be accessed either in this text (see Chapter 3, Travel Vaccines & Malaria Information, by Country) or on the CDC Travelers' Health website (www.cdc.gov/travel) should help with this decision, along with the individual assessment. Chemoprophylaxis recommendations for pilots and air crew include the following:

- **Mefloquine**—The current product label for mefloquine contains a caution against using mefloquine for malaria prophylaxis in pilots.
- **Chloroquine**—There are no contraindications for use of chloroquine in pilots or air crew. Chloroquine may not be the preferred option for many because of the need to continue taking the drug for 4 weeks after the last exposure, thus requiring >4 weeks of drug administration for even a single night of exposure. In addition, in many areas malaria is resistant to chloroquine.
- **Atovaquone-proguanil**—There are no contraindications for use of atovaquone-proguanil in pilots or air crew members. In addition, because of the short-stay nature of their travel, use of atovaquone-proguanil as chemoprophylaxis may be preferred because of the need to take the drug for only 7 days after leaving an area of exposure risk.
- **Doxycycline**—There are no contraindications for use of doxycycline in pilots or air crew. Doxycycline may not be the preferred option for many because of the need to

continue taking the drug for 28 days after the last exposure, thus requiring >4 weeks of drug administration for even a single night of exposure.
- **Primaquine**—There are no contraindications for use of primaquine in pilots or air crew. Like atovaquone-proguanil, use of primaquine as chemoprophylaxis may be attractive because of the need to take the drug for only 7 days after leaving an area of exposure risk. A blood test for the enzyme glucose-6-phosphate dehydrogenase (G6PD) is required before prescribing. CDC recommends primaquine for prevention of malaria in areas with mainly *Plasmodium vivax*.

Additional information on malaria prevention may be found in Chapter 3, Malaria.

Food and Water Precautions and Travelers' Diarrhea

Pilots and air crew members should follow the same safe food and water precautions and prevention and management of travelers' diarrhea as other travelers (see Chapter 2, Travelers' Diarrhea). They should also be well versed in the recognition and self-treatment of travelers' diarrhea to shorten the duration of illness that would affect their job performance.

Bloodborne and Sexually Transmitted Infections

Although these risks and preventions are addressed in more detail in other sections, it is worth reiterating that frequent travelers have an increased likelihood of engaging in casual and unprotected sex. It is common to think that people from Western countries would have the same risk of HIV and other sexually transmitted infections; however, travelers have far higher rates of such infections. The risk of acquisition may be higher not only for diseases such as gonorrhea and chlamydia, but also for chronic illnesses such as hepatitis B and C. Dental procedures and activities such as acupuncture, tattooing, and piercing also are ill-advised during travel to developing countries.

BIBLIOGRAPHY

1. Bagshaw M, Barbeau DN. The aircraft cabin environment. In: Keystone JS, Freedman DO, Kozarsky PE, Connor BA, Nothdurft HD, editors. Travel Medicine. 3rd ed. Philadelphia: Saunders Elsevier; 2013. p. 405–12.
2. Byrne N. Urban malaria risk in sub-Saharan Africa: where is the evidence? Travel Med Infect Dis. 2007 Mar;5(2):135–7.
3. Byrne NJ, Behrens RH. Airline crews' risk for malaria on layovers in urban sub-Saharan Africa: risk

assessment and appropriate prevention policy. J Travel Med. 2004 Nov–Dec;11(6):359–63.
4. CDC. Notes from the field: malaria imported from West Africa by flight crews—Florida and Pennsylvania, 2010. MMWR Morb Mortal Wkly Rep. 2010 Nov 5;59(43):1412.
5. Selent M, de Rochars VMB, Stanek D, Bensyl D, Martin B, Cohen NJ, et al. Malaria prevention knowledge, attitudes, and practices (KAP) among international flying pilots and flight attendants of a US commercial airline. J Travel Med. 2012 Dec;19(6):366–72.

HUMANITARIAN AID WORKERS
Brian D. Gushulak

OVERVIEW

Through organizations and agencies or individual activities, many thousands of people are involved in the delivery of humanitarian aid in diverse locations every year. After large-scale events such as earthquakes or tsunamis, the number of those traveling to provide humanitarian aid and assistance can increase. Maintaining the health of humanitarian aid workers is important to ensure that they are able to deliver care to those in need and avoid additional strain on local health services.

In common with other travelers, people who travel to provide humanitarian aid or disaster relief must first address their personal health and welfare before, during, and after travel. This includes knowledge of and preparation for all the usual elements associated with travel to the area. In addition, aid workers can experience specific risks and situations related to the provision of humanitarian care, such as:

- Exposure to the environment that precipitated or sustains a crisis or event, such as a natural disaster or conflict
- Working long hours under adverse or extreme conditions, often in close contact with the affected population
- Damaged or absent infrastructure, including limits in the availability of food, water, lodging, transportation, and health services
- Reduced levels of security and protection

- Stress, ethical, and moral challenges related to the event and the resource capacities of the situation

Humanitarian service can damage personal health. Studies involving long-term humanitarian workers have noted that >35% report that their personal health status deteriorated during the mission. Accidents and violence are documented risks for humanitarian aid workers and cause more deaths than disease and natural causes. Recent estimates place the risk of violence-related deaths, medical evacuations, and hospitalizations at approximately 6 per 10,000 person-years among aid workers. Conditions and outcomes vary by location, nature of the humanitarian event, and time spent in the field.

A recent study of American Red Cross workers noted a 10% ratio of injury or accident and an exposure to violence of 16%. That study also showed that >40% found the experience more stressful than expected. An earlier study of deaths among Peace Corps volunteers noted that unintentional injuries were the cause of nearly 70% of deaths, followed by homicide at 17%. Illness was responsible for 14% of the Peace Corps fatalities.

However, risks to humanitarian aid workers are not uniformly distributed across the spectrum of humanitarian aid. For example, in 2009 a survey of violence against humanitarian aid workers found that a small number of insecure locations (Afghanistan, Darfur [Sudan], and Somalia) accounted for >60% of these events.

PRE-TRAVEL CONSIDERATIONS
Evaluation and Pre-Travel Medical Care

Giving careful attention to pre-travel evaluation, both medical and psychological, in addition to educating travelers can reduce the likelihood of illness and the need for repatriation. Comprehensive medical examinations can prepare travelers by helping identify previously unrecognized disease and allowing for treatment before travel. Careful evaluation of risk factors (family history, history of alcohol or substance abuse, sexually transmitted diseases, and psychiatric illness) may direct additional evaluation and identify previously unrecognized psychological problems or chronic conditions. Identifying alcohol or substance dependence, depression, or other psychiatric illness is important, as these conditions may be exacerbated by the stress of the mission and are often the reason for emergency repatriation. People planning long-term assignments should have their dental condition assessed and any problems dealt with before departure.

Those who will be providing medical care or participating in clinical research as part of their humanitarian activities should be evaluated in terms of occupational risk and the need for preventive preexposure or postexposure interventions. Humanitarian aid workers destined for areas of active conflict or limited police presence may benefit from specialized security briefings, either provided by the employing agency or private sources. Medical facilities may be compromised by the disaster or overwhelmed in responding to it. Therefore, volunteers with underlying conditions or pregnant women should be counseled against travel and encouraged to support the response in other ways.

Regardless of the area of the world in which the aid worker will be deployed, certain basics should be addressed in the pre-travel encounter, including routine vaccinations, malaria chemoprophylaxis (if appropriate), food and water precautions, self-treatment for travelers' diarrhea, risks from insect bites, and injury prevention.

Counseling and Advice

Predeployment education and training are essential, as personal illness or injury burdens the community the worker has come to support. Injuries and motor vehicle accidents are common risks for travelers anywhere in the world; thus, travelers should be sensitive to their surroundings and carefully select the type of transportation and hour of travel, if possible. In disaster and emergency situations, the traveler should also be aware of physical hazards such as debris, unstable structures, downed power lines, environmental hazards, and extremes of temperature. Although rare, emergency situations in developed nations may involve unusual exposures, such as radiation exposures observed after damage to nuclear facilities in Japan in 2011.

Travelers to conflict areas should be aware of landmines and other potential hazards associated with unexploded ordnance. In situations associated with damage or destruction to local services and facilities, humanitarian aid workers should expect, anticipate, and plan for limited accommodations, logistics, and personal support. Humanitarian aid workers destined for low-resource areas or situations may benefit from pre-travel training and counseling regarding the moral complexities of providing service in these environments.

Preparation
Health Items

The traveler should be advised to prepare a travel health kit that is more extensive than the typical kit and should also be familiar with basic first aid to self-treat any injury until medical attention can be obtained. Aid workers may need to disinfect their own water and may want to carry high-energy, nonperishable food items for emergency use. Humanitarian aid workers should research the available resources in the destination to tailor how extensive their packed supplies should be. People with dental crowns or bridgework may wish to carry temporary dental adhesive for short-term management of a dislodged dental appliance. In addition to a basic travel health kit (see Chapter 2, Travel Health Kits), humanitarian aid workers should consider bringing the following items:

Toiletries
- Toothbrush and toothpaste
- Skin moisturizer
- Soap, shampoo
- Lip balm
- If corrective lenses are used:
  > Extra pair of prescription glasses in a protective case and a copy of the prescription
  > Eyeglasses cleaning supplies and repair kit
  > Extra contact lenses and lens cleaner
- Razor, extra blades[1]
- Nail clippers[1]
- Toilet paper
- Menstrual supplies
- Sewing kit
- Laundry detergent
- Small clothesline and clothespins

Protective clothing
- Comfortable, lightweight clothing
- Long pants
- Long-sleeved shirts
- Hat
- Boots
- Shower shoes
- Rain gear
- Bandana or handkerchief
- Towel (highly absorbent travel towel if possible)
- Gloves (leather gloves if physical labor will be performed; rubber gloves if handling blood or body fluids)

Items for daily living
- Sunglasses
- Waterproof watch
- Flashlight
- Spare batteries
- Travel plug adapters for electronics
- Knife, such as a Swiss Army knife or Leatherman[1]
- If traveling to an area where food and water may be contaminated:
  > Bottled water or water filters/purification system/water purification tablets
  > Nonperishable food items
- If traveling to malaria-endemic areas:
  > Personal bed net (insecticide-impregnated)

Safety and security
- Money belt
- Cash
- Cellular telephone, equipped to work internationally, or satellite telephone (with charger)
- Candles, matches, and lighter in a zip-top bag[2]
- Extra zip-top bags
- Safety goggles

Personal Items

Because of the loss of life, serious injuries, missing and separated families, and destruction often associated with disasters, humanitarian aid workers should recognize that situations they encounter may be extremely stressful. Keeping a personal item nearby, such as a family photo, favorite music, or religious material, can offer comfort in such situations. Checking in with family members and close friends from time to time is another means of support. Satellite telephones are small, can work almost anywhere in the world, and can be rented for <$10 per day.

Important Documents

In uncertain circumstances, extra passport-style photos may be required for certain types of visas or for additional work permits. Travelers should bring photocopies of important documents, such as passports and credit cards, as well as copies of their medical or nursing license, if applicable. Medical information, such as immunization records and blood type, is also helpful to have. The traveler should carry these copies and also leave a copy with someone back home. In addition, they should carry contact information for the person who should be notified in an emergency.

Registration with Embassies

Travelers should register with the US embassy in the destination country before departure, so that the local consulate is aware of their presence, and they may be accounted for and included in evacuation plans. They should also consider supplemental travel, travel health, and medical evacuation insurance to cover medical care and evacuation

---

[1] Pack these items in checked baggage, since they are considered sharp objects and will be confiscated by airport or airline security if packed in carry-on bags.
[2] See www.tsa.gov for restrictions on traveling with lighters and matches.

should they become ill or injured. See the Department of State website for additional information (https://travelregistration.state.gov/ibrs/ui).

POST-TRAVEL CONSIDERATIONS

Returning humanitarian aid workers should be advised to seek medical care if they sustained injuries during their travel or become ill after returning. To ensure proper evaluation, they should advise their providers of the nature of their recent travel.

Depending upon the length of time away or their activities (such as working in health care), returning aid workers may benefit from a complete medical review. Homecoming has also been identified as a risk period for difficulties in psychological adjustment, and treatment or counseling should be sought. Workers who witnessed or were involved in situations of mass casualties, deaths, or serious injuries or who have been victims of violence (assault, kidnapping, or serious road traffic crash) should be considered for referral for critical incident counseling.

Studies have indicated that >30% of aid workers report depression shortly after returning home. The adjustment process can be assisted by a skilled debriefing. Generally, humanitarian aid workers are able to adapt to the acute and chronic stressors of their work and demonstrate considerable resilience, but they will also benefit from proper rest and support to help them fully adjust back into the home environment.

BIBLIOGRAPHY

1. Callahan MV, Hamer DH. On the medical edge: preparation of expatriates, refugee and disaster relief workers, and Peace Corps volunteers. Infect Dis Clin North Am. 2005 Mar;19(1):85–101.
2. Campbell S. Responding to international disasters. Nurs Stand. 2005 Feb 2–8;19(21):33–6.
3. CDC. Coping with a traumatic event: information for the public. Atlanta: CDC; 2009 [cited 2012 Sep 23]. Available from: http://www.bt.cdc.gov/masscasualties/copingpub.asp.
4. Connorton E, Perry MJ, Hemenway D, Miller M. Humanitarian relief workers and trauma-related mental illness. Epidemiol Rev. 2012 Jan;34(1):145–55.
5. Coppola DP. Introduction to International Disaster Management. Amsterdam: Butterworth Heinemann; 2006.
6. Egeland J, Harmer A, Stoddard A. To stay and deliver: good practice for humanitarians in complex security environments. New York: United Nations; 2011 [cited 2012 Sep 23]. Available from: http://ochanet.unocha.org/p/Documents/Stay_and_Deliver.pdf.
7. Gamble K, Lovell D, Lankester T, Keystone JS. Aid workers, expatriates and travel. In: Zuckerman J, editor. Principles and Practice of Travel Medicine. Hoboken, NJ: Wiley; 2001. p. 448–66.
8. Jung P, Banks RH. Tuberculosis risk in US Peace Corps Volunteers, 1996 to 2005. J Travel Med. 2008 Mar–Apr;15(2):87–94.
9. Kortepeter MG, Seaworth BJ, Tasker SA, Burgess TH, Coldren RL, Aronson NE. Health care workers and researchers traveling to developing-world clinical settings: disease transmission risk and mitigation. Clin Infect Dis. 2010 Dec 1;51(11):1298–305.
10. Leaning J, Spiegel P, Crisp J. Public health equity in refugee situations. Confl Health. 2011;5:6.
11. McFarlane CA. Risk associated with the psychological adjustment of humanitarian aid workers. The Australas J Disaster Trauma Stud [serial on the Internet]. 2004 [cited 2012 Sep 23]. Available from: http://www.massey.ac.nz/~trauma/issues/2004–1/mcfarlane.htm.
12. Mitchell AM, Sakraida TJ, Kameg K. Critical incident stress debriefing: implications for best practice. Disaster Manag Response. 2003 Apr–Jun;1(2):46–51.
13. Nurthen NM, Jung P. Fatalities in the Peace Corps: a retrospective study, 1984 to 2003. J Travel Med. 2008 Mar–Apr;15(2):95–101.
14. Pearn J. Pre-deployment education and training for refugee emergencies: health and safety aspects. J Refug Stud. 1997;10:495–502.
15. Peytremann I, Baduraux M, O'Donovan S, Loutan L. Medical evacuations and fatalities of United Nations High Commissioner for Refugees field employees. J Travel Med. 2001 May–Jun;8(3):117–21.
16. Sheik M, Gutierrez MI, Bolton P, Spiegel P, Thieren M, Burnham G. Deaths among humanitarian workers. BMJ. 2000 Jul 15;321(7254):166–8.
17. Stoddard A, Harmer A, Renouf JS. Once removed: lessons and challenges in remote management of humanitarian operations for insecure areas. New York: Humanitarian Outcomes; 2010 [cited 2012 Sep 23]. Available from: www.humanitarianoutcomes.org/resources/RemoteManagementApr20101.pdf.

LONG-TERM TRAVELERS & EXPATRIATES

Rachel B. Eidex, Anne E. McCarthy, Lin H. Chen

The risk of illness or injury increases with duration of travel, so special consideration should be given to travelers who are planning long-term visits (≥6 months is a common definition) to low- or middle-income countries. Points to discuss in the pre-travel consultation include accessing care at the destination, vaccines, infectious diseases not prevented by vaccines, injury, and psychological issues that long-term travelers may encounter.

ACCESSING CARE ABROAD

Before departure, all long-term travelers should undergo an extensive medical and dental examination. Travelers should anticipate that they will need care at some point during their stay, and they should plan where they will get it and how they will pay for it. Those traveling for work or with an organization (such as a university or the Peace Corps) may have a predetermined source of care; other travelers should identify a source in advance (see Chapter 2, Obtaining Health Care Abroad for the Ill Traveler). Long-term travelers should also determine if they will need supplemental travel health insurance and evacuation insurance (see Chapter 2, Travel Insurance, Travel Health Insurance, & Medical Evacuation Insurance).

In some countries, travelers are likely to encounter counterfeit or low-quality medications. Because the pills and packaging may be nearly indistinguishable from their legitimate counterparts, travelers should consider bringing a supply of their routine medications (antihypertensive or antihyperlipidemic drugs, for example) from the United States (see Chapter 2, *Perspectives:* Pharmaceutical Quality & Counterfeit Drugs).

VACCINES

Routine vaccines, including influenza vaccine, should be updated. In addition, long-term travelers should be aware of any vaccine requirements at their destination, either for employment, schooling, or entry.

A number of travel-related vaccines warrant consideration:

- Hepatitis A and typhoid vaccines are appropriate given the cumulative risk, although the traveler should be aware that the latter does not provide full protection.
- Travel-associated hepatitis B infections are rare, but the risk for travelers may be higher than for nontravelers, and the vaccine should be considered for all long-term travelers and expatriates.
- Meningococcal disease is more likely in travelers with prolonged exposure to local populations in endemic or epidemic areas; quadrivalent vaccine should be considered for those at risk.
- According to the Advisory Committee on Immunization Practices recommendations, Japanese encephalitis vaccine is recommended for people living in endemic areas. It is also recommended for travelers who plan to stay ≥1 month during the virus transmission season (see Chapter 3, Japanese Encephalitis).
- Rabies preexposure immunoprophylaxis is an important consideration for people spending a prolonged time in endemic countries, especially in areas where rabies immune globulin is not available. Vaccinating children who will be living in high-risk areas is a priority.
- Yellow fever vaccine should be considered for travelers who will be staying in an endemic area or a country with a vaccine requirement, or who may be traveling to one.

In addition to the intended destination, consider disease risk in surrounding areas, since long-term travelers may be likely to travel locally. For example, a short-term traveler to Seoul would not be considered at risk for Japanese encephalitis, but an expatriate living in Seoul may have opportunities to visit the Korean countryside or other areas in Asia where he or she could be exposed.

INFECTIOUS DISEASES NOT PREVENTED BY VACCINES
Malaria

Data suggest that the incidence of malaria increases and the use of preventive measures decreases with increasing length of stay. For instance, malaria incidence in British travelers returning from West Africa after a stay of 6–12 months was 80 times that of the incidence in travelers who had stayed only 1 week. Expatriates working with the International Committee of the Red Cross who stayed for a mean of 11 months in sub-Saharan Africa were diagnosed with malaria at a rate of 3.81 cases per 1,000 person-months of stay. Expatriate corporate employees in Ghana reported that adherence to malaria chemoprophylaxis deteriorated with increasing duration of stay, and all those who had been on the site for >1 year had abandoned chemoprophylaxis. About half of the cohort used insect repellent only intermittently, and more than one-third never used repellent. Another expatriate cohort living in Nigeria revealed similarly low adherence to chemoprophylaxis; analysis of pharmacy records and household interviews found that only 39% of households were adherent. Given the high relative risk of malaria for travelers in Africa, these data on long-term travelers and expatriates highlight worrisome risks and practices.

A traveler who will be residing in an area of continuous malaria transmission should continue to use malaria chemoprophylaxis for his or her entire stay. It is important to reassure the traveler that the drugs are safe and effective. Doxycycline has been well-tolerated for long-term malaria chemoprophylaxis in the military, and CDC has no recommended limits on its duration of use for malaria chemoprophylaxis. Mefloquine has been well-tolerated during prolonged stays by Peace Corps volunteers, with a discontinuation rate of 0.9%, and showed no evidence of accumulation after long-term use; therefore, mefloquine may be appropriate for long-term chemoprophylaxis for most chloroquine-resistant areas because of its convenient weekly dosing. Atovaquone-proguanil has shown good long-term tolerability in postmarketing surveillance, with a discontinuation rate of only 1% because of diarrhea. Primaquine (in people without glucose-6-phosphate dehydrogenase [G6PD]

deficiency) has been well-tolerated as long-term primary prophylaxis in Japanese transmigrants to Papua New Guinea. A potential concern with chloroquine is retinal toxicity when a cumulative dose of 100 g is reached, which may occur after 5–6 years of weekly dosing. A baseline ophthalmologic examination is recommended, with follow-up every 6–12 months after 5 years of use. Except for ophthalmologic evaluation when taking chloroquine long-term, no specific testing is recommended for the long-term use of other antimalarial drugs.

A consideration for long-term female travelers to malarious areas is pregnancy (see the Pregnant Travelers section earlier in this chapter). Malaria infection during pregnancy can result in potentially severe complications to both mother and fetus. When pregnancy is anticipated, chemoprophylaxis options may need to be adjusted. Ideally, this possibility should be explored before travel with all female long-term travelers of childbearing age. For women who are pregnant or plan to become pregnant during long-term travel, mefloquine is considered safe in all trimesters. Data from published studies in pregnant women have shown no increase in the risk of teratogenic effects or adverse pregnancy outcomes after mefloquine prophylaxis during pregnancy. Chloroquine has also been used long-term without ill effect on pregnancy. If a woman traveling long-term is taking atovaquone-proguanil, doxycycline, or primaquine, she should discontinue her medication and begin weekly mefloquine (or chloroquine in those areas where it remains efficacious) and wait at least 5–6 weeks to conceive so that a therapeutic level of mefloquine can build up in the blood.

Women who become pregnant while taking antimalarial drugs do not need a therapeutic abortion but should be advised during the pre-travel consultation of potential risks. The effect of atovaquone-proguanil on the fetus is unknown, but doxycycline is associated with fetal toxicity in animals and is contraindicated in pregnant women. Primaquine may harm a G6PD-deficient fetus, so it should not be used in pregnancy.

For long-term travelers, also stress the need for adjuncts to chemoprophylaxis, such as personal protection measures to avoid mosquito bites (such as sleeping under a bed net and using screens). Travelers should bring a sufficient supply of antimalarial drugs from the United States, since drugs purchased at the destination may be of poor quality or counterfeit. Even with urging to adhere to personal protective measures and reassurance that long-term chemoprophylaxis is safe and effective, adherence is likely to decline over time. Consequently, the pre-travel consultation for a long-term traveler to a malarious area should stress the severity of malaria, its signs and symptoms, and the need to seek care immediately if they develop. Travelers could consider bringing a reliable supply of drugs to treat malaria if they are diagnosed with malaria. For additional discussion, see the next section in this chapter, *Perspectives*: Malaria in Long-Term Travelers & Expatriates.

Other Diseases

Because diarrhea and gastrointestinal diseases are common in long-term travelers, they should be educated about the management of acute diarrhea, including rehydration, the use of antimotility agents, empiric antimicrobial therapy, and when to seek care.

HIV and sexually transmitted disease risks are increased in travelers and expatriates, and the consistent use of condoms in expatriates is low (approximately 20%). Long-term travelers should be educated about the risk of HIV and sexually transmitted diseases in their destination, as well as preventive measures. The potential for occupational exposure to HIV is important to consider in health care workers; postexposure prophylaxis with highly active antiretroviral therapy and risk avoidance should be included in the pre-travel consultation (see Chapter 2, Occupational Exposure to HIV).

Transfusion is a potential source of hepatitis C infection in expatriates. The risk of hepatitis E, spread by the fecal-oral route, is highest in Asia, although it has been transmitted in many different tropical locations. Pregnant women are at highest risk of fulminant disease.

Other infections vary with location and include schistosomiasis, which may be prevented by not swimming or wading in fresh water. Again, this risk is difficult to communicate to long-term travelers who, for example, may be living in sub-Saharan Africa and who look forward to their vacation at Lake Malawi. The risks of schistosomiasis and screening on return should be discussed. Tuberculosis risk may rise to the level of the local population if the traveler or expatriate has a longer stay and intimate contact with the local population. A baseline tuberculin test and the same test following travel should be considered.

INJURY

Injuries are the leading cause of preventable death in travelers, so long-term travelers should be educated about safety. Road and vehicle safety should be stressed, and travelers should choose the safest vehicle options available. Roads are often poorly constructed and maintained, traffic laws may not be enforced, vehicles may not have seatbelts or be properly maintained, and drivers may be reckless and poorly trained. See Chapter 2, Injuries & Safety, for strategies to reduce the risk of traffic and other injuries.

PSYCHOLOGICAL ISSUES

The stress of long-term travel can trigger or exacerbate psychiatric reactions. A long-term traveler should be assessed for preexisting psychiatric diagnosis, depressed mood, recent major life stressors, and use of medications that may have psychiatric effects. These conditions may suggest a need for further screening. All long-term travelers should be urged to take care of their physical and mental health by exercising regularly and eating healthfully. They should be able to recognize signs of anxiety and depression and have a plan for coping with them. Having photographs or other mementoes of friends and family at hand and staying in close contact with loved ones at home can alleviate the stress of long-term travel. For more information, see Chapter 2, Mental Health & Travel.

BIBLIOGRAPHY

1. Arguin PM, Krebs JW, Mandel E, Guzi T, Childs JE. Survey of rabies preexposure and postexposure prophylaxis among missionary personnel stationed outside the United States. J Travel Med. 2000 Jan;7(1):10–4.

2. Banta JE, Jungblut E. Health problems encountered by the Peace Corps overseas. Am J Public Health Nations Health. 1966 Dec;56(12):2121–5.

3. Berg J, Visser LG. Expatriate chemoprophylaxis use and compliance: past, present and future from an occupational health perspective. J Travel Med. 2007 Sep–Oct;14(5):357–8.

4. Chen LH, Wilson ME, Davis X, Loutan L, Schwartz E, Keystone J, et al. Illness in long-term travelers visiting GeoSentinel clinics. Emerg Infect Dis. 2009 Nov;15(11):1773–82.

5. Chen LH, Wilson ME, Schlagenhauf P. Prevention of malaria in long-term travelers. JAMA. 2006 Nov 8;296(18):2234–44.

6. Cobelens FG, van Deutekom H, Draayer-Jansen IW, Schepp-Beelen AC, van Gerven PJ, van Kessel RP, et al. Risk of infection with *Mycobacterium tuberculosis* in travellers to areas of high tuberculosis endemicity. Lancet. 2000 Aug 5;356(9228):461–5.

7. Cockburn R, Newton PN, Agyarko EK, Akunyili D, White NJ. The global threat of counterfeit drugs: why industry and governments must communicate the dangers. PLoS Med. 2005 Apr;2(4):e100.

8. Correia JD, Shafer RT, Patel V, Kain KC, Tessier D, MacPherson D, et al. Blood and body fluid exposure as a health risk for international travelers. J Travel Med. 2001 Sep–Oct;8(5):263–6.

9. Freeman RJ, Mancuso JD, Riddle MS, Keep LW. Systematic review and meta-analysis of TST conversion risk in deployed military and long-term civilian travelers. J Travel Med. 2010 Jul;17(4):233–42.

10. Guse CE, Cortes LM, Hargarten SW, Hennes HM. Fatal injuries of US citizens abroad. J Travel Med. 2007 Sep–Oct;14(5):279–87.

11. Hillel O, Potasman I. Correlation between adherence to precautions issued by the WHO and diarrhea among long-term travelers to India. J Travel Med. 2005 Sep–Oct;12(5):243–7.

12. Leutscher PD, Bagley SW. Health-related challenges in United States Peace Corps volunteers serving for two years in Madagascar. J Travel Med. 2003 Sep–Oct;10(5):263–7.

13. MacPherson DW, Gushulak BD, Sandhu J. Death and international travel—the Canadian experience: 1996 to 2004. J Travel Med. 2007 Mar–Apr;14(2):77–84.

14. Pandey P, Shlim DR, Cave W, Springer MF. Risk of possible exposure to rabies among tourists and foreign residents in Nepal. J Travel Med. 2002 May–Jun;9(3):127–31.

15. Patel D, Easmon CJ, Dow C, Snashall DC, Seed PT. Medical repatriation of British diplomats resident overseas. J Travel Med. 2000 Mar–Apr;7(2):64–9.

16. Toovey S, Moerman F, van Gompel A. Special infectious disease risks of expatriates and long-term travelers in tropical countries. Part I: malaria. J Travel Med. 2007 Jan–Feb;14(1):42–9.

17. Toovey S, Moerman F, van Gompel A. Special infectious disease risks of expatriates and long-term travelers in tropical countries. Part II: infections other than malaria. J Travel Med. 2007 Jan–Feb;14(1):50–60.

Perspectives

MALARIA IN LONG-TERM TRAVELERS & EXPATRIATES
Lin H. Chen

Long-term travelers and expatriates in malarious areas are at risk for severe malaria throughout their stay, but sometimes they do not recognize the continued need for reducing risk through chemoprophylaxis and personal protective measures. Guidelines for malaria prevention might be interpreted as focusing on preventing *Plasmodium falciparum* malaria in short-term travelers. Optimal malaria prevention in long-term travelers poses dilemmas because of diverse traveler characteristics and itineraries (including traveling in and out of malarious areas), the heterogeneous quality of and access to medical care, and the limited reports on long-term safety and efficacy of antimalarial drugs. Moreover, parasite resistance, seasonality, and the intensity of transmission evolve with environmental and population alterations.

For this discussion, long-term travelers are defined as nonimmune travelers staying in malaria-endemic countries for ≥6 months. A recent review summarized published data on the risk of malaria in long-term travelers, evidence for personal protective measures, and safety and tolerability of malaria chemoprophylaxis during long-term use (Box 8-3).

INDIVIDUALIZED RISK CONSIDERATIONS
Some travelers have preconceived notions about malaria prevention for their long-term journey or stay in an endemic region that may shape their acceptance of standard recommendations. Even when educational efforts appear successful in convincing such travelers to take chemoprophylaxis, they often meet other travelers or locals who convince them that the medication is either not necessary or is in some way detrimental to their health. Nonetheless, assessing their risk may help determine a traveler's likelihood of adherence to preventive actions during long-term travel:

- Traveler's beliefs and practices regarding personal protective measures
- Traveler's knowledge and preferences toward continuous chemoprophylaxis
- Travel characteristics, including the quality of accommodations, activities, and social support and network
- Economic considerations
- Destination-specific infrastructure, including medical service, access to high-quality care, medication supply, and availability of repellents, insecticides, and nets

PRACTICAL RECOMMENDATIONS
Personal Protective Measures
Preventing malaria in all travelers is a complex issue and requires personalized expert advice. For long-term travelers, malaria prevention must stress the role

of personal protective measures as an adjunct to chemoprophylaxis, including adapting behaviors to minimize mosquito exposure, staying in housing with screened windows and doors, using air conditioning, sleeping under an insecticide-treated bed net, applying insecticide sprays in the residence, managing the environment to reduce vector breeding, using effective repellent, and wearing long sleeves and pants when practical (Box 8-4).

Malaria Chemoprophylaxis

Chemoprophylaxis decreases the risk of illness, hospitalization, and death. However, some travelers may disregard chemoprophylaxis recommendations. Working with the traveler to overcome his or her concerns, providing insight into the severity of malaria, and deriving a feasible and sensible chemoprophylaxis plan are recommended (Box 8-5). For example, a long-term traveler or expatriate based in a malaria-endemic country with highly seasonal or geographically focal malaria transmission may rely primarily on personal protective measures at some times and target periods of chemoprophylaxis during the transmission season or when venturing into endemic areas. However, a traveler who will be residing in an area of continuous malaria transmission should continue to use malaria chemoprophylaxis for the entire stay.

Another scenario that may arise and merits discussion with long-term travelers is whether they should continue malaria chemoprophylaxis if they develop fever during travel. Rapid diagnostic tests are unreliable for self-diagnosis in travelers because most travelers are not able to use and read the test correctly. (Rapid diagnostic tests are also not sold to the general public in the United States.) Because fever has numerous possible causes besides malaria, travelers should continue their recommended chemoprophylaxis provided that they are tolerating it well. In addition, they should be tested for malaria, even if taking prophylaxis. Obviously, the possibility of other treatable causes of fever should be explored. However, in addition to continuing chemoprophylaxis, some travelers who will be >24 hours from adequate medical care may be prescribed a full course of malaria medication for emergency self-treatment when malaria is suspected. Travelers who might self-administer treatment should be told that they still require follow-up care as soon as they are able to access it.

Unfortunately, in many countries, malaria is a frequent diagnosis in people who do not have malaria. In addition to receiving unnecessary treatment, long-term travelers who are misdiagnosed with malaria may stop taking their chemoprophylaxis because they erroneously believe that it did not work. It is difficult to relay such a concept during the pre-travel consult, but the attempt should be made.

SUMMARY

Recommendations for malaria prevention in all travelers must be personalized. Tailoring advice by assessing the traveler's preferences and determining the traveler's possible adherence, along with education regarding malaria, will likely result in better adherence than simply prescribing a course of chemoprophylaxis. The following messages should be conveyed to the long-term traveler regarding malaria prevention:

- Adherence to chemoprophylaxis is essential.
- Use of personal protective measures, such as bed nets and screens, is critical (as many will not use repellents long term).
- Reliable medical facilities at the destination should be located as soon as feasible.
- Data support the safety of long-term use of chemoprophylaxis.
- Supplies of antimalarial drugs should be brought from home, because counterfeit and poor-quality drugs are prevalent in malaria-endemic countries.
- Fever is a worrisome sign, and malaria must be considered and ruled out (see Chapter 5, Fever in Returned Travelers).
- A medical evacuation insurance policy should be purchased if the traveler will be in an area with inadequate medical facilities.
- Although individual use of rapid diagnostic tests is not advised, carrying standby treatment with follow-up medical care may be appropriate for some.
- Presumptive antirelapse therapy may be appropriate for exposure in areas with intense P. vivax transmission (after a normal level of glucose-6-phosphate dehydrogenase is documented).
- Misconceptions regarding malaria are pervasive in malaria-endemic countries among expatriates and local residents, and long-term travelers should trust health advice only from reputable and respected sources.

BIBLIOGRAPHY

1. Askling HH, Nilsson J, Tegnell A, Janzon R, Ekdahl K. Malaria risk in travelers. Emerg Infect Dis. 2005 Mar;11(3):436–41.
2. Berg J, Visser LG. Expatriate chemoprophylaxis use and compliance: past, present and future from an occupational health perspective. J Travel Med. 2007 Sep–Oct;14(5):357–8.
3. Chen LH, Wilson ME, Davis X, Loutan L, Schwartz E, Keystone J, et al. Illness in long-term travelers visiting GeoSentinel clinics. Emerg Infect Dis. 2009 Nov;15(11):1773–82.
4. Chen LH, Wilson ME, Schlagenhauf P. Controversies and misconceptions in malaria chemoprophylaxis for travelers. JAMA. 2007 May 23;297(20):2251–63.
5. Keiser J, Singer BH, Utzinger J. Reducing the burden of malaria in different eco-epidemiological settings with environmental management: a systematic review. Lancet Infect Dis. 2005 Nov;5(11):695–708.
6. Leder K, Black J, O'Brien D, Greenwood Z, Kain KC, Schwartz E, et al. Malaria in travelers: a review of the GeoSentinel surveillance network. Clin Infect Dis. 2004 Oct 15;39(8):1104–12.
7. Lengeler C. Insecticide-treated bed nets and curtains for preventing malaria. Cochrane Database Syst Rev. 2004(2):CD000363.
8. Newton PN, Green MD, Fernandez FM, Day NP, White NJ. Counterfeit anti-infective drugs. Lancet Infect Dis. 2006 Sep;6(9):602–13.
9. Pluess B, Tanser FC, Lengeler C, Sharp BL. Indoor residual spraying for preventing malaria. Cochrane Database Syst Rev. 2010(4):CD006657.
10. Toovey S, Moerman F, van Gompel A. Special infectious disease risks of expatriates and long-term travelers in tropical countries. Part I: malaria. J Travel Med. 2007 Jan–Feb;14(1):42–9.

LAST-MINUTE TRAVELERS

Gail Rosselot

Ideally, travelers should seek medical advice at least 4–6 weeks before departure, but clinicians are frequently asked to provide pre-travel care to travelers leaving on short notice, sometimes within days or even hours. "Last-minute travelers" can refer to people who are leaving on short notice (such as some business travelers or immigrants returning to their home country for a family emergency), or it may refer to people who have planned a trip for some time but delayed seeking pre-travel care. Regardless of the reason, clinicians can offer travelers support for their upcoming trip even on short notice. This support could include vaccination with standard or accelerated immunization schedules, health counseling, prescriptions, and referrals to services at the destination.

VACCINATIONS

Consider the traveler's itinerary and activities at the destination when assessing which vaccines might be indicated. Note that immunity generally takes approximately 2 weeks to develop after vaccination, so travelers might not be adequately protected if they are vaccinated immediately before travel. Counsel travelers to adhere to preventive behaviors regarding food, water, and insects (see the Food & Water Precautions and Protection against Mosquitoes, Ticks, & Other Insects & Arthropods sections in Chapter 2) in case they are incompletely protected, as well as to prevent diseases for which no vaccine is available.

Routine Vaccinations

Most travelers who attended school in the United States have received standard routine vaccinations. If the traveler is not completely up-to-date on age-appropriate routine vaccines, administer first or additional doses of measles-mumps-rubella vaccine, polio vaccine, varicella vaccine, tetanus-diphtheria-acellular pertussis vaccine, and the seasonal influenza vaccine. Note that if the traveler needs >1 live-virus vaccine (yellow fever, measles-mumps-rubella, varicella, intranasal

influenza), they must be given on the same day or separated by ≥28 days.

Recommended Vaccinations: Single-Dose Protection

Even when a traveler has limited time before departure, research supports the use of certain single-dose vaccines to initiate protection. These include hepatitis A (monovalent), typhoid (injectable), polio (inactivated), and meningococcal meningitis (conjugate if the traveler is aged 2–55 years) vaccines. The second dose in the hepatitis A vaccine series should be completed ≥6 months after the first dose is administered.

Recommended Vaccinations: Multiple Doses Needed

Last-minute travelers often cannot complete the full course of vaccines that require multiple doses to induce full protection. If a traveler needs protection against hepatitis B, Japanese encephalitis, or rabies, the clinician can consider alternative approaches.

Hepatitis B

As time allows, complete the accelerated monovalent hepatitis B (Engerix-B) schedule (0, 1, and 2 months, plus a 12-month booster) or the super-accelerated combination hepatitis A/B (Twinrix) schedule (0, 7, 21–30 days, plus a 12-month booster). If an accelerated schedule cannot be completed before travel, start the vaccination series and schedule a follow-up visit to complete it, or, for extended-stay travelers or expatriates, help them identify resources at the destination to complete the series.

Japanese encephalitis

No accelerated schedule is available. People who receive only 1 dose may have a suboptimal response and may not be protected. Travelers who cannot complete the primary vaccine series ≥1 week before travel should be counseled to adhere rigidly to mosquito precautions if they will be at risk for Japanese encephalitis.

Rabies

Because of the multiple immunizations required to complete a primary rabies vaccine series (0, 7, and 21 or 28 days), it may be difficult for last-minute travelers to complete the series before departure. A person who starts but does not complete a primary series and is potentially exposed should receive the same postexposure prophylaxis as a completely unimmunized person. Counsel travelers about the importance of avoiding animals, washing any bite thoroughly with soap and water, and seeking immediate medical care. Travelers to developing or remote destinations should consider medical evacuation insurance in case evacuation is needed to receive postexposure prophylaxis.

Required Vaccinations

Documentation of a yellow fever vaccine becomes valid 10 days after administration. If a yellow fever vaccine is required by a country in the traveler's itinerary and the traveler lacks sufficient time, it may be necessary to rearrange the order of travel or reschedule the trip. Otherwise, the traveler risks entry problems at the country's border or risks yellow fever vaccination at the border. Additionally, the traveler who receives the yellow fever vaccine <10 days before entering a yellow fever risk area risks yellow fever infection.

Meningococcal vaccine is required of all adults and children aged >2 years traveling to Saudi Arabia for religious pilgrimage, including Hajj. Hajj visas cannot be issued without proof that applicants received meningococcal vaccine ≥10 days and ≤3 years before arriving in Saudi Arabia.

MALARIA

Effective malaria chemoprophylaxis is possible for the last-minute traveler. The choice of antimalarial agent depends on a number of factors, including itinerary, drug resistance at the destination, medication contraindications and precautions, cost, and patient preference. Chloroquine and mefloquine should be initiated 1–2 weeks before departure, so most clinicians recommend doxycycline or atovaquone-proguanil for travelers who are departing in <1–2 weeks. Both doxycycline and atovaquone-proguanil can be started 1–2 days before arriving in an endemic area. Instruct the traveler to purchase malaria medication before departure and reinforce the importance of minimizing insect bites and of seeking medical care if illness occurs.

HEALTH COUNSELING

Pre-travel counseling is critical for last-minute travelers. Focus on major risks of the trip and deliver simple, customized messages about prevention and self-care. Provide travelers with education and prescriptions for travelers' diarrhea, such as a fluoroquinolone or macrolide, as well as education and prescriptions for altitude illness, if indicated.

Counsel the traveler on these topics (see related in-depth discussions on the following topics in Chapters 2 and 3):

- Unintentional injuries, including motor vehicle accidents (the leading cause of preventable death in healthy travelers), and personal safety
- Accessing health care abroad and the need to consider travel health and evacuation insurance
- Packing a travel health kit that includes an extra supply of usual prescriptions and over-the-counter medications
- Insect precautions
- Rabies avoidance and what to do in the event of an animal bite
- Food and water safety
- Sexually transmitted diseases
- Issues related to long flights, including venous thromboembolism (for at-risk travelers) and jet lag

Clinicians should also encourage last-minute travelers to schedule an appointment after the trip to complete any needed vaccinations and to initiate preparation for the next potential "spur of the moment" trip.

SPECIAL CHALLENGES AND ADDITIONAL CONSIDERATIONS

The Traveler Leaving in a Few Hours: If time does not permit an appointment, the clinician can still provide general prevention messages by telephone or e-mail. Refer the traveler to useful websites such as CDC (www.cdc.gov/travel), the Department of State (www.travel.state.gov), and the International Society of Travel Medicine clinic directory (www.istm.org).

Recommend travel health kit items that can be bought at the airport, if necessary. Many international airports now have travel health clinics; suggest the traveler try to visit one before departure.

The Traveler with Preexisting Medical Conditions: These patients may be at increased risk for travel-related illness if they have inadequate time for preparation. They should consider purchasing travel health insurance, and possibly medical evacuation insurance, and should carry a sufficient supply of all medications and a portable medical record. Emphasize the importance of a pre-travel appointment or conversation with their treating clinician.

The Last-Minute, Extended-Stay Traveler: Advise these travelers to arrange an early visit with a qualified clinician at their destination for additional evaluation and education. A last-minute consultation does not provide an expatriate with adequate time for a full medical and psychological evaluation.

Requests for Off-Label Vaccine Dosing: Because of time constraints, some travelers may ask for a vaccine to be administered off-label (different schedule, double dosing, partial series). Using a vaccine in a nonstandard manner can have consequences that include medical-legal issues and inducing a false sense of protection in the traveler.

Recurring Last-Minute Travelers: Any clinic that frequently sees last-minute travelers may want to address this as a management issue. One option is to build some flexibility into the appointment schedule. Another option, which may be particularly relevant for clinics that are part of a corporation or university, is to attempt early identification of people who are likely to travel internationally and to intervene proactively.

BIBLIOGRAPHY

1. CDC. Epidemiology and Prevention of Vaccine-Preventable Diseases. Washington, DC: Public Health Foundation; 2012 [cited 2012 Sep 24]. Available from: http://www.cdc.gov/vaccines/pubs/pinkbook/index.html.

2. CDC. General recommendations on immunization—recommendations of the Advisory Committee on Immunization Practices (ACIP). MMWR Recomm Rep. 2011 Jan 28;60(2):1–64.

3. Chiodini J. The challenging traveler. Practice Nurse. 2008 Apr 11;35(7):41–8.

4. Connor BA. Hepatitis A vaccine in the last-minute traveler. Am J Med. 2005 Oct;118 Suppl 10A:58S–62S.

5. Lankester T. Health care of the long-term traveller. Travel Med Infect Dis. 2005 Aug;3(3):143–55.

6. Leggat PA, Zwar NA, Hudson BJ, Travel Health Advisory Group A. Hepatitis B risks and immunisation coverage amongst Australians travelling to southeast Asia and east Asia. Travel Med Infect Dis. 2009 Nov;7(6):344–9.

7. Manning SE, Rupprecht CE, Fishbein D, Hanlon CA, Lumlertdacha B, Guerra M, et al. Human rabies prevention—United States, 2008: recommendations of the Advisory Committee on Immunization Practices. MMWR Recomm Rep. 2008 May 23;57(RR-3):1–28.

8. Plotkin SA, Orenstein WA, Offit PA, editors. Vaccines. 6th ed. Philadelphia: Saunders Elsevier; 2012.

9. Ross MH, Kielkowski D, de Frey A, Brink G. Travelling for work: seeking advice in South Africa. Travel Med Infect Dis. 2008 Jul;6(4):187–9.

10. Schuller E, Klade CS, Wolfl G, Kaltenbock A, Dewasthaly S, Tauber E. Comparison of a single, high-dose vaccination regimen to the standard regimen for the investigational Japanese encephalitis vaccine, IC51: a randomized, observer-blind, controlled Phase 3 study. Vaccine. 2009 Mar 26;27(15):2188–93.

11. Shoreland. Travel and Routine Immunizations. 20th ed. Milwaukee, WI: Shoreland Inc.; 2011.

12. Tepper M, Crane F, Schofield S, Anderson J. "I'm leaving tomorrow"—the potential use of partial vaccine series and/or double dosing in adult travellers who present for late consultation, PO02.23 [abstract]. International Society of Travel Medicine Conference 2011 May 8-12 [Internet]. 2011 [cited 2012 Sep 24]. Available from: http://www.istm.org/Documents/Members/MemberActivities/Meetings/Congresses/cistm12/CISTM12-Poster-Abstracts.pdf

13. Zuckerman JN, Van Damme P, Van Herck K, Loscher T. Vaccination options for last-minute travellers in need of travel-related prophylaxis against hepatitis A and B and typhoid fever: a practical guide. Travel Med Infect Dis. 2003 Nov;1(4):219–26.

SPECIAL CONSIDERATIONS FOR US MILITARY DEPLOYMENTS

Alan J. Magill, Michael A. Forgione, Jason D. Maguire, Mark M. Fukuda*

OVERVIEW

The US military, as a matter of policy, follows most of the recommendations in the CDC Yellow Book. However, certain situations apply only to the US military, and some policies or recommendations differ from what is recommended in the Yellow Book for civilian travel. Active-duty military physicians generally manage pre-deployment medicine, but civilian physicians may interact with people who are on reserve status, home on leave, recently discharged from active duty, or veterans. Pre-deployment and post-deployment information, policies, and guidelines for clinicians, service members and their families, and veterans can be found on the Deployment Health Clinical Center website (www.pdhealth.mil). The purpose of this section is to inform US military medical corps officers, who routinely consult the Yellow Book, about these differences and also make civilian clinicians, who frequently see military personnel, aware of them.

In many countries, one of the largest traveling populations is their military personnel. The military should be considered a special population with demographics, destinations, and needs different from those of civilian travelers. This section focuses on the unique aspects of using pre-travel vaccines and malaria chemoprophylaxis in the military population. The specific examples will be from the US military, but the concepts may be applicable to other militaries. In 2012, approximately 1.5 million US military members were on active duty, and approximately 1.0 million were in the reserve forces.

Several characteristics of the military force differ from those of the civilian population (Table 8-7). In general, the active duty military population is younger, in better health than the population at large, and predominately male.

FORCE HEALTH PROTECTION

Force Health Protection (FHP) is an important concept in military medicine. FHP is defined as all measures taken by commanders, supervisors, individual service members, and the military health system to promote, protect, improve, conserve, and restore the mental and physical well-being of service members across the range of military activities and operations. Delivery of vaccines and the use of malaria chemoprophylaxis agents are 2 aspects of FHP.

Medical interventions for FHP are the responsibility of the unit commander, with advice from the unit medical officer. When pre-deployment vaccines or malaria chemoprophylaxis are indicated, the commander includes such requirements in the mission plan. Service members are then required to receive these interventions under proper medical supervision. If a particular vaccine or drug is medically contraindicated, alternative agents may be employed if they are available. The unit medical officer documents which military personnel have not received standard preventive measures, so these people may receive additional monitoring or treatment if they become ill.

FHP policy positions in the Department of Defense (DoD) are issued as directives and instructions. All directives and instructions can be found online at www.dtic.mil/whs/directives. The Policy and Program for Immunizations to Protect the Health of Service Members and Military Beneficiaries is found in directive 6205.02E (September 19, 2006) at www.dtic.mil/whs/directives/corres/pdf/620502p.pdf. Although policy may

---

* The views and opinions expressed in this section are those of the authors and do not represent the official views of the US Department of Defense, The US Army, the US Air Force, the US Navy, the Armed Forces Health Surveillance Center, or the Walter Reed Army Institute of Research.

Table 8-7. Differences between military populations and civilian traveling populations

CHARACTERISTIC	TRAVEL MEDICINE	MILITARY MEDICINE
Primary focus	Individual	Unit
Goal	Optimizing advice and interventions for individual travelers	Ensuring mission success; optimizing advice and interventions for each person is difficult
Adherence	Strongly encouraged but travelers are free to choose	Required; vaccines and malaria chemoprophylaxis are part of Force Health Protection (FHP)
Education	One-on-one encounters	Unit education
Population	Not prescreened; travel health providers see all ages and people with preexisting medical conditions	Prescreened; people with serious medical problems are not allowed to join the military or be deployed
Special populations	Infants, children, pregnant women, elderly people, people with renal or hepatic impairment	Less frequent in military population or deployments
Disease comorbidity	Similar to civilian population	Limited, generally healthy
Gender	50% male, 50% female	85% male
Unusual activities	Adventure activities, such as trekking, climbing, scuba diving, spelunking	Housed in barracks or other group settings, aviators, Special Forces, operating complex weapons systems, hostile and extreme environments, stress of combat operations, night operations, and use of night-vision goggles
Duration of malaria chemoprophylaxis use	Mostly short term, 2–3 weeks	The US military often uses chemoprophylaxis for longer periods of time than do short-term travelers. Many deployments, to Afghanistan for example, are for 1 year or longer.

be made at higher levels in Washington, DC, the final decision to use vaccines or malaria chemoprophylaxis under FHP is made by commanders in the field, guided by their medical staff. In certain circumstances, individual service members may be exempt from vaccination. There are 2 types of exemptions from immunization: medical and administrative. Granting medical exemptions is a medical function that can only be validated by a health care professional. Granting administrative exemptions is a nonmedical function, usually controlled by the person's unit commander. Further information on exemption from vaccination may be found at www.vaccines.mil/documents/969r40_562.pdf#page=9.

ROUTINE AND TRAVEL-RELATED IMMUNIZATIONS

DoD policy states that the recommendations for immunization from CDC and the Advisory Committee for Immunization Practices shall generally be followed, consistent with requirements and guidance of the Food and Drug Administration (FDA) and with consideration for the unique needs of military settings and exposure risks. The Military Vaccine Agency (MILVAX) supports all 5 branches of the US Armed Services to enhance military medical readiness by coordinating DoD immunization (vaccination) programs worldwide. A valuable source of service-specific information on immunizations for all branches of the US military is found at the MILVAX website (www.vaccines.mil).

In particular, the quick reference tab of the MILVAX website (www.vaccines.mil/QuickReference) provides an easily accessible and complete source of information with product specifics and policy documents that both military and civilian providers will find useful. DoD and service-specific policies for vaccines and geographic-specific vaccine recommendations can also be downloaded from this site.

GEOGRAPHIC AREAS OF RESPONSIBILITY

The US military issues FHP recommendations based on geographic areas of responsibility (AOR) (www.vaccines.mil/QuickReference). Command and control over US military personnel in each AOR are under a unified combatant command, which is a joint (all branches of the US military) command that provides recommendations for all service members being deployed to that AOR. For example, Afghanistan is in the Central Command (CENTCOM) AOR. All personnel on orders to deploy or travel to Afghanistan should receive the vaccines listed in the "Vaccine Recommendations" tab of the above quick reference web page unless there is a medical contraindication.

MALARIA CHEMOPROPHYLAXIS

Preventing malaria in military units deployed to endemic areas is an essential objective of FHP. Malaria can be prevented through 1) education and training; 2) use of personal protection measures, which include individual bed nets, permethrin-impregnated uniforms, and insect repellents; and 3) use of chemoprophylaxis where indicated. The joint instruction on immunization and chemoprophylaxis stipulates that medical commanders designate trained staff to provide comprehensive malaria prevention counseling to military and civilian personnel considered to be at risk of contracting malaria and that such counseling "include instruction on how to take prescribed antimalarial medications, the importance of compliance with the prescribed medication schedule, information about potential adverse effects, and the need to seek medical care if these adverse effects occur" (www.vaccines.mil/documents/969r40_562.pdf#page=23).

Malaria cases seen in returning US military personnel reflect the current deployments around the world. In 2011, the highest risk was for people deployed in Afghanistan, with exposures to chloroquine-resistant *Plasmodium falciparum* and *P. vivax* malaria. There is also risk of *P. falciparum* malaria for people with frequent training and development missions to sub-Saharan Africa.

Several features of malaria chemoprophylaxis under FHP that are unique to the US military are derived from the activities and stressors of military deployments. When antimalarial drugs are used for chemoprophylaxis as part of FHP, the military can only use FDA-approved chemoprophylaxis agents in accordance with the specific FDA-approved indications. Off-label use of drugs is not allowed when given under FHP. If off-label use is felt to be in the best interest of the person or unit, trained and knowledgeable clinicians must provide one-on-one medical evaluations, document in the medical record the rationale for such use, and provide a by-name prescription for the drug or vaccine to each person.

In September 2009, the Assistant Secretary of Defense (Health Affairs) issued a policy memorandum on the use of mefloquine for malaria chemoprophylaxis throughout the DoD. In chloroquine-resistant areas in which doxycycline and mefloquine are equally efficacious in preventing malaria, doxycycline is the drug of choice for malarial chemoprophylaxis in personnel with a history of neurobehavioral disorders. Those personnel with a history of neurobehavioral disorders who cannot take doxycycline should be prescribed atovaquone-proguanil for travel to chloroquine-resistant areas.

The rationale for recommending doxycycline over mefloquine is as follows:

- With the increasing recognition of possible neuropsychiatric side effects of mefloquine in some people, new relative contraindications have been added to the product label since 2003. In addition, each person prescribed mefloquine must be given an FDA-approved medication guide. Complying with this guidance requires a one-on-one encounter with a knowledgeable provider, which is not feasible with large deployments.
- Neuropsychiatric side effects may confound the diagnosis and management of posttraumatic stress disorder and traumatic brain injury, which makes the continued routine use of mefloquine less desirable.

In September 2011, United States Africa Command (AFRICOM) issued a policy change recommending atovaquone-proguanil (Malarone) as the recommended malaria chemoprophylaxis option for all personnel for both short- and long-term deployments in high-transmission areas of Africa. High-transmission areas for the purpose of this policy are defined by the National Center for Military Intelligence and can be found at www.intelink.gov/ncmi/index.php (authorization required). For practical purposes, this includes most of sub-Saharan Africa. For people who are unable to receive atovaquone-proguanil because of intolerance or contraindication, doxycycline is the preferred second-line therapy. Use of mefloquine as prophylaxis is a third-line recommendation for those unable to receive either atovaquone-proguanil or doxycycline. Before prescribing mefloquine for prophylaxis, absolute and relative contraindications as described in the approved product label must be considered.

As a matter of policy, the US military routinely uses primaquine for presumptive antirelapse treatment (PART) in returning military populations to prevent the late relapse of P. vivax malaria or P. ovale malaria.

PART is also referred to as "terminal prophylaxis." In PART, primaquine is given to otherwise healthy people on their departure from an endemic area. Primaquine is used for this indication much more frequently in the military than in most civilian travelers.

The FDA-approved regimen for PART is 15 mg (base) given daily for 14 days. This regimen was approved in 1952 and has not been revisited since. In the intervening decades, an overwhelming amount of data has accumulated to show that the total dose of primaquine to eliminate the dormant hypnozoite stages responsible for late relapses is dependent on the infecting P. vivax strain; therefore, the optimal human dose should be based on weight and adjusted for the infecting P. vivax strain.

In 2003, CDC recommended 30 mg (base) of primaquine daily for 14 days based on available evidence, but the FDA-approved regimen remains the lower dose. Adherence to the daily 14-day regimen is poor unless primaquine is given under directly observed therapy, which is rarely done. As a result of noncompliance and subtherapeutic dosing with the 15 mg (base) for 14 days regimen, periodic outbreaks of relapsed P. vivax malaria occur in returning military personnel. Use of the higher-dose primaquine regimen for PART is now recommended for military personnel. This recommendation is consistent with the spirit of DoD issuance 6200.02 (February 17, 2008), in that the higher-dose recommendation for primaquine when used as PART is "standard medical practice in the United States."

The most important risk of using primaquine is hemolytic anemia in those who are deficient in glucose-6-phosphate dehydrogenase (G6PD). Current policy is for all US military personnel to be screened for G6PD deficiency on entry into military service. However, some people, such as reservists, may have deployed without testing, or clinicians may not be able to confirm results for all people in a unit requiring PART. Clinicians should be aware that hemolytic reactions to primaquine may occur in those with unrecognized G6PD deficiency.

A recurrent issue for military medicine is the correct timing of primaquine when given as PART in conjunction with the standard chemoprophylaxis drug being taken. Primaquine can be given at any time after

Table 8-8. Differences between CDC recommendations and US military's use of malaria chemoprophylaxis

	CDC RECOMMENDATION	US MILITARY POLICY
Choice of malaria chemoprophylaxis agent	Chemoprophylaxis guidelines do not recommend one drug versus another, but rather emphasize the goal of individualizing the recommendation for the individual traveler on the basis of past experience, itinerary, possible drug interaction, potential side effects, costs, and medical contraindications such as drug allergies.	Individualizing advice and recommendations for large military deployments is rarely logistically possible or feasible. Recognizing this reality, in September 2009, the US military adopted a new policy on the use of malaria chemoprophylaxis in the US military. Doxycycline is now the drug of choice to prevent malaria in deployed US military forces in all areas other than sub-Saharan Africa. In September 2011, AFRICOM policy changed to recommending atovaquone-proguanil for sub-Saharan Africa.
Doxycycline	An option for chemoprophylaxis in all areas	Recommended first-line chemoprophylaxis in all areas other than sub-Saharan Africa.
Mefloquine	An option for chemoprophylaxis in all areas	Mefloquine is not recommended as a primary option. It should be used only in those whose travel requires malaria chemoprophylaxis, who cannot take either doxycycline or atovaquone-proguanil, and who meet all requirements of the current FDA-approved product label.
Atovaquone-proguanil	An option for chemoprophylaxis in all areas	Atovaquone-proguanil is the drug of choice for sub-Saharan Africa. Atovaquone-proguanil is recommended for those who are intolerant of or who have contraindications to doxycycline in other areas.
Primaquine chemoprophylaxis	CDC recommends the use of primaquine as primary chemoprophylaxis in geographic areas with mainly *P. vivax* malaria.	There is no FDA-approved indication for the use of primaquine to prevent malaria. Therefore, the US military cannot use primaquine as a chemoprophylaxis agent under current FHP guidelines.
PART	Primaquine at 30 mg (base) for 14 days	There is no FDA-approved indication for the use of primaquine at the higher dose of 30 mg (base) for 14 days. However, primaquine is an FDA-approved drug with an indication for PART. The CDC-recommended (higher) dose is recommended, as it is standard of medical practice in the United States.

Abbreviations: AFRICOM, African Command; FDA, Food and Drug Administration; FHP, Force Health Protection; PART, presumptive antirelapse treatment.

leaving an endemic area. For convenience and for enhancing adherence to the 14-day regimen of primaquine, it is often best for military units to prescribe the primaquine in the immediate 2 weeks after deployment. During this time the units are often still at their home base completing their inprocessing before block leave. Once personnel depart on leave, adherence and monitoring for side effects are more difficult.

Under FHP, military personnel are required to take their chemoprophylaxis agents as prescribed to maintain mission readiness. Individual soldiers do not have the right to refuse an order given under FHP. There is great variability in practice as to how seriously individual commanders enforce these policies, however, and continued outbreaks of malaria occur in military populations because of poor compliance.

Differences between civilian and US military use of chemoprophylaxis drugs are summarized in Table 8-8.

UNIQUE NEEDS FOR THE MILITARY

US military personnel may encounter threats, such as biological warfare agents, that are not usually considered for civilian travelers. Vaccines, immunoglobulins, drug prophylaxis, and drug treatment regimens can be given under FHP, but only in accordance with FDA-licensed products and regimens and for FDA-approved indications.

Products not approved by the FDA are given to soldiers only with voluntary informed consent under an institutional review board–approved protocol and in accordance with a current and FDA-approved investigational new drug application.

Only under exceptional circumstances would products not approved by the FDA be given to soldiers without informed consent. This circumstance is governed by emergency use authorization procedures. Section 564 of the Federal Food, Drug, and Cosmetic Act (21 USC 360bbb-3), as amended by the Project BioShield Act of 2004 (Public Law 108–276), permits the FDA commissioner to authorize the use of an unapproved medical product or an unapproved use of an approved medical product during a declared emergency involving a heightened risk of attack on the public or US military forces, or when there is a potential to affect national security.

BIBLIOGRAPHY

1. Armed Forces Health Surveillance Center. Malaria Issue. Medical Surveillance Monthly Report (MSMR) [Internet]. 2012 Jan [cited 2012 Sep 23];19(1). Available from: http://www.afhsc.mil/viewMSMR?file=2012/v19_n01.pdf#Page=01.

2. Brisson M, Brisson P. Compliance with antimalaria chemoprophylaxis in a combat zone. Am J Trop Med Hyg. 2012 Apr;86(4):587–90.

3. Carr ME Jr, Fandre MN, Oduwa FO. Glucose-6-phosphate dehydrogenase deficiency in 2 returning Operation Iraqi Freedom soldiers who developed hemolytic anemia while receiving primaquine prophylaxis for malaria. Mil Med. 2005 Apr;170(4):273–6.

4. Food and Drug Administration. Emergency use authorization of medical products. Rockville, MD: Food and Drug Administration; 2007 [cited 2012 Sep 23]. Available from: http://www.fda.gov/RegulatoryInformation/Guidances/ucm125127.htm.

5. Kotwal RS, Wenzel RB, Sterling RA, Porter WD, Jordan NN, Petruccelli BP. An outbreak of malaria in US Army Rangers returning from Afghanistan. JAMA. 2005 Jan 12;293(2):212–6.

6. Llanos JK. The reporting and recording of unspecified malaria in the military, 1998–2007. US Army Med Dep J. 2009 Apr–Jun:42–5.

7. Office of the Assistant Secretary of Defense. Policy memorandum on the use of mefloquine (Lariam) in malaria prophylaxis. Washington, DC: TRICARE Management Activity; 2009.

8. Townell N, Looke D, McDougall D, McCarthy JS. Relapse of imported *Plasmodium vivax* malaria is related to primaquine dose: a retrospective study. Malaria J. 2012 Jun 22;11(1):214.

9. US Africa Command. Health and medical Force Health Protection procedures for deployment and travel. US Africa Command Manual [Internet]. 2010 [cited 2012 Sep 23]. Available from: http://www.africom.mil/TheaterClearanceCoordCenter/ACM%204200%2003%20%20-%2014%20Apr%2010.pdf.

10. US Department of Defense. Department of Defense directive: Force Health Protection (FHP), no. 6200.04. Washington, DC: US Department of Defense; 2004

[updated 2007 Apr 23; cited 2012 Sep 23]. Available from: http://www.dtic.mil/whs/directives/corres/pdf/620004p.pdf

11. US Department of Defense. Department of Defense instruction: application of Food and Drug Administration (FDA) rules to Department of Defense Force Health Protection programs, no 6200.02. Washington, DC: US Department of Defense; 2008 [cited 2012 Sep 23]. Available from: http://www.dtic.mil/whs/directives/corres/pdf/620002p.pdf.

12. US Department of Defense. Unified combatant commands. Washington, DC: US Department of Defense; 2011 [cited 2012 Sep 23]. Available from: http://www.defense.gov/home/features/2009/0109_unifiedcommand/.

13. Whitman TJ, Coyne PE, Magill AJ, Blazes DL, Green MD, Milhous WK, et al. An outbreak of *Plasmodium falciparum* malaria in US Marines deployed to Liberia. Am J Trop Med Hyg. 2010 Aug;83(2):258–65.

STUDY ABROAD & OTHER INTERNATIONAL STUDENT TRAVEL

Gary Rhodes, Inés DeRomaña, Jodi Ebner

OVERVIEW

Study abroad allows students to complete part of their US degree program outside the United States. International experiences can include classroom study, research, internships, service learning, environmental field studies, and directed travel. Generally, study abroad refers to programs where students earn academic credit for their academic work abroad. However, many students travel abroad for nonacademic programs, which can include athletics, adventure activities, noncredit internships, volunteer or mission groups, and personal international travel.

US student participation in study abroad has more than tripled over the past 2 decades. In the 2009–2010 academic year, 270,604 US students studied abroad for academic credit—an increase of 3.9% over the previous academic year. Although most study in European countries, US students are now spending time in countries all over the world. Fifteen of the top 25 destinations are outside Western Europe. The percentage of students choosing to travel to Africa, Asia, and the Middle East has risen, while the percentage choosing to study in Europe and Oceania has decreased. Substantial numbers of students are now studying in developing countries, where health concerns and endemic infections differ from those in the United States and Western Europe.

Study abroad and international travel can be life-changing and positive experiences for college and university students. However, students and families must take time and effort to plan for study abroad and other international travel to be proactive in supporting health and safety and prepared to respond to incidents abroad. Further resources are included in Table 8-9.

ADMINISTRATION OF STUDY-ABROAD PROGRAMS

Study-abroad program types and administrative structures vary. Some are administered overseas by a local university, with no US staff support onsite. Other US colleges and universities obtain legal status in the country where the program is offered and bring faculty and staff from the United States to run the program. Others hire local staff or resident directors to administer their centers abroad, or partner with nonuniversity, nonprofit or for-profit companies that provide study-abroad programs (often referred to as third-party providers). There are also hybrid versions combining formal connections to international universities with parts of programs administered by the US campus or a third-party provider.

Institutional administrative structures in the United States can vary as well. Some institutions have several study-abroad staff, while others have no full-time staff members. Some universities have specialized professionals to focus on health and safety issues, while others have no staff dedicated to health

Table 8-9. Study-abroad resources

ORGANIZATION	DESCRIPTION
NAFSA: Association of International Educators, www.nafsa.org	Useful information for institutions implementing study-abroad programs, as well as information for students to support their health and safety
www.nafsa.org/uploadedFiles/responsible_study_abroad.pdf	"Responsible Study Abroad: Good Practices for Health & Safety": Advice for developing plans and procedures to implement good practices for program sponsors, students, and parents/guardians/families, especially those pertaining to health and safety issues
Council on Standards for International Educational Travel (CSIET), http://csiet.org/about/standards.html	Standards for exchange programs for US high school students going abroad
http://csiet.org/publications-resources/docs/CSIET_Student_Safety_Guidelines-Final_6–23-09.pdf	Health and safety guidelines
Center for Global Education, SAFETI (Safety Abroad First–Educational Travel Information) Clearinghouse, http://globaled.us/safeti	Resources to support study-abroad program development and implementation, emphasizing health and safety issues and resources for US colleges and universities supporting study abroad
http://globaled.us/SAFETI/program_audit_checklist.asp	SAFETI Program Audit Checklist
http://studentsabroad.com/	Resource website for students that includes a country-specific handbook
Forum on Education Abroad www.forumea.org/standards.cfm	Standards of good practice and a code of ethics for the field of education abroad

and safety support. Some institutions require health insurance that integrates comprehensive medical care, 24-hour assistance, emergency evacuation, and repatriation. Other institutions may recommend obtaining comprehensive health insurance for study abroad but may provide limited or no information about available options.

Some colleges and universities recommend or require that students visit a travel health clinic before travel to specific countries, in addition to obtaining a predeparture health clearance for all countries. Whether or not a university offers pre-travel health clinic support, students should consult with a medical professional as a part of the planning process before study abroad. This consultation should be designed to help students understand what they must do to prepare for a safe and healthy stay in their host country. It should include information on endemic health issues in the host country, availability of medications commonly prescribed in the United States, and information on how to obtain medical care abroad.

PREDEPARTURE PLANNING

Study-abroad program advisors should work with medical professionals to provide the students with a comprehensive pre-travel consultation, including any routine, recommended, and required vaccinations, recommended prophylactic and self-treatment medications, and pre-travel counseling and advice. The pre-travel consultation should also include the following:

- Country- and region-specific health information
- Gender-specific health information
- Advice and resources for students with disabilities
- Information about physiologic and psychological consequences they may encounter as a result of culture shock and changes in their routine, and a specific plan for students with preexisting conditions
- General advice on nutrition and dietary deficiencies
- Cautions about alcohol and drug use and a specific plan for those with preexisting dependency issues
- General instructions for emergency medical situations
- Full health and accident insurance policies and emergency assistance coverage information

The information in the Humanitarian Aid Workers section earlier in this chapter can be useful for students participating in study abroad, internships, or research in the developing world.

Before departure, advisors and professionals should encourage students to learn about their destinations to understand the health and safety issues of the countries they will visit. This also includes reading about the cultural and political climate of those countries.

The Department of State hosts a website specifically for students (http://studentsabroad.state.gov) with direct links to information on passports, visas, crime, safety, security, transportation challenges, and resources for US citizens during international travel. The Department of State provides country-specific information on their website (http://travel.state.gov/travel/travel_1744.html). Students should check on whether there is a travel warning or travel alert providing specific concerns about safe travel to countries they will visit. Travel warnings are issued when long-term, protracted conditions that make a country dangerous or unstable lead the Department of State to recommend that Americans avoid or consider the risk of travel to that country or when the US government's ability to assist

American citizens is constrained. Travel alerts are posted to disseminate information about short-term conditions that pose risks to the security of US citizens. Alerts may be posted for security risks, political or civil unrest, armed conflicts, natural disasters, and terrorist attacks. Before departure, students should consider registering with the Department of State's Smart Traveler Enrollment Program (STEP, available at step.state.gov) to receive updates and information about their host country from the US embassy or consulate and make the process smoother if they need help while abroad or if someone from the United States is trying to contact them.

The CDC Travelers' Health website (www.cdc.gov/travel) contains advice for travelers on the most current health recommendations for international destinations.

HEALTH AND SAFETY WHILE ABROAD
Food and Water Safety

Food and water contamination is one of the leading causes of illness for travelers. Basic precautions can minimize the risk of diarrhea and other illnesses. Specific food and water recommendations depend on the destination country. Consulting with a travel health professional is recommended. Some tips to help students regarding food and water safety include:

- Find out if tap water is safe to drink for non-locals. If it is unsafe—
  > Purify unsafe water before drinking or drink only bottled water, making sure that the seals have not been tampered with. Use only purified or bottled water for brushing teeth. For more information, see Chapter 2, Water Disinfection for Travelers.
  > Avoid ice in drinks, as it may also be unsafe depending on the water used to make it.
- Cooked foods should be eaten hot; raw fruits and vegetables should be eaten only if washed in clean water and then peeled by the traveler.
- Poor refrigeration, undercooked meat, and food purchased from street vendors could pose problems related to food contamination.
- See Chapter 2, Food and Water Precautions for more information.

Adherence to Host Country Laws and Codes of Conduct

Study-abroad professionals and others working with student travelers should advise students about rules and regulations that may differ from those on a home campus, as well as those of the study-abroad program sponsor and the local laws and customs of the countries visited. Students must abide by the legal system of their host country. Additional information on host country laws may be found in the Department of State Consular Information Sheets (www.travel.state.gov/travel/cis_pa_tw/cis/cis_4965.html).

Mental and Physical Health

The NAFSA: Association of International Educators' publication, "Best Practices in Addressing Mental Health Issues Affecting Education Abroad Participants," available at www.nafsa.org/mentalhealth, encourages study-abroad programs "to sensitively offer support that connects the student to professional help before a problem reaches a crisis state or seriously derails the student's academic and career plans." Likewise, students must consider their own mental and physical health issues when applying to a study-abroad program.

US college and university campuses are seeing an increase in the numbers of students with special mental health issues. These issues go abroad with students. Students should be encouraged to disclose any chronic physical and mental health conditions or accommodation needs before departure to the country where they will study. Dealing with stressful situations abroad may be difficult for students away from their familiar support system, which may trigger mental and physical issues. Advisors can encourage students to disclose this information by assuring them that it is meant to maximize their experience while abroad—not to prevent them from going.

Prescription Medication

Students should discuss any existing medical or health issues with their families and health professionals before going abroad. Planning ahead can help them address challenges they may face. Students should not make changes to their medications immediately preceding their time abroad, nor should they discontinue taking prescribed medications while abroad, unless instructed to do so by a health care professional.

Students must travel with a signed prescription for all medications needed while abroad and a letter from the US treating physician explaining the recommended dosage, the student's diagnosis, and the treatment. In most countries, arriving with quantities exceeding the limits set for personal use is prohibited.

Generally, US prescriptions are not accepted by host country pharmacies and cannot be filled without visiting a local medical practitioner first. Students must check first whether the US prescription will be readily accepted by a local pharmacy abroad. Students are highly recommended to fill prescriptions in the United States before departure, reducing the need to purchase medication overseas and decreasing potential exposure to counterfeit and poor quality medications (see Chapter 2, *Perspectives:* Pharmaceutical Quality & Counterfeit Drugs).

Medications commonly prescribed in the United States may not be available or legal in the host country. It is vital for students to research the availability and legality of their prescription medications before traveling, discuss with their health care providers whether some medications should be changed, and allow sufficient time to make adjustments before study abroad.

Shipping or mailing medications may not be a viable option because many countries' laws prohibit the mailing of drugs, including prescription medicines, to individuals.

Emergency Contacts

Students should print and fill out an emergency information card (http://studentsabroad.com/emergencycard.asp) with important contact numbers and personal information and carry a copy with them at all times. Students should share a copy of all important contact information while abroad with their emergency contacts in the United States, as well as share information for emergency contacts in the United States with the study-abroad program and the host school.

Students should keep both their program staff and their emergency contacts at home well informed of their whereabouts and activities and provide them with copies of their travel documents (passport, visa, plane tickets, and prescriptions) and itinerary.

Transportation

Traffic crashes are a major cause of injury to students while traveling abroad. It is imperative for students to understand what safe and legitimate modes of travel are available in their host country. A good source of information is the Association for Safe International Road Travel at www.asirt.org.

Alcohol and Drugs

The misuse and abuse of alcohol and drugs abroad can increase the risk of accidents, injury, unwanted attention, and theft. Being in a foreign environment requires the ability to respond to new and changing circumstances, which is impaired under the influence of drugs or alcohol. Many students are not of legal drinking age in the United States but are in the host country. Many do not receive adequate alcohol- and drug-prevention education explaining the consequences of risky drinking and drug abuse before departure. Violating drug laws abroad may result in serious consequences. In some countries, being found guilty of violating drug laws can lead to life in prison or the death penalty. Study-abroad professionals should conduct a proper orientation about the risks associated with drinking and abusing drugs abroad.

BIBLIOGRAPHY

1. Gore J, Green J. Issues and advising responsibilities. NAFSA's Guide to Education Abroad for Advisors and Administrators. 3rd ed. Washington, DC: NAFSA Association of International Educators; 2005. p. 261.
2. Institute of International Education. Americans study abroad in increasing numbers. New York: Institute of International Education; 2009 [cited 2012 Sep 24]. Available from: http://www.iie.org/en/Who-We-Are/News-and-Events/Press-Center/Press-Releases/2009/2009-11-16-Americans-Study-Abroad-Increasing.
3. Institute of International Education. Host regions of US study abroad students, 1999/00–2008/09. Open Doors report on international educational exchange. New York: Institute of International Education; 2011 [cited 2012 Sep 24]. Available from: http://www.iie.org/en/Research-and-Publications/Open-Doors/Data/US-Study-Abroad/Host-Regions/2000–10.
4. Interorganizational Task Force on Safety and Responsibility in Study Abroad. Responsible study abroad: good practices for health and safety.

Washington, DC: NAFSA: Association of International Educators; 2002 [cited 2012 Sep 24]. Available from: http://www.nafsa.org/knowledge_community_network.sec/education_abroad_1/developing_and_managing/practice_resources_36/policies/guidelines_for_health/.
5. NAFSA: Association of International Educators. Best practices in addressing mental health issues affecting education abroad participants. New York: NAFSA: Association of International Educators; 2006 [cited 2012 Sep 24]. Available from: http://www.nafsa.org/mentalhealth.
6. Pedersen ER, LaBrie JW, Hummer JF. Perceived behavioral alcohol norms predict drinking for college students while studying abroad. J Stud Alcohol Drugs. 2009;70(6):924–8.
7. The Forum on Education Abroad. Code of ethics for education abroad. Carlisle, PA: Dickinson College; 2008 [cited 2012 Sep 24]. Available from: http://www.forumea.org/documents/ForumonEducationAbroadCodeofEthics.pdf.

TRAVEL TO MASS GATHERINGS
C. Virginia Lee, Gary W. Brunette, Nancy M. Gallagher

OVERVIEW

Every year, millions of people travel internationally for mass gatherings that range from major sports events to fairs, festivals, concerts, or political rallies. These mass gatherings pose special risks for travelers, because large numbers of people in small areas can facilitate the spread of infectious diseases or increase the risk of injury. These issues should be considered when providing pre-travel consultations.

A mass gathering is usually defined as more than a specified number of people (which may be as few as 1,000 people, although 25,000 people is most commonly used), at a specific location, for a specific purpose, for a defined period of time. The World Health Organization defines a mass gathering as "an event [where] the number of people attending is sufficient to strain the planning and response resources of the community, state, or nation hosting the event." Although mass gatherings can be spontaneous events, such as a funeral for a head of state, or a form of political expression, such as a rally or march, most are planned events. Some mass gatherings occur regularly at different locations (such as the Olympic Games or the FIFA World Cup), and others recur in the same location (such as the Hajj or Wimbledon).

Mass gatherings can be characterized by purpose, location, participants, and duration. The reason for the gathering will often set a predictable tone for the event. Rock concerts are expected to be loud and boisterous, and segments of the crowd will engage in more risky behaviors. On the other hand, a religious event, such as a papal visit, would have other predictable characteristics. The purpose often influences the characteristics of the participants (age, origin, culture, homogeneity). For example, religious and family-oriented events tend to have participants at the extremes of age, who may have increased susceptibility to certain diseases.

The location will determine the climate and weather and will give some indication of social and political stability in that area. There will be diseases endemic to that area, and there may be specific disease outbreaks occurring that could affect the health of visitors. Geography (particularly altitude) and climate can predispose visitors to problems such as altitude sickness, heat-related illnesses, and dehydration. The actual venue can be fixed (stadium, open space) or mobile (procession, pilgrimage). Some gatherings are indoors or in protected spaces that can shield against the elements, while others are completely exposed. The health infrastructure at the event and in the area will determine the ability to respond to both anticipated and unanticipated incidents. Facilities for food, water, and sanitation can affect the health of attendees. Often these facilities are temporary, recently erected, and may not meet the needs of the population.

The density of the crowd influences the potential risks, such as problems with crowd control, disease transmission, and injury. Large crowds can quickly overwhelm facilities. Crowd characteristics, such as age, mood, and availability of drugs or alcohol, will influence whether violence is a risk. Densely packed crowds are more likely to be violent. Events with large numbers of international participants tend to have increased risk of infectious disease outbreaks. This is in part related to differences in patterns of endemic diseases and levels of vaccinations between host and home countries. The longer an event lasts, the more likely that stresses to facilities, organizers, and participants will occur.

The most common health problems reported at mass gatherings are injuries, respiratory and cardiac issues, heat-related illness, alcohol or drug effects, and gastrointestinal illnesses. These problems can typically be addressed by either on-site clinics or nearby health facilities. However, circumstances leading to mass casualties have occurred at many different types of events.

Although communicable diseases are an understandable concern for organizers of large gatherings, they have historically not been a major cause of adverse health events. For example, infectious diseases contributed to <1% of health care visits during the 1996 Atlanta Olympic Games and the 2000 Sydney Olympic Games. Furthermore, illnesses such as influenza may be difficult to definitively attribute to attendance at an event. On the other hand, meningococcal meningitis transmission during the Hajj not only caused illness but also resulted in changes in requirements for Hajj pilgrims (see Chapter 4, Hajj Pilgrimage, Saudi Arabia).

Mass gatherings held in the context of an outbreak or pandemic pose additional risks for travelers and the population of host countries. International attendees bring to the gathering their cultures, languages, social and health behaviors, and disease susceptibilities, all of which may affect the course of the outbreak. Organizers of these events, in cooperation with local officials and health authorities, should strongly consider these factors when conducting a risk assessment for the event. If a decision is made to continue with the event while the outbreak is ongoing, special precautions might be recommended for attendees.

GUIDANCE FOR INTERNATIONAL TRAVELERS TO MASS GATHERINGS

All travelers to international mass gatherings should be evaluated by a travel health provider, ideally 4–6 weeks before travel, to assess the level of risk faced by the traveler and to take steps to manage the risk. Travelers should take precautions to mitigate risks associated with mass gatherings:

- Be aware of the most likely health risks associated with the particular event they are attending and what they can do to stay healthy and safe.
- Be up-to-date with all routine immunizations, including influenza vaccine, when available.

- Maintain vigilance at gatherings where drug and alcohol use could contribute to dangerous behavior.
- Avoid gatherings where political or religious fervor may contribute to violence, or where inadequate facilities may contribute to an unhealthy environment.
- Try to avoid densely congested areas with limited egress.
- Be aware of emergency precautions and locate exit routes and medical facilities.

Knowledge of the country or region being visited is essential. Country information can be obtained from destination pages on the CDC Travelers' Health website (wwwnc.cdc.gov/travel/destinations/list.aspx), which provides destination-specific information and will often post specific guidance for major events. The Department of State website (http://travel.state.gov/travel/travel_1744.html) may provide additional information about countries and specific events.

BIBLIOGRAPHY

1. Emergency Management Australia. Safe and healthy mass gatherings: a health, medical and safety planning manual for public events. Commonwealth of Australia; 1999 [cited 2012 Sep 23]. Available from: www.dh.sa.gov.au/pehs/publications/ema-mass-gatherings-manual.pdf.
2. Fapore D, Lurie P, Moll M, Weltman A, Rankin J. Public health aspects of the Rainbow Family of Living Light annual gathering—Allegheny National Forest, Pennsylvania, 1999. MMWR Morb Mortal Wkly Rep. 2000;49(15):324–6.
3. Kaiser R, Coulombier D. Epidemic intelligence during mass gatherings. Euro Surveill. 2006;11(12):E061221.3.
4. Lombardo JS, Sniegoski CA, Loschen WA, Westercamp M, Wade M, Dearth S, et al. Public health surveillance for mass gatherings. Johns Hopkins APL Technical Digest. 2008;27(4):1–9.
5. Milsten AM, Maguire BJ, Bissell RA, Seaman KG. Mass-gathering medical care: a review of the literature. Prehosp Disaster Med. 2002 Jul–Sep; 17(3):151–62.
6. World Health Organization. Communicable disease alert and response for mass gatherings: key considerations. Geneva: World Health Organization; 2008 [cited 2012 Sep 23]. Available from: http://www.who.int/csr/Mass_gatherings2.pdf.

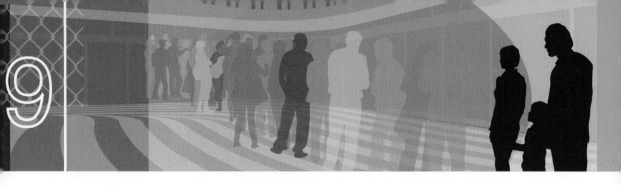

Health Considerations for Newly Arrived Immigrants & Refugees

INTRODUCTION

Christine K. Olson, Mary P. Naughton, Luis S. Ortega

According to the Department of Homeland Security, approximately 73,000 refugees were admitted into the United States during fiscal year (FY) 2010 (October 1, 2009, through September 30, 2010). In addition, >1 million immigrants obtained legal permanent resident status during FY 2010; 566,000 of these were already living in the United States and 476,000 came directly from overseas. Map 9-1 shows countries of origin for refugee and new immigrant arrivals in FY 2010.

A medical examination is mandatory for refugees and applicants for US immigration. Refugees undergo the examination overseas, whereas immigrants are examined in the United States or overseas, depending on their place of residence. CDC's Division of Global Migration and Quarantine (DGMQ) provides panel physicians and civil surgeons with technical instructions for conducting the medical examinations. A panel physician is an experienced medical doctor practicing overseas who has an agreement with a local US embassy or consulate general to perform overseas examinations. A civil surgeon is a US physician who is designated to perform immigrant medical examinations. DGMQ works closely with the Department of State, which has agreements with panel physicians, and US Citizenship and Immigration Services within the Department of Homeland Security, which approves physicians to serve as civil surgeons.

BIBLIOGRAPHY

1. CDC. Technical instructions for civil surgeons. Atlanta: CDC; 2010 [cited 2012 Sep 26]. Available from: http://www.cdc.gov/immigrantrefugeehealth/exams/ti/civil/technical-instructions-civil-surgeons.html.
2. CDC. Technical instructions for panel physicians. Atlanta: CDC; 2012 [cited 2012 Sep 26]. Available from: http://www.cdc.gov/immigrantrefugeehealth/exams/ti/panel/technical-instructions-panel-physicians.html.
3. US Department of Homeland Security, Office of Immigration Statistics. Yearbook of Immigrant Statistics: 2010. Washington, DC: US Department of Homeland Security; 2011 [cited 2012 Sep 26]. Available from: http://www.dhs.gov/xlibrary/assets/statistics/yearbook/2010/ois_yb_2010.pdf.

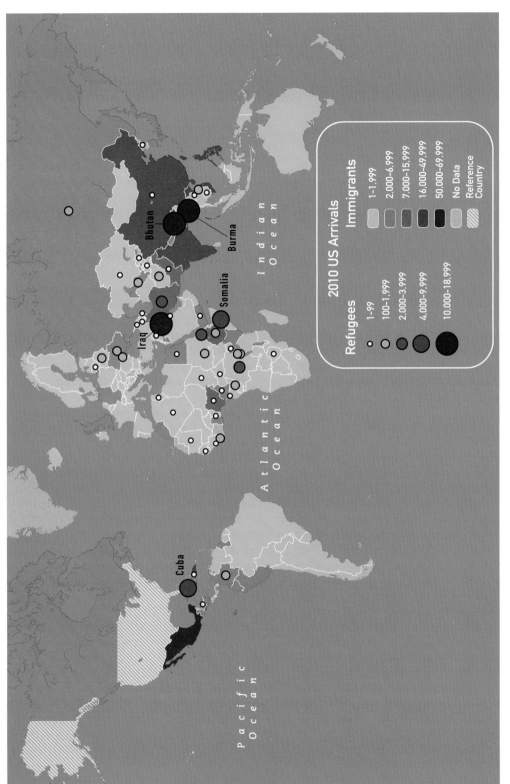

MAP 9-1. US REFUGEE AND NEW IMMIGRANT ARRIVALS BY COUNTRY OF ORIGIN, FISCAL YEAR 2010[1]

[1] Data from Office of Immigration Statistics, US Department of Homeland Security.

BEFORE ARRIVAL IN THE UNITED STATES: THE OVERSEAS MEDICAL EXAMINATION

Christine K. Olson, Mary P. Naughton, Luis S. Ortega

BACKGROUND

The Immigration and Nationality Act (INA), which relates to the immigration, temporary admission, naturalization, and removal of foreigners, mandates that all refugees and applicants for US immigration undergo an overseas medical screening examination performed by a panel physician to screen for inadmissible conditions. A panel physician is a medically trained, licensed, and experienced medical doctor practicing overseas who has an agreement with a local US embassy or consulate general. More than 760 panel physicians perform overseas medical examinations in accordance with requirements referred to as technical instructions.

MEDICAL EXAMINATION AND TREATMENT

CDC is responsible for providing the technical instructions to the panel physicians and for monitoring the quality of the overseas medical examination process through its quality assessment program. The technical instructions give specific requirements for the screening performed during the medical examination and are periodically updated to reflect current medical practice. The purpose of the mandated medical examination is to detect inadmissible conditions of public health significance. These medical conditions include infectious diseases such as tuberculosis, Hansen disease, and sexually transmitted diseases; mental disorders associated with harmful behavior; and substance abuse or addiction (www.cdc.gov/immigrantrefugee health/exams/ti/panel/technical-instructions-panel-physicians.html).

The testing modalities required for the medical examination include a physical examination, mental health evaluation, syphilis serology, review of vaccination records, and chest radiography, followed by acid-fast bacillus smears and sputum cultures if the chest radiograph suggests tuberculosis. Treatment is also required for certain conditions, such as tuberculosis, specified sexually transmitted diseases, and Hansen disease.

In 2007, CDC began implementation of the Culture and Directly Observed Therapy (DOT) Tuberculosis Technical Instructions (www.cdc.gov/immigrantrefugeehealth/pdf/tuberculosis-ti-2009.pdf) in some countries. Priority for implementation is assigned on the basis of the country's tuberculosis prevalence, volume of US-bound immigrants or refugees, and contribution to tuberculosis prevalence in the United States. These technical instructions require *Mycobacterium tuberculosis* culture, drug susceptibility testing, and directly observed therapy throughout the course of treatment, before immigration. As of July 2012, approximately three-quarters of US-bound immigrants and refugees are being screened by using the Culture and DOT Tuberculosis Technical Instructions. Since these technical instructions have been implemented in 3 major immigrant source countries, California has reported a decline from 4.2% to 1.5% in the proportion of immigrants with tuberculosis-suspect classifications who were identified with active tuberculosis within the first 6 months of US arrival. CDC is working to complete worldwide implementation of the Culture and DOT Tuberculosis Technical Instructions by 2014.

The required examination also includes evaluation of mental disorders with associated harmful behaviors and substance-related disorders. Inadmissibility based on a physical or mental disorder is limited to applicants with associated harmful or potentially harmful behavior.

For specific refugee populations, the visit to the panel physician additionally provides an opportunity for preventive medical interventions, such as immunizing against vaccine-preventable diseases and administering presumptive therapy for parasitic or other infectious diseases, including nematode infections and malaria, that may be affecting the population at the time of migration.

PROOF OF VACCINATION

In 1996, a subsection was added to the INA requiring that people seeking immigrant visas for permanent residency show proof of receipt of all vaccination series recommended by the Advisory Committee on Immunization Practices (ACIP) (www.cdc.gov/vaccines/recs/acip). In 2009, CDC adopted revised vaccination criteria to determine which vaccines recommended by ACIP should be required for immigrant visa applicants. These criteria allow CDC the flexibility to adapt vaccination requirements according to public health needs (www.cdc.gov/immigrantrefugeehealth/laws-regs/vaccination-immigration/revised-vaccination-criteria-immigration.html). The vaccination criteria state that the vaccine must:

- Be age-appropriate
- Protect against a disease that has the potential to cause an outbreak
- Protect against a disease that has been eliminated or is in the process of being eliminated in the United States

These requirements apply to all adult immigrants and most immigrant children. However, internationally adopted children who are aged ≤10 years may obtain a waiver of exemption from the immunization requirements. Refugees are not required to meet the INA immunization requirements at the time of entry into the United States. Instead, they must show proof of vaccination at the time they apply for permanent US residence, typically 1 year after arrival. Updated instructions regarding vaccination requirements are available on the CDC website (www.cdc.gov/immigrantrefugeehealth/exams/ti/panel/vaccination-panel-technical-instructions.html).

CLASSIFICATION OF APPLICANTS

To determine the inadmissibility of an applicant, the medical conditions of public health significance are categorized as class A or B. Class A conditions are defined as those that preclude an immigrant or refugee from entering the United States. An immigrant or refugee who has an inadmissible condition may still be issued a visa after the illness has been adequately treated or after a waiver of the visa ineligibility has been approved by the United States Citizenship and Immigration Services. Class B conditions are defined as physical or mental abnormalities, diseases, or disabilities serious enough or permanent in nature as to amount to a substantial departure from normal well-being. Follow-up evaluation soon after US arrival is recommended for immigrants or refugees with class B conditions. For more information, see Arrival in the United States: Health Status & Screening of Refugees, Immigrants, & International Adoptees later in this chapter.

NOTIFICATIONS AND FOLLOW-UP

The Department of State forms completed by panel physicians are collected at US ports of entry when immigrants and refugees arrive. These forms summarize the results of the overseas medical examination and include classification of health conditions. On the basis of this information, CDC notifies state or local health departments of all arriving refugees, immigrants with class A conditions (with waiver), and immigrants with class B tuberculosis classifications who are resettling in their jurisdictions and need follow-up evaluation and possible treatment. The notification and Department of State form data are transmitted to state or local health departments electronically through CDC's Electronic Disease Notification System (EDN).

State and local health departments are asked to report to CDC through EDN the results of these US follow-up evaluations, as well as any serious public health conditions identified among recently arrived immigrants and refugees. Reporting allows a better understanding of epidemiologic patterns of disease in recently arrived immigrants and refugees and is a way of monitoring the quality of the overseas medical examination.

REGULATIONS

In 2008, CDC amended the regulations that govern the required overseas medical examination for immigrants and refugees by adding the following disease categories to those already specified in the INA: 1) quarantinable diseases designated by presidential executive order (www.cdc.gov/quarantine/About LawsRegulationsQuarantineIsolation.html) and 2) diseases that meet criteria of public health emergency of international concern and require notification of the World Health Organization under the revised International Health Regulations (2005). This change allows CDC the flexibility to determine which diseases are included in the medical screening and testing of immigrants and refugees in areas of the world that are experiencing outbreaks of specific diseases. These changes

reduce the health risk to the United States from emerging diseases, without imposing undue burden on either the immigrants and refugees or the US health care system.

As of January 4, 2010, testing for HIV is no longer a required part of the US immigration medical screening process. HIV infection is no longer an inadmissible condition that prevents non-US citizens from entering the United States (www.cdc.gov/immigrantrefugeehealth/laws-regs/hiv-ban-removal/final-rule.html and www.cdc.gov/immigrantrefugeehealth/exams/ti/hiv-guidance-panel-civil.html).

BIBLIOGRAPHY

1. CDC. Technical instructions for panel physicians. Atlanta: CDC; 2012 [cited 2012 Sep 26]. Available from: http://www.cdc.gov/immigrantrefugeehealth/exams/ti/panel/technical-instructions-panel-physicians.html.

2. Lowenthal P, Westenhouse J, Moore M, Posey DL, Watt JP, Flood J. Reduced importation of tuberculosis after the implementation of an enhanced pre-immigration screening protocol. Int J Tuberc Lung Dis. 2011 Jun;15(6):761–6.

3. Maloney S, Ortega L, Cetron M. Overseas medical screening for immigrants and refugees. In: Walker PF, Barnett ED, editors. Immigrant Medicine. Philadelphia: Saunders Elsevier; 2007. p. 111–22.

4. Maloney SA, Fielding KL, Laserson KF, Jones W, Nguyen TN, Dang QA, et al. Assessing the performance of overseas tuberculosis screening programs: a study among US-bound

immigrants in Vietnam. Arch Intern Med. 2006 Jan 23;166(2):234–40.

5. US Department of Homeland Security. Immigration and Nationality Act. Washington, DC: US Department of Homeland Security; 1952 [cited 2012 Sep 26]. Available from: http://www.uscis.gov/portal/site/uscis/menuitem.f6da51a2342135be7e9d7a10e0dc91a0/?vgnextoid=fa7e539dc4bed010VgnVCM1000000ecd190aRCRD&vgnextchannel=fa7e539dc4bed010VgnVCM1000000ecd190aRCRD&CH=act.

6. US Department of Homeland Security. Title 8 of Code of Federal Regulations (CFR). Washington DC: US Department of Homeland Security; 1938 [cited 2012 Sep 26]. Available from: http://www.uscis.gov/portal/site/uscis/menuitem.f6da51a2342135be7e9d7a10e0dc91a0/?vgnextoid=fa7e539dc4bed010VgnVCM1000000ecd190aRCRD&vgnextchannel=fa7e539dc4bed010VgnVCM1000000ecd190aRCRD&CH=8cfr.

ARRIVAL IN THE UNITED STATES: HEALTH STATUS & SCREENING OF REFUGEES, IMMIGRANTS, & INTERNATIONAL ADOPTEES

Patricia F. Walker, William M. Stauffer, Elizabeth D. Barnett

OVERVIEW

There is great diversity among immigrant and refugee populations arriving in the United States each year, with a concomitant wide spectrum of health needs. Some immigrants

and refugees arrive with infectious diseases of personal or public health significance; others with untreated chronic conditions, such as vitamin deficiencies, diabetes, or hypertension; and many with both infectious and chronic disease issues.

Although an overseas medical examination is mandatory for all immigrants and refugees before admission to the United States, the purpose of this examination is primarily to identify applicants with inadmissible health-related conditions for the Department of State and US Citizenship and Immigration Services (for more information, see the previous section in this chapter, Before Arrival in the United States: The Overseas Medical Examination). Medical screening after arrival in the United States is recommended but not required for all refugees and international adoptees (a category of immigrants). This postarrival screening is a more comprehensive examination that provides not only an opportunity to screen for communicable and noncommunicable diseases, but also to provide preventive services, including immunizations and initiation of treatment for latent tuberculosis, individual counseling (such as nutritional and mental health), and an opportunity to establish ongoing primary care. Immigrants with medical conditions requiring follow-up (class B conditions) are also recommended to be evaluated after their arrival; however, these evaluations are targeted for particular conditions such as tuberculosis. Ideally, all these evaluations should be done within 30 days of US arrival.

Postarrival medical screenings are often conducted at state or local health departments, as well as private clinics and community health centers. Many clinicians are unfamiliar with screening recommendations and diseases endemic to immigrants' countries of origin and may feel unprepared to deal with medical issues affecting these populations. In addition, clinicians and health systems are frequently unprepared to cope with language, social, and cultural barriers in caring for new arrivals. Further, refugees and immigrants often have other priorities related to their new environment, such as English classes, schooling, housing, and work, that take precedence over accessing health care services.

Refugees and internationally adopted children have a more formal, organized resettlement process and, as a result, have more health information available than other groups. Therefore, data and recommendations have largely focused on these populations.

This section outlines the recommended components of the postarrival health assessment, as well as available resources for refugees, immigrants, and internationally adopted children after arrival.

MEDICAL SCREENING FOR NEWLY ARRIVED REFUGEES

Many refugees and immigrants originate from countries with a high prevalence of tropical and other infectious diseases that may present a threat to individual or public health. In addition, untreated chronic health conditions, such as hypertension, diabetes, and obesity, are becoming increasingly common. Infectious diseases with long latency periods, including tuberculosis, hepatitis B, and certain intestinal nematodes, such as *Schistosoma* spp. and *Strongyloides stercoralis*, can be particularly challenging. Recommendations for this postarrival medical evaluation should be tailored to the specific population and based on such factors as country of origin; race; receipt of predeparture interventions, including vaccinations and presumptive therapy for malaria and intestinal parasites; and epidemiologic risks in the country of origin, as well as the country or countries of first asylum.

Medical screening should include a detailed medical and social history, as well as a physical examination. Evidence-based screening guidelines for refugees have been developed by CDC in collaboration with Office of Refugee Resettlement (ORR), the basic components of which are outlined in Box 9-1. Full guidelines, as well as a summary checklist of the components and recommended testing, are available at www.cdc.gov/immigrantrefugeehealth/guidelines/domestic/domestic-guidelines.html. Currently, population-specific guidelines do not exist, emphasizing the importance of acquiring local epidemiologic data.

An additional function of the postarrival medical screening is to arrange and coordinate ongoing primary care. Many refugees have not had age-appropriate cancer screening, such as a Papanicolaou test, mammography, and colon cancer screening, and these needs should be addressed at early follow-up visits. Clinicians should be aware of cancers with a higher prevalence in many immigrant populations, such as cervical, liver, stomach, and nasopharyngeal cancer.

BOX 9-1. RECOMMENDED COMPONENTS OF REFUGEE DOMESTIC HEALTH ASSESSMENTS[1,2]

- Review all available records, including chest radiograph (ask for overseas records).
- Complete a history and physical examination, including vision, hearing, and dental evaluation.
- Conduct mental health screening and, when clinically indicated, a more detailed social history, including any history of trauma/torture or rape.
- Evaluate for infectious disease, including tuberculosis, HIV and other sexually transmitted infections, and malaria and other parasitic infections (schistosomiasis and intestinal nematodes, including *Strongyloides*), depending on local epidemiology.
- Review overseas records for presumptive therapy for strongyloidiasis, schistosomiasis, or malaria, depending on point of departure.
- Evaluate for chronic diseases, including obesity, hypertension, diabetes, and nutritional deficiencies, such as vitamin B12 deficiency in select populations.
- Perform age-appropriate cancer screening, such as mammography, colonoscopy, or Papanicolaou test.
- Update immunizations as needed.
- Complete laboratory testing (hematologic testing, urinalysis, lead (as appropriate), HIV testing, hepatitis B serology for those arriving from countries with prevalence >2%, specific sexually transmitted infection testing, or other screening, such as basic metabolic panel and liver function testing, when clinically appropriate).

[1] A more detailed discussion of the medical examination of immigrants and refugees is available at www.cdc.gov/immigrantrefugeehealth/guidelines/refugee-guidelines.html.
[2] Full refugee health domestic screening guidelines are available at www.cdc.gov/immigrantrefugeehealth/guidelines/domestic/domestic-guidelines.html.

HIV testing was removed from the requirements for US admission in January 2010, which has implications for providers seeing patients from higher-prevalence countries. *HIV screening is highly encouraged in all newly arriving immigrants and refugees.* Culturally sensitive counseling regarding HIV testing is critical.

Nutritional deficiencies occur more commonly in refugee populations, a recent example being B12 deficiency in Bhutanese Nepali new arrivals. Prevalences ranged from 64% in people tested before migration to 27%–32% in people tested in the United States after arrival. Clinicians should be aware of the possibility of micronutrient deficiencies and screen and treat accordingly.

In areas of the world from which many refugees originate, potential lead exposures include lead-containing gasoline combustion; burning of fossil fuels and waste; and lead-containing traditional remedies, foods, ceramics, and utensils. Ongoing lead exposure among refugee children in the United States has also been well documented. For these reasons, CDC recommends checking blood lead levels of all refugee children 6 months to 16 years of age at the time of arrival, with follow-up blood lead testing to be done 3–6 months after settling into a permanent residence.

In addition to CDC's postarrival domestic medical screening guidelines for refugees, other published resources are available to the clinician. Most recently, the Public Health Authority of Canada has produced consensus documents on evidence-based screening for newly arriving refugees to Canada. The following section of this chapter, Migrant Health Resources, includes a list of clinical resources for providers and organizations.

Refugees may qualify for state Medicaid programs to cover this medical screening and any needed ongoing medical care. Refugees determined ineligible for Medicaid are eligible for Refugee Medical Assistance, which provides for their medical care needs for up to 8 months from the date of arrival in the United States. For more information, clinicians and refugees can contact their state health departments and can also access more information through the ORR, which administers this program (www.acf.hhs.gov/programs/orr/programs/cma.htm).

MEDICAL SCREENING FOR IMMIGRANTS AND INTERNATIONAL ADOPTEES

For immigrants, no formal mechanism or funding source is available for medical screening; therefore, immigrants, with the exception of international adoptees, do not routinely receive any postarrival medical screening beyond the recommended evaluation for class B conditions. All newly arrived immigrants, however, would benefit from comprehensive postarrival health screening.

Formal postarrival medical examination is recommended for internationally adopted children. There are many similarities in health conditions on arrival between international adoptees and refugees. An important distinction is that refugees generally remain within their own cultural group for some time after arrival and may have limited interactions with the wider community, whereas international adoptees frequently enter into households and communities that are naive to infections common in resource-poor settings. This distinction is particularly pertinent for conditions that may continue to be infectious for weeks to months after arrival (such as hepatitis A or B and *Giardia*). The American Academy of Pediatrics offers guidance in the Red Book: Report of the Committee on Infectious Diseases for clinicians who will serve this population after their arrival in the United States; the Red Book may be accessed at http://aapredbook.aappublications.org. For more information, see Chapter 7, International Adoption.

CONCLUSION

Limited health interventions are provided to immigrants and refugees before they enter the United States. Points of contact during the migration process, such as overseas examination, transit stops, and postarrival medical visits offer opportunities to intervene to improve the health status of the person, as well as to minimize any public health risk.

BIBLIOGRAPHY

1. Avery R. Immigrant women's health: infectious diseases. Part 1: clinical assessment, tuberculosis, hepatitis, and malaria. West J Med. 2001 Sep;175(3):208–11.

2. Barnett ED. Immunizations and infectious disease screening for internationally adopted children. Pediatr Clin North Am. 2005 Oct;52(5):1287–309, vi.

3. Barnett ED. Infectious disease screening for refugees resettled in the United States. Clin Infect Dis. 2004 Sep 15;39(6):833–41.

4. Barnett ED. Immunizations for immigrants. In: Walker PF, Barnett ED, editors. Immigrant Medicine. Philadelphia: Saunders Elsevier; 2007. p. 151–70.

5. CDC. Final rule removing HIV infection from US immigration screening. Atlanta: CDC; 2010 [cited 2012 Sep 26]. Available from: http://www.cdc.gov/immigrantrefugeehealth/laws-regs/hiv-ban-removal/final-rule.html.

6. CDC. Notice of revised vaccination criteria for US immigration. Atlanta: CDC; 2010 [cited 2012 Sep 26]. Available from: http://www.cdc.gov/immigrantrefugeehealth/laws-regs/vaccination-immigration/revised-vaccination-criteria-immigration.html.

7. CDC. Vitamin B12 deficiency in resettled Bhutanese refugees—United States, 2008–2011. MMWR Morb Mortal Wkly Rep. 2011 Mar 25;60(11):343–6.

8. Chen LH, Barnett ED, Wilson ME. Preventing infectious diseases during and after international adoption. Ann Intern Med. 2003 Sep 2;139(5 Pt 1):371–8.

9. Geltman PL, Brown MJ, Cochran J. Lead poisoning among refugee children resettled in Massachusetts, 1995 to 1999. Pediatrics. 2001 Jul;108(1):158–62.

10. Ivey SL, Faust S. Immigrant women's health: screening and immunization. West J Med. 2001 Jul;175(1):62–5.

11. Miller LC. International adoption: infectious diseases issues. Clin Infect Dis. 2005 Jan 15;40(2):286–93.

12. Minnesota Department of Health. Lead poisoning in Minnesota refugee children, 2000–2002. Disease Control Newsletter [Internet]. 2004 [cited 2012 Sep 26];32(2). Available from: http://www.health.state.mn.us/divs/idepc/newsletters/dcn/2004/0402dcn.pdf.

13. Posey DL, Blackburn BG, Weinberg M, Flagg EW, Ortega L, Wilson M, et al. High prevalence and presumptive treatment of schistosomiasis and strongyloidiasis among African refugees. Clin Infect Dis. 2007 Nov 15;45(10):1310–5.

14. Pottie K, Tugwell P, Feightner J, Welch V, Greenaway C, Swinkels H, et al. Summary of clinical preventive care recommendations for newly arriving immigrants and refugees to Canada. CMAJ. 2010 Jul 26.

15. Seybolt L, Barnett ED, Stauffer W. US Medical screening for immigrants and refugees: clinical issues. In: Walker PF, Barnett ED, editors. Immigrant Medicine. Philadelphia: Saunders Elsevier; 2007. p. 135–50.

16. Stauffer WM, Kamat D, Walker PF. Screening of international immigrants, refugees, and adoptees. Prim Care. 2002 Dec;29(4):879–905.

17. Stauffer WM, Maroushek S, Kamat D. Medical screening of immigrant children. Clin Pediatr (Phila). 2003 Nov–Dec;42(9):763–73.

MIGRANT HEALTH RESOURCES

William M. Stauffer

Historically, the Yellow Book has addressed travel health issues for US residents visiting countries outside the United States. In this increasingly mobile world, the discipline of travel medicine is evolving to recognize nontraditional groups who cross international boundaries into and out of the United States. One such group includes people who originate in other countries and migrate to the United States, either temporarily or permanently. Recognized migrants to the United States include immigrants (documented and undocumented), refugees, asylum seekers, and international adoptees. In addition, students and corporate workers are frequent visitors to the United States. Many clinics serving the traditional travel population also function as contact points with the US medical system for these populations, particularly for immigrants and refugees. This section provides resources to assist clinicians and organizations that serve these populations to access up-to-date patient-care guidelines, online education materials, and print resources.

CLINICAL REFERENCES
Organizational Guidelines
- **Centers for Disease Control and Prevention:** predeparture and postarrival presumptive treatment and medical screening guidelines for refugees relocating to the United States, available at www.cdc.gov/immigrantrefugeehealth/guidelines/refugee-guidelines.html
- **American Academy of Pediatrics:** guidance on medical screening and vaccination issues in adoptees, refugees, and immigrants, available in the online Red Book at http://aapredbook.aappublications.org
- **Canadian Collaboration for Immigrant and Refugee Health:** clinical preventive guidelines for primary care for newly arriving immigrants and refugees, available at www.ccirh.uottawa.ca

Websites
- **Centers for Disease Control and Prevention**
  > Immigrant and Refugee Health: information on immigrants and refugees who are resettling in the United States and resources, at www.cdc.gov/immigrantrefugeehealth/index.html
  > Travelers' Health: health information for international travelers, at www.cdc.gov/travel
  > Division of Parasitic Diseases and Malaria: clinical and public policy information on parasitic diseases, at www.cdc.gov/parasites AND www.cdc.gov/malaria
  > International Emergency and Refugee Health: health information pertaining to complex humanitarian emergencies, at www.cdc.gov/globalhealth/ierh
- **Refugee Health Technical Assistance Center:** multiple refugee resources and online education, at www.refugeehealthta.org
- **Minnesota Department of Health:** multiple resources for clinicians in refugee health at www.health.state.mn.us/divs/idepc/refugee/hcp/index.html, as well as refugee topics, at www.health.state.mn.us/divs/idepc/refugee/topics/index.html

- **Healthy Roads Media:** health education materials, including video, in a variety of languages, at http://healthyroadsmedia.org
- **EthnoMed:** information about cultural beliefs, medical issues, and other related issues pertinent to the health care of recent immigrants, at http://ethnomed.org/ethnomed
- **Health Information Translations:** common hospital signs with multiple translations, at www.healthinfotranslations.com
- **Medical Leadership Council on Cultural Proficiency:** database of patient information resources in a variety of languages and organizations providing services in languages other than English, at www.medicalleader ship.org/resources/patient_education.shtml
- **Refugee Health Information Network:** multilingual information for clinicians, refugees, and asylum seekers in print, audio, and video formats, at www.rhin.org
- **US Committee for Refugees and Immigrants:** toolkits on multiple health issues for clinicians, migrants, and communities in multiple languages, at www.refugees.org
- **US Citizenship and Immigration Services:** information regarding adjustment of status, at www.uscis.gov
- **United Nations High Commissioner for Refugees, Health Information System (HIS):** information about health issues in specific refugee camps or populations where refugees are originating, at www.unhcr.org/pages/ 49c3646ce0.html

Reference Books
Textbooks with a Focus on Migrant Health
- **Immigrant Medicine.** Walker PF, Barnett ED, editors. Philadelphia: Saunders Elsevier; 2007.
- **Migration Medicine and Health: Principles and Practice.** Gushulak BD, MacPherson D, editors. Hamilton, ON: BC Decker; 2006.
- **Travel Medicine and Migrant Health.** Lockie C, Walker E, Calvert L, Cossar J, Knill-Jones R, Raeside F, editors. Edinburgh: Churchill Livingstone; 2000.
- **Refugee and Immigrant Health. A Handbook for Health Professionals.** Kemp C, Rasbridge LA, editors. New York: Cambridge University Press; 2004.

Textbooks with a Focus on Tropical Diseases
- **Atlas of Tropical Medicine and Parasitology. 6th ed.** Peters W, Pasvol G, editors. Edinburgh: Mosby; 2007.
- **Mandell, Douglas, and Bennett's Principles & Practice of Infectious Diseases. 7th ed.** Mandell GL, Bennett JE, Dolin R, editors. Philadelphia: Churchill Livingstone; 2010.
- **Hunter's Tropical Medicine and Emerging Infectious Diseases. 9th ed.** Magill AJ, Ryan ET, Hill D, Solomon T, editors. Philadelphia: Saunders Elsevier; 2012.
- **Manson's Tropical Diseases. 22nd ed.** Cook GC, Zumla AI, editors. Edinburgh, UK: Saunders Ltd; 2008.
- **Tropical Infectious Diseases: Principles, Pathogens and Practice. 3rd ed.** Guerrant RL, Walker DH, Weller PF, editors. Philadelphia: Churchill Livingstone; 2011.

GENERAL RESOURCES
Reading Lists
- **Global Health Education Consortium's Global Health Bibliography:** bibliography of selected citations for use by students and faculty in global health, at http://globalhealthedu.org/resources/Pages/GlobalHealthBibliography.aspx
- **University of Minnesota reading list on refugee and immigrant health:** comprehensive reading list for people interested in refugee and immigrant health, at www.globalhealth.umn.edu/residenttraining/reading/home.html

Educational Opportunities
- **University of Minnesota/CDC:** American Society of Tropical Medicine and Hygiene (ASTMH)-accredited course in global health—open access to lectures and online content with a focus on immigrant and refugee health, at www.globalhealth.umn.edu.
- **ASTMH-accredited courses in tropical and travel medicine:** list of ASTMH-accredited tropical and travel medicine courses, at www.astmh.org/Approved_Diploma_Courses/2867.htm
- **Harvard Program in Refugee Trauma:** http://hprt-cambridge.org

Organization Websites with Migrant Information
- **US Department of Health and Human Services**

- > Office of Refugee Resettlement: www. acf.hhs.gov/programs/orr
- > Office of Global Health Affairs: www. globalhealth.gov
- **Centers for Disease Control and Prevention, Immigrant and Refugee Health:** www.cdc. gov/immigrantrefugeehealth/index.html
- **United Nations High Commissioner for Refugees:** www.unhcr.org/cgi-bin/texis/vtx/ home
- **World Health Organization refugee page:** www.who.int/topics/refugees/en
- **American Society of Tropical Medicine and Hygiene:** www.astmh.org
- **International Organization for Migration:** www.iom.int
- **International Society of Travel Medicine, Health of Migrants and Refugees Commitee:** www.istm.org/WebForms/Members/ Member Activities/VolunteerActivities/inter est_groups/migrants.aspx
- **Global Health Education Consortium:** http://globalhealtheducation.org
- **Global Health Council:** www.globalhealth.org
- **Consortium of Universities for Global Health:** www.cugh.org

Other Resources

- **Pre-travel handouts for non-English-speaking patients** (multiple topics in over 15 languages): www.tropical.umn.edu/ TTM/VFR/index.htm
- **The Providers' Guide to Quality and Culture:** http://erc.msh.org/mainpage.cfm? file=1.0.htm &module=provider&language= English

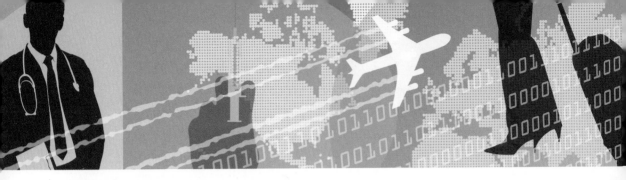

Appendices

APPENDIX A: PROMOTING QUALITY IN THE PRACTICE OF TRAVEL MEDICINE
Stephen M. Ostroff

Travel medicine remains a young area of medical practice, but even as the field continues to mature based on a growing body of scientific and medical information, there remains no recognized specialty or subspecialty of travel medicine anywhere in the world, including the United States. Clinicians offering travel medicine services are not "board certified" in travel medicine. Instead, travel medicine physicians generally have credentials in other disciplines, usually infectious diseases, internal medicine, or family practice. The same applies to nurses, pharmacists, and other allied health professionals. Clinics in the United States that offer travel medicine services are also not specifically credentialed for this purpose.

Given these circumstances, how can travelers maximize the likelihood their provider will deliver quality travel-related medical care and that the advice, preventive measures, and treatment services they are given fall within accepted standards? Similarly, how can providers assure patients they have sufficient knowledge of the subject matter relevant to travel medicine?

Research into the quality of travel health care is limited, but several studies suggest that travelers who visit a clinician with training in travel medicine are more likely to receive pre- and post-travel advice and care than if they see other clinicians for such services. Similarly, 2006 guidelines on travel medicine published by the Infectious Diseases Society of America (Box A-1) recommend that pre- and post-travel care be obtained from a clinician with expertise in travel medicine. This is especially relevant for travelers going to exotic destinations, or engaging in adventure travel or who have special needs or medical problems.

Below is a partial list of resources for clinicians who wish to enhance their knowledge of travel medicine. People seeking travel-related medical services may want to inquire about whether their provider or clinic participates in these organizations or activities.

TRAVEL MEDICINE–RELATED PROFESSIONAL ORGANIZATIONS
International Society of Travel Medicine (ISTM)
Founded in 1991, ISTM (www.istm.org) is the preeminent multinational organization dealing exclusively with travel medicine. ISTM has about 3,000 members worldwide, slightly fewer than half of whom are located in the United States.

ISTM activities include the following:

- *Journal of Travel Medicine*
- An active listserv (TravelMed) where members share information and can ask questions
- Special-interest groups that include travel medicine nurses and travel medicine pharmacists
- A biennial travel medicine meeting and annual regional submeetings
- A directory of domestic and international travel clinics affiliated with ISTM members in 80 countries
- An annual examination leading to a Certificate of Knowledge in Travel Medicine, available to physicians, nurses, pharmacists, and other professionals offering travel advice
- ISTM Travel Medicine Continuous Professional Development Program

The Certificate of Knowledge in Travel Medicine has been administered by ISTM since 2003. The Body of Knowledge, which covers the scope of the specialty of travel medicine, forms the basis for examination questions. It was last updated in 2006 and is published in the *Journal of Travel Medicine*. Content areas in the Body of Knowledge include the following:

- Epidemiology related to travel medicine
- Immunology and vaccinology (including travel- related vaccines)
  - Pre-travel consultation and management
  - Patient evaluation
  - Travelers with special needs
  - Special itineraries
  - Prevention and self-treatment
  - Precautions
- Diseases contracted during travel
  - Vectorborne diseases
  - Diseases transmitted from person to person
  - Foodborne and waterborne diseases
  - Diseases related to bites and stings
  - Diseases due to environmental hazards
- Other conditions associated with travel
  - Conditions occurring during or after travel
  - Conditions due to environmental factors
  - Threats to personal safety and security
  - Psychocultural issues
- Post-travel management
- General travel medicine issues
  - Medical care abroad
  - Travel clinic management
  - Travel medicine information resources

Since it was introduced, the Certificate of Knowledge in Travel Medicine examination has been taken by more than 2,000 practitioners in 60 countries. The society hosts a periodic 2-day intensive exam preparation course. Those who are successful in the examination are awarded a Certificate in Travel Health (CTH). Beginning with CTHs awarded in 2011, the Certificate is good for 10 years and the awardee must be recertified either through professional development activities or by retaking the examination. Practitioners offering travel medicine services or interested in the subject should strongly consider membership in ISTM. ISTM practitioners are listed on the organization's website, and those who have the CTH are designated as such.

ISTM also offers research programs. These include research grants, travel awards, and support for such efforts as the GeoSentinel Surveillance Network (see Chapter 1, Travel Medicine Data Collection: GeoSentinel & Global TravEpiNet)

American Society of Tropical Medicine and Hygiene (ASTMH)

Formed in 1951 through the merger of predecessor organizations dating back to 1903, ASTMH (www.astmh.org) has a subsection that deals exclusively with tropical and travel medicine, known as the American Committee on Clinical Tropical Medicine and Travelers' Health.

ASTMH activities include the following:

- *The American Journal of Tropical Medicine and Hygiene*
- An annual meeting
- An electronic distribution list
- A tropical and travel medicine consultant directory
- A biennial examination leading to a Certificate of Knowledge in Clinical Tropical Medicine and Travelers' Health, available to those who have passed an ASTMH-approved tropical medicine diploma course or have sufficient tropical medicine experience

The content areas of the ASTMH Certificate of Knowledge in Clinical Tropic Medicine and Travelers' Health are as follows:

- Basic science and fundamentals
- Infectious and tropical diseases (including parasites, bacteria, fungi, and viruses)
- Other diseases and conditions
- Diagnostic and therapeutic approach to clinical syndromes
- Travelers' health
- Public health in the tropics
- Epidemiology and control of disease
- Laboratory diagnosis

Almost 700 people who have passed the ASTMH examination are listed on the ASTMH website. The society offers an annual intensive update course in clinical tropical medicine and travelers' health, which is in part designed to prepare those planning to take the Certificate of Knowledge examination.

Wilderness Medical Society

Organized in 1983, this society (www.wms.org) focuses on adventure travel, including wilderness travel and diving medicine. Its activities include the following:

- The journal *Wilderness and Environmental Medicine*
- Practice guidelines for emergency care in wilderness settings
- An annual world congress and subspecialty meetings
- Courses leading to certification in advanced wilderness life support
- A wilderness medical curriculum that, when successfully completed, qualifies members for fellowship in the Academy of Wilderness Medicine

Infectious Diseases Society of America (IDSA)

IDSA (www.idsociety.org) is the largest organization representing infectious diseases clinicians in the United States. Although IDSA does not deal exclusively with travel medicine, it has many active members with expertise in tropical and travel medicine and has strong interests in these disciplines. In 2006, IDSA published extensive evidence-based guidelines on the practice of travel medicine in the United States (Box A-1). An update of the guidelines, which are available on the IDSA website, is underway. IDSA also publishes travel-related research in its 2 journals: *The Journal of Infectious Diseases* and *Clinical Infectious Diseases*.

International Society for Infectious Diseases (ISID)

ISID (www.isid.org) was formed in 1986 and has approximately 20,000 members in 155 countries around the world. Like IDSA, ISID does not specifically focus on travel medicine. However, its international reach, particularly in low-resource countries, makes travel medicine an important topic in ISID and a valuable source of information for infectious diseases clinicians in many overseas travel destinations. Activities relevant to travel medicine that are supported by ISID include the following:

- *International Journal of Infectious Diseases*
- The biennial meeting International Congress on Infectious Diseases

- The Program for Monitoring Emerging Diseases (Pro-MED), an open-source electronic reporting system for reports of emerging infectious diseases and toxins, including outbreaks (www.promedmail.org)

Aerospace Medical Association

This organization (www.asma.org) represents professionals in the fields of aviation, space, and environmental medicine who deal with air and space travelers. Its activities include the following:

- The journal *Aviation, Space, and Environmental Medicine*
- An annual meeting
- Continuing medical education in topics related to aerospace medicine

FINDING CARE WHILE TRAVELING OUTSIDE THE UNITED STATES

Both the ISTM and ASTMH websites contain the names of non-US-based clinics and health care providers affiliated with members of these organizations. Travelers are advised to review these lists before departure to identify health care resources at their travel destination. A number of countries or national travel medicine societies have websites related to travel medicine that also provide access to clinicians, including the following:

- Canada: Health Canada (www.phac-aspc. gc.ca/tmp-pmv/yf-fj/index-eng.php)
- Great Britain: National Travel Health Network and Centre (www.nathnac.org) and British Global and Travel Health Association (www. bgtha.org)
- South Africa: South African Society of Travel Medicine (www.sastm.org.za)
- Australia: Travel Medicine Alliance (www. travelmedicine.com.au)
- China: International Travel Healthcare Association (http://en.itha.org.cn)

Emergency travel-related medical care and medical evacuation may be accessed through a number of private companies. One example is International SOS, which operates throughout the world. Provider locations and details may be found at www. internationalsos.com.

BIBLIOGRAPHY

1. Boddington NL, Simons H, Launders N, Hill DR. Quality improvement in travel medicine: a programme for yellow fever vaccination centres in England, Wales and Northern Ireland. Qual Prim Care. 2011;19(6):391–8.
2. Hill DR, Ericsson CD, Pearson RD, Keystone JS, Freedman DO, Kozarsky PE, et al. The practice of travel medicine: guidelines by the Infectious Diseases Society of America. Clin Infect Dis. 2006 Dec 15;43(12):1499–539.
3. Kozarsky P. The body of knowledge for the practice of travel medicine—2006. J Travel Med. 2006 Sep–Oct;13(5):251–4.
4. LaRocque RC, Jentes ES. Health recommendations for international travel: a review of the evidence base of travel medicine. Curr Opin Infect Dis. 2011 Oct;24(5):403–9.
5. Ruis JR, van Rijckevorsel GG, van den Hoek A, Koeman SC, Sonder GJ. Does registration of professionals improve the quality of travelers' health advice? J Travel Med. 2009 Jul–Aug;16(4):263–6.
6. Schlagenhauf P, Santos-O'Connor F, Parola P. The practice of travel medicine in Europe. Clin Microbiol Infect. 2010 Mar;16(3):203–8.
7. Spira A. Setting the standard. J Travel Med. 2003 Jan–Feb;10(1):1–3.

APPENDIX B: ESSENTIAL ELECTRONIC RESOURCES FOR THE TRAVEL MEDICINE PRACTITIONER

David O. Freedman, Katherine J. Johnson

SELECTED ELECTRONIC RESOURCES IN TRAVEL MEDICINE

A variety of electronic resources is available for practitioners who provide pre- and post-travel medical care for international travelers (Table B-1). Checking >1 authoritative website on a specific issue is always recommended. Authoritative recommendations may contain some element of opinion, and some sites are updated more frequently than others. Practitioners should check the indicator at the bottom of each page stating when the last update was done.

ELECTRONIC NOTIFICATION AND DISCUSSION FORUMS

Electronic distribution lists (such as Listserv) use e-mail with or without a browser-based interface. Some lists are set up to provide information only. Others promote active discussion among members, whereby anyone who has joined a particular group can e-mail a posting to a central server, which is then disseminated to all members who have subscribed to the same list. On a moderated list, each posting is reviewed and accepted by a moderator or editor, while unmoderated lists disseminate each posting instantly to all other subscribers. TravelMed is an example of an unmoderated list, which focuses on issues related to the practice of travel medicine (see www.istm.org/WebForms/Members/MemberActivities/listserve.aspx for further information). CDC's website provides an information-only e-mail notification system called GovDelivery on a variety of health topics, including updates to the CDC Travelers'

Health website. For more information or to subscribe, see www.cdc.gov/emailupdates/index.html.

Another common form of electronic notification is RSS (Really Simple Syndication). Many websites provide RSS feeds that instantly inform users when updates are made. To receive feeds, users must have an RSS reader on their computer or mobile device. Readers are commonly available as embedded features of most web browsers and e-mail applications or can be downloaded from commercial organizations. Users can customize notification settings to send multiple feeds directly to their e-mail account, or they can view feeds through their web browser, desktop, or mobile device.

Many of the resources below provide RSS feeds. CDC Travelers' Health generates feeds on 2 topics: travel notices and updates to the Yellow Book. For more information, see wwwnc.cdc.gov/travel/contentRss.aspx. Table B-2 highlights a subset of primary resources that provide RSS feeds that may be useful to travel medicine practitioners. Check the resources in Table B-1 for more information or updates through e-mail lists and other social media.

Note: Tables B-1 and B-2 provide a representative but by no means exclusive sampling of resources that may be useful to the travel medicine practitioner. Brief descriptions of selected websites have been included to highlight resources that may be of particular interest. Please be advised that website URLs and content may change at any time.

Table B-1. Selected websites for the travel medicine practitioner

Authoritative Travel Medicine Recommendations

CDC Travelers' Health homepage *Includes current travel health notices, disease- and destination-specific health recommendations, and guidance on a variety of topics in travel medicine*	www.cdc.gov/travel
CDC Travelers' Health Yellow Book homepage *Includes a searchable version of CDC Health Information for International Travel 2014 ("The Yellow Book") and a list of any updates occurring between print editions*	www.cdc.gov/yellowbook
US Department of State Bureau of Consular Services	www.travel.state.gov
US Department of State country-specific information, travel warnings, and travel alerts	http://travel.state.gov/travel/cis_pa_tw/cis/cis_4965.html
WHO international travel and health homepage *Includes the current edition of the International Travel and Health ("Green Book") publication, disease updates for travelers, International Health Regulations documents, and other disease-specific information*	www.who.int/ith/en
The Practice of Travel Medicine: Guidelines by the Infectious Diseases Society of America	cid.oxfordjournals.org/content/43/12/1499.full
US Department of Transportation aircraft disinsection requirements	http://ostpxweb.dot.gov/policy/safetyenergyenv/disinsection.htm

Emerging Diseases and Outbreaks

WHO Global Alert and Response (GAR) homepage *Includes current Disease Outbreak News and outbreaks sorted by country, disease, and year*	www.who.int/csr/en
CDC Health Alert Network message archive	www2a.cdc.gov/HAN/ArchiveSys
GeoSentinel Surveillance Network of the International Society of Travel Medicine and CDC	www.geosentinel.org
ProMED-mail: program for monitoring emerging diseases *Includes moderated reporting of global infectious diseases and acute exposure to toxins*	www.promedmail.org

continued

TABLE B-1. SELECTED WEBSITES FOR THE TRAVEL MEDICINE PRACTITIONER (continued)

HealthMap: Global Disease Alert Map	www.healthmap.org/en
Global Health Facts (Kaiser Family Foundation portal for information on the US role in global health)	www.globalhealthfacts.org
Surveillance and Epidemiologic Bulletins	
CDC MMWR Weekly, Recommendations and Reports, and Surveillance Summaries	www.cdc.gov/mmwr
WHO Weekly Epidemiological Record	www.who.int/wer/
PAHO list of links to National Bulletins in the Americas	www.paho.org/English/DD/AIS/vigilancia-en.htm
PAHO list of Ministries of Health in the Americas	www.paho.org/English/PAHO/MOHs.htm
WHO list of links to national travel and health websites	www.who.int/ith/links/national_links/en/index.html
Zoonotic disease surveillance: World Organisation for Animal Health	www.oie.int
Eurosurveillance	www.eurosurveillance.org
ECDC Communicable Disease Threat Report (weekly)	http://ecdc.europa.eu/en/publications/surveillance_reports/Communicable-Disease-Threats-Report/Pages/Communicable-Disease-Threats-Report.aspx
Caribbean Epidemiology Centre	www.carec.org
ReliefWeb: administered by the UN Office for the Coordination of Humanitarian Affairs *Includes information on humanitarian emergencies and natural disasters from a variety of UN agencies and other sources*	www.reliefweb.int
WHO Crises and Emergencies: health-related situational updates	www.who.int/hac/crises/en
EpiNorth Europe	www.epinorth.org
EpiSouth Europe	www.episouthnetwork.org

continued

TABLE B-1. SELECTED WEBSITES FOR THE TRAVEL MEDICINE PRACTITIONER (continued)

Vaccine Resources

US Advisory Committee on Immunization Practices (ACIP): recommendations on individual vaccines	www.cdc.gov/vaccines/pubs/ACIP-list.htm
CDC vaccine information statements (VIS) for patients: fact sheets to download	http://www.cdc.gov/vaccines/pubs/vis/default.htm
CDC information on vaccination shortages	http://www.cdc.gov/vaccines/vac-gen/shortages/default.htm
American Academy of Pediatrics table on status of licensure and recommendations for new vaccines	http://aapredbook.aappublications.org/news/vaccstatus.shtml
CDC Pink Book: Epidemiology and Prevention of Vaccine-Preventable Diseases *Includes an online version of the current edition, updates to the print edition, slide sets, and selected chapters from earlier editions*	www.cdc.gov/vaccines/pubs/pinkbook/index.html
Immunization Action Coalition—Directory of Vaccine Resources	www.immunize.org/resources
Translation of international vaccine-related terms into English	www.immunize.org/izpractices/p5121.pdf
Vaccine-preventable disease terms in multiple languages	www.immunize.org/izpractices/p5122.pdf
Vaccine information from the Immunization Action Coalition	www.vaccineinformation.org
WHO immunization, vaccines, and biologics *Includes links to national, regional, and international resources providing immunization information*	www.who.int/immunization/en
WHO country-specific routine immunization schedules	http://apps.who.int/immunization_monitoring/en/globalsummary/ScheduleSelect.cfm
Program for Appropriate Technology in Health (PATH) vaccine resource library	www.path.org/vaccineresources

continued

TABLE B-1. SELECTED WEBSITES FOR THE TRAVEL MEDICINE PRACTITIONER (continued)

Consumer-Oriented Travel Health Information and Products

High Altitude Medicine Guide	www.high-altitude-medicine.com
Travel Health Online	www.tripprep.com
MDTravelHealth.com	www.mdtravelhealth.com
Chinook Medical Gear, Inc.	www.chinookmed.com
Magellan's Travel Supplies	www.magellans.com
Travel Medicine, Inc.	www.travmed.com

Overseas Medical and Safety Assistance

US Department of State medical information for Americans abroad	http://travel.state.gov/travel/tips/brochures/brochures_1215.html
International Association for Medical Assistance to Travelers	www.iamat.org
International SOS: medical and security solutions, products, and assistance	www.internationalsos.com
MEDEX: worldwide travel assistance and international medical	www.medexassist.com

Maps and Country Information

US Overseas Security Advisory Council Includes current US Department of State travel alerts, travel warnings, embassy Warden Messages, and safety and security resources	www.osac.gov
US Central Intelligence Agency: The World Factbook	https://www.cia.gov/library/publications/the-world-factbook
US Department of State Background Notes	www.state.gov/r/pa/ei/bgn
US Federal Aviation Administration data on air safety standards in foreign countries	www.faa.gov/about/initiatives/iasa
European Commission Air Safety portal	http://ec.europa.eu/transport/air/index_en.htm

continued

TABLE B-1. SELECTED WEBSITES FOR THE TRAVEL MEDICINE PRACTITIONER (continued)

Falling Rain global gazetteer and place name altitude finder	www.fallingrain.com/world
Association for Safe International Road Travel	http://asirt.org
UN maps	www.un.org/Depts/Cartographic/english/htmain.htm
Perry-Castañeda Library map collection	www.lib.utexas.edu/Libs/PCL/Map_collection/map_sites/map_sites.html
Nations Online: destination guide to countries and nations	www.nationsonline.org
GeoNames geographic database	www.geonames.org
Lonely Planet travel information	www.lonelyplanet.com

Disability Information

MossRehab ResourceNet: accessible travel	www.mossresourcenet.org/travel.htm
US Department of Transportation Aviation Consumer Protection and Enforcement	http://airconsumer.ost.dot.gov/publications/disabled.htm
Society for Accessible Travel and Hospitality	www.sath.org
Mobility International USA	www.miusa.org

Professional Medical Societies with a Focus on Travelers' Health

International Society of Travel Medicine	www.istm.org
American Society of Tropical Medicine and Hygiene	www.astmh.org
Infectious Diseases Society of America	www.idsociety.org
Pediatric Infectious Diseases Society	www.pids.org
Divers Alert Network	www.diversalertnetwork.org
Wilderness Medical Society	www.wms.org
Undersea and Hyperbaric Medical Society	www.uhms.org

continued

TABLE B-1. SELECTED WEBSITES FOR THE TRAVEL MEDICINE PRACTITIONER (continued)

American Travel Health Nurses Association	www.athna.org
Christian Medical and Dental Associations	www.cmda.org
Disease Information	
CDC diseases and conditions: A–Z list	www.cdc.gov/DiseasesConditions
WHO health topics: A–Z list	www.who.int/topics/en
PAHO health topics: A–Z list	http://new.paho.org/hq/index.php?option=com_joomlabook&Itemid=260
Oxford Malaria Atlas Project	www.map.ox.ac.uk
CDC Malaria Map Application	www.cdc.gov/malaria/map/index.html
CDC influenza homepage *Includes information about seasonal influenza, avian influenza, and others*	www.cdc.gov/flu
US Tropical Medicine Central Resource Tropical Radiology Atlas	http://tmcr.usuhs.mil/toc.htm#
WHO Rabies Bulletin: Europe	www.who-rabies-bulletin.org
WHO water supply and sanitation assessment	www.who.int/water_sanitation_health/monitoring/globalassess/en
WHO Global Schistosomiasis Atlas	www.who.int/schistosomiasis/epidemiology/global_atlas/en/index.html
Global Polio Eradication Initiative	www.polioeradication.org
General Travel Aids	
Embassies in the United States	www.state.gov/s/cpr/rls
Embassies in the United States web links	www.embassy.org/embassies/index.html
Times around the World	www.timeanddate.com/worldclock
Tourism Offices Worldwide Directory	www.towd.com

continued

TABLE B-1. SELECTED WEBSITES FOR THE TRAVEL MEDICINE PRACTITIONER (continued)

Visa/Plus ATM locator	http://visa.via.infonow.net/locator/global/jsp/SearchPage.jsp
MasterCard/Cirrus ATM locator	www.mastercard.com/cardholderservices/atm
US Organizations Offering Training in Travel Medicine	
International Society of Travel Medicine	www.istm.org
American Society of Tropical Medicine and Hygiene	www.astmh.org
Gorgas Memorial Institute	www.gorgas.org
Tulane Department of Tropical Medicine	www.sph.tulane.edu/tropmed
University of Washington School of Medicine	http://depts.washington.edu/cme/home
University of Minnesota Department of Medicine	www.globalhealth.umn.edu

Abbreviations: WHO, World Health Organization; MMWR, Morbidity and Mortality Weekly Report; PAHO, Pan American Health Organization; ECDC, European Centre for Disease Prevention and Control; UN, United Nations; ATM, automated teller machine.

Table B-2. Selected travel medicine resources providing RSS feeds

CDC Travelers' Health *Feeds include travel notices, updates to the Yellow Book*	wwwnc.cdc.gov/travel/content/rss.aspx
CDC (agency-wide) *Feeds on a variety of health topics*	www2c.cdc.gov/podcasts/rss.asp
US Department of State *Feeds include travel warnings, travel alerts, country-specific information, country background notes*	www.state.gov/misc/echannels/66791.htm
World Health Organization *Feeds include emergencies and disasters news, disease outbreaks, avian influenza*	www.who.int/about/licensing/rss/en
Pan American Health Organization *Feed for the latest news headlines from the organization*	www.paho.org/english/dd/pin/rssfeed.htm

continued

TABLE B-2. SELECTED TRAVEL MEDICINE RESOURCES PROVIDING RSS FEEDS (continued)

CDC MMWR Weekly, Recommendations and Reports, and Surveillance Summaries *Feed for current MMWR headlines*	www.cdc.gov/mmwr/rss/rss.html
Zoonotic disease surveillance: World Organisation for Animal Health *Feeds for subscribers to receive Immediate Notifications and Follow-up Reports for animal and disease categories of interest*	www.oie.int/en/animal-health-in-the-world/the-world-animal-health-information-system/info-list-rss/
ProMED-mail *Feeds from ProMED monitoring emerging diseases*	http://ww2.isid.org/rss/
Eurosurveillance *Feed for website updates*	www.eurosurveillance.org/Public/RSSFeed/RSSFeed.aspx
US Central Intelligence Agency (CIA): The World Factbook *Feeds on various topics, including CIA press releases and statements, featured stories, careers, library, kids' page updates*	https://www.cia.gov/news-information/your-news/index.html
ReliefWeb: administered by the United Nations Office for the Coordination of Humanitarian Affairs *Feeds of new website content for user-selected topics*	http://reliefweb.int/rss
Divers Alert Network *Feeds include news items, upcoming events, and medical frequently asked questions*	www.diversalertnetwork.org/rss/index.asp
International Association for Medical Assistance to Travelers *Feed including recent blog posts*	www.iamat.org/blog/rss.cfm

Abbreviations: MMWR, Morbidity and Mortality Weekly Report.

BIBLIOGRAPHY

1. Freedman DO. Sources of travel medicine information. In: Keystone JS, Freedman DO, Kozarsky PE, Connor BA, Nothdurft HD, editors. Travel Medicine. 3rd ed. Philadelphia: Saunders Elsevier; 2013. p. 25–30.

2. Keystone JS, Kozarsky PE, Freedman DO. Internet and computer-based resources for travel medicine practitioners. Clin Infect Dis. 2001 Mar 1;32(5):757–65.

APPENDIX C: TRAVEL VACCINE SUMMARY TABLE

David R. Shlim

Table C-1 is a quick reference for administering or prescribing travel-related vaccines. Before administering any vaccine, please pay particular attention to the dose and whether it is to be administered intramuscularly or subcutaneously. Also review detailed instructions, contraindications, precautions, and side effects under the specific vaccines discussed in this book or in the manufacturer's package insert. For other immunizations, refer to the corresponding disease section in Chapter 3.

Table C-1. Travel vaccine summary

VACCINE	BRAND NAME	DOSE	ROUTE	SCHEDULE	BOOSTER	AGE
Hepatitis A (adults)	Havrix	1.0 mL (1,440 ELISA units)	IM	0 and 6–12 months	None	≥19 years
	Vaqta	1.0 mL (50 units)	IM	0 and 6–18 months	None	≥19 years
Hepatitis A (pediatric)	Havrix	0.5 mL (720 ELISA units)	IM	0 and 6–12 months	None	1–18 years
	Vaqta	0.5 mL (25 units)	IM	0 and 6–18 months	None	1–18 years
Combined hepatitis A and hepatitis B	Twinrix	1.0 mL (20 µg of hepatitis B antigen and 720 ELISA units of hepatitis A antigen)	IM	0, 1 month, and 6 months; accelerated schedule: days 0, 7, and 21–30, with a fourth dose at 12 months	None	≥18 years
Hepatitis B (adult)	Engerix-B	1.0 mL (20 µg)	IM	0, 1 month, and 6 months; can be given on an accelerated schedule of 0, 1 month, 2 months, and 12 months	None	≥20 years
	Recombivax HB	1.0 mL (10 µg)	IM	0, 1 month, and 6 months	None	≥20 years
Hepatitis B (pediatric)	Engerix-B	0.5 mL (10 µg)	IM IM IM	0, 1 month, and 6 months; can be given on an accelerated schedule of 0, 1 month, 2 months, and 12 months. If using an accelerated schedule, give 0.5 mL (10 µg) for ages birth through 10 years and 1.0 mL (20 µg) for ages 11–19 years	None	≤19 years
	Recombivax HB (primary)	0.5 mL (5 µg)		0, 1 month, and 6 months	None	≤19 years
	Recombivax HB (adolescent accelerated)	1.0 mL (10 µg)		0, 4–6 months	None	For ages 11–15 years

Vaccine	Trade name	Dose	Route	Primary series	Booster	Age
Japanese encephalitis	Ixiaro	0.5 mL	IM	0 and 28 days	≥1 year after primary series[1]	≥17 years[1]
Meningococcal conjugate (MenACWY)	Menactra (MenACWY_D)	0.5 mL	IM	2-dose primary series separated by 3 months	See Chapter 3, Meningococcal Disease	9–23 months
	Menactra (MenACWY_D)	0.5 mL	IM	1 dose	See Chapter 3, Meningococcal Disease	2–55 years
	Menveo (MenACWY_CRM)	0.5 mL	IM	1 dose	See Chapter 3, Meningococcal Disease	2–55 years
Meningococcal polysaccharide (MPSV4)	Menomune	0.5 mL	SC	1 dose	See Chapter 3, Meningococcal Disease	≥2 years
Inactivated polio (adult)	Ipol	0.5 mL	SC or IM	1 dose at ≥18 years, if patient has already had an acceptable polio vaccine series	None	≥18 years[2]
Rabies	Imovax	1.0 mL	IM	Preexposure series: days 0, 7, and 21 or 28	See Chapter 3, Rabies	No age restrictions
	RabAvert	1.0 mL	IM	Preexposure series: days 0, 7, and 21 or 28	See Chapter 3, Rabies	No age restrictions
Typhoid capsular polysaccharide	Typhim Vi	0.5 mL	IM	1 dose	Every 2 years	≥2 years
Typhoid oral, live, attenuated	Vivotif	1 pill	Oral	1 pill every other day for 4 doses	Every 5 years	≥6 years
Yellow fever	YF-Vax	0.5 mL	SC	1 dose	Every 10 years	≥9 months, same dose for children and adults[3]

Abbreviations: ELISA, enzyme-linked immunosorbent assay; IM, intramuscular; SC, subcutaneous.

[1] See Chapter 3, Japanese Encephalitis. Data on the response to a booster dose administered ≥2 years after the primary series are not available. Data on the need for and timing of additional booster doses are also not available. Ixiaro may be approved for use in children when studies are completed.

[2] For catch-up immunization in pediatric population, see Table 7-2.

[3] Special considerations apply in deciding whether to administer yellow fever vaccine. Please review Chapter 3, Yellow Fever before administration. Yellow fever vaccine is never given to infants <6 months and is given with precaution and only under special circumstances for ages 6–8 months. There is also a precaution for its use in patients aged ≥60 years.

TRAVEL VACCINE SUMMARY TABLE

APPENDIX D: THE HEALTHMAP SYSTEM

Amy L. Sonricker Hansen, Clark C. Freifeld, John S. Brownstein

SYSTEM OVERVIEW

Over the past 15 years, internet technology has become an integral part of public health surveillance. Information about infectious disease outbreaks is disseminated not only through online communications by government agencies but also through informal channels, ranging from media reports to blogs to chat rooms. Collectively, these sources provide a view of global health that is fundamentally different from that of traditional public health infrastructure. Web-based sources provide valuable epidemic intelligence by disseminating current, highly localized information about outbreaks, especially in areas that have limited public health capacity.

HealthMap (www.healthmap.org) was developed with the aim of creating an integrated global view of emerging infectious diseases, based not only on traditional public health reports but also on a broad range of available information sources, including these informal Internet channels. HealthMap is a publicly available online resource that collects, filters, and visualizes disease outbreak reports in real time, by means of a series of automated text-processing algorithms. Sources include online news through aggregators such as Google News, expert-curated discussion such as ProMED-mail, and validated official reports from organizations such as the World Health Organization (WHO). Disease outbreak reports are collected in 9 languages (Arabic, Chinese, English, French, German, Korean, Portuguese, Russian, and Spanish) classified by disease and location, and then mapped to a user-friendly, interactive display (see Figure D-1).

The system also allows disease experts, public health professionals, and the general public to submit reports of events not collected by the automated system, through both the web interface and by mobile applications (www.healthmap.org/outbreaksnearme). The "Outbreaks Near Me" mobile application uses GPS technology to show health alerts and ongoing outbreak news in the vicinity of the user.

The application also allows users to search for outbreaks in any location worldwide.

Currently, HealthMap serves as a direct information source for over a million visitors per year and serves as a resource for physicians, local health departments, governments, and multinational agencies (such as WHO), which use the HealthMap data stream for day-to-day surveillance activities. CDC has a relationship with HealthMap that includes a specific layer of the map used to geolocate travel-related illness detected by the GeoSentinel Surveillance Network. Also, in collaboration with CDC, HealthMap hosts an interactive map of global dengue activity (www.cdc.gov/dengue). HealthMap extracts data and provides a user interface that is particularly focused on providing users with news of immediate interest, while reducing information overload.

HEALTHMAP DATA VISUALIZATION AND DISSEMINATION

The HealthMap site presents users with a customizable map view of worldwide infectious disease alerts. An advanced search area allows users to control the map view, including the ability to filter by source, date, disease, and region. "Full screen" mode expands the map to cover the full browser window, allowing richer visual display and navigation. The "Local" tab on the HealthMap site automatically detects the location of the user and displays disease alerts within a user-selected radius (see Figure D-2).

Automated e-mail alerts of infectious disease reports are also available from HealthMap. As with the website, users may customize these e-mails to receive only information corresponding to specific parameters, such as diseases, locations, or sources of interest.

Overall, automated surveillance of Internet information sources provides a method for creating a timely, sensitive, and comprehensive view of worldwide emerging infectious diseases. Mining the web is a valuable new approach that plays a useful role in

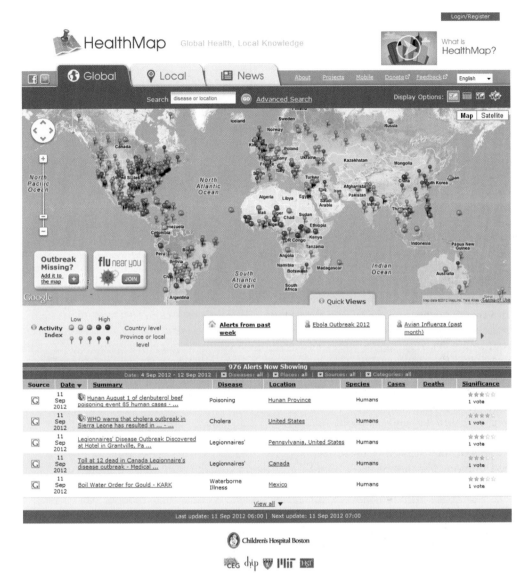

FIGURE D-1. SCREENSHOT OF HEALTHMAP

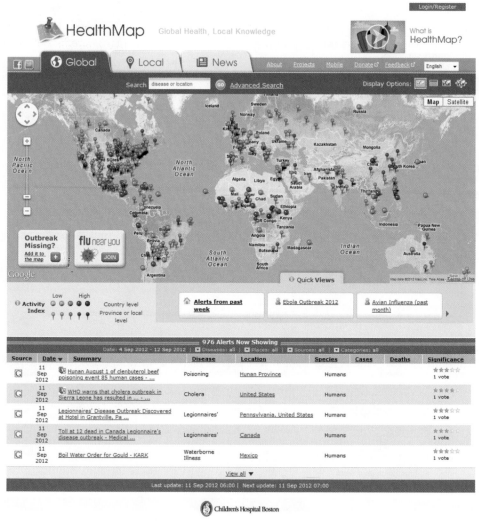

FIGURE D-2. SCREENSHOT OF HEALTHMAP'S LOCAL PAGE VIEW

the efforts of public health practitioners and clinicians. Ultimately, HealthMap's integration of real-time, web-based infectious disease surveillance works to augment epidemic intelligence with information from outside the traditional public health infrastructure to enhance situational awareness of disease threats.

BIBLIOGRAPHY

1. Brownstein JS, Freifeld CC, Madoff LC. Digital disease detection—harnessing the web for public health surveillance. N Engl J Med. 2009 May 21;360(21):2153–5, 7.
2. Brownstein JS, Freifeld CC, Reis BY, Mandl KD. Surveillance sans frontières: internet-based emerging infectious disease intelligence and the HealthMap project. PLoS Med. 2008 Jul 8;5(7):e151.
3. Freifeld CC, Mandl KD, Reis BY, Brownstein JS. HealthMap: global infectious disease monitoring through automated classification and visualization of Internet media reports. J Am Med Inform Assoc. 2008 Mar–Apr;15(2):150–7.

Index

Note: Page numbers followed by the letter b refer to boxes; those followed by the letter f refer to figures; those followed by the letter m refer to maps; and those followed by the letter t refer to tables.

violence, 111–3
viral hemorrhagic fevers (VHFs), 326–8
Virgin Islands, British
  dengue distribution in, 167*m*
  no reported cases of rabies, 271*t*
  vaccine considerations for, 403
Virgin Islands, US
  dengue distribution in, 167*m*
  no reported cases of rabies, 271*t*
  vaccine considerations for, 403
viruses, size and susceptibility to filtration, 88*t*
visceral leishmaniasis (VL), 224–5
visiting friends and relatives (VFRs), 11, 569–72
  Global TravEpiNet, 12–3
  returning to malarious country, 236
  typhoid fever, 320
vitamin A, 250

W
Wake Island (US), 403
Wales. *See* United Kingdom
Wallis and Futuna Islands (France), 403
water disinfection, 86–91
water injuries, 111
water precautions, 81–5, 86–91, 111, 122
Western Pacific Islands, risk for Japanese encephalitis in, 219*t*

Western Sahara
  malaria information for, 230*m*, 403
  vaccine considerations for, 403
  yellow fever information for, 403
Western Samoa. *See* Samoa
West Nile virus, traveler's role in translocation of, 16
whipworm, 181

Y
Yangtze River, cruising, 440*b*
Yap Islands. *See* Micronesia
The Yellow Book
  history and role of, 2–3
  recommendations, 21
yellow fever, 329–40
  contact information, 4
yellow fever vaccine, 24–5, 30*t*, 40*t*, 47*t*, 332–42, 346, 633*t*
  breastfeeding and, 535
  categories of recommendations for, 347*t*
  history of vaccination requirements, 344–5
  immunization of children, 532
  immunization of immunocompromised adults, 545*t*, 550–2
  immunization of pregnant women, 565
  International Certificate of Vaccination or Prophylaxis (ICVP), 337–9, 338*f*

  last-minute travelers, 590
  medical waivers, 339*f*, 339
  yellow fever vaccine-associated neurologic disease (YEL-AND), 333
  yellow fever vaccine-associated viscerotropic disease (YEL-AVD), 333–4
Yemen
  malaria information for, 230*m*, 403–4
  onchocerciasis, 261
  vaccine considerations for, 404
  yellow fever information for, 403
yersiniosis, 119, 345–6

Z
Zambia
  African trypanosomiasis in, 308
  Lujo virus in, 327
  malaria information for, 230*m*, 404
  vaccine considerations for, 404
  yellow fever information for, 330*t*, 341*m*, 404
zanamivir, 209, 210*t*
Zimbabwe
  malaria information for, 230*m*, 404
  Marburg hemorrhagic fever in, 326
  vaccine considerations for, 404
  yellow fever information for, 404

Photography Credits

FRONT COVER IMAGES
Lanterns: Cần Thơ B, Vietnam
Market: Beijing, China
Photos by BK Kapella

BACK COVER IMAGE
Budapest, Hungary
Photo by Andor Kovács

BANNER IMAGES FOR SELECT DESTINATIONS
from left to right

East Africa: Safaris (p. 407): Emily S. Jentes/Personal Collection, Michelle Russell/Personal Collection, Huong McLean/Personal Collection

Tanzania: Kilimanjaro (p. 411): all photos, Michelle Russell/Personal Collection

South Africa (p. 414): Mark Sotir/Personal Collection, Rebecca Myers/Personal Collection, Rebecca Myers/Personal Collection

Argentina/Brazil: Iguassu Falls (p. 417): iStockphoto, Mercedes Carnethon/Personal Collection, iStockphoto

Guatemala & Belize (p. 420): Fiona Genasi/Personal Collection, Stephen N. Molnar/Personal Collection, Fiona Genasi/Personal Collection

Jamaica (p. 424): Megan Crawley O'Sullivan/Personal Collection, Jinan N. O'Connor/Personal Collection, Adrienne Dukes/Personal Collection

Mexico (p. 428): all photos, Deron Pardue/Personal Collection

Peru: Cuzco–Machu Picchu (p. 431): all photos, Kelly Holton/Personal Collection

Cambodia: Angkor Wat (p. 435): David Snyder/CDC Foundation, Michelle Russell/Personal Collection, David Snyder/CDC Foundation

China (p. 439): BK Kapella/Personal Collection, Mark Sotir/Personal Collection, BK Kapella/Personal Collection

India (p. 444): all photos, Ann M. Woodward/Personal Collection

Nepal (p. 449): Dénes Egervari/Personal Collection, Dénes Egervari/Personal Collection, iStockphoto

Thailand (p. 453): BK Kapella/Personal Collection, Gabrielle A. Benenson/Personal Collection, Stephen N. Molnar/Personal Collection

Vietnam (p. 457): all photos, BK Kapella/Personal Collection

Saudi Arabia: Hajj Pilgrimage (p. 461): all photos, Tahseen Choudhry/Personal Collection

Egypt & Nile River Cruises (p. 465): all photos, Fiona Genasi/Personal Collection